GATEWAY
TO
SUCCESS IN SURGERY

GATEWAY TO SUCCESS IN SURGERY

**(Long and Short Cases, Commonly Asked
Questions and Answers, Short Notes and Viva Tips)**

MD Ray
MBBS (Cal) MS (Surgery) DU
Senior Research Fellow (Oncosurgery) ICMR
Assistant Professor
Army College of Medical Sciences
New Delhi, India

Forewords
Sanjay Kapoor VSM
AN Sinha

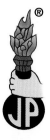

JAYPEE BROTHERS MEDICAL PUBLISHERS (P) LTD

New Delhi • Panama City • London

Jaypee Brothers Medical Publishers (P) Ltd.

Headquarter

Jaypee Brothers Medical Publishers (P) Ltd
4838/24, Ansari Road, Daryaganj
New Delhi 110 002, India
Phone: +91-11-43574357
Fax: +91-11-43574314
Email: jaypee@jaypeebrothers.com

Overseas Offices

J.P. Medical Ltd.
83 Victoria Street, London
SW1H 0HW (UK)
Phone: +44-2031708910
Fax: +02-03-0086180
Email: info@jpmedpub.com

Jaypee-Highlights Medical Publishers Inc.
City of Knowledge, Bld. 237, Clayton
Panama City, Panama
Phone: + 507-301-0496
Fax: + 507-301-0499
Email: cservice@jphmedical.com

Website: www.jaypeebrothers.com
Website: www.jaypeedigital.com

Inquiries for bulk sales may be solicited at: jaypee@jaypeebrothers.com

This book has been published in good faith that the contents provided by the author contained herein are original, and is intended for educational purposes only. While every effort is made to ensure accuracy of information, the publisher and the author specifically disclaim any damage, liability, or loss incurred, directly or indirectly, from the use or application of any of the contents of this work. If not specifically stated, all figures and tables are courtesy of the author. Where appropriate, the readers should consult with a specialist or contact the manufacturer of the drug or device.

Gateway to Success in Surgery
First Edition: **2012**

ISBN: 978-93-5025-224-6

Printed at Ajanta Offset & Packagings Ltd., New Delhi

Dedicated to

My Parents and Guides
Teachers, Friends, Followers and Students
Present, Past and Future

Foreword

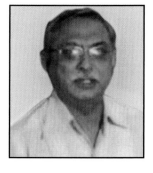

It is heartening to see Dr MD Ray, compiled the book *Gateway to Success in Surgery* for the surgery residents and MBBS students as well. It is one of the greatest moments of my life, as he has been my student, and I feel really proud of him. Even at this young age, he has done what many of us want to do, but do not, since we suffer from a writer's block.

Academics has three stages, learning, teaching and writing and it is great to see him reach the third and final stage, so soon and I am sure that the book, meant for surgery residents and medical students, will be highly useful.

These three years of PG in the life of a surgeon are the most important, tough and full of struggle, long working hours and the pressure of work is killing, but most come out of it brilliantly, in spite of repeated thought of quitting on innumerable occasions. Resident means one who lives, and a resident practically has to live under the roof of the hospital during this period.

Postgraduation is multitasking. We have to learn many things. To assess a patient and reach a diagnosis, learn to operate and to study to pass examinations while working gives experience, but that is never enough. To pass examinations and even for assessing patient, one needs to know theory, studies are mandatory, as the eyes do not see what the mind does not know. I have innumerable books, but much of what we need in practice is not mentioned in it, and much of what is written is not practised, hence a balanced blend of work and reading are essential to pass examinations and to be a good surgeon—what this book is.

We may know the latest article and the most recent advances in a subject, but we fumble at the basics and these can only be cleared by bedside clinics, and I am really happy to see, that the short book has those simple, but important and commonly asked questions and answers and other tips to present a case successfully and to pass exams which are very useful for undergraduate and postgraduate students too.

Knowing theory is like making a skeleton, practices add flesh, but it is only experience that puts the soul. So learning is an ongoing process. First we learn when and how to operate, but we become good surgeons, only when we can also decide when not to operate.

I wish Dr Ray, the book and all the budding surgeons, who read this, all the best.

Brigadier Sanjay Kapoor VSM
Consultant, Professor
Surgery and Surgical Oncology
Indian Army

Foreword

It is my pleasure to write a foreword for Dr (Major) MD Ray's book *Gateway to Success in Surgery*. I know him for a couple of years but I feel, I know him for more than a decade. He worked with me for a few months and proved his worth.

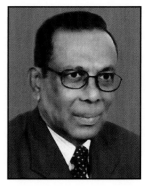

I have gone through the proof of the book. I am very much sure that the book will help a lot both the undergraduate and postgraduate students. It is really a fantastic book for case presentation and truly it is the *Gateway to Success in Surgery* to pass out the surgery examinations, i.e. MBBS, MS, DNB, BAMS, BHMS, etc.

I also believe that general practitioners and surgeons will also be benefited to assess different common cases effectively.

I am sure that his book will be highly appreciated by the entire community of medical students and medical faculties too.

Professor (Dr) AN Sinha MS FAIS FICS
DNB Examiner
Senior Consultant Surgeon and
Former Head, Department of Surgery
VMMC and Safdarjung Hospital, New Delhi, India

About the Principal Editors of the Book

The principal editor of the book Dr (Colonel) Chandra Kishor Jakhmola, MBBS, MS, GI Surgery from AIIMS. He is one of the renowned GI surgeons of Indian Army. He is the most senior advisor in GI Surgery in the Army Medical Corps.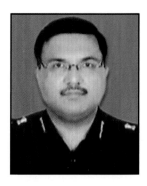

He has performed maximum number of advanced laparoscopic surgeries in Armed Forces. He has got more than 22 years vast experience in the surgical field, especially in GI surgery, advanced laparoscopic surgery, emergency and trauma surgeries.

He has also published a lot of papers in national and international journals. He is a renowned DNB teacher and examiner for the long time. He has been awarded different prestigious awards like Army Commander Award, VSM for his excellence in works.

Presently, he is working as a Professor, Army College of Medical Sciences and as a Senior Advisor, GI Surgery, Base Hospital, Delhi, India.

Despite of his busy schedule, he took a great interest to edit the book sincerely. The writer is ever grateful to him for his kind attention to make this book more rational and useful.

Dr GC Bhattacharya, MD (Pathology) 83 years old, a renowned pathologist, served Indian Air Force for decades. My recent friendship with Dr MD Ray, is an episode of "Love at first sight". In age he is slightly elder than my grandson, but in professional knowledge he appears to be my "grandpa". I pray his potential genius blossom into a future a Dr Bidhan Chandra Roy. In my versatile experience in every field of medical sciences and extraordinary knowledge of human physiognomy as a first pilot Doctor of Indian Air Force have been of some help to encourage him as a friend, philosopher and guide. I shall consider myself fortunate.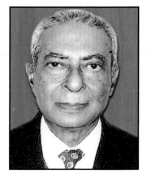

The book is a product of a genius, first of its kind in my knowledge. This is a pioneer venture with all sincerity and dedication under Dr MD Ray's command. I feel the name *Gateway to Success in Surgery* coined by him is appropriate and suitable. I prophecy and forecast that many many budding surgeons, medical students will feel fortunate to enter through this gateway into the kingdom of surgery.

Preface

Most people, the vast majority in fact, lead the lives that circumstances have thrust upon them, and though some repine, looking upon themselves as round pegs in square holes and think that if things had been different they might have made a much better showing, the greater part accept their lot, if not with serenity, at all events with resignation, I think they are like tram, cars travelling for ever on the self same rails. They go backwards and forwards inevitably, till they can go no longer and then are sold as a scrap iron.

My sincere effort to write the book is to make you an exceptional personality in the field of surgery through this *Gateway to Success in Surgery*. I feel the book will help all the medical students both undergraduates and postgraduates to present cases, better in examination and which is very very important to get through the exam door; I mean that is the *Gateway to Success in Surgery*.

I have also tried to include all the possible examination type questions and answers which will help the students to get through the exam very much. I will tell, there is no alternate way of hard work. So keep studying standard textbooks, and try to understand the subject and learn little but learn accurately forever.

Lastly, I will say, prove William Shakespeare's word in Macbeth wrong "it (life) is a tale told by an idiot, full of sound and fury, signifying nothing".

Say with me, life is a tale told by a wise full of joy and merry signifying many things. Welcome for constructive criticism always.

All the best always.

MD Ray
dr_mdray@yahoo.com

Acknowledgments

I am ever and ever grateful to the following personalities for this book and for my career forever:

1. Brigadier (Dr) Professor Sanjay Kapoor, a great Oncosurgeon. He is overall a super human being and my research guide in Oncosurgery under ICMR, New Delhi and he is my teacher always. His valuable lecture, notes are included in the book. Without his writing the book would have never been completed. He is a man of confidence in his professional as well as personal front of life too. He knows how to become an ideal guide always in life.

2. Professor (Dr) AN Sinha, Senior Consultant Surgeon, and former Head, Department of Surgery, VMMC and Safdarjung Hospital, New Delhi, India, one of the editor of the book and my well-wisher all the way.

3. Colonel (Dr) CK Jakhmola, GI Surgeon, the Principal Editor of this book who took a great pain to correct the book all the aspects. The way he encouraged for the book it showed his greatness and great heartedness. As a surgeon as well as a human he is really a big man. I am ever grateful to him.

4. Professor (Maj General) RP Choubey, GI Surgeon, my MS guide and teacher. He was literally excited to see the publishing of my book. I am ever grateful to him also.

5. Dr Amar Bhatnagar, MCh (Oncosurgery), Senior Consultant and Head, Department of Cancer Surgery, VMMC and Safdarjung Hospital, New Delhi, India, an excellent cancer surgeon, my teacher and guide in my path of career.

6. Group Capt (Dr) Sharan Choudhuri, a great Oncosurgeon. To tell the truth, I have never seen such type of marvelous surgeries in my life. I am very much grateful to him for his exceptional teaching of standard surgery in my PG days and early days in Army College of Medical Sciences, New Delhi, India.

7. Dr Pinaki Ranjan Debnath, Pediatric Surgeon, my constant inspiration to do well in life.

8. Dr Suddhaswatya Chatterjee, Physician, who took special interest to complete this book at the earliest by guiding his wife to get the book typed very sincerely and Dr Sanjiv Kumar Gupta, Laparoscopic Surgeon, who took pain to correct the proofs of the book many times.

9. Base Hospital, New Delhi, India, I am thankful to Col CK Jakhmola, Col SS Jaiswal, Wing Commander P Chatterjee, Maj Amit Agarwal, Lt Col Manoj Talreja, Col BC Nambiar, OT Metron, Capt Pactesia and specially Lt Col (Dr) Manish Nakra, Anesthesiologist and Intensivist, for their enthusiasm towards my book and me. I must give special thanks to them.

10. Dean, Brig SS Anand, Dr Dibyajyoti Bora, Dr Prakash Rana, Dr Mitalee, Dr Sindhu, Dr Chitralekha, Lt Col S Ghatak, Dr Lalit Garg, Lt Col D Bandopadhyay, Lt Col Shusil Sharma, Dr SK Sharma, Dr Dayal, Dr Revthy, Dr Suchi, Dr Paras Gupta, Dr S Mata, Army College of Medical Sciences, New Delhi, India for their ever encouragements in all of my social and academic activities. Lab Assistant, Mr Gulav for assisting in paper work.

11. Recently, a surprise fatherly figure joined in the list of friends mentioned above and became my friend, philosopher and guide all the way, he is Dr Gopal Chandra Bhattacharya, a renowned pathologist, a young man of 82 years who loves to encourage with all his versatile experiences in all field of life to all the talented persons he meets. His constant companionship was a welcome help to me in the publication of the book. I cannot but remember him forever.

My sincere thanks to Dr Garima Kapoor, Dr Sindhu Chandra (Gynecologists), Assistant Professors, ACMS for their contribution in the chapter 'Pelvic Mass' and Dr Amit Goyel for contributing in the short note 'Laparoscopic Surgery – Recent Trends.' My sincere thanks to all of my Doctors' friends, Baljinder Kaur, Himanshu, VK Mishra, Abhijit, Mohan, Sanjoy, Biswajit (Bishu), Manoj, SR Sahoo, Akash for their ever encouragements in all of my social and academic activities.

I am very thankful to my loving mother Saralashree Ray and my beloved wife Anisha Ray, Graded Classical Artist, All India Radio, for their constant sufferings and support to make this hard work possible. I am also very much thankful to my seven-year-old naughty son Mayukhraj, who is my astrologer and guide all the time. He always gives a positive astrology to get my every hardwork done. And definitely I am thankful to all of my family members and relatives, especially Mr PK Das,

Mrs Urmimala Das, Amit Da, Boudi, Sima Das and elder sisters Mrs Kavita Bhattacharya, Kalpana, Suparna, Archana, Bandana, sisters Munny, Alpana, Dhriti, Chandrima, Sampa, Pampa, Tumpa, Tunu, Dr PK Chakraborty, Biswajit, Uttam, Sasanka, Subhas Da, Sibu, Subho, Santu, Tutun, Veltu, Swachhatoya, Munai, Diya, Kakima Sipra and Masima Partima Mukherji, Dr Narayyan Bhattachaya for their ever encouragements in all events in my life.

I am very much thankful to Mr BC Dey more than my elder brother and Mrs Panchali Chatterjee, Mrs Bhawna Sharma, PK Yadav, Biswas Da, Mr Partha Gupta, who took a great pain to type this book very sincerely. Mr Swadhin Roy, artist and my students of ACMS especially Nandishwar, Rahul Ranawat, Pankaj Tiwary, Sumit Sachan, Pawan Kumar Gaba, Elly Verma put their sincere efforts in linediagrams and various aspects to complete the book. Without their sincere efforts the book cannot be handed over to the publisher.

My sincere thanks to Shri Jitendar P Vij (Chairman and Managing Director), Mr PG Bandhu (Senior Director–Sales), Mr Tarun Duneja (Director-Publishing), Mr KK Raman (Production Manager), Seema Dogra, Sunil Dogra (Production Executive), Neelambar Pant (Production Coordinator), Ms Samina Khan (PA to Director-Publishing), Akhilesh Kumar Dubey, Sarvesh Kumar Giri, Ankit Kumar, and Hemant Kumar of M/s Jaypee Brothers Medical Publishers (P) Ltd, for bringing this book to light. I will always welcome all the constructive criticisms from the sincere readers of this book.

Overall I am deeply indebted to all of my patients—present, past and future.

Thank you all very much.

Contents

SHORT CASES

PEDIATRICS CASES

Basic Tips for Viva

1. Proper dressing, simple, sober clothes
   Full sleeve apron—well written Exam Roll No over it, and don't forget to wear **SMILE AND CONFIDENCE** always, Think at the exam hall "I tried my level best—nothing to get tense. I know better than anyone else". Take long breaths frequently to avoid anxiety and fear.
2. Take the following things in exam hall:
   - Two pens
   - Stethoscope, Sphygmomanometer
   - Measuring tape
   - Torch
   - Gloves and Lignocaine Gel
   - Roll made X-ray film
   - 4 tourniquets
   - Hammer
3. Be gentle and polite in exam hall. **Never argue with the examiners—never and never**. Not only in examination it is applicable in all the fields of life too.
4. When you are given a case, go to the patient smiling and introduce yourself. Give him/her a packet of biscuit and tell "this is my very important exam. Cooperate with me and don't get annoyed please". Make him/her comfortable and friendly. Take relevant history. Request him/her; tell the same story/words to the examiner also, if he/she is asked by the examiner please.
5. Take proper history. You know, perfect history taking will take you through the *Gateway to Success in Surgery*. Remember the points for the specific case and write down the long case till case summary and provisional/differential diagnosis.
6. Examination of patient and its findings should be perfect. Don't try to make it as per book, make it whatever it is. Examiners like the truth, not the bookish knowledge or the manipulation. You know he is more than hundred times experienced than you.
7. Be confident to see the examiners. Say 'Good morning sir', 'Thank you sir', etc.
8. If examiner asks to tell history it is always better to speak history without seeing case sheet. Have eye-to-eye contact with examiner. If he asks the summary /diagnosis tell that thing only. First you listen what examiner is asking you. Take a pause then start speaking—speak in proper speed, not very fast, not too slow. Give a common diagnosis first. Remember diagnosis of a rare disease will be rarely correct.
9. Always avoid speaking uncommon words, uncommon terms or syndromes.
10. Think for a second which you are going to tell. In exam hall each word is important which takes you through or may not take you through the 'Gateway'.
11. **Maintain basic things**. If you don't know the answer, say, 'I don't know sir'. Never stand dumb. And never try to fool examiner by giving irrelevant answers. If required quote a standard textbook not any guidebook or note Pl.
12. Lastly I would say the same, '**practice makes perfect**.' Practice case presentation in Clinical Meeting, in front of teachers, friends and above all at home in front of a mirror repeatedly.

Wish you easy overcome the
Gateway to Success in Surgery
All the best
-ever and always.
MD Ray

Concise Information About Health

ACCORDING TO WHO

"Health is a state of complete physical, mental and social well-being and not merely an absence of disease or infirmity".

Physical dimension: Physical health implies the notion of perfect functioning of body. Signs of physical health—a good complexion, a clear skin, bright eyes, lustrous hair with a body well clothed, firm fresh not toe fat, a sweet breath, a good appetite, sound sleep, regular activity of bowels and bladder and smooth easy coordinate bodily movements.

Mental dimension: It is a state of balance between individual and the surrounding world, a state of harmony between oneself and other with coexistence between the realities of the self and that of other people of that of the environment.

Signs of mental health: Free from internal conflicts, he is not at 'war' with himself.

- He is well adjusted; he is able to get along well with others. He accepts criticism and is not easily upset.
- He searches for identity
- He has a strong sense of self-esteem
- He knows himself; his needs, problems and goals
- He has a good self control—balances rationality and emotionality.

He faces problems and tries to solve them intelligently, i.e. coping with stress and anxiety.

Social dimension: It is quantity of quality of an individual interpersonalities of the extent of environment with the community. Social dimensions include the level of social skills one possesses, social functioning and the ability to see one self as a member of a large society.

Well-being—indicates standard of living and lifestyle.

Maintain your perfect health and be happy forever.

SUGGESTIONS FOR SUCCESS

- Marry /keep constant relation with the right person. This one decision will determine 90% of your happiness or misery.
- Give people more than they expect and do it cheerfully.
- Be forgiving to yourself and others
- Be generous
- Have a grateful heart
- Persistence
- Discipline yourself to save money on even the most modest salary
- Treat everyone you meet like you want to be treated
- Commit yourself to quality
- Be loyal
- Be honest
- Be a self stater
- Stop blaming others. Take responsibility in every area of your life
- Take good care of those you love.
  The basic triad of success:
  i. Exercise
  ii. Meditation
  iii. Study

What is Surgery?

Surgery is an art of learning not only when to cut but it is more important to learn when not to cut.

Surgery is such an act which once done, cannot be reversed.

Surgery is a science as well as an art. Try to be artistic in surgery and life too.

Surgical triad   i. Measure thrice
                 ii. Think twice
                iii. Cut once.

The lesser the indication, the greater the complication.

In surgery as well as life too there is no question of 'Short Cut'.

Many very skillful operators are not good surgeons.

HOW TO START THE STUDY

1. Start practicing meditation before you start studying, i.e. concentrate your mind first please.
2. Start with anatomy of specific topic you are going to read. I will advise the following anatomy books—BD Chaurasia's Human Anatomy/Lee McGregor's Surgical Anatomy/Snel's Anatomy and Last's Anatomy, etc. for reference.

REMEMBER ONE THING

If you know the road map you can drive properly.

You know the anatomy, you do the surgery perfectly.

1. Go through the standard **textbook** for same topic which you are going to read
    i. Bailey and Love's Short Practice of Surgery (the book is enough for undergraduate students)
   ii. Schwartz's principle of surgery or
  iii. Sabiston textbook of surgery
   iv. Maingot's abdominal operations.
2. Read Clinical Surgery—Dr S Das—A Manual on Clinical Surgery/Dr ML Saha's—Bedside Clinics in Surgery/SRB's—Bedside Clinics in Surgery.
3. Read this book *Gateway to Success in Surgery* for case presentation and questions-answers for the same topic.
4. Read Nyhus Mastery of Surgery or at least Farquharson's Textbook of Operative General Surgery for Operative Steps.
5. If you make notes on specific topic, get it attached in your textbook in the same page of the topic or right down in your textbook about the notes where it is written. Try to study the notes in the same time when you feel required.

I can assure you will cross the *Gateway to Success in Surgery* very easily without any doubt.

How to take History in Surgical Cases?

History taking is an art that helps you to reach the diagnosis in more than 90% cases. History taking in the surgical cases is slightly different from medical history taking. You have to give importance to special important points in surgical cases as below.

1. **Patient's particulars**
   i. *Name:* Ask the patient by name. Patient will always be happy. He/She will feel that, "my doctor knows my name like my relatives".
   ii. *Age:* Age is important aspect to establish the diagnosis. Examples: congenital anomalies appear usually since birth like cleft palate, phimosis, cystic hygroma, etc.

      Solitary nodular, multinodular colloids goiter occurs in 20–30 years. Papillary carcinoma in young girl. Follicular carcinoma in middle aged women, medullary carcinoma 58–70 years.

      Sarcoma in younger age group, i.e. teenagers and early third decade people are usually the victim. Choledochal cysts usually in young adults around 20 years of age.

      Carcinoma usually occurs in the elderly after 50 years, so many exceptions are there like Wilms' tumor occurs at the age of 2–4 years.

      Few disease are bimodal e.g. Hodgkin's lymphoma occurs pick at around 20 years and another pick at 50 years and above. Benign breast disease occurs below 35 years and another pick is above 60 years. Carcinoma breast occurs in 45–55 years.

      So from the age you can have a primary idea about the disease which helps you to reach the diagnosis.
   iii. *Sex:* Few diseases are very common in male like lung, kidney, stomach diseases, carcinoma lip, tongue, etc. Few diseases are very common in female like thyroid, breast, Raynaud's disease, varicose vein, cystitis, urinary tract infection, pyelonephritis, etc.
   iv. *Residence:* Residence is important aspect of history taking. Few diseases predominantly occurs in certain areas like gallbladder diseases are common from Delhi to Patna belt, Southern and Eastern regions of our country especially in Gangetic belts.

      Thyroid disorders like goiter are common in rocky mountains area, i.e. Himalayas, Vindhyas belts known as goiter belts in India.

      Urinary bladder stone disease is common in Punjab and Rajasthan. Other examples are Kangri Cancer in Kashmiri people due to carrying burning charcoal (Kangri) at their abdomen to keep them warm during cold. Chronic pancreatitis is more common in Kerala, Karnataka. In Tamil Nadu, practice of reverse smoking (burning site of *bidi/* cigarette inside the mouth) causes palatal cancer.
   v. *Occupation:* Occupation plays an important role to cause different diseases like—Varicose vein is very common in tram on driver, traffic police, rickshaw puller, bus conductors where job demands for a long standing.

      Housemaid knee (prepatellar bursitis) common in housemaid as the work involves kneel down position to clean the floor.

      Bladder cancer is common in the factory workers who are working with aniline dye, gas, printing, rubber, textile, leather, etc.

      Thyroid disease is commonly associated with stress and strain

      Carcinoma lip is commonly seen in a man of outdoor activities, that's why it is called 'Countryman lip'.

Peptic ulcer is commonly seen with the business executives, civil servants, clerks, and those who are habituated to take tea, coffee frequently and smoke excessively.

(Other points you have to highlight when required in surgical cases like)

vi. Religion in case of carcinoma penis; as carcinoma penis commonly occur in Hindus, not commonly in Jews and Muslims owing to their religious custom of circumcision in infancy and early childhood.

vii. Social status—Carcinoma breast, appendicitis are common in high social status people; whereas tuberculosis, portal hypertension, renal, vesicle calculus, peptic perforation, etc. usually common in low social status group.

viii. Bed number and

ix. Date of admission, etc.

2. **Chief complaints:** Write patient's main complaints in brief and in patient's own language. If multiple complaints are there, write it in a chronological order, i.e. longer duration to shorter duration.

If the problems start simultaneously write it in order of severity.

Minor complaints should not be mentioned in chief complaints.

Examples are given in subsequent disease presentation part.

3. History of present illness (the sequence of events from the time of onset of the chief complaints to the time of patient's visit to the doctor)

Starts like this way my patient was apparently symptomatic 6 months/1 year back then, describe the details of chief complaints with OPD.

i. O–Onset

ii. P–Progress

iii. D–Duration (Remember OPD).

If patient complains of pain, describe onset, progress, duration site, nature, radiation/referred ,aggravating, relieving factors, etc.

Describe the treatment part related with the disease. Exclude the expected symptoms (related with the disease) by asking gastrointestinal, respiratory, cardiovascular, urinary, neurological or muscular skeletal systems. These are called negative history (i.e. these symptoms may be present with the disease but not present in this case).

4. **Past history:** Mention all the major disease that patients are suffering from and major disease in the past like hypertension, diabetes, tuberculosis, chronic obstructive pulmonary disease (COPD). Others like jaundice, autoimmune disease psychiatric illness, if any.

History of similar disease in the past.

History of any significant operation and its complications in the past.

Past history of any allergy to any drug, etc.

5. **Personal history:** Dietary habits

Addiction to alcohol, cigarette/bidi, tobacco, betel, betelnut, etc. Marital status, socioeconomic background, bowel, bladder and sleep habits.

In case of female along with the above—menstrual history is very important (like breast carcinoma details menstrual history is important) Menarche cycle, duration, amount of blood loss, LMP (Last menstrual period), etc.

6. **Family history:** Ask about the same and any significant illness his/her family especially in patients, siblings, children and first/second degree relatives.

Examples: Carcinoma breast is familial—Fissure in ano, hemorrhoids are familial also.

7. **Physical examination:** Physical examination includes:

i. *General Survey:* Write like this way—The patient is cooperative, comfortable looking having smiling/anxiety/ (faces), average build, well/averagely/ poorly nourished.

Next comment on pallor, icterus, edema and generalized lymphadenopathy (clubbing, cyanosis, pigmentation, neck vein engorgement, etc. if these are prominently marked only)

Next Pulse—details only in specific cases like thyrotoxicosis, etc.

Blood pressure right arm spine .

Temperature Respiration

ii. *Local examination:* It includes—(i) Inspection, (ii) Palpation, (iii) Percussion and (iv) Auscultation

Example—In lump abdomen—On inspection you have to mention, shape of abdomen—scaphoid/flat/protruded, any obvious swelling/bulge is there or not.

Position of umbilicus—central/deviated.

Movements of abdomen—all quadrants move with respiration or not.

Skin over the abdomen—any venous engorgement, scar marks, pigmentation.

Flanks/Renal angle are full or not .

Hernial sites, external genitalia are normal or any abnormality is there.

On Palpation: Temperature (first), tenderness of the lump and describe the lump in details—Site, size, surface, consistency margins, movement with reception, relation with underlying or overlying structures, etc.

Liver, spleen palpable or not, fluid thrill, renal angle, and palpation of lymph nodes.

Percussion: Very important like supraclavicular lymph nodes.
–   General note over the abdomen—tympanitic/dull
–   Shifting dullness
–   Upper border of liver dullness, etc.

Auscultation:
–   Bowel sounds (see for one minute)
–   Any added sound, etc. Next do not forget .
–   Digital per rectal examination (DRE) and paravaginal examination in case of female.

(In exam hall, ask the examination when it is very much essential, at least try to do DRE)

iii. *Systematic examination*
a. Respiratory—write bilateral air entry equal. Bronchovesicular sounds breath sound, there is no adventitious sound heard.
b. CVS—SI, SII (normal) no murmur heard
c. Neurological examination—higher motor functions are normal, no neurodeficit is found. Other examinations are essentially normal.

(Mind that if any abnormality is detected in above system, write in details please).

Summary of the case:

Write in two paragraphs: First paragraph—brief history, Second paragraph—only positive clinical findings to reach the diagnosis.

Provisional diagnosis: From history and clinical examination which you think is the most possible disease. Next differential diagnosis, i.e. other possibilities think why you are thinking the other possibilities. What are the positive points in favor of them and what are points not in favor.

It is always better to tell the history to the examiner without seeing the casesheet, so practice case presentation repeatedly and you know it is the *Gateway to Success in Surgery*.

LONG CASES

You know, long case is very important part in surgery examination. Time is allotted 45 minutes only.

Practically, it is very much applicable if you are the first candidate for the examination. In this fixed time you have to write down the case sheet, history, general examination, local examination and systemic examination in details.

To tell the truth, until or unless you practice case presentation properly and repeatedly it's very difficult to manage whole thing in the examination hall. If you practice case presentation as per the guideline of this book, all points will come across in your inner vision and you can cope up with the stressful situation very easily and you know if you manage long case examination properly you are almost through the *Gateway to Surgery*.

In postgraduate, MS or DNB examination long cases are usually lump abdomen and to some extent peripheral vascular disease (PVD).

But for undergraduates any case, example—hernia, breast lump, thyroid, is given as a long case. Examiner will come and ask.

i. **Start your case:** Then you have to start from the beginning, my patient, Ravi Shanker a 60 years old male presented with so and so complaints, etc.

    Up to the provisional diagnosis (on history, general examination and local, and systemic examination, the diagnosis which comes in your mind first)

    Keep relevant differential diagnoses in your mind.

ii. If examiner ask, what is your case? Then you say the summary of the case (presentation, positive general survey , and positive local and systemic examination) and ending by giving provisional diagnosis.

iii. If examiner asks 'what is your diagnosis' ?

    Then you straight way give the complete diagnosis. In Hernia case you tell.

    Example—My diagnosis is right-left sided indirect/direct inguinal hernia which is incomplete/complete, reducible/ irreducible, complicated/uncomplicated and containing intestinal loop/Omentum–like this way. Other examples are written in concerned cases.

For clinical purpose, abdomen is divided into nine regions in the following way:

Basically two horizontal and two vertical lines divide the abdomen into nine regions.

1. *Horizontal line:*
   i. The upper horizontal line, also called transpyloric line is the midway between suprasternal notch and the symphysis pubis.

   Usually the line comes in between xiphisternum and umbilicus. But always mention the bony points which are fixed points in the body.
   ii. The lower horizontal line, also called transtubercular line, connecting two tubercles of the iliac crest (the tubercles are usually 5 cm behind the anterosuperior iliac spine).
2. *Vertical line:* The right vertical line is the line passing through the midpoint of right anterosuperior iliac spine and symphysis pubis and connecting right midclavicular point.

   Left vertical line is the line through the midpoint of left anterosuperior iliac spine and symphysis pubis connecting the left midclavicular point above.

   Otherway you can say two vertical lines, each passing through midclavicular point to mid inguinal point [the mid inguinal point is the middle point between symphysis pubis and anterosuperior iliac spine which is different from midpoint of inguinal ligament, i.e. midpoint between anterosuperior iliac spine and pubic tubercle].

   The nine regions of abdomen are:
1. Right hypochondrium
2. Epigastrium
3. Left hypochondrium
4. Right lumbar
5. Umbilical region
6. Left lumbar
7. Right iliac fossa
8. Hypogastrium
9. Left iliac fossa.

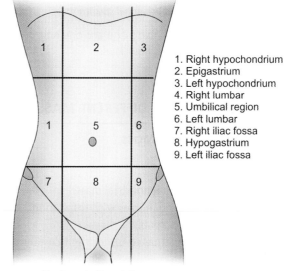

1. Right hypochondrium
2. Epigastrium
3. Left hypochondrium
4. Right lumbar
5. Umbilical region
6. Left lumbar
7. Right iliac fossa
8. Hypogastrium
9. Left iliac fossa

Regions in the abdomen

- Upper horizontal or transpyloric line midway between symphysis pubis and suprasternal notch.
- Lower horizontal line is at the levels of two tuberles of liac crest, i.e. transtubercular line.
- The vertical lines are drawn on either side through the midpoint between anterosuperior liac spine and symphysis pubis connecting corresponding midclavicular point.

The present concept of dividing abdomen is more practical.

For clinical examination, abdomen is presently divided into four quadrants by drawing:
a. Vertical line—in the mid plane and
b. Horizontal line—at right angle to the vertical line crossing at the umbilicus.

The four quadrants are:
1. Right upper quadrant.
2. Left upper quadrant.
3. Right lower quadrant.
4. Left lower quadrant.

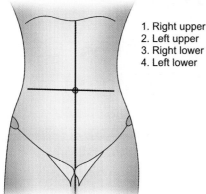

1. Right upper
2. Left upper
3. Right lower
4. Left lower

Present concept of abdominal quadrants

- One vertical line through mid plane and one horizontal line at right angle though the umbilicus.
- This is more practical.

CHARACTERISTICS OF DIFFERENT MASS

Right Hypochondrial Mass

Liver Mass

Intra-abdominal right hypochondrial mass.
- It is horizontally placed, moves with respiration.
- Upper border is not palpable.
- Fingers cannot be insinuated under right costal margin and the mass.
- Dull on percussion.

In hydatid cyst
- Soft, smooth, nontender liver.
- Well localized.
- Hydatid thrill may be palpable.
- Usally nontender, unless it is infected [infected cyst can be tender].

In hepatoma like HCC or solitary secondary in liver
- Hard mass.
- Usually smooth surface.
- May be tender [due to tumor necrosis often and as a result of stretching of liver capsule.
- Vascular bruit may be heard.
- Usually occurs in cirrhotic liver, hence features of cirrhosis may be there.

In multiple secondaries
- Hard in consistency.
- Multinodularity with central umbilication.
- Amoebic liver abscess—smooth tender mass.

Gallbladder Mass

- Intra-abdominal right, hypochondrial mass.
- Pyriform shaped.
- It is located right-to-right rectus muscle below right costal margin or below the lower margin of palpable liver.
- Usually smooth or soft in benign enlargement but hard and irregular in carcinoma—Gallbladder.
- It moves side-to-side, i.e. horizontally—it is a very important characteristic in GB mass. [But in malignancy this feature may be absent].
- It moves with respiration.
- Fingers cannot be insinuated between the lump and costal margin. [Except benign lesion like mucocele of gallbladder where you can insinuate your fingers].
- Dull on percussion.

In carcinoma gallbladder
- Hard gallbladder
- Irregular surface.
- Nontender
- Usally fixed and nonmobile.

Mucocele in GB/enlarged GB in obstructive jaundice—Soft, nontender, smooth.

Empyema GB: Tender and irregular wall.

Other lumps at right hypochondrium are:

Right kidney lump like RCC /hydronephrosis arising from upper pole of right kidney.

Features of kidney lump
- Lumbar region
- Bean/reniform in shape
- Bimanually palpable
- Ballotable
- Can insinuate fingers in between lump and costal margin
- Moves with respiration
- Renal angle fullness
- Band of colonic resonant infront [in case of large lump the colon may be displaced from the front of the lump, so dull note is palpable over the mass].
- The lump usually does not cross the midline.

Suprarenal tumor
- Deeply placed, nodular
- Nonmobile
- Not moving with respiration
- Often crosses the midline
- Resonant on percussion (because of colon infront).

Lump of hepatic flexure of the colon
- Hard, irregular.
- Restricted movement or no movement.
- Retroperitoneal lump, so it does not fall forward in knee elbow position.

MASS IN EPIGASTRIUM

Left lobe of liver mass → Secondary
                             → Hepatocellular carcinoma (HCC)
                             → Hydatid cyst
                             → Amoebic liver abscess.

- Intra-abdominal
- Upper border not felt
- Epigastric mass
- Extends towards right hypochondrium
- Moves with respiration
- Dull on percussion.

Stomach mass
- Intra-abdominal epigastric lump.
- Mass better felt on standing position.
- Nodular hard in consistency.
- Usually mobile—smooth, firm in leiomyoma.
- Moves with respiration.
- Mass in the body—placed horizontally without any features of obstruction.
- Mass in pylorus—margins are well felt, mobile with features of gastric outlet obstruction (GOO).
- Resonant or impaired resonance on percussion.
- Succussion splash in pyeloric mass.

Pancreatic cyst:
(Pseudocyst or cystic adenoma)
Epigastric lump—retroperitoneal
- Smooth, soft cystic lump.
- Does not move with respiration.
      (Pseudocyst may move with respiration when it is attached with stomach, liver or organs moving with respiration).
      [Remember large retroperitoneal lump may be have like an intra-abdominal lump].
- Lower margins usually felt well but not upper border.
- It is not mobile usually.
- Retroperitoneal mass, so it does not fall forward in knee elbow position.

Baid test
If you put a Ryles tube in stomach it is felt per abdomen as the stomach is pushed front by the cyst.

Transverse Colon Mass (Carcinoma Transverse Colon)

- Intra-abdominal epigastric lump.
- Placed horizontally.
- Nodular, hard in consistency.
- Does not move with respiration.
- Tympanic or impaired resonant on percussion.
- Cephalocaudally mobile whereas restricted mobility horizontally.

Lymph nodal mass
Due to   → Secondaries
          → Lymphoma
          → Tuberculosis
- Retroperitoneal epigastric mass.
- Vertically placed, above the umbilicus.
- Nonmobile.
- Not moving with respiration.
- Resonant on percussion [due to over lying gas filled bowel loops].

Aortic aneurysm
- Pulsatile [even in knee elbow position expansile pulsation is felt].
- Vertically placed.
- Smooth, soft.
- Nonmobile.
- Not moving with respiration.
- Resonant on percussion.

Retroperitoneal sarcoma/teratoma:
- All features of retroperitoneal solid lumps like—large mass usually.
- Does not fall forward on knee elbow position.
- Fixed/not mobile.
- Not moving with respiration.
- Hard, ill defined margin.
- Tympanic note on percussion (because of bowel infront).

LEFT HYPOCHONDRIAL MASS

a. Enlarged spleen:
   - Clinically palpable when it enlarges three times or more).

- Direction of enlargement is towards right iliac fossa, i.e. downward, forward and inward.
- Splenic swelling is usually smooth, uniform and anterior border is sharp with one or more notches.
- Splenic swelling moves well with respiration.
- Fingers cannot be insinuated in between swelling and left costal margin called +ve 'Hook sign'.
- Dull on percussion.
- No fullness in renal angles.

b. Splenic flexure or colon mass:
   In carcinoma colon
   - It is mobile slightly.
   - It does not move with respiration.
   - It has a nodular consistency on palpation.
   - Resonant on percussion.
   - Fingers can be insinuated between the lump and costal margin.

c. Left renal mass from upper pole
   - Features as described earlier.

d. Left adrenal mass:
   - It is retroperitoneal.
   - Not mobile.
   - It may move with respiration [as it is in contact with diaphragm]
   - Often crosses the midline.
   - It mimics renal mass.
   - Resonant on percussion.
   - Does not fall forward in knee elbow position.

e. Mass from tail of pancreas:
   (Pseudocyst or cyst adenoma)
   - Retroperitoneal lump.
   - Usually does not fall forward on knee elbow position.
   - Not mobile.
   - Does not move with respiration.

Mass in Right and Left Lumbar Region

- **Kidney mass:** → As described
- **Colonic mass:** → Right sided ascending colonic mass
  → Left sided descending colonic mass.

Features as described
- **Adrenal mass** as described.
- **Retroperitoneal tumors** → Sarcoma
  → Teratoma
  → Lymph nodal mass.

Mass in Umbilical Region

- Carcinoma stomach, duodenum—as described.
- Transverse colonic growth—as described.
- Omental cyst
  - Smooth
  - Soft, nontender
  - Mobile in all direction
  - Moves with respiration
  - Dull on percussion
- Mesenteric cyst:
  - Soft, intra-abdominal fluctuating mass.
  - Moves perpendicular to the root of mesentery.
  - Resonant all around the cyst and over the cyst it is dull.

This triad of signs is called Tillard's triad
- Lymph nodal mass
- Pancreatic mass
- Aortic aneurysm
- Retroperitoneal connective tissue tumor.

Right Iliac Fossa Mass

Appendicular Lump
- Most common swelling in right iliac fossa (RIF).
- Firm, smooth swelling – margins are well felt.
- May be tender
- Notmobile
- Not moving with respiration.
- Resonant on percussion.

Iliocecal TB
- Firm, smooth.
- Nontender.
- May be slightly mobile.
- Does not move with respiration.
- Resonant on percussion.

Crohn's disease
- Clinical features are stage related.
- Lump is firm, smooth.
- Tenderness may be present.
- Nonmobile.

Carcinoma cecum
- Hard, nodular mass
- Mobile, mobility becomes restricted when it gets adherent to psoas muscles.
- Does not move with respiration.

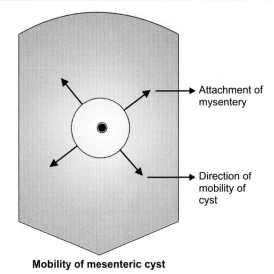

Mobility of mesenteric cyst

- Tympanic or impaired resonant on percussion.
  Lymph nodal mass:
  Mesenteric lymph nodes
  External iliac, lymph nodes
  Features of different lymph nodal mass—as described.

Mass in Hypogastrium

Bladder mass
- Hard, nodular midline mass.
- All margins palpable except lower margin.
- May be mobile on horizontal direction.
- Size may be reduced after emptying the bladder.
- Can be felt on per rectal examination.

Uterine mass
- Firm to hard midline mass
- Globular in shape
- Smooth
- Lower border not felt
- Can be felt on pervaginal examination
- Ballotable.

Ovarian mass/Tubo-ovarian mass
- The swelling appears to be arising from the pelvis and can be pushed into the pelvis.
- Palpable mass at right iliac fossa. Ovoid in shape and have side-to-side mobility.
- Ovarian mass can be bimanually papable and ballotable.
- Pervaginal examination—ovarian mass can be felt through one of the fornices with a finger in the vagina.
- Cystic ovarian mass have a characteristic pattern of percussion note—dullness infront and resonant at the flank, where the bowel loops are pushed.

Left Iliac Fossa Mass

Lower part of descending/sigmoid colon mass:
- Palpable mass–hard
- Movable, well defined margin
- Does not move with respiration
- Tympanic note on percussion

Retroperitoneal lymph nodes:
→ Lymphoma
→ Metastatic
→ Retroperitoneal soft tissue sarcoma
  – Liposarcoma
  – Malignant fibrous histiocytoma.

Ovarian mass/Tubo-ovarian mass: as described above

Unascending Kidney

- The pathological unascended left kidney might be palpable in the iliac fossa.
  Pathology may be hydronephrosis or malignancy.
- Retroperitoneal lump.
- Reniform shape.

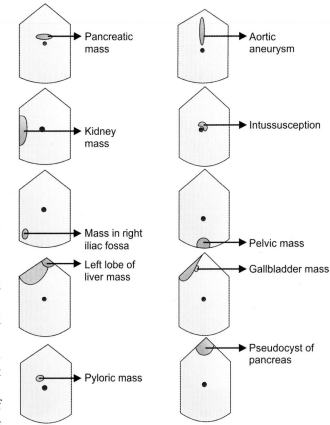

Mass in defferent regions of abdomen

7

- Ballotability may be present but difficult to elicit in the iliac fossa.

Undescended Testicular Mass

- History of absence of testis in the scrotum since birth. Young males are affected.
- The undescended testes is not palpable unless pathological in the iliac fossa.
- The scrotum examination reveals—no testes in the hemiscrotum, the hemiscrotum is undeveloped and devoid of Rougies, then the lump in the iliac fossa to be considered as malignant testes.
- It is retroperitoneal.
- Usually, it is fixed in retroperitoneum.

Differentiation between parietal, intra-abdominal and retroperitoneal lump.

In any abdominal lump—first you decide whether it is parietal or intra-abdominal.
↓
Do Carnett's test also called leg lifting test. Ask the patient to raise both extended legs without bending knees, from the bed.
↓
In parietal swelling—it will be more prominent.

It will be easily movable over the taut muscle, if the swelling is subcutaneous but won't move while it is fixed to the muscle.

In intra-abdominal swelling—it will either disappear or become less prominent in Carnett's test.

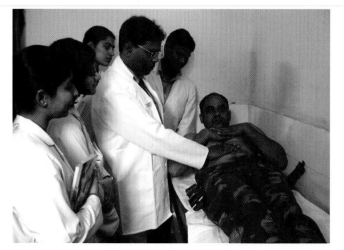

Rising test

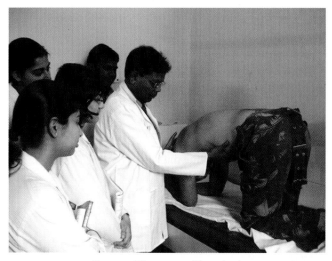

Knee—Elbow position test

Another Differentiating Point

Move the swelling vertically with respiration
↓
If it moves—it is obviously an intra-abdominal swelling

You can do also 'rising test'—which the patient raises his shoulder from the bed with arms are kept over the chest. The features will be same as Carnett's test.

To differentiate retroperitoneal and intra-abdominal swelling.
↓
When you confirm it is an intra-abdominal swelling- do *'knee elbow'* position test to differentiate between intra-peritoneal and retroperitoneal lump.

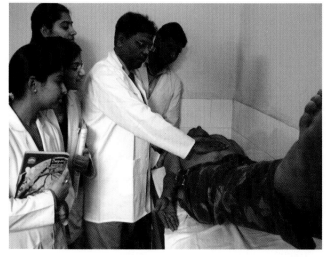

Carnett's test (leg lifting test)

On knee elbow position, if the lump falls forward—it is intraperitoneal: so called intra-abdominal.

If does not fall forward it is retroperitoneal lump.

How abdominal lump is related to leg lifting test?

1. Both rectus muscles fixe the pelvis when legs are being raised, this causes construction of both recti and they become taught thus abdominal lump becomes less prominent.

2. The fascia lata of thigh is attached to inguinal ligament. So extension of thigh pulls the abdominal wall downwards and makes it tense in which the parietal lump will be more prominent and intra-abdominal lump will either become less prominent or disappear.

CASE 2   Surgical Obstructive Jaundice

My patient, Kusumkali, a 65-year-old female, factory worker, resident of UP, presented to this hospital with chief complainants of:

- Yellowish discoloration of eyes and urine for last 4 months.
- Itching all over the body for last 2 months.
- Passing whitish color stool for last 1 month.

HISTORY OF PRESENT ILLNESS

(No need to utter heading in front of examiner).

My patient was apparently well 4 months back when she started developing yellowish discoloration of her eyes and urine which was gradually progressive without any history of pain abdomen.

She has got a history of progressive itching all over the body for last 2 months which disturbs her sleep. She is passing clay color stools for last 1 month. She has also got a history of unquantified weight loss and loss of appetite for last 2 months.

But there is no history of:

i. Fever, nausea, retching, vomiting (prodromal symptoms for viral hepatitis).
ii. No history of hematemesis, malena (suggestive of malignant infiltration to duodenal/gastric mucosa or a result of ruptured fundal varices due to splenic vein thrombosis (development of portal hypertension).
iii. No history of urinary disturbances (involvement of kidney) but urine color is gradually deepening.
iv. No history of alteration of bowel habit or large bulky stool (steatorrhea).
v. No history suggestive of gastric outlet obstruction (GOO) (Tumor can press gastric outlet).
vi. No history of cough, chest pain, hemoptysis. No history of bone pain, etc. (to exclude metastasis).
vii. No history of primary silvery colored stool followed by remission in jaundice (suggestive of sloughing of ampullary growth).

PAST HISTORY

i. No history of hypertension. Tuberculosis (co-morbidity).
ii. There is a history of diabetes for last 2 years and she is on regular medicine (this is hereditary type of diabetes which is related to carcinoma, head of pancreas).
iii. No history of blood transfusion or prolonged hospitalization.
iv. No history of drug allergy in past.
v. No history of long-term drug ingestion which may cause cholestatic jaundice (H$_2$ blockers, clavulanic acid, etc.)
No history of significant operation in the past.

PERSONAL HISTORY

She is a factory worker (carcinoma head of pancreas related with beta naphthalene and benzidine). She smokes 10-15 bidi/day for last 15 years. No history of alcoholism as such.

Family History

Family history is not contributory (though hereditary pancreatitis related with carcinoma head of pancreas).

On General Examination

Patient is cooperative, ill looking, average built and averagely naurished.

Pulse 64/min   BP- 110/70 mm Hg

Pallor +, Icterus +

No edema or generalized lymphadenopathy noticed.

But scratch marks present all over the body.

No features suggestive of chronic hepatic insufficiency like confusion, spider telangiectasia, [gynecomastia bilateral testicular atrophy (in male)], palmer erythema, tremor, loss of pubic and axillary hairs, etc.

Systemic Examination

Abdomen

On inspection
- Abdomen scaphoid/bulky/any obvious visible lump
- Umbilicus center
- All quadrants move with respiration
- No visible scar, swellings, prominent veins or peristalsis
- Flanks are not full
- Hernial sites and external genitalia appear normal.

On palpation (Before palpation, kindly warm heads)
- Local temperature not raised
- Nontender abdomen
- Abdomen is soft
- There is a 6 × 3 cm piriform shaped, intra-abdominal mass at right hypochondrial region quaclrant of abdomen.
- Nontender
- Firm in consistency
- Well defined margin except upper margin which is merged with liver
- Surface–smooth, moves with respiration and side-to-side mobility is there present
- Fingers can be insinuated in between costal margin and the mass (In gallbladder lump, one can insinuate the fingers if it is not infiltrating to the liver benign lump like mucocele, gallbladder but when it gets fixed to the liver, e.g. in case of carcinoma gallbladder one can- not insinuate the fingers between costal margins and the mass)
- No other lump palpable
- No hepatosplenomegaly (if hepatomegaly is present than as follows describe – 3 cm on mid clavicular line. Hepatic dullness at 5th intercostall space, etc.).
- No free fluid
- Hernial sites and external genitalia are normal
- No supraclavicular lymph nodes palpable
- Digital per rectal exam (DKE)
  - No 'Blumer self' palpable

Auscultation – Bowel Sound+ (head)

Others Systemic Exam:
- Respiratory system–bilateral air entry+, no adventitious sound heard.
- Musculoskeletal system–no bony tenderness, swelling noticed. [To exclude bone mets].

- CVS—S1, S2 Normal. No murmur.
- CNS—Higher motor function- normal. No neurodeficit.

Summary

My patient, a 65-year-old female, factory worker, presented with complaints of yellowish discoloration of eyes and urine for last 4 months, itching all over the body for last 2 months and passing clay color stool for last 1 month.

There was no history of fever, pain abdomen, hematemesis, malaena. There is no history suggestive of gastric outlet obstruction and metastasis.

On Examination

Patient has pallor and icterus, scratch marks all over the body.

Abdomen-soft, there is 6 × 3 cm palpable GB lump, well defined, firm in consistency, smooth surface, side-to-side mobility present. No other organomegaly present or supraclavicular lymph node palpable.

So my provisional diagnosis is—this is a case of obstructive jaundice, most probably *due to periampullary carcinoma,* i.e. lower end of cholangiocarcinoma, carcinoma head of pancreas, ampullary carcinoma, carcinoma duodenum, etc. (carcinoma duodenum usually present with gastric outlet obstruction).

Why do you say this jaundice is due to periampullary carcinoma?
- Elderly patient having progressive pain less jaundice (pain in obstructive jaundice radiating to back suggestive of carcinoma head of pancreas).
- Most common cause of obstructive jaundice, is peri-ampullary carcinoma [carcinoma head of pancreas (29%)].
- History of malaise, loss of weight, loss of appetite also suggestive of malignancy.
- Gallbladder well palpable.l
- Jaundice is not waxing and waning type (seen in ampullary carcinoma).
- No history suggestive of silvery stool to exclude ampullary carcinoma.
  - *Differential diagnoses:* Carcinoma gallbladder (11.5%)—Gallbladder is a smooth, firm usually not started with progressive painless jaundice. Jaundice appears later.
  - Lower end cholangiocarcinoma 10%.
  - Ampullary carcinoma 7%.
  - Periampullary lymphadenopathy.

How will you investigate the case?

Sir, I will confirm my diagnosis first

I will do - i. *Liver function tests*—in obstructive jaundice.

Conjugated bilirubin is increased

Alkaline phosphatase ≥6 times of its normal value. [Normal value 60 or 170 IU/L]

AST (SGOT) ≤3 times

ALT (SGPT) ≤3 times

GGT – increased

Albumin – may decrease

Coagulation profile may be deranged particularly PT (Prothrombin time)

ii. *Tumor markers* – CEA, CA 19-9 may be increased

iii. *Stool for occult blood* test may be positive.

USG ABDOMEN

To see

- IHBR dilatation which is the hallmark of surgical obstructive jaundice (SOJ).
- Organ of origin of the lump.
- Site of obstruction – dilated duct system.
- CBD dilatation till lower end with abrupt cut off (suggestive of periampullary pathology).
- Type of mass-solid or cystic.
- Ascites present or not.
- Lymph node—if any
- Any impacted stone, stone in CBD, condition of GB (calculus/distention).
- Hepatic metastasis—USG can be repeated to count the number of metastasis in follow-up.

CECT ABDOMEN

As USG has observer bias and CT film is more accurate in detecting:

- Site of obstruction
- Extent of disease
- Involvement of superior mesenteric vessels/ portal vein/ IVC/celiac trunk, etc.

[If any doubt about the vessels involvement CDFI (color Doppler flow imaging) can be done followed by angiography].

- Hepatic metastasis.
- Lymph nodes involvement. In a word, CT scan helps to stage the disease.

Along with triple phase CECT we see the involvement of portal vein, hepatic artery, hepatic veins, etc.

UPPER GI ENDOSCOPY

- To see esophageal varices.
- Site viewing endoscopy to see ampullary growth duodenal carcinoma or carcinoma head of pancreas infiltrating duodenum/ampulla.

How to treat the patient?

If the tumor is operable, baseline investigations to be done followed by Whipple's pancreaticoduodenectomy which consists of:

- Resection of head and neck of pancreas, duodenum and up to 10 cm of jejunum.
- Partial gastrectomy, removal of 30-40% of distal stomach.
- Cholecystectomy.
- Excision of CBD.
- Lymph nodes dissection and reconstructive surgery
- Surgical obstructive jaundice
- Pancreaticojejunostomy
- Gastrojejunostomy
- Hepaticojejunostomy

(Jejunojejunostomy is done only when Roux En Y anastomosis is used for pancreaticojejunostomy and hepatico- jejunostomy. Other wise it is a single jejunal loop).

What is jaundice?

Jaundice is yellowish discoloration of skin and/or mucous membrane due to increase level of circulating bilirubin in the blood.

(Normal level of bilirubin is 0 .2- 1.2 mg%, latent jaundice 1.3-2mg% and clinical jaundice in greater than 2 g%. Remember clinical jaundice is well marked when bilirubin is more than 3 mg% practically. In obstructive jaundice if bilirubin is 4-6 mg% the mucous membrane, hard palate will be yellowish. When nail bed and palm are yellowish it is around 8 mg% and when the sole and generalized body skin involved then the bilirubin is > 8 mg%).

What are the types of jaundice?

There are three types of jaundice:

i. *Hemolytic (Prehepatic):* Unconjugated bilirubin increased in the blood due to hemolysis in the body as with hemolytic anemia.

ii. *Hepatocellular:* Both conjugated and unconjugated bilirubin are increased as in viral hepatitis.

iii. *Obstructive jaundice:* Conjugated bilirubin increases in the blood due to hepatobiliary out flow tract obstruction.

What is acholuric jaundice?

Clinical jaundice with absence of bile pigment in urine. It is found in hemolytic jaundice as unconjugated bilirubin is not water soluble and cannot be filtered through kidney.

What are the tests for bile pigment, bile salt and urobilinogen?

In obstructive jaundice conjugated bilirubin is increased in the blood which is water soluble and thrown out from urine. If urine is tested for bile salts and bile pigment it will be positive.

For bile pigment – Fouchet's test (remember PF. P for Pigment and F for Fouchet) 10 ml of urine + 5 ml of BaCl 2+ pinch of $MgSO_4$ – causes of formation of $Ba SO_4$ which is filtered over a filter paper - add few drops of Fouchet's reagent – green/blue color appear in urine in presence of bile pigments.

Hay's test for bile salt (remember HS) 2 ml of urine + sprinkle sulfur – bile salt settle in the bottom.

Ehrlich's test for urobilinogen—5 ml fresh voided urine + 1 ml Ehrlich's reagent → wait for 5 minutes – formation of red color indicates urobilinogen in urine.

Is malignant obstructive jaundice painless all the time?

No sir, in case of carcinoma head of pancreas patient may experience pain if:
1. It is the consequence of chronic pancreatitis.
2. Pancreatic duct obstruction causing stasis which may give rise pain.
3. Involvement of retropancreatic nerve plexus may cause pain.

Tell me the conditions where pruritis appear first then jaundice?

1. Cholangiocarcinoma—peripheral type.
2. Sclerosing cholangitis.
3. Cholestasis during pregnancy.
4. Cholestatic phase of chronic hepatitis.

What is periampullary carcinoma?

Any malignant tumor arising within 2 cm from ampulla, i.e. radius is 1 cm.

Carcinoma arising periampullary regions are:
1. Adenocarcinoma head of pancreas 50-60%.
2. Ampullary tumor arising from ampulla of Vater itself- up to 30- 40% cases.
3. Distal CBD carcinoma- 10%.
4. Carcinoma arising from adjacent duodenum 5-10%.
5. Adjacent Lymph node enlargement.

What are the special characteristics of ampullary carcinoma?

1. Waxing and waning type of jaundice. [As (i) Necrosed tissue is being sloughed off intermittently from the obstructive tumor mass, (ii) Fistulas track may form between the growth and the adjacent gut].
2. Melena is one of the important features of ampullary carcinoma.
3. Silvery paint stool (clay stool mixed with blood).
4. Dilatation of the pancreatic duct.

How will you differentiate between Medical and Surgical Jaundice?

Medical jaundice	*Surgical jaundice*
1. Prodromal symptoms like nausea, may be vomiting, retching and fever present. Most of the time, by the time clinical jaundice appears the prodromal symptoms disappear.	1. Prodromal symptoms absent. Fever with chill, and rigor, pain abdomen suggestive of cholangitis.
2. Rapidly progressive deep jaundice. Without any features of obstruction.	2. Features of obstruction like purities and clay color stool, etc. along with gradually progressive jaundice.
3. LFT: ALP< 6 times of its normal value. (Normal value of Alkaline phosphate 60-170 IU/L. It may vary from lab to lab.) Gamma glutamyl transferase (GGT) within normal limit. SGOT, SGPT> 3 times of their normal value. SGPT>SGOT	3. ALP> 6 times of its normal value. SGOT, SGPT< 3 times of its normal value. Gamma glutamyl transferase (GGT) increased.
4. USG—No IHBR dilatation. There may be features of increased echogenicity of liver and hepatomegaly.	4. IHBR dilatation is most important finding of obstructive jaundice. [Intrahepatic biliary radicles (IHBR)]. Hepatomegaly is late features of obstruction.

What is the rate of fall of bilirubin level after biliary drainage/decompression?

Bilirubin level falls at an average rate of 8% per day, so the value will be 25% of the preoperative value by day 10 and about 10% of preoperative value 2 weeks after operation.

What is Courvoisier's law and its exceptions?

"In obstruction of the common bile duct due to a stone, distention of the gallbladder seldom occurs; the organ usually is already shrivelled."

Exceptions:

1. Double stone impaction- one in CBD, another one in cystic duct.
2. Oriental cholangiohepatitis. [Endemic in far east, the fluke – clonorchis- in habits in bile duct- causing fibrous thickening of the duct wall – leads to distended gallbladder- usually asymptomatic, but may cause biliary pain, stones, cholangitis, cirrhosis, bile duct carcinoma.
3. Pancreatic calculus obstructing the ampulla.
4. Distended gallbladder (mucocele) due to large stone impaction in the cystic duct.
5. Palpable gallbladeler, i.e. in carcinoma gallbladeler (due to blockage of cystic duct owing to infiltration/lymph nodal compression).

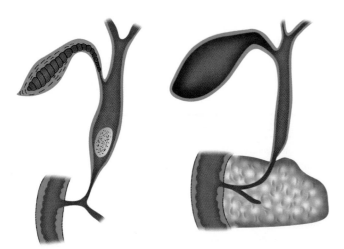

[Diagrammatic presentation of Courvoisier's law in a case of jaundice due to stone in CBD, distention of gallbladder seldom occurs, as the organ is already shrivelled.
- If there is a stone in CBD, gallbladder is usually not distended owing to previous inflammatory fibrosis.
- If CBD is obstructed due to periampullary growth, the gallbladder becomes distended due to back pressure changes (as in hydronephrosis due to ureteric stone)].

6. Mirizzi syndrome – Type I.

Why spleen is enlarged in obstructive jaundice?

Prolonged unrelieved obstructive jaundice causes secondary biliary cirrhosis and then splenomegaly due to portal hypertension.

Portal hypertension which is due to obstruction in portal vein or due to splenic vein thrombosis may cause splenomegaly.

What are the causes of hepatomegaly in obstructive jaundice?

Hepatomegaly is due to:

1. Prolonged stasis of bile causes back pressure changes and hepatomegaly.
2. Metastasis in the liver.
3. Hepatocellular carcinoma.

Why prothrombin time (PT) is increased in obstructive jaundice?

Vitamin K is required for synthesis of coagulation factors. As vitamin K is fat soluble vitamin and fat is soluble only in bile but as bile is absent in GI tract lumen, all fat soluble vitamins (ADEK) absorption gets hampered. So there is impaired synthesis of coagulation factors. So prothrombin time is increased in obstructive jaundice.

NB- PT correction- Inj. vit. K 10 mg IM (K1 may be given IV) for 5-7 days.

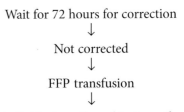

Wait for 72 hours for correction
↓
Not corrected
↓
FFP transfusion
↓

In normal individual prothrombin time, the difference between the controls and tests should be ≤4 sec and more than 5 sec is considered abnormal

What are the indications of endoscopic retrograde cholangiopancreatography (ERCP)?

ERCP is a therapeutic and diagnostic procedure.

Diagnostic: Diagnostic of all periampullary carcinoma biopsy, cholangiogram, pancreaticogram, brush cytology, etc.

Therapeutic: Endoscopic papillotomy.
CBD/Pancreatic duct stone extraction stenting, etc.

Indications:

1. With side view, ampulla of Vater can be seen directly. Biopsy can be taken from the visible growth, if any. (Side viewing endoscopy is only diagnostic procedure).
2. To visualize both bile duct and pancreatic duct.
3. Site of obstruction, proximal dilatation of CBD may be observed.
4. Brush-cytology can be taken for the diagnosis of cholangio carcinoma or bile is collected for exfoliative cytology.
5. Stenting can be done when bilirubin is >15 mg%.
6. Bile sampling for neoplastic cells (as 40% of carcinoma gallbladder, bile will be positive for malignant cells).

What are the indications of MRCP?

- To see the biliary tree and pancreatic duct as it has got better delineation of biliary and pancreatic duct.
- When bilirubin is <15 mg% and stenting is not contemplated.
- To avoid unnecessary invasive procedure like ERCP. (Only disadvantage is that it cannot be used as therapeutic procedure like ERCP).

How barium meal X-ray help in diagnosis of obstructive jaundice?

- In ampullary growth 'Rose thorn' appearance due to mucosal irregularity. Inverted '3' sign due to filling defect in the region of ampulla.
- In carcinoma head of pancreas widening of C-loop- (*Pad sign*)
- Gastric distention due to gastric outlet obstruction (GOO).

What is hypotonic duodenography?

It is the pathological change and deformity of duodenum owing to pathology in pancreas.

Procedure: Duodenum is made atonic by giving Antrenyl injection or dicyclomin hydrochloride injection.
↓
Hypotonic barium is pushed through gastroduodenal tube.
↓
Duodenum is distended with air.
↓
Observations are: in periampullary carcinoma- Rose thorn, inverted '3' sign.
In carcinoma head of pancreas: Pad sign- widening C loop, others like diverticula, papilloma are clearly seen.

What are the determining factors for resectibility?

Involvement of superior mesenteric vessels, portal vein, IVC, celiac axis, etc. suggestive of inoperability of the growth.

Para-aortic lymph node/celiac lymph node or mesenteric lymph node involvement are also suggestive of inoperability.

What is double duct sign?

It is seen in periampullary carcinoma where both the bile duct and pancreatic duct are dilated as a result of constriction of both the ducts in the region of pancreatic head. Double duct sign is detected by either ERCP or MRCP.

How are left supraclavicular lymph nodes involved in GI malignancy like carcinoma pancreas?

Left supraclavicular lymph nodes involvement in abdominal malignancy is through thoracic duct which drains in the junction between the left subclavian and left internal jugular vein.

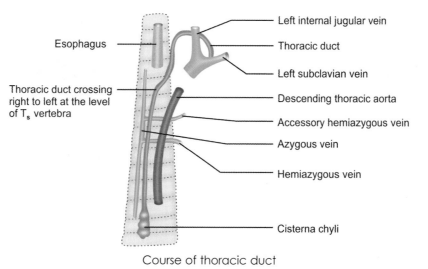

Course of thoracic duct

The hypothesis is:
I. During sudden increase of intrathoracic pressure like coughing, sneezing, the tumor cells reflux back and invade the lymph nodes.
II. Tumor cells deposit in the small lymphatics, draining the lymph nodes, resulting in obstruction and subsequently leading to lymphadenopathy.

COURSE OF THORACIC DUCT

The thoracic duct—The largest lymphatic vessels in the body. 45 cm long, beaded appearance because of the presence of many valves in its lumen.

Course: Thoracic duct begins as continuation of upper end of cisterna chyli near the lower border of 12th thoracic vertebra and enters the thorax through the aortic opening of the diaphragm (T12). It ascends through posterior mediastinum crossing from the right to left side at the level of 5th thoracic vertebra. Along the edge of esophagus it runs through the superior mediastinum and reaches the neck.

In the neck: It arches laterally at the level of transverse process of 7th cervical vertebra and then descends in front of 1st part of left subclavian artery and ends into the junction of left subclavian and left inernal jugular vein.

Right lymphatic duct: The right jugular, subclavian and bronchomediastinal trunks which drain the right side of head and neck, right side of thorax, respectively, may join to form the right lymphatic duct. This is approximately ½ inch (1.3 cm) long and opens into the beginning of the right brachiocephalic vein. Alternatively, the trunks open independently into the great veins at the root of neck.

What are the preoperative preparation in obstructive jaundice?

Problem of surgery in jaundice patients are:
• Obstruction and sepsis.
• Impaired clotting.
• Risk of renal disorder due to hepatorenal syndrome.
• Impaired resistance to infection.

So patients to be given:
• Antibiotic prophylaxis.
• Maintain hydration (Intake output chart to be maintained).
• Inj vit K 10 mg IM OD, 5-7 days to improve clotting factors.
• Correct malnutrition- high protein diet.
• Correction of anemia by blood transfusion and to make Hb% > 10 gm%.
• Dehydration to be corrected (hyperosmolarity of blood due to increase level of conjugated bilirubin and low

intake of fluid and food due to associated anorexia caused by malignancy).

What is extended Whipple's operation?

This is called Fortner's operation. When growth involves superior mesenteric vessels and adjacent lymph nodes, a wider clearance can be done by resecting a segment of superior mesenteric vessels with bypass graft. Adjacent lymph nodes to be cleared.

What all to study in this case?

• Anatomy and blood supply of hepatobiliary system.
• Blood supply of CBD.
• Bilirubin metabolism/hepatobiliary circulation.
• Carcinoma pancreas.
• Choledochal cyst.
• Cholangiocarcinoma.
• Carcinoma gallbladder.
• Periampullary carcinoma.

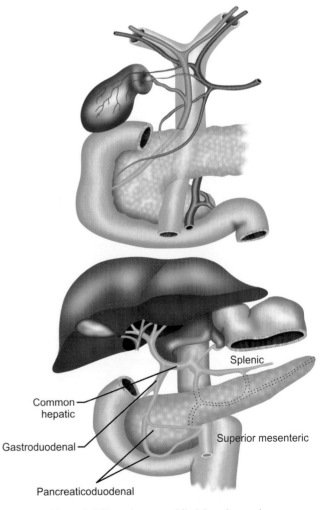

Hepatobiliary tree and its blood supply

SHORT NOTE ON SURGICAL OBSTRUCTIVE JAUNDICE

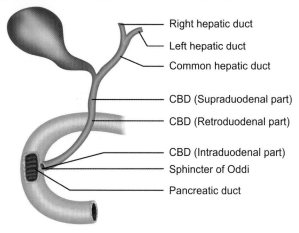

- Right hepatic duct
- Left hepatic duct
- Common hepatic duct
- CBD (Supraduodenal part)
- CBD (Retroduodenal part)
- CBD (Intraduodenal part)
- Sphincter of Oddi
- Pancreatic duct

Anatomy of hepatobiliary tree

BILIRUBIN METABOLISM

Destruction of senescent RBC in the RE system 80-85%
Marrow destruction of matured RBC (15-20%)

Heme containing protein (liver turnover)- minimal
↓
Hemoglobin
↓
↓ Heme oxygenase
Biliverdin
↓ Biliverdin reductase
Bilirubin
↓ binds with albumin
Bilirubin albumin complex transported to the liver
↓
Liver takes up bilirubin
↓
Conjugate with glucuronic acid and forms
monoglucuronide and diglucuronide
By UDP Glucuronyl transferase
↓
After deconjugation, bilirubin is absorbed at terminal
ilium, ileocecal junction
↓
Free bilirubin
↓ Reduction
Urobilinogen 20% (gives urine color) and
Stercobilinogen 80% (gives stool color)
↓
Oxidized and re-entered into enterohepatic circulation (13%)
Excreted through urine (4-7%)

Bilirubin is produced from the destruction of senescent RBC's by the removal of the iron by the action of the enzyme heme oxygenase; the reaction liberates carbon monoxide, the only reaction in the body releasing carbon monoxide. The intermediate product being biliverdin.

Bilirubin a water insoluble compound is transported to the liver bound to albumin.

In the liver the bilirubin is taken up activity by two mechanisms. The first being a membrane bound carrier protein and the second being by two cytoplasmic proteins namely protein Y and Z. These proteins pick up the bilirubin diffusing into the cytoplasm.

Once in the hepatocyte the bilirubin is bound to glucuronic acid thus forming bilirubin mono and di glucuronide by the enzyme UDP glucuronyl transferase. The enzyme reduced products get excreted as stercobilinogen. The kidneys excrete a part of the absorbed bilirubin as urobilinogen and the rest enters the enterohepatic circulation.

CLASSIFICATION

Obstructive jaundice can be classified as:

- Complete
- Intermittent
- Chronic intermittent
- Segmental

There are many classification systems available for obstructive jaundice. The most common one in use is the *Benjamin classification*.

Etiology of obstructive jaundice:

Benign	38%
CBD stone	32%
Post-cholecystectomy biliary structure (approximate 0.4% biliary injury occurs in laparoscopic cholecystectomy)	3%–4%
Intrabiliary rupture of hydrated cyst	2%
Misccllaneous	3%
Malignant	62%
Carcinoma head of pancreas	29%
Periampullary	7%
Extrahepatic bile duct carcinoma	10%
Carcinoma gallbladder	12%
Secondaries in porta	4%

Type I Complete obstruction (produces jaundice)	Tumors specially pancreatic head, ligation of CBD Cholangiocarcinoma- complete type Parenchymal liver tumors primary, secondary
Type II Intermittent obstruction (produces symptoms and biochemical changes of obstruction but may or may not produce jaundice)	Choledocholithiasis Periampullary carcinoma Choledochal cyst Intrabiliary parasites
Type III Chronic incomplete obstruction (with or without symptoms or biochemical changes but will eventually produce pathological changes in the liver, ducts)	Strictures of CBD Stenosed biliary enteric anastomosis Chronic pancreatitis Cystic fibrosis Stenosis of sphincter of Oddi
Type IV Segmental obstruction (one or more anatomical segments are involved with either of the above types)	Traumatic Hepatodocholithiasis Sclerosing cholangitis Cholangiocarcinoma

CONSEQUENCES OF BILIARY OBSTRUCTION

Proximal dilatation of the biliary tree. It is more marked in acute complete obstruction and may be completely reversible.

Increased secretory pressure of bile. (N=120-250 mm water.) Stabilizes at around 300 mm of water in biliary obstruction. Ultimately secondary biliary cirrhosis sets in unrelieved obstructive jaundice. Patient may present with features of portal hypertension.

In cirrhotic patient usually there is no intrahepatic biliary radicles dilatation.

Prolonged obstruction leads to fibrosis of the biliary tract and the dilatation may not be evident. This is a Grave sign and fibrosis makes anastomosis difficult.

Cholesterol and phospholipid secretions are reduced more than bile acids thus less lithogenic bile. Later bile acid secretion reduces.

Cyto P450 is converted it to inactive form cyto P420.

A serum bilirubin higher than 12 mg% significantly increases risk of surgical complications.

Hepatorenal syndrome: In severe liver disease, renal failure appears where there are no intrinsic renal disturbances. Kidney function is usually promptly improved if hepatic dysfunction is reversed.

Here renal perfusion pressure decreases followed by renal vasoconstriction.

Concentrate urine is retained, oliguria with a hyperosmolar urine which is devoid of proteins and low sodium is surprisingly characteristic features.

PATHOLOGICAL EFFECTS OF BILIARY OBSTRUCTION

Liver

- Dilated biliary canaliculi (centrilobular) with swollen, tortuous villi
- Bile thrombi
- Inflammatory reaction around the canaliculi due to recurrent cholangitis which may further aggravate the obstruction.

Kidney

- Causes renal failure the reasons for which are:
  i. Direct toxic effect of elevated bilirubin
  ii. Endotoxemia
  iii. Absence of bile acid from the small intestine
  iv. Alteration in mitochondrial oxidative phosphorylation
  v. Renal vascular fibrin deposition
  vi. Decreased sensitivity of α-adrenergic effects of noradrenaline.
- Incidence: 3-50%
- Mortality: 25-80%
- Endotoxin causes renal vasoconstriction and redistribution of internal blood flow away from the cortex.
- Hence, aim for urine drainage does not reduce mortality from ARF following surgery for obstructive jaundice.

Wound Healing

Wound healing will be delayed:
- Wound dehiscence in 2-4%.
- Incisional hernia in 10-12.5% cases as skin prolyl hydroxylase activity is low.

(Except where cause is not known whether this is due to malnutrition or hyperbilirubinemia).

Endotoxemia

- Absence of bile salts encourages the endotoxin production by loss of specific binding function of bile salts and alteration of small bowel microflora.
- Depressed hepatic RE cell function and thus decreased clearance of endotoxins.
- Cimetidine prevents endotoxin absorption.
- A direct anti-endotoxic effect of lactulose has been proposed (indirect effect by altering the gut flora).
- Kaolin, pectin and cholestyramine have been shown to bind endotoxins in animal models.
- There is an increase in the incidence of infection of bile. It ranges from 36% in the case of malignant obstruction to 80% in benign biliary strictures.

Coagulation Defects

- There is a decrease in the levels of vit K dependent coagulation factors synthesis (II, VII, IX, X) and also fibrinogen, prothrombin and factor XI.
- There is reduced synthesis of coagulation inhibitors like protein C, S and antithrombin C.
- There is failure to clear activated coagulation factors from circulation. This along with endotoxemia probably predisposes to a higher incidence of DIC.

Hemodynamic Changes

- Decreased systemic arterial pressure.
- Decreased peripheral vascular resistance.
- Decreased responsiveness to norepinephrine (noradrenaline).
- Increased atrial natriuretic peptide.
- These patients have a reduced interstitial volume and marginally reduced plasma volume.

CLINICAL MANIFESTATIONS

- Ductal stones are more common in females and cancers common in males.
- Pain, a continuous dull boring pain in the upper abdomen. Usually precedes the onset of jaundice. *Pain before jaundice is more common in benign obstruction than in malignancies.* Pain radiating to back is seen in chronic pancreatitis and pancreatic cancers.
- Icterus (may or may not be present- see classification). The level may fluctuate as seen in CBD stones, ampullary tumors where it is due to sloughing of a part of the tumor. This may be accompanied by an intermittently palpable gallbladder. Scleral icterus begins to appear with a serum bilirubin of 2.5-3 mg% and yellowing of skin and mucosa does not appear until the serum bilirubin is around 6 mg%.
- Pruritus (irritation of cutaneous nerve ending by bile salts).
- Weight loss is frequent and results from sitophobia, malabsorption and effects of cancer.
- Clay colored stools due to absence of bile from, intestine.
- Cholangitis, i.e. fever with chills and rigor. Usually occurs in benign conditions and is rare in malignant obstruction. (As the malignant obstruction is usually a complete block). The chills and rigors are due to a cholangiovenous and cholangiolymphatic reflux of bacteria from the obstructed and infected ducts.
- **Courvoisier's law:** "In obstruction of the common bile duct due to a stone distention of the gallbladder seldom occurs; the organ usually is already shrivelled." Gallbladder is usually thickened and nondistensible due to recurrent attacks of cholecystitis).
- **Chung law:** The palpable GB simply represents a chronically elevated ductal pressure which is more likely to result from a high grade malignant obstruction.
- Deficiency of fat soluble vitamins ADEK.
- Malena.
- **Charcot's triad:** Abdominal pain, jaundice and fever suggestive of cholangitis.
- **Reynold's pentad:** Alongwith Charcot's triad, i.e. abdominal pain, jaundice and fever. There will be mental obtundation and shock. This suggestive of severe cholangitis with septicemia.

INVESTIGATION PROTOCOL FOR A JAUNDICE PATIENT

Biochemical Parameters

Serum Bilirubin (0.2-1.2 mg%)

There is an increase in the conjugated bilirubin. The increase may be marginal especially in incomplete or intermittent obstruction. It can be very difficult to differentiate between obstructive and hepatocellular jaundice solely on the basis of serum bilirubin.

Alkaline Phosphate (60-170 IU/ L; 3-13 KAU/mL)

This enzyme is elevated in SOJ. The enzyme is actively secreted into the biliary canaliculi. Increased levels in obstruction are due to back diffusion or leak from the ducts. The level of rise is not proportional to the degree of obstruction. The levels of enzyme start to reduce after the relief of obstruction but it may take time. The measurement of the biliary isozyme (the other being the hepatic) may allow for a better differentiation between complete or minimal biliary obstruction.

Gamma glutamyl transferase (GGT) is more specific. Normal value is 10–48 IU/L. Highest activity occurs in biliary obstruction and markly increase in any form of hepatic parenchymal damage.

Transminases (3-48 IU/L)

These are elevated initially even before the rise of serum bilirubin and ALP but return to normal later. In prolonged obstruction they may get elevated again and this is a poor prognostic factor.

Serum Albumin (TP 6-8 g/dL; Alb: 3.8-5 g/dL; Glb: 1.8-3.5 g/dL)

Used as an indicator of hepatic synthesis. But due to its long half-life it is not a very useful measure of acute hepatic dysfunction. Decreased levels are commonly seen in malignant obstruction. Half-life of albumin is 20 days. Lack of prealbumin indicates hepatic deficiency.

Coagulation Profile

There is deranged prothrombin time, INR which promptly returns to normal after administration of vitamin K (as opposed to hepatocellular jaundice when the PT shows poor response to vit K).

Urinary Bilirubin and Urobilinogen

There is absence of urinary urobilinogen and there may be bilirubinuria.

Increased gamma glutamyl transpeptidase (GGT) itself confirms liver involvement.

Radiological Investigations

Plain X-ray abdomen has limited role if any value. Calcified stones may be seen in 10-20% of choledocholithiasis. Speckled calcification in the region of the head of pancreas may be seen in chronic pancreatitis.

Hypotonic Duodenography

As described earlier.

Done using a double lumen derringer tube. Rarely used now. Gives a mucosal relief and can be used to pick up periampullary tumors.

Abdominal USG

Noninvasive and free of risk.

Defines the *presence of a dilated biliary tree*, calculi, abnormal hepatic anatomy and pancreatic abnormality in pancreas.

Can determine the site of obstruction in 60-80% and the cause of obstruction in 50% but it cannot reliably exclude extrahepatic obstruction.

More sensitive than CT for detecting cholelithiasis.

Endoscopic USG

May be more accurate than combined ERCP and CT scan in defining the nature and extent of biliary obstruction. The more specific to periampullary carcinoma. During the procedure one can take FNAC from the liver.

CECT Scan

Can establish the level of obstruction in 90% cases and the cause, in 75-94%.

The dilated biliary system is divided into four parts:
- Hepatic.
- Suprapancreatic
- Pancreatic
- Ampullary

An abrupt change in caliber of a grossly dilated CBD is indicative of malignancy. The terminal end of the CBD may be irregular, rounded or nipple shaped but the end is always abrupt.
- Calculi are visible in 80-90%.
- More sensitive than USG in detecting choledo-cholithiasis.
- Can visualize small (1-2 cm) hepatic parenchymal lesions.
- Assesses the distal CBD which cannot be done by USG.
- Can evaluate inflammatory process.

MRCP/MRI: It has got several advantages over CT in hepatobiliary disease.
  i. MRI to be offered in patience with allergy to iodine containing dye.

An Algorithm for management of obstructive jaundice

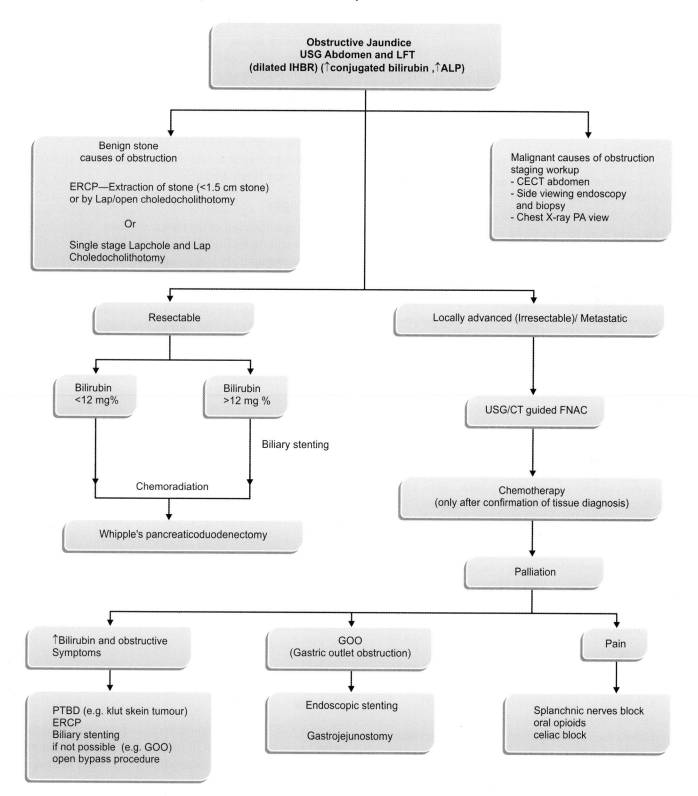

Obstructive Jaundice
USG Abdomen and LFT
(dilated IHBR) (↑conjugated bilirubin ,↑ALP)

Benign stone
causes of obstruction

ERCP—Extraction of stone (<1.5 cm stone)
or by Lap/open choledocholithotomy

Or

Single stage Lapchole and Lap
Choledocholithotomy

Malignant causes of obstruction
staging workup
- CECT abdomen
- Side viewing endoscopy
  and biopsy
- Chest X-ray PA view

Resectable

Locally advanced (Irresectable)/ Metastatic

Bilirubin
<12 mg%

Bilirubin
>12 mg %

Biliary stenting

USG/CT guided FNAC

Chemoradiation

Whipple's pancreaticoduodenectomy

Chemotherapy
(only after confirmation of tissue diagnosis)

Palliation

↑Bilirubin and obstructive
Symptoms

GOO
(Gastric outlet obstruction)

Pain

PTBD (e.g. klut skein tumour)
ERCP
Biliary stenting
if not possible (e.g. GOO)
open bypass procedure

Endoscopic stenting

Gastrojejunostomy

Splanchnic nerves block
oral opioids
celiac block

ii. MRCP has excellent delineation of biliary tree and pancreatic duct as a non-invasive procedure. Any pathology in biliary tree and pancreatic duct is easily picked up.

Percutaneous Transhepatic Cholangiogram (PTC)
(Rarely used nowadays as a diagnostic procedure as MRCP being a non-invasive and more specific investigation).

Technique
Now done with a thin flexible CHIBA needle 22-gauge.

A brisk puncture is more likely to be successful than intermittent advance.

When the needle enters the duct the contrast moves slowly away from the needle tip unlike the washout seen in the puncture of the vessels.

If the contrast is outside the duct and tracks along the duct then the margins are not sharp and well defined.

Lymphatics appear as irregular linear structures which do not washout form a organized branching pattern.

Results
In dilated systems up to 99% success.

In nondilated system up to 80% success.

Complications: 5% serious complications like sepsis, hemorrhage, etc.

Precautions
Antibiotic coverage especially in the presence of cholangitis.

In the presence of cholangitis aspirate some bile before injecting the contrast and inject a small amount.

Advantages
Accurate preoperative delineation of structure.

Can play good role in surgery, i.e. reduce complications.
Percutaneous needle biopsy under fluoroscopic guidance.
Therapeutic placement of stent, draining catheters.

PTC Pictures in Various Diseases
Sclerosing cholangitis: alternate dilatations and strictures throughout the biliary tree intraluminal filling defects.

Ascaris: Long linear filling defects, beaded appearance.
Echinococcus: Large grape like filling defects.
Hemobilia: Large irregular filling defects.
Caroli's disease: Multiple contrast filled spaces in line with the intrahepatic ducts. Fluffy contrast collections in the ends of the ducts are seen in absence of complicating cholangitis.
Calculus: A steeply curved margin or claw shaped end.

Malignant obstruction: A sharp cut off below a grossly dilated duct or irregular stricture.

Benign stricture: Incomplete obstruction. Long narrowing with smooth margins.

Extrinsic compression: Extrinsic scalloped margin with forward displacement.

Endoscopic Retrograde Cholangiopancreatography (ERCP)
- Shows the distal part of obstructive lesions.
- Success ranges from 60-92%.
- Should be carried out with preparedness to do a laparotomy if required.

Advantages

Frequent opacification of the pancreatic duct.
Direct visualization of stomach and duodenum.
Can biopsize ampullary lesion and obtain fluid for cytology.
Therapeutic applications.
Endoscopic sphincterotomy.
External drainage of obstructed bile ducts through nasobiliary duct.
Internal biliary stents.
Complications of ERCP:
   i. Cholangitis
   ii. Pancreatitis
   iii. Perforation
   iv. Bleeding.

TREATMENT

The treatment of obstructive jaundice depends on the specific condition causing it. The perioperative morbidity and mortality for surgery in patients with obstructive jaundice approaches 50% and 25%, respectively.

The basic considerations in the management of obstructive jaundice are:
   Establishing a diagnosis.
   Amelioration of symptoms.
   Relief of the obstruction.

Amelioration of Symptoms

Pruritis

There is a distressing symptom mediated centrally through opioid receptors agonism. It may be due to deposition of bile pigments in the skin. Establishment of a biliary drainage best relieves pruritis.

Cholestyramine may be effective in reducing pruritis due to partial biliary obstruction. It has no effect in complete biliary obstruction.

Drugs used include the anion exchange resins, cholestyramine and colestipol, and hepatic enzyme inducing drugs, such as rifampicin, phenobarbital, etc. More invasive examples include plasmapheresis, charcoal hemoperfusion, and partial external diversion of bile.

Antihistamines are often administered. However, no skin changes consistent with histamine-mediated effects are found and antihistamines do not appear to be efficacious.

Sedatives, such as phenobarbital, benzodiazepines, and antihistamines may have a nonspecific beneficial effect by facilitating sleep, but may impair activities that require mental concentration.

Miscellaneous therapies that have been tried include ultraviolet light, lignocaine, androgens, and hydroxyethylrutosides. None of these therapies have a clear rationale and none have been shown convincingly to be efficacious.

Other drugs used include naloxone and glucagon on experimental basis.

Relief of Obstruction

The ideal situation is to provide internal drainage.

The factors to be considered are:
- Nature of the underlying problem/lesion.
- Biliary and GI anatomy.
- Desired goal.
- Local expertise.

It can be done by the following methods:
- Radiological and percutaneous drainage techniques (PTBD).
- Endoscopic techniques.
- Surgery.

All the techniques are complementary to each other.

Patients are best managed by a multidisciplinary approach.

When a procedure is being done as a palliative measure then the nonsurgical methods are preferred.

Factors associated with poor risk are:
1. Clinical:
   Depth of jaundice.
   Cholangitis.
   Malignancy.
   Malnutrition.
   Deranged renal function.
2. Laboratory:
   Hyperbilirubinemia.

Immune suppression.
Prothrombin time impairment.
Delayed antipyrine clearance.
GTT (linear GTT curves have a poorer prognosis as compared to parabolic curves).

RADIOLOGICAL AND PERCUTANEOUS DRAINAGE TECHNIQUE

PTC

- It is imperative to drain the system completely to avoid acute supprative cholangitis.
- Technique as described earlier.
- Antibiotics for 24-48 hours.
- After the cholangiogram a guidewire can usually be passed through the obstruction and in most cases a Cope loop type self-retaining catheter can be passed to provide internal drainage.
- Balloon dilatation can be done and an endoprosthesis can then be passed (the common self-expanding ones being Gianturco Z or Wallstents stents). These stents have a maximum life of up to 15 months.

Percutaneous Transhepatic Biliary Drainage (PTBD)

External drainage – when stricture is non-negotiable. Internal drainage – when stricture can be dilated and stent can be put to across the stricture.

Indications of percutaneous transhepatic biliary drainage (PTBD)
- Decompression of biliary tract in cases of tumor obstruction.
- Permits biopsy and scraping for cytological study.
- Procedure of choice in patients with proximal tumors who are poor candidates for surgery due to high operative risk or unresectability.

Contraindications of PTC/PTBD.
   i. Ascites
  ii. Deranged coagulations profile.

ROLE OF PREOPERATIVE PERCUTANEOUS BILIARY DRAINAGE

Controversial more studies have shown that it has no effect and the few study has shown that though as a procedure it is useful but the effect is offset by the drainage related complications.

Complications of Transhepatic Intubation

1. Sliding of tube (less common if secured below the obstruction).
2. Hemorrhage.
3. Sepsis.
4. Irritative skin lesion.
5. Tumor invasion.

Endoscopic Technique

Endoscopic sphincterotomy with or without placement of stents.
- Use of 10F (external diameter 3.4 mm) tube as the smaller 1.7 mm tube gets blocked early.
- Papillotomy prior to insertion.
- If the tube gets blocked then it can be easily changed.
- It is done as an emergency procedure when patient is not fit for ERCP stenting.

Nasobiliary drainage: Useful for short-term drainage.
- Done using a 250 cm long WURB's tube external diameter 1.7 or 2.2 mm. It has a preformed tip which prevents slipping.
- Tube is passed through the instrumentation channel of a side viewing endoscope after carrying out a papillotomy and advanced proximal to the obstruction and the scope is then removed. The tube is then taken out through the nose and fixed to the cheek.

SURGERY

A. Curative surgery
B. Palliative surgery

Curative Surgery

- Radical cholecystectomy
- Hemihepatectomy
- Whipple's procedure, etc.

Palliative Surgery

- Cystojejunostomy
- Gastrojejunostomy
- Roux en Y hepaticojejunostomy
- Segment III bypass.

Surgery for Benign Lesions

1. Choledocholithiasis .... choledocholithotomy/ Choledoduodenostomy (open/laparoscopic).
2. Hepatolithiasis .... hepaticolithotomy

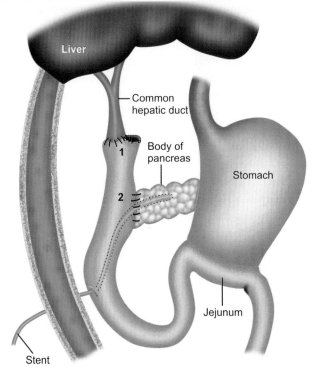

Reconstructions after Whipple's procedure, Hepaticojejunostomy, Pancreaticojejunostomy and Gastrojejunostomy

3. Chronic calculus pancreatitis .... pancreaticojejunostomy
4. Biliary strictures .... choledochoduodenostomy/ hepaticojejunostomy
5. Pancreatic pseudocyst .... cystogastrostomy/ cystojejunostomy.
6. Intrabiliary ruptures of hydatid cyst .... drainage of liver cyst.
   i. Choledochotomy
   ii. T tube drainage of CBD.

NOTES ON CONGENITAL NONHEMOLYTIC ANEMIA

Types

A. Unconjugated hyperbilirubinemia
B. Conjugated hyperbilirubinemia.

Unconjugated Hyperbilirubinemia

1. Gilbert syndrome:
   - Autosomal dominant
   - Young adult
   - Mild severity
   - Deficiency glucuronyl transferase

Etiology of cancer induced weight loss:

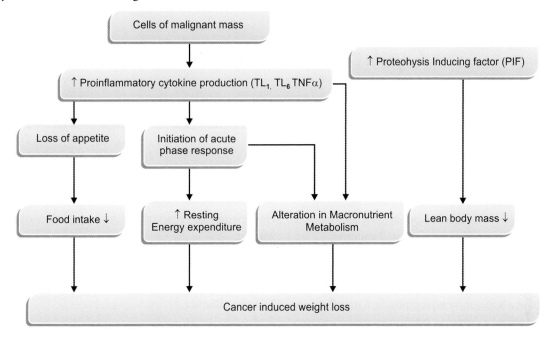

- Pathology -defective bilirubin uptake
- Fasting test +ve
2. Crigler-Najjar:
   Type- I
   - Autosomal rececive
   - Neonate
   - Glucuronyl transferase either absent or reduce
   - No f=binding to bilirubin
   - Very severe.
   - Kernicterus- death.
   Type-II
   - Autosomal dominant
   - Neonate
   - Glucuronyl transferase reduced
   - Moderate to severe
   - Can survive up to adulthood.

Treatment can be offered in severe cases:
- Phenobarbitone
- UV rays
- Liver transplantation.

Conjugated Hyperbilirubinemia

1. Dubin Johnson:
   - Autosomal rececive
   - Reduction of canalicular excretion of bilirubin
   - Mild at any age
   - Normal lifespan
   - None.

2. Rotor:
   - Autosomal dominant
   - Defective hepatic uptake of bilirubin and binding
   - Mild
   - Treatment none.

Mirizzi Syndrome

It is an unusual complication of gallstone disease.

Type 1: External compression of the common hepatic duct by the calculus impacted in the cystic duct/neck of gallbladder.

Type 2: Where the calculus has eroded into the bile duct creating cholecystocholedochal fistula and cholecystobiliary fistula is present with less than one-third of the circumference of the bile duct.

Type 3: Cholecystobiliary fistula involves up to 2/3rd of its circumference.

Type 4: Cholecystobiliary fistula with complete destruction of the entire wall of the common bile duct.

Treatment: In type 1 MS, cholecystectomy is adequate but fundus first approach is favored over the conventional Calot' first dissections.

In types 2 and 3 MS, partial cholecystectomy is a prudent approach using gallbladder cuff for choledochoplasty.

In type 4 MS, Roux-n Y hepaticojejunostomy is the procedure of choice.

CASE 3   Cystic Lump Abdomen

My patient, Radhika, a 50-year-old lady resident of Jabalpur, MP, presented to this hospital with complaint of:
- Lump in her upper middle part of abdomen for last 6 months.
- Pain off and on over the lump for last 2 months.

HISTORY OF PRESENT ILLNESS

- My patient was apparently asymptomatic 6 months back since she noticed a lump in her upper mid abdomen which is gradually progressive to attain its present size approximatlly 6 × 5 cm from its initial size of approximatlly 2 × 1 cm.
- Initially for 4 months the lump was painless but for last 2 months she has been having dull aching pain off and on over the lump.
- Pain is diffused in character.
- Nonradiating.
- No relieving or aggravating factors as such.
- There is no history of trauma.
- No history of acute pain abdomen, vomiting, distention of abdomen (GOO/ Intestinal obstruction).
- No history of alteration of bowel habit (to exclude gut mass).
- No history of urinary disturbance (to exclude hydronephrosis)
- No history of hematemesis, malena (to exclude growth like GIST).
  - Jaundice (Pressure on CBD).
  - No features suggestive of tuberculosis. (Encysted-peritoneal tuberculosis).

PAST HISTORY

No history of HTN, DM, TB.
No significant past history of operation.
No past history of any drug allergy.
No past history of any significant surgery.

PERSONAL HISTORY

Housewife, non-vegetarian. She is non-alcoholic and non-smoker.

FAMILY HISTORY

Not contributory.

GENERAL SURVEY

- Patient cooperative, average built and nourished.
- No pallors, icterus, edema or generalized lymphadenopathy.
- P-70/min, BP- 110/70 mm Hg. Temperature normal, respiratory rate 16 per min.

On Examination

Abdomen Inspection:
- Abdomen scaphoid
- Umbilicus center
- All quadrants move with respiration
- No obvious swelling noticed
- No visible pulsation or peristalsis noticed, no visible veins
- There is no scar mark
- Flanks appear normal
- External genitalia and hernial sites appear to be normal

Palpation: Abdomen soft, no rasied temperature, nontender. There is a 6 × 5 cm, intra-abdominal, spherical mass, soft cystic in nature, diffuse margin, mobile and fluctuation positive, resonant all around the cystic lesion. Mobile straight angle of mesenteric root, not along the line of mesenteric attachment.

No organomegaly, no free fluid in abdomen, no supraclavicular lymphadenopathy noticed.

Percussion: Dull note over the lump and tympanic note all around the cystic lump.

Auscultation: Bowel sounds heard.

Digital per rectal examination: Nothing abnormal detected.

Other systemic examination:

1. **Respiratory:** Bilateral air entry equal, no adventitious sound heard.
2. CVS- $S_1 S_{11}$ (N) no murmur.

Other examinations are essentially normal.

Summary of the case: My patient Radhika, a 50-year-old lady presented with a lump in epigastrium for last 6 months and diffuse pain over the lump for last 2 months. General examination is essentially normal.

On abdominal examination: There is a 6 × 5 cm intra-abdominal mass, spherical in shape, soft cystic in nature, diffuse margin, mobile and fluctuant cyst and dull note over the cystic mass but tympanic all around the cystic swelling mobility is right angle to the mesenteric root, not along the line of mesenteric attachment. So my provisional diagnose is, this is a case of mesenteric cyst without any features of complications.

Why do you say it is a mesenteric cyst?

It is mesenteric cyst: Painless intra-abdominal fluctuant mass, moves at the right angle to the mesenteric root. Resonant all around the cyst. (But cyst is dull on percussion) **called Tillaux triad**, age 20-30 years usually.

DIFFERENTIAL DIAGNOSIS

1. **Omental cyst:** Smooth, soft, nontender. Rolled up mass, placed transversely, moves with respiraton, mobile in all directions, dull on percussion.
2. **Encysted tubercular peritonitis:** Above the age of puberty, loculated mass, history of TB or features suggestive of TB.
3. **Rare causes:** Hydatid cyst of mesentery, aortic aneurysm, etc.

DIFFERENTIAL DIAGNOSIS OF EPIGASTRIC INTRA-ABDOMINAL SOFT MASS

1. Mass arising from left lobe of liver.
2. Mass arises from transverse colon.
3. GIST—usually from stomach, intra-abdominal epigastric mass, smooth, firm, moves with respiration, mass better felt at standing or walking, mobile (may be fixed if it gets adherent posteriorly).
4. Pylorus mass- all margin well felt with features of gastric outlet obstruction (GOO), mass from the body of the stomach is placed horizontally (like transverse colon mass) without any features of obstruction.

DIFFERENTIAL DIAGNOSIS OF RETROPERITONEAL CYSTIC LUMP

1. Pseudocyst of pancreas—Typical history of pancreatitis, epigastric mass, smooth, soft, nontender, mobility restricted or nonmobile, does not fall forward on knee elbow position. Lower border well felt, but upper border not clear, tympanic note on percussion.

   [*Remember:* Large retroperitoneal cyst behaves like an intra-abdominal cyst. Pancreatic cyst can be moved with respiration when it is in contact with liver/ stomach].

   [*Baid test:* Ryle's tube can be felt easily on palpation if pseudocyst pushes the stomach forwards].
2. Cystic abdomen/ cyst adenocarcinoma- smooth, firm mass, does not move with respiration, patient presents with mass with back pain, no history suggestive of pancreatitis.
3. Hydronephrosis—typical history, Dietl's crisis, changes in size (described in the topic of hydronephrosis).

How will you proceed?

Sir, I will confirm my diagnosis first by doing:

1. USG abdomen.
2. Upper GI endoscopy.
3. USG guided FNAC.

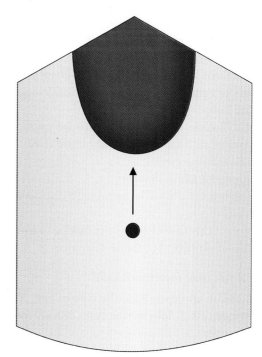

Pseudopancreatic cyst

4. Barium meal follow through (Nowadays rarely done as CECT scan is available as better modality of investigation).
5. CT scan is done in all cases after initial USG abdomen.
    a. Metastatic work up.
        1. Chest X-ray PA view.
        2. Liver function test.
    b. Baseline investigations for anesthetic purpose.
        1. Total hemogram
        2. Platelet count.
        3. Random blood sugar level.
        4. Renal function test.
        5. Chest X-ray PA view.
        6. ECG.
        7. Urine –routine and microscopic.
        8. Coagulation profile.
        9. Tubercular work up: ESR, Mantoux, PCR, Quantiferon gold (IgG, IgM, IgA, etc.).

REASONS BEHIND INVESTIGATIONS

1. *Straight X-ray abdomen:* To exclude tubercular calcified lymph nodes.
2. *Ultrasound abdomen:* Initial diagnostic imaging of choice—it shows origin of solid or cystic mass or cystic changes in a solid mass. Involvement of lymph nodes, presence of cyst in front of the intestine suggest omental cyst.
3. *Upper GI endoscopy:* To rule out associated ulcer, gastric erosion, gastric compression, etc.
    Biopsy from the ulcer can be taken. Done only earlier history of hematemesis or malena or USG suggestive of gastric lump.
    [In GIST endoscopic biopsy cannot be informative as mucosa usually appears normal; biopsy from the ulcer may be informative].
4. *Barium meal follow through:*
    The hollow viscera will be found to be displaced around the cyst.
    Portion of the lumen of intestine may be narrowed.
5. *USG guided FNAC:* For tissue diagnosis.

How will you treat mesenteric cyst?

Surgical treatment depends on the type of cyst. The most common variety is chylolymphatic cyst. [Types of mesenteric cyst-Remember CUTE].

C- Chylolymphatic cyst
U- Urogenital
T- Teratomatous
E- Enterogenous

Most common variety—Chylolymphatic cyst.

Characteristics:
- Almost solitary.
- Arises mostly in mesentery of the ileum (small intestine 60%, colon- 40%).
- It has got its own blood supply.

Open Surgery or Laparoscopic Surgery

For Chylolymphatic Cyst

Enucleation of the cyst is the treatment of choice without resecting gut as the cyst has got its own blood supply, independent of that of the adjacent intestine.

Enterogenous Cyst

Characteristics
- Derived from the diverticulum of the mesenteric border of the intestine.
- Cyst got thicker wall than chylolymphatic cyst.
- Blood supply from the mesenteric border of intestine.
- Surgical resection of the cyst along with resection of related portion of intestine followed by intestinal anastomosis is the treatment of choice.

Urogenital cyst: Resection of the cyst either open or laparoscopic.
Teratomatous cyst: Resection is the treatment of choice.

What is the treatment for omental cyst?

Omental cyst: Omentectomy is the treatment of choice.

How will you manage encysted form of peritoneal tuberculosis?

Treatment: Laparotomy or laparoscopic evacuation of fluid -> abdomen is closed-> antitubercular therapy to be completed.

What is pseudomesenteric cyst?

Most often caseating tubercular material collects between the layers of mesentery and *forming cold abscess*, mimicking like a mesenteric cyst called pseudomesenteric cyst.

[For the case presentation see the chapter Carcinoma colon (See case 11)]

You know, left iliac fossa refers to the left lower quadrant of the abdomen. The differential diagnoses of left iliac fossa masses include relatively limited pathology but require careful history taking, clinical examination and investigations for their work up to establish the diagnosis.

The pathological conditions arising from the structures in the left iliac fossa are the followings:

1. Carcinoma descending or sigmoid colon, i.e. portion of the large bowel. The lower part of descending colon and the entire sigmoid colon lie in relation to the left iliac fossa. Malignancies of this part of the colon may give rise to a palpable mass.

   Other rare pathologies leading to masses in left iliac fossa include tuberculosis of descending colon, diverticulitis, pericolic abscesses, etc.

2. **Retroperitoneal tumors** like liposarcomas and malignant fibrous histiocytomas are significant.

3. *Lymph nodal mass involving retroperitoneal lymph nodes:* The retroperitoneal lymph nodes in the left iliac fossa lie along the common iliac and external iliac vessels. More commonly, the retroperitoneal lymph nodes enlarge in malignant processes, i.e. lymphomas and become palpable in left iliac fossa. Rarely, testicular tumors may metastasize to left iliac lymph nodes although para-aortic lymph nodes are generally palpable.

4. **Ovarian cysts/tumors:** Both benign and malignant ovarian cysts and inflammatory tubo-ovarian masses arising from the left ovary and fallopian tube can be palpated in the left iliac fossa and form important differential diagnoses in female patients. Thouth these are usually asymptomatic initially.

5. *Ectopic left kidney:* The embryonic kidney arises from the metanephros in the sacral region and then ascends cranially to its final position in the retroperitoneum in the lumbar region. Failure of ascent of the kidney gives rise to a pelvic ectopic kidney (incidence 1:1000) which, reasons not clearly understood, is usually left-sided. Any pathology in this kidney, e.g. hydronephrosis or malignancy can produce a left iliac fossa mass.

6. *Undescended left testis:* The testes develops from the germinal epithelium on the posterior abdominal wall and then subsequently descends down to the scrotal sac by the ninth month of intrauterine life. An arrest in the normal descent of the testis, any enlargement in such a testis (most commonly by a malignancy) produces a mass in the left iliac fossa.

7. *Psoas abscess:* Tubercular infection affecting the lumbar vertebral bodies, manifests in the iliac fossa/inguinal region as a result of the pus traveling down below the sheath of the psoas muscle to the most dependent area giving rise to a psoas abscess; appears as left iliac fossa mass.

8. *Rare lesions:* Include aneurysms. AV fistula in relation to the iliac vessels; may also give rise LIF mass.

HISTORY

The following section highlights the important points in history –taking that must be elicited in a patient presenting with a lump in the left iliac fossa.

1. A left iliac fossa mass may present as an asymptomatic mass or lump or with nonspecific symptoms of anorexia and weight loss.

2. *Bowel complaints:* A patient with suspected bowel pathology may present with one or more of the following complaints:
   - Alteration of bowel habits- usually alternating diarrhea and constipation
   - Hematochezia (Merun color stool)
   - Colicky abdominal pain and distention of abdomen
   - Tenesmus and spurious diarrhea.

3. High-grade fever, drenching night sweats and significant weight loss (> 10% in the last 6 months) constitute the B

symptoms of lymphomas and hence must be elicited in case a lymph node mass is suspected.

Other relevent history that might be excluded include pruritis, alcohol-induced pain and bone pains. Sometimes, back pain by massive retroperitoneal nodal involvement can be a presenting complaint.

4. Urinary symptoms like colicky pain, hematuria or burning sensation during micturition can be felt in left iliac fossa with pathologies in unascended left kidney. These symptoms might be seen in hydronephrotic kidney with stone disease. A renal malignancy should be suspected in patients presenting with rapidly enlarging mass in left iliac fossa with history of painless hematuria. This can be associated with significant weight loss.

5. History of painful swelling in the left iliac fossa along with restricted mobility at the hip joint, hip will be in position of flexion, on the same side gives an indication towards a psoas abscess. The reason for this is the flexation spasm of the psoas muscle because of the inflammatory process in the muscle.

6. Congenital absence of testes can be an important part of history in patients with a left iliac fossa swelling.

7. Pressure effects of the mass in left iliac fossa can be a presenting compliant, e.g. left sided lower limb edema due to the presence of enlarged iliac group of lymph nodes causing extrinsic compression and hampering venous drainage.

8. History of recurrence of swelling in left iliac fossa should be elicited as retroperitoneal tumors and can have recurrences even after several years of previous surgery.

EXAMINATION

General Examination

1. Cachexia or malnutrition is usually obvious at first look and mandates a search for a debilitating illness like tuberculosis or malignancy, etc.

2. Significant pallor even without history of overt blood loss especially in elderly patients should be investigated for underlying malignancy like large bowel malignancy, malignant ovarian tumors or renal cell carcinoma in unascended left kidney, etc.

3. Lymphadenopathy is important for diagnosis and also for staging of malignant tumors:
   - *Generalized lymphadenopathy:* Patients present with generalized lymphadenopathy or the presence of any other lymph node group involvement along with left iliac fossa mass (lymph node mass-external iliac group

of lymph nodes), the diagnosis of lymphoma is to be considered.
   - Presence of left supraclavicular lymph node mass in a setting of left iliac fossa mass, malignant pathology should be considered like left ovarian malignancy or large bowel malignancy.
   - The presence of generalized lymphadenopathy and a cold abscess or psoas abscess in left iliac fossa, the diagnosis of tuberculosis should be considered.
   - Splenomegaly with lymphadenopathy may be suggestive of lymphoma.

4. Pedal edema: A unilateral pedal edema can be because of pressure effect from the left iliac fossa mass (lymph node mass); if bilateral, this could be a manifestation of hypoproteinemia associated with florid tuberculosis or underlying malignancy.

5. An abnormal posture like a painful flexion deformity at the hip joint could be because of a psoas abscess.

LOCAL EXAMINATION

The following points have to be kept in mind while performing a detailed physical examination.

Inspection

- Shape and extent of the swelling: For example, reniform swelling-ectopic kidney, Visible pulsations, Visible peristalsis, Cough impulse.

Palpation

Confirm if lump is parietal or intra-abdominal (Leg by lifting test or Rising test).

Temperature and tenderness-to rule out an inflammatory cause.

Fluctuation or specifically cross-fluctuation, if elicited, is diagnostic of a psoas abscess. As the psoas muscle crosses deep to the inguinal ligament before its insertion, a part of the swelling may be palpable below the inguinal ligament and cross fluctuation with the swelling above can be elicited.

In an intra-abdominal lump, an effort should be made to find out if the lump is intraperitoneal or retroperitoneal.
- Fixity/ Mobility
- Examination in knee elbow position to see retroperitoneal lump (does not fall forward)
- Pulsatile or not
- consistency, etc.

Digital Rectal Examination (DRF)

A large sigmoid malignancy may be palpable in the pouch of Douglas or metastatic deposits in the pouch of Douglas may be palpable.

Bimanual Examination

Bimanual palpation in left iliac fossa masses is especially useful where swelling is arising from pelvic structures, e.g. adnexal tumors. Abdominorectal (bimanual) palpation is useful in sigmoid or descending colon mass. (Ideally best elicited under general anesthesia.) This procedure not only enables to know the extent of the tumor but also the fixity to the surrounding structures and thus indicates the resectability of the tumor.

Per Vaginal Examination (PVE)

This is important for ovarian tumors as the masses can be felt through one of the fornices with a finger in the vagina. Also the swelling arising from the pelvis can be pushed inside the pelvis and examined through the vagina.

Ballotability

Ballotability is a feature found on bimanual palpation and when elicited using a digital examination in the vagina or rectum, it usually indicates adnexal tumors.

Percussion

To elicit the presence of ascites. Cystic ovarian tumors have a characteristic pattern of percussion note. There is dullness in front of abdomen and resonant areas in the flanks where the bowel loops are pushed, whereas in ascites the flanks are dull because of fluid in the flanks.

Auscultation

The left iliac fossa masses should be auscultated for presence of abnormal sounds, e.g. increased bowel sound proximal to a constricting malignancy of large bowel is because of presence of obstruction.

INVESTIGATIONS

The aim of investigating the patient is:
- To establish the diagnosis (both anatomical and pathological)
- To assess the extent of disease
- To assess fitness for surgery.

Diagnostic Investigations

1. Ultrasonography of the abdomen – first investigation to be done for a left iliac fossa mass because:
   - It is noninvasive and cost-effective procedure.
   - May be the only investigation required to establish diagnosis. For example, hydronephrotic ectopic kidney, psoas abscess, etc.
   - May indicate the organ of origin to decide the further line of investigation- Renal, bowel or adnexal lump.
   - USG is important for documenting minimal amount of free fluid where is not clinically detectable.
   - Lymph nodes greater than 2 cm can be documented by USG but it is not a good modality for staging of tumors as smaller lymph nodes can be missed.
   - Bowel gas hampers the assessment of USG abdomen since it is not a very good modality for detecting bowel pathology.

2. *Proctosigmoidoscopy/Colonoscopy*—In the cases of suspected bowel pathology, the next line of investigations is to visualize the lower gastrointestinal tract.
   - Proctoscopy in left iliac fossa masses is of very little consequence, as lumps of rectum and anal canal usually do not extended to reach up to the left iliac fossa.
   - Sigmoidoscopy (flexible) can visualize up to 60 cm of the large bowel and can be used to visualize any growth or pathology. It can also give us tissue for histological diagnosis.
   - Colonoscopy is mandatory in all patients with a suspected large bowel malignancy in order to visualize the growth, to assess for the the presence of synchronous lesions or polyps in the rest of the large bowel and therapeutic for biopsy and polypectomy.
   - The further line of investigation of a patient large bowel malignancy is discussed in the chapter of Carcinoma colon (See case 11).

3. *Intravenous urography:* In the patients where the diagnosis is suspected to be an ectopic kidney, an intravenous urography should be done to assess the presence of pathology in the ectopic kidney and its function and also to assess the function of the contralateral kidney, in case, a nephrectomy is required.

4. *Computerized tomography (CT scan):* CT scan of the abdomen is useful when
   - Ultrasound is unable to give an accurate diagnosis
   - Mass appears to be retroperitoneal in origin, e.g. retroperitoneal lymph nodal mass, as ultra-

sonography is not a good modality for imaging the retroperitoneum.

- The work up of a patient with lymphoma is discussed in the chapter of cervical lymph adenopathy.

5. *Magnetic resonance imaging (MRI):* Although not routinely used, MRI can be useful in the following situations:

- Useful for soft tissue enhancement especially where tissue invasion is not distinct by CT scan.
- Useful in delineation of malignancies of pelvic organs, where staging is done better with MRI as compared to CT scan.
- No radiation hazard, no risk of reaction with contact agents.

IMPORTANT DIFFERENTIAL DIAGNOSES

Parietal Swellings

Parietal lesions are common swellings present elsewhere in the body like sebaceous cysts, lipomas, and abscess, etc.

Psoas abscess is a cold abscess arising from the lumbar vertebra and tracking down the psoas sheath. On the left side it can present in the left iliac fossa as a soft swelling, mildly tender but no obvious signs of inflammation. It is a retroperitoneal swelling. Characteristic feature is a psoas spasm on same side. Sometimes another swelling is palpated below the inguinal ligament with cross fluctuation with the above swelling. This occurs when psoas abscess tracks along the psoas sheath till its level of insertion. The diagnosis might require an USG examination and X-ray of dorsolumbar spine. Sometimes in diagnostic dilemma a CT scan might be helpful. Match with other evidences of tuberculosis like chest X-ray, ESR, ELISA, PCR for TB.

Unascended Left Kidney

Urinary complaints like colicky pain, hematuria, burning micturation, may be present. The pathological unascended left kidney might be palpable in the left iliac fossa; pathology may be hydronephrosis or malignancy. It is reniform in shape, retroperitoneal.

Bimanually Palpable

Ballotability might be present though this might be difficult to elicit in the left iliac fossa. It is to be confirm by USG abdomen. Presence of hydronephrosis and size of the kidney or any space-occupying lesion in the kidney can be assessed on USG.

An intravenous pyelogram or a CT scan might be required for confirmation of diagnoses. A space-occupying lesion is diagnosed by CT scan as exact nature of lesion and its staging can be effectively done. Also the function of the contralateral kidney can be assessed in case nephrectomy is required.

Undescended Testes

History of testis being absent in scrotum since birth, young males are affected. The undescended testes is not palpable, unless pathological, in the left iliac fossa.

The scrotum should be examined for position of testes and if missing the lump should be considered to be malignant testis. It is retroperitoneal, might not confirm to any shape and usually fixes in retroperitoneum. Confirmation by USG, but CT scan is usually required for staging of the disease.

Lymph Nodes

History of fever, weight loss, unilateral or bilateral edema of leg may be seen especially with lymphomas. Usually middle aged males. Retroperitoneal swelling in the left iliac fossa can be a lymph nodal mass.

This could be part of iliac group of lymph node involvement in carcinoma testis or part of generalized lymphadenopathy of lymphomas.

No specific shape. Fixed in retroperitoneum. Confirmation usually by CT scan as staging of tumor of lymphoma is accurate with CT scan and the follow-up is accurate with CT scan. For carcinoma testis, the tumor markers are alpha fetoproteins, LDH (Lactate dehydrogenase) and beta-hCG (human chorionic gonadotropin). These tumor markers and the CT scan should be repeated in timely follow-up.

Retroperitoneal Tumors

History is not specific. History of weight loss may be there. Any age group may be involved. Besides lymph nodes, retroperitoneal swellings can be derived from the soft tissue in the retro- peritoneum. They are usually malignant unless proved otherwise. The tumors include retroperitoneal lipomas, liposarcomas, malignant fibrous histiocytoma, rhabdomyosarcomas, etc.

Diagnosis is confirmed by CT scan. This not only confirm diagnosis but also define the extent of the tumor the relation to vital structures like vessels, e.g. external iliac or common iliac, the degree of invasion into adjacent structures and if to define resectable or not.

Aneurysms of external or common iliac are rare but presence of expansile pulsation in the swelling usually indicates an Aneurysm. Diagnosis is made by Doppler, USG and confirmed by Angiography.

Ovarian Cysts/Tumors

Both benign and malignant tumors can be palpated in the left iliac fossa and hypogastrium. The patients might be completely asymptomatic except for mass. Malignant masses might present with cachexia and sometimes with menstrual irregularities and edema of leg. The swelling are ovoid in shape and have side-to-side mobility. The upper and lateral margins are well palpable but inferior margin is ill defined. The swelling appears to be arising from the pelvis and can be pushed into the pelvis. A bimanual palpation with a finger in the vagina, the tumor can be pushed in the pelvis and palpated between the finger in the vagina and the abdominal hand. Percussion shows dullness in the center and tympanic note in the flanks. Diagnosis is confirmed by USG of the pelvis and abdomen though large complex masses usually requiring a CT scan for confirmation to know the nature of the tumor and if malignant then to assess the extent of the lesion and its resectability.

Left Sided Bowel Malignancy

This is usually an annular constricting presenting with chronic intestinal obstruction history of:

1. Alteration in bowel habits, a history of increasing constipation occurs in a patient with previously normal bowel habit. The patient has to take increasing amounts of purgatives. Because of excessive amounts of purgative causing excessive secretion of mucus above the constricting neoplasm, attacks of constipation are followed by diarrhea. This is more obvious in left sided large bowel malignancy because the lesions tend to be constricting in nature.

2. *Bleeding per rectum:* Although relatively uncommon in descending colon and sigmoid colon malignancy. Bleeding occurs when there is an ulcerating lesion and passage of hard stool damages the friable mucosa. It can also occur by the necrotic process of the malignancy. The bleeding of malignancy of descending and sigmoid colon is characteristically painless and usually mixed with stools unlike that of hemorrhoids where the bleeding occurs at the end of defecation as a spurt of bleeding.

3. *Abdominal pain:* The characteristic of the pain may be colicky pain which is relieved on passing of flatus or stools or a constant pain due to local extension and fixity of the mass.

4. *Spurious diarrhea and tenesmus:* This is characteristics of proliferative growths in the sigmoid colon which give rise to a feeling of the urge to evacuate, which results in tenesmus accompanied by the passage of mucus and blood, especially in early morning. There can be a sense of incomplete evacuation, where the patient has his bowels open but feels that there are more feces to be passed, but this is more characteristic features of lower rectal malignancies. The patients might use to evacuate his bowels several times a day (*spurious diarrhea*), often with passage of flatus and blood stained-mucus (bloody lime).

5. Palpable abdominal lump in the left lower abdomen may be a presenting feature on rectal or bimanual palpation. It is sometimes the impacted feces and not the tumor that is palpable (which indents on pressing). When tumor is situated in the pendulous pelvic colon a hard movable mass might be palpable. Visible peristalsis can sometimes be seen above the swelling or in the swelling itself.

   Digital rectal examination – can detect 10% of the colorectal malignancies. Either the tumor of the rectosigmoid may be palpable by a bimanual examination or in advanced stage; metastatic deposits in the pouch of Douglas rectovasical pouch may be palpable.

Diagnostic Evaluation

1. *Fecal occult blood testing:* This is done using stool guaiac test or *orthotolidine* test. A positive test is an indication for a patient to undergo colonoscopy. Fecal occult blood test is shown to be positive in 50-60% of patients with colorectal cancer.

2. Full lenath colonoscopy is considered the diagnostic study of choice for carcinoma colon. It allows an evaluation of the lesion and biopsy from the lesion and from any suspicious lesions. It is also important to examine the rest of large bowel for any polyps or synchronous lesions and allows biopsies from any synchronous lesions before definitive surgery is planned.

   Synchronous lesions are defined as other lesions which are present at the time of primary tumor assessment or diagnosed within a period of 6 months of diagnosing the primary lesion. The histology of both the primary and the synchronous lesion are same. The histological grade of both the lesions should be same.

   The limitation of colonoscopy is failure to visualize the entire colon in 10-15% or missing a lesion in 10-20% and a perforation rate of 0.1-0.3%.

3. Sigmoidoscopy and biopsy only if constricting lesion prevents a colonoscopy.
4. *Double contrast barium enema:* This is especially useful in constricting lesion. In such cases, synchronous lesions and polyps can be picked up by barium enema. If the entire large bowel is to be scrutinized by colonoscopy barium enema need not be done. It is nontherapeutic, does not provide a tissue diagnosis and has a false positive rate of up to 25% especially in the presence of diverticular disease.
5. *Virtual colonoscopy* is a new technique for noninvasive examination of the colon. Instead of an endoscope being manipulated inside of the patient, the colon is inflated with air and the patient is imaged in a CT scan. It is then possible to generate a similar view to the endoscope by using virtual reality techniques to fly through the resulting. Three-dimensional image – virtual colonoscopy may provide a useful screening tool for patients with suspected cancer of the colon especially in the presence of a constricting lesion where visualization of the proximal bowel is not possible by usual colonoscopy.

Staging Evaluation

- Assessment of local extent of disease
- Detection of synchronous lesions
- Detection of metastasis.

Staging of Colorectal Cancer

Modified Duke Staging System: (Astler Coller Modification).

Modified Duke A
Tumor penetrates into the mucosa of the bowel wall but no further invasion.

Modified Duke B
B1: Tumor penetrates into, but not through the muscularis propria of the bowel wall.
B2: Tumor penetrates into and through the muscularis propria of the bowel wall.

Modified Dukes C
C1: Tumor penetrates into, but bit through the muscularis propria of the bowel wall: there is pathologic evidence of colon cancer in the lymph nodes.
C2: Tumor penetrates into and through the muscularis propria of the bowel wall: there is pathologic evidence of colon cancer in the lymph nodes.

Modified Dukes D
Tumor which has spread beyond the confines of the lymph nodes to different organs such as the liver, lung or bone.

TNM Staging System
Tumor
- T1: Tumor invades submucosa.
- T2: Tumor invades muscularis propria
- T3: Tumor invades through the muscularis propria into the subserosa or into the perirectal tissues.
- T4: Tumors directly invades other distant metastases organs.

Stage Grouping
- Stage 1 – T1 No Mo T2 No Mo
- Stage 2 – T3 No Mo: T4 No Mo
- Stage 3 – any T, N1-2, Mo
- Stage 4 – any T, any N, M1

Nodes
- No: No regional lymph node metastasis
- N1: Metastasis in 1 to 3 regional lymph nodes.
- N2: Metastasis in 4 or more regional lymph nodes.

Metastasis
- Mo: No regional lymph node metastasis
- M1: Distant metastasis present.

Lymphoma (see Case 20—Cervical Lymphadenopathy)

Lymphadenopathy in left iliac fossa can be, because of lymphoma but is usually a generalized lymphadenopathy rather than just being restricted to left iliac fossa.

Signs and Symptoms

1. Painless lymphadenopathy is the chief complaint in both Hodgkin's disease (HD) and non-Hodgkin's lymphoma (NHL).
2. Systemic symptoms (B called symptoms): Fever with chills, drenching night sweats and significant weight loss (>10% in past 6 months).
3. Purities often intense may be the presenting complaint in HD, especially nodular sclerosis subtype.
4. Pain
   1. Alcohol induced pain in areas of involvement is infrequent but when present, is pathognomic of HD.
   2. Bone pain may reflect areas of localized areas of bone destruction or diffuse marrow involvement.
   3. Neurogenic pain is caused by spinal cord compression, plexopathies, nerve root infiltration,

involvement of meninges and complicated varicella zoster, etc.

4. Back pain suggests massive retroperitoneal nodal involvement.

Physical Examination

Should include evaluation for hepatosplenomegaly, the presence of effusion, evidence of neuropathy, and signs of distal obstruction (e.g. edema limbs, superior vena cava syndrome, spinal cord compression, and hollow visera involvement).

Lymph nodes to be *examined include Waldeyer's ring* (including complete evalution of naso, oro- and hypopharynx by endoscopy), submental, supraclavicular, infraclavicular, epitrochlear, iliac, femoral, and popliteal nodes.

The lymph nodes are examined for size, multiplicity consistency and tenderness. Lymph nodes involved are typically a rubbery in consistency.

Investigations

When the patient presents with intra-abdominal nodes as the only presentation, the series of investigation planned are.

1. Ultrasound of the abdomen for the site of the lymph nodes to confirm that these are solid lesion and for USG guided FNAC.
2. Biopsy of any peripheral enlarged lymph node.
3. Chest X-ray and CT scan chest for mediastinal and hilar lymphadenopathy.

4. Iliac crests bone marrow aspiration, but preferably a bone marrow biopsy to rule out bone marrow involvement.
5. CT scan of the abdomen and pelvis useful in delineating abnormal enlargement of nodes in retroperitoneal, mesenteric, portal and other lymph node sites. It also detects splenomegaly and may define space-occupying lesions in liver, spleen and kidney.
6. If only iliac group of lymph nodes is clinically enlarged, a USG guided trucut biopsy is useful for typing of lymphoma and avoids laparotomy or laparoscopic biopsy.
7. If the lymph nodes are so placed that an USG guided or blind trucut biopsy can injure vital structure like sigmoid colon and no other lymph nodes are available for biopsy a laparoscopic biopsy is preferable and avoids a staging laparotomy. Laparoscope procedure gives information about all the lymph nodes involved and biopsy from them and decreases morbidity as compared to staging laparotomy.

CT scan is best for staging lymph nodes in lymphomas and has replaced staging laparotomies in most of the stages. Ideally a two monthly scan after completion of primary therapy for the first-two years. Followed by three monthly scans for next two years and then every 6 to 12 months. The risk of relapses is maximum in the first-two years.

CT scan has made bipedal lymphangiogram almost obsolete as better information is available with CT scan. *Staging laparotomy:* The main purpose of staging laparotomy and splenectomy was to save patients with a truly supradiaphragmatic disease from the long-term complications of alkylator based chemotherapy. Patients with a negative laparotomy or limited upper abdominal disease would be treated by radiation alone.

The current possible indications of staging laparotomy include patients with limited supradiaphragmatic disease (CS IA, IB and IIA) or equivocal stage IIIB disease, particularly if chemotherapy is to be avoided. The operative mortality should be <0.5% and the significant morbidity <5% to justify the procedure. Nowadays **laparoscopy is being used as staging modality rather than laparotomy**.

Definition of an Adequate Staging Laparotomy

- Wedge and needle biopsies of both lobes of liver.
- Splenectomy with removal of splenic hilar lymph nodes.
- Biopsies of random celiac, iliac, portal and mesenteric nodes; and node that is enlarged or feels abnormal, and equivocal or abnormal nodes on lymphangiography.

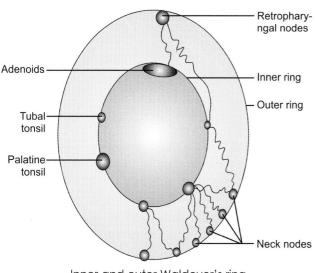

Inner and outer Waldeyer's ring

Retropharyngeal nodes

Adenoids

Inner ring

Outer ring

Tubal tonsil

Palatine tonsil

Neck nodes

- Open iliac creast bone biopsy
- Oophoropexy in young women.

Staging

The Ann Arbor staging system was previously universally being used but now has been modified by *Cotswold*. This is used for the noth Hodgkin's and non-Hodgkin's lymphoma although the histological subtype is the prime determinant of survival in NHL.

COTSWOLD STAGING CLASSIFICATION OF LYMPHOMA

Classification Description

Stage I—involvement of a single lymph node region or lymphoid structure.

Stage II—involvement of two or more lymph node regions on the same side of the diaphragm (the mediastinum is considered as a single site; here hilar lymph nodes are lateralized). The number of anatomical structures should be indicated by a subscript (e.g. II_3).

Stage III—involvement of lymph node regions or structures on both sides of the diaphragm.

III (a)—with involvement of splenic hilar, portal or celiac nodes.

III (b)—with involvement of para-aortic, iliac and mesenteric nodes.

Stage IV—involvement of one or more extranodal sites in addition to a site for which the designation 'E' has been used.

Designations applicable to any disease stage.

A-Absent symptoms

B-Fever (temperature>38° C) drenching night sweats, unexplained loss of >10% of body weight within the preceding 6 months.

X-Bulky disease (a mediastinal mass exceeding one-third the maximum transverse diameter greater than 10 cm).

E-involvement of a single extranodal site that is contiguous or proximal to a known nodal site:

CS-clinical stage

PS-pathological stage.

Right Iliac Fossa Mass

A PATIENT OF ILEOCECAL TUBERCULOSIS

My patient Pradipta, a 25-year-old boy, resident of Bihar, MBA student. Present with complaints of:

- Pain right lower part of abdomen for last 1½ years.
- Lump in right lower abdomen for last 6 months.

My patient was apparently asymptomatic 1½ years back since when he started having pain in right lower abdomen, the pain was mild, colicky in nature, insidious onset, non-radiating, accompanied by nausea and occasionally by vomiting and it was relieved by medication.

Initially the pain was off and on and for last 6-8 months, he has a frequent colicky pain.

In one of such attack, he was diagnosed as a case of acute appendicitis and appendicectomy was performed 6 months back but there is still no improvement of pain rather nowadays, the pain is dull aching in nature and almost continuous which is temporarily relieved by analgesics.

Since last 5-6 months he has noticed a lump in his right lower quadrant of abdomen which is gradually increasing in size and nowadays, it is accompanied by evening rise of temperature, loss of appetite, weight loss and frequent diarrhea. But there is no history of subacute intestinal obstruction, cachexia, jaundice (to exclude advanced carcinoma cecum).

No history of recurrent intestinal obstruction (Crohn's disease).

No history of any urinary complaint (to exclude unascended kidney).

(In a case of female – ask about gynecological complaints to exclude ovarian mass).

Past History

Patient is not a known case of tuberculosis, diabetes or hypertension.

He has got a past history of appendicectomy for right sided pain abdomen.

Personal History

MBA student, staying in hostel. Smoker smokes 5-10 cigarrates per day for last 4/5 years.

No history of alcohol intake as such.

Family History

His grantmother has abdominal tuberculosis, treated surgically along with antitubercular therapy (ATT).

General Survey

Patient is cooperative, looking anxious on average built, averagely nourished. Pallor present. No icterus, no edema or generalized lymphadenopathy.

Pulse – 80/min, temperature not raised, BP 118/76 mm Hg right arm supine, respiratory rate 16/min.

Systemic Examination

On inspection:

- Abdomen is scaphoid shaped.
- No obvious swelling is noticed.
- All quadrants move with respiration.
- Umbilicus central.
- No visible peristalsis or pulsation noticed.
- No visible veins.
- There is an oblique scar mark through McBurney's point.
- Flanks are not full.
- External genitalia and hernial sites appear to be normal.

On Palpation

Abdomen soft
    Temperature not raised
    Nontender

There is an intra-abdominal mass in right iliac fossa. 5 × 3 cm in size.

The mass is firm, irregular, nontender and fixed.

It is immobile but there is slight side-to-side movement observed. External genitalia and hernial sites are normal.

No free fluid in abdomen.

No hepatosplenomegaly.

No supraclavicular lymphadenopathy.

On percussion: Tympanic note is heard on percussion over the lump.

On auscultation: Bowel sound normal (may be hyperperistaltic).

No borborygmi. No bruits heard over the lump.

Digital rectal examination (DRE): NAD.

Other Systemic Exams

1. Respiratory—Bilateral air entry equal, No adventitious sounds heard.
2. CVS—S1, S2 (Normal)

   No murmur heard.

   Other examinations are essentially normal.

Summary of the Case

My patient Pradipta, a 25-year-old student present with dull aching colicky pain at his right lower quadrant of abdomen for last 1½ years and lump at the region for last 6 months along with evening rise of temperature, weight loss and frequent diarrhea.

On Examination

He is mildy anemic.

There is 5 × 3 cm intra-abdominal lump in right iliac fossa, firm, nontender, irregular, not moving with respiration and more or less it is fixed but slightly side- to-side movement is there. Tympanic note on percussion.

So, on the basis of history and clinical examination this is most probably a case of *ileocecal tuberculosis.*

Why you are telling it is a case of ileocecal tuberculosis?

From history—25 years student from Bihar present with dull aching colicky pain abdomen and firm lump at right iliac fossa.

From Clinical Features

Along with weight loss, anemia, loss of appetite and evening rise of temperature.

- History of diarrhea – (it is only 10-20% cases of ileocecal tuberculosis).
- Fever is associated with (50-70% cases).
- Mass in right iliac fossa (35%) firm, irregular, nontender, nonmobile, tympanitic note on percussion.

All of the above features suggestive of ileocecal tuberculosis.

Then why you are telling the word most probably?

Sir, I have told, most probably it is a case of ileocecal tuberculosis because there are few other conditions also mimic this case like.

- Carcinoma cecum
- Crohn's disease
- Appendicular lump, etc.

Ok, can you tell me why ileocecal junction is the common site of tuberculosis?

Sir, the causes are:

1. Physiological stasis
2. Abundant Peyer's patches – prone to get infected
3. As the surface area is more, the bacterial contact to mucosa is more.
4. Liquid content in the region.
5. 'M' Cells of Peyer's patches phagocytose bacilli and transfer to host cells.

How will you proceed in the case?

Sir, I will confirm my diagnosis first. For this why I will do

1. USG abdomen to see
   - Organ of origin of the lump–cecal thickening.
   - Nature of the swelling – cystic or solid.

   Others like—Nodal status, ascites, etc.

What are the USG Features of Abdominal Tuberculosis?

- Thickened bowel wall, mesentery, omentum, and peritoneum.
- Loculated ascites and or inter loop ascites with alternate echogenic and echofree areas–Club–sandwich appearance.
- *Stellate sign:* Bowel loops radiates from its mesenteric root.
- Mesenteric thickness more than 15 mm.
- Lymph nodal enlargement
- Hepatosplenomegaly, etc.

2. I will do

Chest X-ray and Barium Study X-ray

Chest X-ray to exclude pulmonary TB. If pulmonary TB is diagnosed we can safely treat this case as hyperplastic ileocecal tuberculosis.

Barium study: X-ray (Enteroclysis followed by barium enema or barium meal follow through) may reveal.

i. Obtuse ileocecal angle but remains in the same line.
ii. Pulled up cecum (by scarring).
iii. Long narrow constricted loop of ileum with thickned ileocecal valve looks like an inverted umbrella called **Fleischner sign**.
iv. Incompetent ileocecal valve.
v. Napkin lesions: Ulcers and stricture in the terminal ileum and cecum.
vi. **Stierlin's sign:** Hurrying of barium due to rapid flow.
vii. Calcifications may be found.

FNAC from palpable mass—USG guided FNAC is better for tissue diagnosis.

Colonoscopy

Most direct method to establish the diagnosis.

- It can rule out ca-cecum, biopsy can be taken from suspected lesion.
- It excludes other pathology like Crohn's disease to exclude ulcers, skipped lesions, etc.

CT Scan Abdomen

- Also better and more reliable to the diagnosis.
- It can show the extension of disease, involvement of lymph nodes, etc.

Diagnostic Laparoscopy:

Very useful method of investigation.

- A mass of terminal ileum and cecum are glued together.
- Inflamed segment is covered with fibrinous exudate and inflexible narrow lumen appears like a '**Hose pipe**'.
- Wall of intestinal segment is thickened and lumen narrowed.
- Serosal surface is granular, and grayish.
- Mesentery is thickened; numerous tubercles can be seen on the mesentery.
- Enlarged lymph nodes are visible.
- Biopsy can be taken from enlarged lymph nodes, omentum, peritoneum and suspected areas. Ascitic fluid can be collected for analysis.
- Polymerase chain reaction (PCR) can be assessed from biopsy tissue or from ascitic fluid and ADA (adenosine deaminase) also from ascitic fluid.

Other Tests

- Hb%, ESR, Mantoux
- Adenosine deaminase (ADA) activity in ascitic fluid which is 95% specific for tuberculosis and 98% sensitive for it.
- Plain X-ray abdomen to exclude intestinal obstruction it can show calcifications.
- Tuberculer work up—ESR, Mantoux, PCR, Quantiferon gold (IgG, IgM, IgA).

How will you treat this case?

Sir, after confirming my diagnosis.
I will start antitubercular drugs

i. INH (isoniazid), rifampicin, Ethambutol and pyrazinamide in a proper dose.
   (Details written in the chapter of cervical lymphadenopathy).

If the patient goes in for intestinal obstruction (due to fibrosis or stricture formation) segmental resection and end-to-end or side-to-side anastomoses to be done.

- Rarely hemicolectomy is required, e.g. when ileocecal, junction is involved.
- **Stricture plasty** is also very useful procedure.

Temporary ileostomy – in case of moribund patient who presents with obstruction.

What are the complications of ileocecal tuberculosis?

The complications are:

i. Intestinal obstruction
ii. Blind loop syndrome – anemia. Weight loss, steatorrhea, etc.

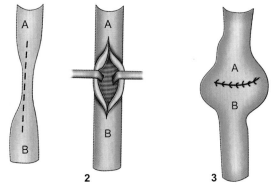

Stricture plasty:

1. **A strictured length of intestine is incised along its length.**
2. **The bowel is opened and the walls are retracted as shown.**
3. **The bowel is sutured transversely to widen the narrowed segment.**

iii. Malabsorption
iv. Dissemination of tuberculosis
v. Cold abscess formation
vi. Fecal fistula formation
vii. Rare complication are hemorrhage, perforation, etc.
viii. Interbowel fistula.

Can you tell me what are the indications for steroid therapy in tuberculosis?

Yes Sir,

The indications of steroids are:
i. Miliary tuberculosis
ii. Tubercular meningitis
iii. Tubercular pericarditis
iv. Adrenal tuberculosis
v. Pleural and endobronchial tuberculosis
vi. To prevent fibrosis in extensive pulmonary TB
vii. To prevent adhesions in abdominal TB
viii. Rapidly progressive tuberculosis, mediastinal lymph nodes involvement.
ix. Ocular tuberculosis.

What is abdominal cocoon?

In a case of peritoneal tuberculosis there is a dense adhesion in peritoneum and omentum with content inside, it looks like a cocoon called abdominal cocoon.

From where from the tubercular infection come to abdomen?
• May be directly from the ingestion of sputum, in sputum positive case of pulmonary TB.
• Systemic hematological spread from lung.

What is tuberculosis?

This histological term used to describe granulomatous lesion in tuberculosis.

The essential features are:
i. Central caseating necrosis
ii. Surrounded by epithelioid cells (Hallmarks) and Langerhans gaint cells.
iii. Surrounded by lymphocytes and fibroblasts.

What is the prognosis of abdominal tuberculosis?

Prognosis is very good. Medical treatment followed by surgery if required or surgery in between medical treatment cure the patient completely.

SHORT NOTE ON
RIGHT ILIAC FOSSA MASS

Right iliac fossa refers to right lower quadrant of abdomen. The different diagnosis of right iliac fossa masses include few pathologies but require careful clinical examination and investigations to establish the diagnosis.

The pathological conditions arising from the structure of right iliac fossa are the following:

1. Ileocecal tuberculosis
2. Appendicular lump
3. Carcinoma cecum
4. Crohn's disease (Regional ileitis)
5. Lymph nodal mass involving right iliac group
6. Retroperitoneal tumors
7. Tubo-ovarian mass
8. Ectopic right kidney
9. Undescended right testis
10. Psoas abscess

Ileocecal Tuberculosis

Usually hypertrophic ileocecal tuberculosis (types of ileocecal TB are ulcerative, hypertrophic and ulcerohypertrophic).

Tuberculosis manifests as a right iliac fossa mass tuberculars infection starts at lymphoid follicles and then spread to submucosa and subserous plane. The intestinal wall becomes thickend with narrowing of its lumen. There will be early involvement of regional lymph nodes which becomes matted along with involvement of terminal part of ileum and cecum to produce the lump.

Clinical Features

- Usually young individual with good body resistance and less virulent organism but it may occur at any age group.
- Patient presents with dull aching constant abdominal pain. The pain is described as wind moving around the umbilicus.
- Recurrent attack of abdominal pain with diarrhea.
- Features of blind loop syndrome manifested as anemia, loose motion, weight loss, even diarrhea, usually foul smelling (dilated lumen above the obstruction leads to infection in the lumen, leading to diarrhea).
- There may be episode of severe abdominal pain; abdominal distention and vomiting indicate subacute intestinal obstruction.

- Patient may present with right iliac fossa mass with ill health and evening rise of temperature.
- On examination: The lump is smooth hard, nontender, tympanic note on percussion, does not move with respiration.

Investigations

- *Plain X-ray abdomen:* Air fluid levels in dilated bowel loops in presence of obstruction.
- *Chest X-ray PA view:* To exclude pulmonary tuberculosis
- USG abdomen:
  - An empty right iliac fassa due to upward displacement of contracted cecum.
  - Bowel wall-thickening looks like another kidney called 'Third Kidney Sign'.
  - Enlarged lymph nodes my be visible.

Barium meal follow through and barium enema—May show:

- Mucosal ulcerations, strictures, deformed cone shaped, retracted cecam with incompetent ileocecal *valve.*

Fleischner sign: A wide gap between thickened ileocecal valve and a narrowaed ileum.

Stierlin sign: A fibrotic ileum that empties into a rigid, contracted cecum.

CT scan abdomen shows:

- Mural thickening affecting the ileocecal region either only terminal ileum or cecum or both. Mural thickening is usually concentric
- Enlarged hypodense nodes in the adjacent mesentery
- Skip areas of concentric thickening seen in ileal loops
- Luminal narrowing with or without proximal dilatation.

Drawback of CT scan is the failure to accurately define stenosis in the bowel in patients with threatened obstruction.

Colonoscopy

- Direct visualization of the lesion
- Biopsy can be taken from the lesion
- Mucosal nodules, ulcers, strictures
- Deformed, patulous, edematous ileocecal valve
- Even ileum (15-20 cm) can be seen.

Treatment

A. *Conservation:* Antitubercular drugs (Details written in cervical lymphadenopathy).

B. *Surgical:*
- Resection and anastomosis, i.e. resection of diseased segment and anastomosis done and to continue antitubercular drugs.
- Strictureplasty: Often strictureplasty is beneficial if there is a single stricture.

Appendicular Lump (Appendicular Phlegmon)

- Most common swelling in the right iliac fossa. Appendicular lump usually appears 3 days after an attack of acute appendicitis.
- There may be rigidity of abdominal muscle, thereby; the tender mass may not be felt easily.
- The mass consists of inflamed appendix, greater omentum, edematous cecal wall, surrounded by coils of small intestine matted together with lymph nodes.
- The lump is tender smooth, firm, irregular and fixed, well localized and tympanic note on percussion.
- Appendicular lump should note not be confused with appendicular abscess where variable constitutional features like fever, unwellness along with redness and edematous abdominal wall.

Investigations

- TLC will be increased
- USG abdomen shows the appendicular mass

  Treatment: (A) Conservative

  (B) Surgery

Conservative

Ochsner-Sherren regimen
  i. IV fluid, nasogastric aspiration.
  ii. Observation of pulse, BP, temperature and respiration.
  iii. Mark the mass to see the regression.
  iv. *Antibiotics:* Like ampicillin, cephalosporin, metronidazole, and gentamicin in appropriate doses.
  v. Analgesics
     - Patient usually improves by 72 hours. Temperature, pulse are settled, mass redues in size.
     - Contraindications of Ochsner - Sherren regimen are:
       – When diagonosis is in doubt
       – In acute appendicitis in children and elderly

– In gangrenous appendicitis, burst appendicitis, etc.
– Appendicitis with diffuse peritonitis when formed abscess bursts into peritoneal cavity.

Surgery Laparoscopic Open

Interval appendicectomy after 6 weeks of an acute attack.

Carcinoma cecum

Patients above 40 years may present with:
- Anemia-moderate to severe unresponsive to treatment.
- Palpable mass at right iliac fossa only in 10% cases is the first sign.
- Unexpected discovery at operation for acute appendicitis or appendicular abscess failing to resolve.
- Carcinoma cecum can be the apex of intussusception presenting with symptoms of intermittent obstruction.
- Dull, nagging pain in right iliac fossa.
- Anorexia, weight loss, easy fatiguability may be the only symptoms.
- Cachexia, jaundice, hepatomegaly are the features of an advanced disease.
- There may not be any change of bowel habit.

Investigations

  i. Occult blood test from stool
  ii. **Barium meal X-ray:** A tumor of cecum is more likely to be discovered by barium meal X- ray which will show 'fillings defect' in the cecum–is the main diagnostic feature of this condition.
  iii. **Colonoscopy:** Occult blood in the stool is the diagnostic point for special investigations.
     With fiberoptic colonoscope, the whole of the colon up to cecum can be viewed for practical purposes.
- Biopsy can be taken under direct vision through colonoscope. Sometimes in carcinoma cecum biopsy is difficult through colonoscopy, in such situation a wash specimen or brushing may be obtained through colonoscope for cytological study.
- To identify synchronous growths in the colon.

Treatment

Operable case: Right hemicolectomy is the answer which includes whole cecum along with mass, ascending colon, right 1/3rd of transverse colon and up to 10 cm of terminal ileum to be taken off.

Inoperable case: Adjuvant chemotherapy-ileotransverse anastomosis is done as a by pass procedure/loop ileostomy/ end ileostomy and mucous fistula.

Palliative chemotherapy

Cyclophosphamide + 5 FU are beneficial.

or cisplatin/oxaliplatin + 5 FU is the present day's therapy.

Crohn's Diseases or Regional Ileitis

In chronic ileitis – pain in right lower abdomen is the most frequent symptom and this is due to partial obstruction of the lumen and increase motilities proximal to the site of obstruction.

In advanced cases pain is constant aching type:

- Tender and palpate mass near always accompany this type of pain.
- Diarrhea is the next most frequent symptoms. Frothy and foul smelling stool without mucous, pus or blood are characteristics.
- Fever is present in about 1/3rd of patients.
- Weight loss, anemia, hypoproteinemia are the manifestations of malnutrition.
- **Extraintestinal manifestations are:**
  Skin—Erythema nodosum
  Eye—Uveitis, iritis
  Joint—Arthritis
  Mouth—Aphthous ulcer, etc.
  May be seen in one way or the other in late cases.

Investigations

Barium study usually barium enema is useful diagnostic procedure for Crohn's diseases.

i. **In nonstenosing stage** it shows:
   - *Cobblestone pattern:* Ulcers combined with submucosal edema, produce a coarse nodularity
   - Straightening of valvulae conniventes
   - Raspberry or rose thorns appearance.
   - Ulceration tends to take the form of sharp 'fissures' passing from the lumen into the lower wall shows as spikes.
   - Filling defect may be the neoplastic consequence of a chronic disorder.
   - Skip lesion with apparent normal intervening mucosa is the hallmark of the disease.
   - Fistula formation between adjacent organs like bowel, bladder, uterus, etc.

ii. **In stenosing stage:**
   String sign of Kantor: There is gross irregular narrowing of the terminal ileum.
   Stricture formation is the end result of fibrosis.

Endoscopy: Direct visualization of the pathology of Crohn's disease is very helpful in diagnosis of this disease

- It is more useful in case of colonic affection.

To follow-up the course of disease and response to therapy are well looked after by endoscope.

iii. A rectal biopsy is frequently, done to establish the diagnosis.

Through colonoscope, biopsy may be taken form sigmoid colon or descending colon.

Treatment

1. Conservative
2. Surgical.

Conservative—Medical Therapy

- Steroids are the mainstay of treatment
- Relapse being treated with up to 40 mg prednisolone orally daily.

  In colonic involvement 5ASA compounds along with prednisolone are suitable.
- Azathioprine is used for its additive and steroid sparing effect.

  Infliximab—a monoclonal antibody, has shown much promise as a new treatment for Crohn's disease.

  Apart from the above, nutritional support is essential. Anemia, hypoproteinemia, electrolytes, metabolic bone problems must be taken care of.

Surgical Treatment

Indications for surgery

- Recurrent intestinal obstruction
- Recurrent bleeding
- Perforation
- Unresponsive to medical therapy
- Malignant changes
- Fulminant colitis
- Intestinal fistula
- Perianal disease, etc.

Surgery

1. Ileocecal resection is the usual procedure for ileocecal disease with primary anastomosis between the ileum and the transverse colon.
2. Segmental resection of involved segment and restoration of continuity.
3. Colectomy with ileorectal anastomosis in case of widespread colonic disease.

Remember the differene between Crohn's disease and ulcerative colitis

Crohn's disease (CD)	Ulcerative colitis (UC)
1. Usually it is know as regional ileitis. It can affect any part of GI tract	• UC affects the colon, sigmoid and rectum (95% cases rectum is involved usually)
2. CD affects the full thickness of bowel wall	• UC is a mucosal disease
3. CD has characteristics skip lesions	• UC produces confluent disease of the colon
4. CD more commonly causes stricture and fistula	• Stricture and fistula formations are less common in UC
5. Granulomas may be found in CD	• Granuloma is not found in UC
6. Perianal disease is common with CD	• Perianal disease is very unusual in UC
7. CD affects terminal ileum and produces symptoms like appendicitis	• UC dose no affect terminal ileum and dose not produce such symptoms but back wash ileitis may be features
8. Recurrence is very common after resection of CD segment	• In UC, resection can cure the patients
9. Mesenteric fat creeping over the serosa	• Uncommon mesenteric fat creeping over serosa
10. Pseudopolyp not seen	• Pseudopolyp formation common

4. Temporary loop ileostomy in case of acute distal disease allowing remission and later restoration of continuity.

5. Proctocolectomy with permanent ileostomy in a case of widespread colon, rectum and anal disease.

6. Strictureplasty is a local widening procedure to avoid excessive small bowel resection.

7. Anal disease is simple treated by drainage of abscess, placing Setons around fistula, etc.

Lymph Nodal Mass

Enlargement of exeranal iliac group and mesenteric lymph nodal mass produce lump in this region.

Causes are lymphoma, secondaries, tuberculosis, filariasis are the main causes.

Lymphosarcoma gives rise to rapid enlargement of the node without any other ailment usually young individual gets affected.

Secondary- there may be known primary. Here nodes are fixed, hard and nodular.

Tubercular and filarial lymph nodal mass may be associated with typical features of TB and filaria.

Mesenteric Tuberculous Lymphadenitis

• Tabes mesenterica massive enlargement of mesenteric lymph nodes due to tuberculosis.

• Acute or chronic tuberculous adenitis present as lymph nodal mass in right iliac fossa (Acute nonspecific mesenteric lymphadenitis is called **Nurse's syndrome).**

Klein's sign: Shifting tenderness may be elicited on palpation in supine and left lateral position called Klein's sign.

[Know the attachment of mesenteric root- which is 15 cm] long and it extends from the duodenojejunal flexure on the left side of L2 vertebra to the upper part of right sacroiliac joint.

Surface marking: The starting point is the point 1 cm below the transpyloric plane and 3 cm from midplane of abdomen then it extends 15 cm obliquely downwards towards the right iliac fossa].

Treatment of the lymph nodes depends on primary cause and extension of the disease.

It is due to infection, like tuberculosis, filariasis, etc. and treat the cause primarily.

Surgical removal of tubercular lymph nodes are indicated:

• Residual lymph nodal mass following completion of ATT course.

• Non-responding cold abscess.

• When the sinus persists.

Treatment of secondaries depending on the stage and site of primary malignancy.

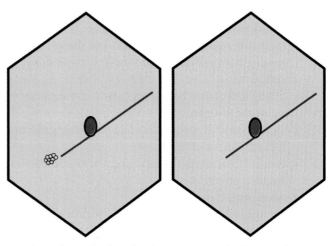

Lymph nodes involve in nurse's root of mesentery

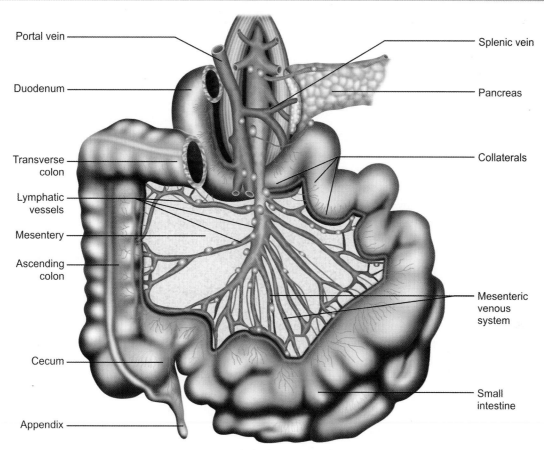

Portal vein

Duodenum

Transverse colon

Lymphatic vessels

Mesentery

Ascending colon

Cecum

Appendix

Splenic vein

Pancreas

Collaterals

Mesenteric venous system

Small intestine

Mesenteric lymphadenitis

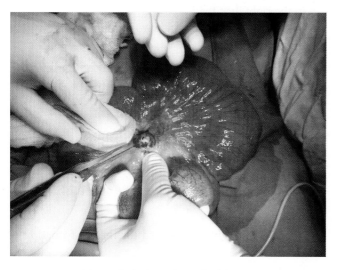

Mesenteric lymph node biopsy

Treatment of tubercular mesenteric lymphadenitis-antitubercular drugs.

Surgery—laparoscopy and proceed.

Diagnostic laparoscopy to see mesenteric lymph nodes, omental and peritoneal vicinity.

RETROPERITONEAL TUMORS

Nonspecific history. History of weight loss may be there. Any age group is involved besides lymph nodal mass retroperitoneal swelling can be derived from retroperitoneal soft tissue structure. They are usually malignant unless proved otherwise.

The tumors include retroperitoneal lymphomas liposarcomas, malignant familial histiocytoma, rhabdomyosarcomas, etc.

Clinical Feature:
- Usually large
- Fixed, thereby nonmobile
- Not moving with respiration
- Does not fall forward on knee elbow position
- Resonant on percussion as the bowel lies infront.

Specific Features for Retroperitoneal Sarcoma:
- Mass can be felt per abdomen
- Back pain and compressive features are the presentations.
- Organ specific complications are:
  GI tract obstruction especially by leiomyosarcoma hydronephrosis due to compression over the ureter, varicose veins due to compression over major veins, arterial compression is usually rare.
- Liver, lung secondaries to be looked for.
  Note: Retroperitoneal cyst and sarcoma are usually smooth but lymphoma is firm and nodular.
- Most common retroperitoneal benign tumor is lipoma [*Sites where lipomas more prone to turn into malignancy are* retroperitoneal lipoma, lipoma in the shoulder region (subcutaneous) and intramuscular lipoma in the thigh].
- Liposarcoma is the most common malignant retroperitoneal tumor in India but worldwide, malignant fibrous histiocytoma is the most common.
  Diagnosis:
  Confirm the diagnosis by:
  – USG abdomen
  – CECT abdomen for staging—USG/CT guided FNAC.
  – MRI to exclude neurovascular bandle involvement.

Treatment of Retroperitoneal Tumors

i. Wide local excision with minimum 1 cm free margin is ideal. Often part of adjacent structure to be removed to give a proper clearance.
ii. Palliative debulking surgery is indicated for an extensive disease.
iii. Chemotherapy (like Adriamycin) and radiotherapy are palliative procedures. Neoadjuvant CT/RT can be given to down grade the tumor before surgery.
  Retroperitoneal NHL is treated by chemotherapy.
  Usually surgery is required to give symptomatic relieve like relieve from obstruction, etc.
  Enucleation through pseudocapsule not advisable as recurrence rate is too high.
iv. Right ovarian mass
  - Both benign and malignant swellings can be palpable at right iliac fossa.

- Patients might be asymptomatic except the mass.
- Malignant swelling may present with anemia, cachexia, menstrual irregularities, edema of the leg, etc.
- Ovoid shaped swelling and has got side-to-side mobility.
- The upper and lateral margins are well palpable but inferior margin is ill defined.
- The swelling appears to be arising from the pelvis and can be pushed into the pelvis.
- A bimanual palpation with a finger in the vagina, the tumor can be pushed in the pelvis and thereby palpable between the finger in the vagina and abdominal hand.
- Percussion shows dullness in the center and resonance in the flanks.

Diagnosis:
- USG abdomen and pelvis.
- CT scan is required for large and complex masses. It can confirm the nature and extent of tumor and its resectability.

Treatment:
- Benign lesion-excision.
- Malignant lesion debulking surgery with omentectomy.
- Neoadjuvant and adjuvant chemotherapy has got definite role to control the tumor.

Unscended Right Kidney
- Urinary complains like colic pain, hematuria, burning micturtion, may be present.
- Pathological unascended right kidney might be palpable in the right iliac fossa.
- Pathology may be hydronephrosis or malignancy.
- It is retroperitoneal.
- Reniform in shape.
- Usually does not cross the midline.
- Bimanually palpable and or ballotable but might be difficult to elicit in the right iliac fossa.

Diagnosis
USG abdomen shows:
- Size of the kidney
- Space occupying lesion in the kidney
- Hydronephrosis.

CECT or IVP might be required for the confirmation of diagnosis.
- Status of the kidney, i.e. functional capacity, abnormality, etc.

- Any space occupying lesion if it is malignant and it's staging
- Function of contralateral kidney can be assessed, if nephrectomy is planned in the diseased kidney.

Treatment: Partial or radical nephrectomy depends on the nature and extent of disease.

Undescended right testis:
- Right hemiscrotum undeveloped.
- History of testis being absent in right sided hemiscrotum since birth.
- Young male are usually affected.
- The undescended testis is not palpable unless pathological in right iliac fossa.
- Usually it is fixed in retroperitoneum.

Diagnosis
- USG abdomen to localize the tumor.
- CT scan to stage the disease.
- Laparoscopy both diagnostic and therapeutic.
  The different sites of undescended testis are:
  i. Retroperitoneal at the site of RIF
  ii. Just above the internal rings; extraperitoneal
  iii. In inguinal canal
  iv. In superficial inguinal pouch.

Treatment: Always Surgery
Between 2 and 4 years of age. Principles of surgery are mobilization of cord, repair associated hernia, adequate scrotal fixation without tension.
  [Details written in the chapter of undescended testis].

Psoas Abscess at Right Iliac Fossa
Psoas abscess is commonly due to tuberculosis of spine (T10) and lymph nodes.
  It may be a pyogenic abscess.

Clinical Features
- Back pain, fever are the presenting complaints.
- Swelling in the iliac fossa.
- Swelling is smooth, nontender, nonmobile, not moving with respiration.
- Spinal tenderness, paraspinal spasm and restricted spine movement may be associated.
- Psoas abscess may extend across the groin and below the inguinal ligament so, **cross fluctuation** across the inguinal ligament will be present.
- Patient is able to flex his hip but finds difficult to extend the hip.

Investigations
- X-ray spine and chest
- Mantoux test, ESR, ADA, PCR for TB
- USG abdomen
- Peripheral smear
- CT scan
- MRI dorsolumbar spine, etc.

Treatment
- ATT to be started immediately
- Surgery under GA. Through lateral loin incision, the psoas abscess is drained extraperitoneally and wound to be closed.
- Pus to send for culture, sensitivity and culture for acid fast bacilli.
- All caseating material and disease part of vertebra should be removed.

My patient, Bhusan Bhat, a 30-year-old man, resident of Punjab, complaint of:

- Pain at upper mid abdomen for last 3 months, and
- Swelling at the same site for last 2 months.

My patient was apparently asymptomatic 3 months back when he had a sudden attack of abdominal pain after consumption of 6 large pegof alcohol in a party. He underwent conservative treatment for his agonizing pain of abdomen but having dull ache at upper abdomen regularly thereafter.

Pain is usually dull aching, sometimes severe and radiates to back, pain is relieved with bending forward position. He underwent conservative management like IV fluid, analgesic, etc. twice within last 3 months.

He noticed a swelling two months back which is gradually progressive and attained its present size approximately 12 × 10 cm from a lemon size swelling (approx 3 × 2 cm).

History of unquantified weight loss and anorexia present but there is no history of alcoholism, gallstone disease. He has got no history of similar type of abdominal pain before 3 months back and no history of hematemesis and melena.

Past history: No history of hypertension, diabetes, TB or any past history of long-term drug intake. No past history of any significant operation.

Personal history: He is a serving army soldier, non- smoker, takes alcohol occasionally.

Family history: It is not contributory.

General survey: Patient is cooperative but having anxious facies. He has an average built and averagely nourished.

Pallor, icterus, edema, generalized lymphadenopathy are not there.

Pulse—80/min, BP—120/80 mm Hg, right arm supine. Respiration—18/min. Temperature is normal.

LOCAL EXAMINATION

Abdomen

On Inspection

Abdomen is scaphoid except there is an obvious bulge in the epigastrium.

- Umbilicus is pushed downwards and slightly stretched.
- All quadrants move with respiration (equally).
- No visible scar, prominent veins, peristalsis noticed.
- Flanks are not full.
- Hernial sites and external genitalia appear normal.

On Palpation

Temperature not raised, nontender. There is a retroperitoneal swelling in the epigastric region extending into umbilical and both hypochondrial regions which is hemispherical in shape.

- Soft cystic swelling.
- Smooth surface.
- Upper margin is diffuse, lower margin is well defined.
- Not mobile.
- Not moving with respiration.
- Transmitted pulsation is felt (To be confirmed by knee-elbow position as it disappears in this position).

   Baid test + ve (Remember? I have already written before. Once more, if you put a Ryle's tube in stomach it is felt per abdomen as the stomach is pushed infront by the cyst).

- No other swelling palpable in the abdomen.
- No hepatosplenomegaly.
- No free fluid in abdomen, hernial sites and external genitalia appear normal.
- No supraclavicular lymphadenopathy noticed.

On Percussion

There will be tympanic or impaired resonant sound over the swelling.

Other Systemic Examination

Respiratory: Bilateral air entry equal. No adventitious sounds heard. (vs: $S_1 S_{11}$ (N) No murmur heard. Others systems are essentially normal.

Summary of the Case

My patient a 30-year-old man, presented with pain upper mid abdomen for last 3 months and swelling at the same site for last 2 months following an attack of pain in abdomen after consumption of a large amount of alcohol. Pain is dull aching peritoneal usually, sometimes pain is severe and radiates to back. The retroperitoneal swelling is gradually progressive and attained it's present size 12 × 10 cm. Upper margin is diffused but lower margin is well defined, swelling does not move with respiration.

Transmitted pulsation felt over the swelling. Baid test positive.

So, this is a case of pseudopancreatic cyst based on history and clinical examination.

What are the other possibilities?

The other possibilities are:
   i. Cystadenoma or cystadenocarcinoma of pancreas
  ii. Simple cyst of pancreas
 iii. Aortic aneurysm
  iv. Mesenteric cyst
   v. Omental cyst.

Cystadenoma or Cystadenocarcinoma of Pancreas

- Female predominant
- No history suggestive of previous attack of pancreatitis
- Patient presents with vague abdominal pain and backache
- In case of cystadenocarcinoma there may be history of weight loss, anorexia
- There may be features of gastric outlet obstruction due to compression by the cystic mass
- May present with epigastric lump which is slowlly progressive.
  On examination—it is a lobulated cyst.
  Smooth, soft cystic swelling, does not move with respiration, nonmobile, does not fall forward on knee-elbow position, resonant on percussion.

USG/CT scan shows central "*Sunburst*" calcification in the cyst or its wall in case of serous cystadenoma and in case of mucinous cystadenoma or adenocarcinoma there is "*Rim calcification*" in the wall, encasement of neighboring vessels is the surest sign of adenocarcinoma.

Pancreas appears normal.

ERCP shows there is no duct communication with the cyst).

Simple Cyst of Pancreas

- Patients are usually asymptomatic, may have vague pain abdomen
- Swelling appears in epigastrium
- All features of retroperitoneal cyst like it does not move with respiration, does not fall forward in knee, elbow position, etc.

USG and CT Scan are Diagnostic: CT scan is always better diagnostic tool for pancreatic swelling:
- Smooth wall
- Well capsulated/encapsulated
- Arising from pancreatic body or tail
- No sunburst or rim calcification, etc.

Aortic Aneurysm

- \> 50 years
- Male > female
- Most patients are asymptomatic
- May presents with pulsatile epigastric swelling
- May have back pain when it is progressive.
  On clinical exam the swelling is usually around umbilicus felt at epigastrium and mostly left to the midline (Abdominal aorta is in left side).
- Expansile pulsation present all the time even on knee-elbow position.
- USG abdomen, CT scan, angiogram are important diagnostic modalities.

Mesenteric Cyst

- Intra-abdominal cystic lump
- Swelling more in the umbilical region
- Smooth, fluctuant, not moving with respiration
- Moves side-to-side and in the direction perpendicular to the line of mesentery, not vertically
- Zone of resonance around the cyst
- Intra-abdominal swelling falls forward on knee-elbow position.
  (Details written in the chapter—Cystic Swelling Abdomen).

How will you differentiate between pseudocyst and cystic neoplasm (cystadenoma) of pancreas?

S.no	Subject	Pseudocyst	Cystic neoplasm
1.	History	Pancreatitis present	No history suggestive of pancreatitis
2.	Clinical exam	Clinically epigastric cystic lump, unilobulated	Epigastric cystic lump, may be multilobulated
3.	USG/CT findings	Uncapsulated, thin wall cyst	Well capsulated glistening surface
		Saponification, peripancreatic adhesion, fluid may be present	Not adhered to surrounding
		Suggestive of pancreatitis	Pancreas appears normal except the cyst
		Cyst wall lining is by granular tissue	Epithelial lining is there
		No neovascularization on cyst wall	Neovascularization is there
		Fluid serous in nature	cystic fluid may be hemorrhagic or mucinous
4.	Fluid for amylase	Fluid contains high level of amylase	No amylase is in the cystic fluid
5.	Cytology	No malignant cells on frozen section biopsy or histopathology examination	Malignant cells may be present in case of cyst-adenocarcinoma

How will you differentiate between malignant and benign lesions?

S.no	Subject	Benign	Malignant
1.	Age	Usually occurs at younger age group	Usually malignant lesion occurs in elderly though it may occur in younger age
2.	Symptoms	(i) Slow growing painless	Usually rapid growing pain at late stage
		(ii) No history of loss of weight	Loss of weight is common associated feature
3.	Signs	(i) Swelling is usually firm, smooth, mobile not fixed to underlying structure or overlying skin	Usually hard or variegated consistency, irregular restricted mobility or fixed
		(ii) Anemia, cachexia weight loss are absent	Anemia, cachexia weight loss are usual features
		(iii) Pressure effects, secondary changes like venous engorgement, color changes local infiltration are absent	Pressure effects, secondary changes, local infiltration changes are usual features
		(iv) Lymph nodes are not enlarged	Lymph nodes involvement and enlargements are important features
4.	Histology	Characteristic cell differentiation without loss of polarity, no anaplasia are features of benign growth, nuclei are same as parent tissues and are without mitosis	Characteristic cell differentiation, undifferentiation loss of polarity, anaplasia are common features of malignant growth neucle becomes larger hyperchromatic with mitosis.

How will you proceed in this case?

I will confirm my diagnosis first. I will do USG abdomen to see the cyst and it's relation to the pancreas.

I will look for features of chronic pancreatitis and exclude any intraductal calculi in the pancreas.

What is the role of CT scan in this case?

CT scan is more sensitive and specific to diagnose pseudocyst:

- It confirms USG findings
- It shows the extension of the cyst
- It shows the relation of cyst to pancreas, adjacent structure, like stomach, bowel loop, etc.
- It can clearly differentiate between pseudocyst and cystic adenoma.
- To see the wall thickening of the cyst, etc.

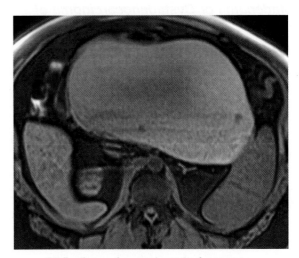

CT findings of pseudocyst of pancreas

What is the role of ERCP in this case?

Endoscopic retrograde cholangiopancreaticography (ERCP) is indicated in:

- Pancreatic ascites—for stenting the pancreatic duct
- When there are intraductal stricture or calculi is present
- It shows the communication between duct and cyst, ductal calcification, etc. prominently.
- When internally drained cyst leading intrapancreatic fistula formation owing to duct cyst communication.

(But before performing ERCP one has to be very clear about it's requirement in that case as because ERCP may aggravate pancreatitis and it introduces infection into the pseudocyst).

What other tests will you do in this case?

I will do, liver function test, serum amylase to exclude persistent pancreatitis and I will do all the baseline investigations to make the patient fit for anesthesia and surgery.

What surgery will you perform in such a case?

Sir, before performing surgery, I will see the size of the cyst, location as well thickness of the cyst. If the cyst is medium to large size, confined in epigastric region only and adherent to stomach, I will do cystogastrostomy.

Cystogastrostomy involves an anterior gastrostomy along the long axis of the stomach and when the cyst is very large, extending beyond epigastrium, cystojejunostomy with Roux-en-Y loop of jejunum, to be the preferred method.

OK, what's about the wall thickness of the cyst?

Sir, wall thickness is very important to do cystogastrostomy or cystojejunostomy. The chance of anastomotic leak is high if wall thickness of the cyst is 5 mm or less. Thin wall will not hold sutures effectively. Cyst wall should be minimum 6 mm for effective anastomosis.

Suppose the pseudocyst is in the head of pancreas or in relation with body and tail of pancreas what will you do?

As the head of pancreas comes in relation with second part of duodenum so, the pseudocyst is best drained by cystoduodenostomy. Thick rim of parenchyma should not come in between the cyst and duodenal wall.

If the cyst is in the relation with body and tail of pancreas, cystojejunostomy with Roux-en-Y loop is preferable as the cyst does not come in relation with stomach usually. So cystogastrostomy is not preferable.

Suppose the pseudocyst is very large and it is adherent to stomach wall, will you prefer to do cystogastrostomy in such a case?

No sir, cystogastrostomy is not a preferred procedure in such a large cyst though the cyst is adherent to stomach because.

No (i) there will be a difficult drianage of gastric and pancreatic secretions from the dependent part of the cyst. Stasis may result in an abscess formation.

No (ii) gastrostomy opening is more prone to be sealed off within a short duration so, large cyst cannot be drained properly. As a result, cyst will recure and may be infected easily. However, it is preferable to drain large pseudocyst with Roux-en-Y loop of jejunum.

What are the indications for drainage of pseudocyst?

i. Symptomatic cyst—pain, vomiting, discomfort, etc.
ii. Cyst with pressure symptoms—obstructive jaundice, gastric outlet obstruction, etc.
iii. Gradually increasing cyst in serial follow-up.

What are the drainage procedures for pseudocyst?

i. Open drainage—internal drainage and external drainage. External drainage is done by insertion of pig tail. In 20-30% cases pig tail causes pancreatic fistula formation.
ii. Endoscopic drainage—the cyst is connected either into stomach or duodenum.
iii. Laparoscopic drainage.

How will you manage a pseudocyst associated with chronic pancreatitis?

When pseudocyst is associated with chronic pancreatitis with dilated pancreatic duct with calculi—a lateral pancreaticojejunostomy (Fray's procedure) to be done along with cystojejunostomy with Roux-en-Y loop.

Which types of pseudocysts are most likely to resolve and which do not?

The pseudocysts are **most likely** to be resolved are:
i. Small cyst usually less than 5 cm.
ii. Thin wall cyst with an indistinct interface between the cyst wall and the adjacent structure.
iii. Pseudocyst is not associated with chronic pancreatitis.
iv. Nontraumatic pseudocyst.

Pseudocysts which are **not likely** to resolves are:
i. Large cyst; usually more than 5 cm.
ii. Thick wall (>6 mm) cyst.

   iii. Post-traumatic pseudocyst.

   iv. Associated with chronic pancreatitis.

   v. Size is increasing even after 4 weeks.

Can you tell me in what conditions early interventions are required for a pseudocyst?

   i. Infected cyst.

   ii. Rupture of the cyst.

   iii. Rapidly increasing in size and discomfort of the patient.

   iv. Large cyst which has got pressure effects like.

      a. Pressure on duodenum causing gastric outlet obstruction.

      b. Pressure on CBD causing obstructive jaundice.

What are the other drainage procedures for a pseudocyst?

- *Endoscopic drainage:* Where cystogastrostomy or cystoduodenostomy is done through endoscope. Here the cyst is punctured endoscopically through the stomach or duodenal wall approx 1-2 cm by using a diathermy.

- *Percutaneous drainage:* Where a catheter is placed into the pseudocyst, under USG/CT guidance, percutaneously.

What are the indications of endoscopic drainage of a pseudocyst?

Indicated when:

   i. Patient is unable to tolerate surgical procedure, i.e. patient is not fit for surgery.

   ii. Where debridement is not required along with drainage peocedure.

The drawbacks of endoscopic drainage are:

   i. Debridement not possible.

   ii. Bleeding is more from cut margin.

   iii. Cystic fluid may leak into the peritoneal cavity.

   iv. Chances of infections are more.

What are the indications of percutaneous drainage (external drainage) of pseudocyst?

   i. Infected pseudocyst.

   ii. Rapidly increasing cyst causing pressure effect.

   iii. Pseudocyst in rare location which is not suitable for internal drainage, like pseudocyst in pelvis, mediastinum.

   iv. Critically ill patient and patient not fit for surgery.

   v. Cyst associated with hemorrhage where clot may block the drainage tube.

Drawbacks of percutaneous drainage are:

   i. Pancreatic fistula formation as a result of catheter placement into the cyst. It usually closes within few months.

   ii. Pancreatic duct obstruction and dilatation along with pseudocyst remain untreated.

   iii. Recurrence of pseudocyst when it is particularly, communicated with the duct.

What are the essential procedures to be undertaken during internal drainage surgery?

During cystojejunostomy or cystogastrostomy procedure:

   i. Cystic fluid to be sent for cytology.

   ii. Cyst wall to be sent for cytological examination.

   iii. The septae of the cyst to be broken and cyst cavity to be irrigated with normal saline.

How hematemesis—melena occur in pseudocyst?

In a case of pseudocyst:

   i. If enterocystic fistula formation is there, the fluid of the cyst irritates gastric mucosa and forms ulcer which may cause bleeding.

   ii. Splenic vein thrombosis cause portal hypertension leads to esophageal varices and bleeding.

   iii. Pseudocyst of body and tail of pancreas may erode splenic artery and may cause hemorrhage.

What is pseudo-pseudopancreatic cyst?

Sometimes in acute pancreatitis a large soft mass is formed which consists of edematous pancreas, peripancreatic swelling of omentum and retroperitoneal tissue, which is called pseudo-pseudocyst.

SHORT NOTE ON EPIGASTRIC LUMP

PSEUDOCYST

A collection of pancreatic fluid surrounded by a nonepithelialized wall of granulation tissue and fibrosis is called pseudocyst. It is pseudo as no epithelial lining is there in the cyst like a true cyst.

Characteristics of Pseudocyst

Cyst appears following an acute attack of pancreatitis. The cyst is extrapancreatic.

Common sites are lesser sac commonest, others in relation to duodenum, jejunum, etc.

- Pancreatic duct anatomy usually normal
- There is persistent hyperamylasemia and cystic fluid is rich in amylase.
- ERCP may reveal duct-cyst communication
- Cyst has no epithelial lining
- Acute pseudocyst may resolve up to 50% cases over a course of 6 weeks and 50% cases it does not resolve, thereby drainage is required to resolve it.

Causes of Pseudocyst

Pseudocysts occur in up to 10% of patients with acute pancreatitis and 20 to 40% of patients with chronic pancreatitis.

Mechanism

In acute pancreatitis fluid collection occurs rapidly in lesser sac due to duct disruption with leakage of pancreatic juice. In chronic pancreatitis pancreatic duct leak, with extravasation of pancreatic juice and results in a pancreatic fluid collection in the surrounding area like lesser sac. Up to 50% cases pseudocysts are resolved in the following ways:

i. Spontaneous transperitoneal resorption
ii. Spontaneous fistula formation with adjacent structure like cystogastric or cystojejunal fistula.
iii. Cystic fluid decompression through pancreatic duct.
iv. Spontaneous rupture of the cyst into peritoneal cavity.

Clinical Presentations

A patient is diagnosed with acute pancreatitis and the symptoms do not resolve with conservative management and persisting for more than 10 days or the patient deteriorated after an initial recovery, is suspected to have a pseudocyst

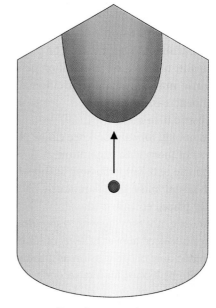

Pseudopancreatic cyst

formation. About 60% patients present with epigastric cystic lump. Persistent hyperamylasemia following an acute pancreatitis suggests development of pseudocyst.

Diagnosis

- USG
- CT scan abdomen
- ERCP
- Liver function tests, amylase, etc. as described above.

Treatment

Internal drainage is preferred to external drainage (Details are described above).

INTRA-ABDOMINAL SOLID SWELLINGS IN THE EPIGASTRIUM—DIFFERENTIAL DIAGNOSIS

i. **Liver mass:** Especially from left lobe enlargement of liver is determined by palpating its lower border and percussing its upper limit. Upper border cannot be felt— Hepatic swellings are continuous with the liver dullness and move up and down with respiration.
- Dull on percussion.

53

ii. **Transverse colon mass—as in carcinoma.**
- Horizontally placed mass
- Hard, nodular, moves above downwards, restricted side ways movement
- Moves with respiration
- Cecum will be dilated and may be palpable
- Tympanic or impaired resonant on percussion.

iii. **Pancreatic mass:** Cystadenocarcinoma, carcinoma head of pancreas.
- Epigastric firm mass
- Does not fall forward on knee elbow position
- Does not move with respiration
- Tympanic note on percussion as intestine infront.

iv. **Lymph nodal mass:** Like para-aortic LN mass.
- Deeply placed epigastric mass
- Nonmobile, not moving with respiration
- Vertically placed above the level of umbilicus
- Tympanic note on percussion as intestine infront
- Causes to be looked for like secondaries from testis, lymphoma, tuberculosis, etc.

v. **Retroperitoneal mass:** Like sarcoma, teratoma, etc.
- Deeply placed mass
- Usually smooth and hard
- Does not fall forward in knee elbow position
- Nonmobile, does not move with respiration
- Tympanic note on percussion.

IMPORTANT SHORT NOTE ON PANCREAS

Pancreas is known as abdominal trigger.

Anatomy: Retroperitoneal organ, 15-20 cm in length, lies against T1-T2 vertebra, lies posterior to stomach, separated by lesser sac.

Parts: Divided into head, neck, body and tail. Head lies in the concavity of duodenum and tail in the hilum of spleen. Posterior surface of neck is related to terminal part of superior mesenteric vein and the beginning of portal vein.

Ducts
i. Main pancreatic duct (duct of Wirsung). It begins in the tail of pancreas and runs on the posterior surface of the body and head of pancreas, receives numerous tributaries at right angle along its length (Herring bone pattern). It joins to the lower end of CBD at second part of duodenum to form ampulla of Vater and opens on the summit of major duodenal papilla (8-10 cm from pylorus).

ii. Accessory pancreatic duct (duct of Santorini). It begins in the lower part of head and opens into the duodenum at minor duodenal papilla.

Blood Supply
i. Pancreatic branches of splenic artery.
ii. Superior pancreaticoduodenal artery—branch of gastro-duodenal artery.
iii. Inferior pancreaticoduodenal artery—branch of superior mesenteric artery.

Nerve supply: Parasympathetic supply from vagus. Sympathetic innervations from splanchnic nerves.

Annular pancreas: This is as a result of failure of complete rotation of the ventral pancreatic bud during its development. So a ring of pancreatic tissue surrounds the second and third part of duodenum.

Acute pancreatitis: This is defined as acute abdominal condition presenting with characteristics abdominal pain and is usually associated with raised pancreatic enzymes level in the blood.

May occur at any age but common in young men and elderly women.

Etiology: Major causes are: (i) Biliary calculi 50-70%, (ii) Alcohol abuse 25%. Third important cause is, (iii) Traumatic/ Post ERCP. Other causes are, (iv) Drug induced pancreatitis—the drugs are:

Definite: 6 Mercaptopurine, azathioprine, asparginase, didanosine.

Other suspected drugs are:
- 5 aminosalicylate, valproic acid
- Cytosine arabinoside
- Diuretics, estrogen, frusemide
- Tetracycline, metronidazole, acetominophen, methyldopa, INH, etc.

v. Ischemia
vi. Metabolic cause—Hyperparathyroidism
- Hypercalcemia
- Hyperlipidemia (Where amylase not raised in blood as it cannot be measured in hyperlipidemia).
vii. Mechanical obstruction—ductal hypertension and disruption.

Other rare causes are:
viii. Autoimmune
ix. Hereditary
x. Infection—Mamas, coxiella
xi. Malnutrition

xii. Scorpion bite—causes painless pancreatitis

xiii. Idiopathic.

Pathology: Pancreatitis is primarily due to intracellular alteration of trypsinogen to trypsin by numerous stimuli.

Clinical features: Pain is the cardinal symptom. Pain characteristically develops quickly reaching maximum intensity within minutes and persists for hours or even days. Constant agonizing pain initially in epigastrium, may be localized to either upper quadrant or felt diffusely throughout the abdomen. There is radiation of pain to back in about 50% cases. Some patients may gain pain relief by sitting or leaning forward position (as peritoneum gets detached from inflamed pancreas).

i. Dramatic onset of pain is seen in:
   - Acute pancreatitis (Others perforated peptic ulcer and ruptured aneurysm).

ii. Nausea, vomiting and retching are usually marked accompaniments, vomiting is often frequent and persistent retching may persist, despite the stomach being kept empty by nasogastric aspiration.

iii. Hiccoughs may be troublesome and may be due to gastric distention or diaphragmatic irritation.

On Examination

- Patients look ill to gravely ill may be with profound shock.
- Tachypnea is very common.
- Tachycardia and hypotension may be present.
- Temperature initially normal or even subnormal but gradually temperature rises as inflammation develops.
- Mild icterus can be caused by biliary obstruction in gallstone pancreatitis.
- Acute swinging temperature suggests cholangitis.
- **Gray Turner sign:** Bleeding into facial planes can produce bluish discoloration of the flanks (Remember— Grant Feast, i.e. (G) Gray Turner (F) Flank.
- **Cullen's sign:** Bleeding into facial planes can produce bluish discoloration around umbilicus called Cullen's sign (Remember CU—Calcutta University, i.e. (C) Cullen's sign (U) Umbilicus).
- **Fox sign:** Sameway if the bluish discoloration is at the hypogastrium which is called fox sign.
  (But above three signs are not pathognomic of acute pancreatitis. Infact Cullen's sign was first described with rupture of an ectopic pregnancy. Bluish discoloration is due to liberated proteolytic and circulating enzymes gain access to body fluid and act on hemoglobin giving rise this discoloration).

- Red, tender nodules on the skin of the legs may be found due to subcutaneous fat necrosis.
- Abdominal examination may reveal distention due to ileus. A mass can be felt at epigastrium—called pseudo-pancreatic cyst (described above).
- Pleural effusion is observed in 10-20% of patients.

Investigations

i. **Serum amylase** level usually elevates four times above of its normal value.

   Normal value is 16-108 U/L

   Or 200-250 somogyi unit

   Half-life in 24 hours

   It is not very specific but definitely sensitive along with the characteristic features of pancreatitis. Amylase may be high in following conditions:
   - Salivary gland diseases
   - Mesenteric ischemia
   - Intestinal obstruction
   - Perforated duodenal ulcer
   - Ruptured aortic aneurysm.

   Others

   Ectopic gestation, salpingitis, etc.

ii. Serum lipase will increase.

iii. CRP, LDH will increase (CRP-C-reactive protein).

   Remember: Amylase isoenzyme-P is specifically increased in pancreatitis in other condition amylase isoenzyme-S is commonly increased. It can be analyzed with other proteolytic enzymes like lipase, elastase which are more relevant.

   Amylase level of peritoneal fluid is more than serum.

   Amylase is significant for pancreatitis.

iv. Straight X-ray abdomen may reveal generalized or local ileus (*sentinel loop*).

   Sentinel loop—air in the proximal loop of jejunum due to localized ileus.

   Colon cut off sign—due to ileus of spasm of distal part of transverse colon.

   Renal halo sign. Occasional findings are pancreatic calcification, calcified gallstones. Pleural effusion present in about 20% cases.

   USG abdomen: Swollen pancreas may be detected but gland is poorly visualized in 25-50% cases but it is valuable to detect.

   Free peritoneal fluid, gallstones, dilatation of the common bile duct, etc.

CT scan is investigation of choice for acute pancreatitis to exclude pancreatic necrosis which usually starts after 36-48 hours after onset. Otherwise in critically ill patients who do not improve within 24-36 hours CT is warranted.

It confirms the findings of ultrasound abdomen more accurately.

Balthazar classification of acute pancreatitis as on CT scan findings:

A—Pancreas is normal

B—Focal or diffuse enlargement of gland

C—Peripancreatic edema or intrinsic abnormality of A and B

D—Single ill defind fluid collection, phlegmon

E—Two or more fluid collection or presence of gas.

CT Severity Index (CTSI) of Acute Pancreatitis

CT Grading

i. Focal /diffuse enlargement of pancreas-1

ii. Pancreatic and peripancreatic edema-2

iii. Peripancreatic one collection-3

iv. Peripancreatic collection two or more-4.

Degree of Necrosis

- No necrosis—O.
- Necrosis in 1/3rd of pancreas—2
- Necrosis in 1/2 of pancreas—4
- Necrosis involvement is > ½ of pancreas—6.

CTSI= CT grading + degree of necrosis

   Mild pancreatitis 0-5

   Moderate pancreatitis-5-7

   Severe pancreatitis > 7.

CECT: IV contrast is essential, particularly in case of severe pancreatitis to enable visualizating of pancreas and differentiation of the gland from heterogeneous collection or fluid and peripancreatic inflammatory tissue. Pancreatic necrosis is seen as area of nonenhancement. In clinical practice all the heterogeneous areas of peripancreatic collections are considered area of fat necrosis unless proved otherwise.

Most important CT finding is diffuse pancreatic necrosis and demonstration of gas in pancreatic or peripancreatic region which is produced by gas forming bacteria. If gas is not present and patient has high persistent fever and high leukocyte count, USG/ CT guided aspiration of the collection is essential. To conclude, CECT is the imaging modality of choice to stage the severity of inflammatory process, detect pancreatic necrosis to predict local complications and the incidence of mortality.

Nonsurgical intervention can be performed under USG/ CT guidance with reduced mobility and mortality. CECT has become an intergral part and almost indispensible in assessing the initial injury and thus to help in proper management of the patient.

Laparotomy: Misdiagnosis of acute pancreatitis is very common as because the presentation is very much variable. Characteristic appearance, bulky, edematous pancreas, peripancreatic fluid collection, widespread fat necrosis of omentum, mesentery, etc.

Atlanta classification of acute pancreatitis:

- Acute edematous pancreatitis 80%
- Acute peripancreatic milder fluid collection 10%
- Acute necrotizing pancreatitis 20%. Characterized by pancreatic and peripancreatic necrosis mortality is 15%.
- Postpancreatitis pseudocyst
- Pancreatic abscess.

Scoring system to predict severity of pancreatitis:

- Ranson score for **alcoholic pancreatitis.**

On admission

   Age > 55 years

   WBC > 16000/cumm

   Blood glucose > 10 mmol, i.e. 200 mg%

   LDH > 350 IU/L

   AST > 250 IU/L

   (SGOT)

Within 48 hours

   Blood urea nitrogen rise > 5 mg%

   Atrial oxygen saturation (PaO_2) < 60 mm Hg

   Serum calcium <2 mmol/L, i.e. 8 mg/dl

   Hematocrit—Altered by 10%

   Base deficit > 4 meq/liter.

   Fluid sequestration > 6 liters.

   (Remember – 4, 5, 6, 8, 10 and 60)

   Score up to 5 – Relatively better prognosis

          5-7 – Equivocal, prognosis poor

   7 or more   – Prognosis very poor

Pancreatitis is considered to be severe when three or more factors are present. **Total score is 11.**

Drawbacks of Ranson scoring system are:

i. It has got only good negative predictive valve.

ii. It is ment for alcoholic pancreatitis mainly.

Ranson score for gallstone pancreatitis

On admission	Within 48 hours
Age > 70 years	Hematocrit altered by 10%
WBC > 18000/cumm	Blood urea nitrogen rise > 5 mg%
Blood glucose > 200 mg%	Serum calcium < 8 meq/L
LDH > 400 IU/L	Base deficit > 5 meq/L
AST (SGOT) > 250 IU/L	Fluid sequestration > 4L

Glassgo Scale

On admission

Age > 55 years

WBC > 15000/cumm

Blood glucose> 10 mmol/L, i.e. >200 mg% (Without any history of diabetes).

Serum urea > 16 mmol/L (no response to IV fluid)

Arterial O_2 saturation (PaO_2) <60 mm Hg.

Within 48 Hours

Serum albumin <2 mmol/L, i.e. <8 mg%

Serum albumin < 3.2 gm/dl

LDH > 600 U/L

AST/ALT >600 U/L

AST—Aspartate aminotransferase; ALT—Alanine aminotransferase; LDH—Lactate dehydrogenase.

Remember: Decrease serum calcium level is worst prognostic indicator of pancreatitis.

APACHE II (Acute physical and chronic health evaluation) scoring system can be applied. It consists of:

a. *Vitals*
    i. Respiratory rate
    ii. Heart rate
    iii. Mean BP
    iv. Rectal temperature
b. *Monitor*
    i. Oxygenation, i.e. SPO_2
c. *Lab tests*
    i. Hematocrit
    ii. WBC
    iii. Serum electrolytes (Na, K) and creatinine.

A score of 9 or more indicates a severe attack. A patients having APACHE II sore 6 or more, are prone to develop (>95%) complications.

Treatment: (a) Conservative mainly, (b) Invasive procedure, (c) Surgery where indicated.

a. **Conservative:** Remember—PANCREAS
    P – Pain relief by NSAIDs (morphine, dicyclomine or atropine, etc.) as it causes relaxation of sphincter of Oddi. Pethidines usually causes sphincter spasm so it is better to avoid. Protease inhibitors like aprotinin, plasma, etc. are used.
    A – Antibiotics—cephalosporin group of antibiotic like cefuroxime, cefotaxime, cefipime, etc. Anticholinergic—may be used to reduce sphincter pressure.
    N – Nasogastric aspiration, urinary catheterization, nasal O_2, i.e. oxygen inhalation.
    Nutritional support like total parenteral nutrition (TPN).
    C – Calcium gluconate 10% when calcium level is <8 mg%
    Calcitonin
    CVP line
    R – Rehydration by IV fluids, plasma, blood.
    Resuscitation
    Respiratory support (ventilatory support if PaO_2 is not maintained), Ranitidine 50 mg IV 12 hourly.
    E – Endotracheal intubation, electrolyte management
    A – Analgesics, antacids
    S – Swan Ganz catheter/central line for CVP and TPN, somatostatin and its analog (Octreotide).

b. **Invasive procedures:** If gallstones are the etiology of severe pancreatitis, urgent ERCP (preferable within 36 to 48 hours) is indicated to exclude the presence of a struck stone in the ampulla of Vater. The presence of cholangitis with abnormal LFT, urgent endoscopic intervention is indicated like endoscopic sphincterotomy should be performed.

c. **Surgery**
    Indications:
    • Patients deteriorates inspite of good conservative treatment
    • When infected necrosis is established or suspected
    • Pancreatic abscess formation
    • And as diagnostic laparoscopy/laparotomy where
    • Diagnosis is in doubt.

Principles of Surgery

i. **Percutaneous drainage:** Infected pancreatic necrosis to be removed through percutaneous drainage with a rigid scope.

ii. **Laparotomy:** If CT guided aspirate is infected and patient is deteriorating, a laparotomy with debridement of the dead tissue around the pancreas is essential.

iii. **Beger's procedure:** Continuous postoperative closed drainage of the lesser sac. Lavage is carried out through several double lumen or single lumen catheter. Each time 1 liter of saline is infused through and drained over a period of hours and the process repeated, i.e. in 24 hours 24 liters can be infused and drained the same.

iv. **Bradley's procedure:** Here repeated laparotomies are suggested until there is a clean granulating cavity around the pancreas.

v. **Necrosectomy:** By high pressure jet of water or by blunt side of the knife.

Prognosis of Acute Pancreatitis

Mild pancreatitis mortality is less than 1%. Severe pancreatitis mortality rate 20-25%. Pancreatitis with infected necrosis mortality is up to 50%.

Few Important Things in Pancreatitis

How alcohol causes pancreatitis?

i. Alcohol has direct toxicity on the pancreatic cells as it is a cellular metabolic poison and it causes damage of parenchymal cells.

ii. It causes spasm of sphincter of Oddi causing obstruction of the flow of pancreatic juice.

iii. It causes precipitation of proteins and calcium in the pancreatic duct resulting in ductal obstruction.

iv. It increases permeability of the pancreatic duct as a result leakage of enzymes from damage pancreatic tissue.

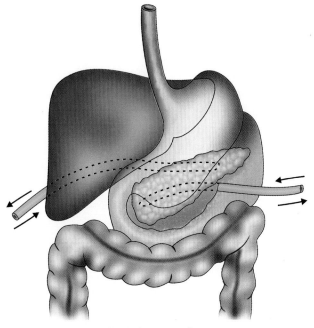

Beger's procedure

v. Alcohol reduces the blood supply to pancreas thereby, may cause ischemic damage to pancreas.

vi. Alcohol is the cause of malnutrition, by hyperlipidemia, hypersecretion which may cause pancreatitis.

How gallstones cause pancreatitis?

i. **Common channel hypothesis:** In which blockage by gallstones below the junction of biliary and pancreatic ducts would cause bile to flow into the pancreas which could then be damaged by the detergent of bile salt.

   Important objection to this theory—Majority individuals have such a short common channel anatomically that a stone located here would block both the pancreatic and biliary ducts, effectively isolating two system, further more, hydrostatic pressure in the biliary tract is lower than in the pancreas, a condition that would favor abnormal flow of pancreatic juice into the bile duct rather than in the opposite direction.

ii. **Reflux of activated enzymes and infected fluid:** Passage of gallstone through sphincter of Oddi renders it momentarily incompetent, permitting the reflux of duodenal juice containing activated digestive enzymes into pancreatic ductal system reflux of infected bile into the pancreatic duct causes activation of pancreatic enzymes, leading to pancreatitis.

   Objection to the theory: Procedures designed to render the sphincter incompetent such as sphincterotomy do not routinely cause pancreatitis.

iii. **Other theories of developing pancreatitis are:** Pancreatic duct obstruction and hypertension. Pancreatic duct may get obstructed by helminthic infestation or its blockage by tumors, produce ductal hypertension resulting from ongoing exocrine secretion into an obstructed pancreatic duct leading to pancreatitis.

iv. **Colocalization theory:** (Steer and Saluja theory) highly accepted theory as it explains cellular mechanism of acute pancreatitis. In response to ductal obstruction, the lysosomal hydrolases are improperly colocalized in a vacuolar structure unlike in normal situation within pancreatic acinar cell. Trypsinogen may colocalize with cathepsin-B to produce activated trypsin which in turn activates the other digestive zymogens. These activated digestive enzymes then begin autodigestion within the pancreas.

CHRONIC PANCREATITIS

Definition: It is chronic inflammatory disease of pancreas which causes persistent progressive and irreversible damage of pancreatic tissue.

Etiology: Most common cause of chronic pancreatitis is high alcohol consumption. Other important causes are.

Pancreatic duct obstruction by:

- Stricture
- Postacute pancreatitis
- Pancreatic carcinoma
- Stones in biliary tree
- Hereditary pancreatitis
- Post-traumatic pancreatitis
- Idiopathic
- Congenital anomaly like pancreatic divisum, etc.

Idiopathic groups are those who live in warm climates such as **Kerala in southern India** and appear to have a high incidence of pancreatitis. In such a case pancreatitis begins at young age and associated with high incidence of diabetic mellitus and stone formation is frequent.

Pathology

- Segmental or diffuse fibrosis
- Focal necrotic changes
- Parenchymal calcification or ductal stones
- Stricture or obstruction of the duct
- Dilatation of the duct.

Classification of Chronic Pancreatitis

Singer and Chari classification:

i. Chronic calcific pancreatitis due to alcohol, hereditary, topical, hyperlipidemia, hypercalcemia, etc.

ii. Chronic obstructive pancreatitis—due to pancreatic tumor, ductal stricture, gallstone, pancreatic divisum, etc.

iii. Chronic inflammatory—Idiopathic.

iv. Chronic autoimmune pancreatitis associated with primary sclerosing cholangitis, primary biliary cirrhosis, etc.

v. Asymptomatic pancreatitis associated with pancreatic fibrosis, chronic alcohol, i.e. endemic in tropical climates.

Clinical Features

i. **Pain epigastric region:** Most common. Up to 60% cases mild to moderate or even severe pain may radiate to back off and on. Pain is due to irritation of retropancreatic nerves, ductal dilatation or stasis or due to chronic inflammation itself. Right or left subcostal pain depending on the part of pancreas involved. Nausea, vomiting are common during attacks.

Characteristics of pain: It is dull and gnawing. Both continuous and episodic. Severe bouts of pain may occur.

ii. **Exocrine dysfunction:** Loss of weight, anorexia, asthenia, malabsorption, diarrhea, steatorrhea (signifies severe pancreatic insufficiency), creatorrhea.

iii. **Endocrine dysfunction:** Increasing incidence of diabetes mellitus with time.

iv. **Mild jaundice:** May be there due to narrowing of retro-pancreatic bile duct and cholangitis.

v. **Mass upper abdomen:** Just above the umbilicus. Tender hard, nodular, not moving with respiration, nonmobile, does not fall forward on knee elbow position, tympanic note on percussion. Mass is felt due to pseudocyst formation or due to neoplastic change.

vi. **Mallet Guys sign:** In right knee chest position if left hypochondrium is palpated, tenderness can be evoked in a case of chronic relapsing pancreatitis. In such a position bowel loops are shifted to right so, pancreas become palpable directly.

Chronic pancreatitis may lead to carcinoma pancreas.

Complications of Chronic Pancreatitis

i. Pseudocyst which may cause:
- Duodenal or gastric obstruction
- Biliary stricture as lower end of CBD gets compressed.
- Thrombosis of splenic vein
- Abscess
- Perforation, etc.

ii. Inflammatory mass in head of pancreas:
- Bile duct stenosis
- Portal vein thrombosis
- Duodenal obstruction
- Colonic stricture as inflammatory process spreads to adjacent colon.

iii. Ductal strictures and/or stones
- Ductal hypertension and dilatation

iv. Pancreatic carcinoma

v. Extrapancreatic complications
- Pancreatic duct leak with ascites or fistula
- Pseudocyst extension beyond lesser sac into mediastinum
- Pancreatoenteric fistula.

Investigations

i. Serum amylase: Only in the early stages of pancreatitis serum amylase is raised.

ii. Plane X-ray abdomen shows calcification is about 65% cases.

iii. USG abdomen—to see
- Duct dilatation (Normal duct diameter is 3 mm)
- Stones in CBD, pancreatic duct, gallbladder
- Pancreatic parenchyma, liver status
- USG guided FNAC if suspected mass lesion is there.

iv. CT scan abdomen is the investigation of choice. It also shows the outline of the gland, the main area of damage and the possibilities for surgical correction.

v. ERCP—may show
- Abrupt obstruction of main duct
- Encasement of pancreatic duct
- Parenchymal filling with necrosis
- Double duct sign
- Scrambled egg appearance
- Pancreatic juice cytology or brush biopsy is done through ERCP.

vi. Glucose tolerance test
- Fecal chymotrypsin and elastase analysis
- Pancreatic function test merely confirm the diagnosis as the test is affected only when more than 70% of the gland has been destroyed.

vii. CA 19-9 is useful tumor marker (Details written in obstructive jaundice).

Treatment

a. Conservative
b. Surgery

Advice

- Low fat, high protein, high carbohydrate diet with no alcohol, tobacco smoking.
- Small meal frequently.

Medicine

- H_2 blockers or proton pump inhibitors which are very effective. (The drugs reduce the secretion of HCl, thereby make a alkaline media in which pancreatic enzymes and supplementary pancreatic enzymes act only).
- Pancreatic enzymes supplements, vitamins, minerals, etc.
- Pain relief analgesics, splanchnic or celiac plexus block.
- Diabetic control.

- Somatostatin and its analogs like octreotide to prevent complications.
- Others symptomatic measurements like ascitic tap, etc.

Surgery

Indications to relieve:
- Persistent pain
- To overcome obvious obstruction
- To remove mass lesion
- To releive from complications like malabsorption, multiple relapses, etc.

Commonly offered surgeries for pancreatitis are:

i. **Beger procedure:** If there is a mass in the head of pancreas, where duodenal preserving pancreatic head coring, infront of portal vein, with jejunal loop anastomosis.

ii. **Frey's procedure:** When duct is dilated markedly, lateral pancreaticojejunostomy with partial excision of pancreatic head to improve drainage.

iii. **Whipple's procedure:** If the disease mainly involves head of pancreas and a mass lesion is there at the head Whipple's procedure (already described in obstructive jaundice) is preferable.

iv. **Duval procedure:** Resection of body and tail of pancreas with retrograde pancreaticojejunostomy done when the disease involves body and tail of pancreas.

v. **Total pancreatectomy:** When the disease involves entire gland aiming to relieve pain and to avoid development of malignancy.

SHORT HISTORY OF INITIAL OPERATIONS

Initially Puestow started the operation for chronic pancreatitis. In such cases where the duct dilatation is more than 8 mm, duct can be easily opened longitudinally. Ducts anastomized to the jejunum as Roux-en-Y after removing the stones along with splenectomy. This operation is slightly modified by Partington Rochelle where splenectomy was not to be done.

CARCINOMA HEAD OF PANCREAS

Eighty five percent cases are duct cell adenocarcinomas. Tobacco smoking and chronic pancreatitis are the most common predisposing factors.

Clinical Features

Most common—epigastric discomfort.

- Ampullary tumors usually present with jaundice and weight loss.
- Carcinoma head and neck of pancreas patients present with weight loss and jaundice.
- Cystadenocarcinoma patients present with pain in back, weight loss and mass in epigastrium.
- **On examination:** Scratch marks all over the body, evidence of weight loss, palpable gallbladder, hepatomegaly and metastatic lymph nodes in the neck.
- Superficial migratory thrombophlebitis (**Trousseau's sign**) can be seen. This is due to release of platelet aggregating factors from the tumor and or its necrotic materials.

Investigations

Liver function test (LFT): Direct serum bilirubin is increased, serum albumin is decreased with altered A: G ratio.

Prothrombin time is widened. Serum alkaline phosphates (ALP) of its normal value (20-90 IU/L).

- **USG abdomen:** To see the origin of growth
  - Gallbladder, liver, CBD diameter
  - Lymph nodes, portal vein, ascites, etc.
- **Barium meal:**
  Pad sign
  - Widened duodenal 'C' loop in a head of pancreas.
  - Reverse '3' sign in periampullary carcinoma.
- **CECT:** To stage the disease.
  - For example, size and extension of growth
  - Portal vein infiltration
  - Involvement of superior mesenteric vessels
  - Lymph nodes involvement, ascites, etc.

ERCP – may show
- Abrupt obstruction of main duct
- Encasement of pancreatic duct
- Parenchymal filling with necrosis
- Double duct sign
- Scrambled egg appearance
- Pancreatic juice cytology or brush biopsy is done through ERCP.

CA 19-9 is useful tumor marker (Details written in obstructive jaundice).

Treatment

Seventy to eighty percent cases are inoperable by the time patient is kept ready for surgery.

Criteria for surgery
- Tumor is relatively smaller (4 cm)
- Growth not adherent to superior mesenteric vessels.
- No para-aortic or mesenteric lymphadenopathy.
- There should be no hepatic metastases.
  Preoperative preparation: Injection mannitol (to prevent hepatorenal syndrome).
- Antioxidants
- Vitamin K 10 mg IM for 5-7 days
- Correction of anemia, malnutrition, etc.
  (Details is written in obstructive jaundice).
- Prophylactic antibiotics, etc.

Surgery Operable cases: (i) Whipple's operation—The resection includes:
- Tumor along with head, neck of pancreas, i.e. division at the neck of pancreas.
- 'C' loop duodenum and proximal jejunum up to 10 mm/cm.
- Distal part of stomach 30-40%.
- Lower end of CBD, gallbladder
- Lymph nodes.
  Continuity is maintained by: (i) pancreaticojejunostomy, (ii) hepaticojejunostomy and (iii) gastrojejunostomy

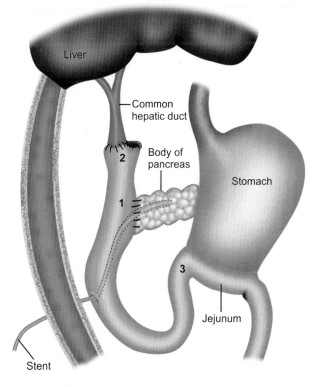

Post Whipple's (i) Pancreaticojejunostomy, (ii) Hepaticojejunostomy and (iii) Gastrojejunostomy

(Jejunojejunostomy done only when Roux' loop pancreati-cojejunostomay done).

   i. Pylorus preserving pancreatectomy.

  ii. **Fortner's regional pancreatectomy:** Includes recreation of tumor with C loop of duodenum with segment of superior mesenteric vein which is anastomosed with portal vein with clearance of lymph nodes in the region. This extensive procedure is rarely done nowadays.

Inoperable Cases

   i. In case of severe jaundice (bilirubin > 15 mg%). ERCP stenting or cholecystojejunostomy is required to be done to reduce jaundice.

  ii. Endoscopic duodenal stenting in case of gastric outlet obstruction.

 iii. PTBD where ERCP stenting is not possible.

 iv. Choledochojejunostomy with jejunojejunostomy and gastrojejunostomy are done as palliative procedures to drain bile into small bowel and to prevent gastric outlet obstruction, respectively.

ERCP and stenting where possible as an alternative good palliative procedure.

Adjuvant Therapy

- Radiotherapy
- 5 FU may be useful chemotherapeutic agent
- Gemcetabine is a newer useful drug
- Chemotherapy provides 10-15% overall survival benefit up to 55 years

Pain control in carcinoma pancreas:

- USG/CT guided ethanol (50% of 20 mg) injection into celiac ganglion
- Epidural analgesia
- Palliative radiotherapy
- Video assisted transthoracic splanchnicectomy

Prognosis: Despite of all sorts of therapy and surgery mentioned above, mean survival is 6-9 months only.

Ampulla of Vater carcinoma—who underwent resection, 5 years survival is up to 40% but in a case of ductal carcinoma the survival rate is 20% maximum.

CASE 7

Hepatic Mass

My patient, Jeet Singh, a 57-year-old male, resident of Rajasthan, presented with complains of:

- Lump at right upper quadrant of abdomen for last 6 months.
- Pain over the lump for last 1 month.

My patient was apparently asymptomatic 6 months back when he noticed a lump at his right upper abdomen which is gradually painlessly progressive and attained its present size approximately 8 × 10 cm from its initial size of a lemon, approximately 3 × 2 cm.

It was slowly progressive for initial 6 months but for last 2 months the lump is rapidly increasing in size.

Initially the lump was painless but for last 1 month he has been having pain over the lump off and on.

The pain is dull aching in nature, insidious in onset.

Sometimes, it disturbs his daily activities, aggravated with exhaustion and relieved on lying down after taking rest.

There is history of weight loss approximately 10-12 kg for last 6 months.

History of anorexia is there for last 2/3 months.

Bowel, bladder habit is more or less normal.

There is no history of fever, jaundice or blood transfusion (to exclude viral hepatitis).

No history of vomiting, hematemesis, malena, no history of urinary symptoms.

No history of cough, chest pain, hemoptysis or bone pain, etc. (to exclude mets).

Past history: He is not a known case of HTN, DM, TB, IHD, etc.

No history of long stay in hospital.

Personal history: He is farmer by occupation

Nonvegetarian

Alcoholic for last 10/15 years; 3/4 pegs per day.

Chronic smoker. 1 bundle per day for 20 years.

Family history: Not significant.

General survey: Patient is cooperative anxious facies, average built, poorly nourished.

Pulse 80/min, afebrile, BP 120/70 mm Hg right arm supine.

No pallor, icterus, edema or generalized lymphadenopathy noticed.

No scratch marks over the body, no feature suggestive of chronic liver insufficiency.

System examination:

GIT: Abdomen scaphoid but there is an obvious right upper abdominal visible swelling, umbilicus central, all quadrants move with respiration.

No visible veins, no scar marks, no other lump visible.

Flanks are not full, hernial sites and external genitalia appear normal.

On palpation: There is an intra-abdominal lump at right hypochondrium and epigastrium extending towards right lumbar region.

The lump is 8 × 10 cm well circumscribed, firm, and irregular surface, nontender, nodular somewhere.

Upper margin merged with liver, fingers cannot be insinuated in between the lump and costal margin, lower medial and lateral margins are well defined.

Moves with respiration craniocaudally but not mobile side-to-side (side-to-side mobility is a special characteristic of GB mass).

The mass is nontender

No other lump or organomegaly palpable.

No free fluids

Hernial sites, testes are normal.

No supraclavicular lymphadenopathy noticed.

On percussion: Liver dullness starts at right 5th intercostal space and it enlarged 3 fingers (4.5 cm) on midclavicular line.

On auscultation: No bruit heard over the swelling.

DRE : Blumer shelf- not palpable.

Other systemic examination:

Respiratory: Bilateral air entry equal no adventitious sound heard.

CVS: S1 S2 (N), no murmur.

CNS: Higher motor function normal, no neurodeficit.
Others are essentially normal.

Summary

My patient, Jeet Singh, a 57-year-old male presented with a progressive lump at his right upper quadrant of abdomen for last 6 months and pain over it for last 1 month, along with significant weight loss and anorexia without any history of fever, jaundice, hematemesis, malena, cough, hemoptysis, etc.

On examination: General survey is essentially normal.

On systemic examination there is 8 ×10 cm intra-abdominal lump, firm, irregular nodular surface, moves with respiration but does not move side-to-side, well defined all margins, except upper margin which is merged with liver and finger cannot be insinuated in between the lump and costal margin.

So my provisional diagnosis is: a hepatic mass most probably due to secondaries.

Why do you say so?

- Clinically it is a hepatic mass
- Well defined irregular margin
- Palpable liver which is hard, multinodular with umbilication.
- Most common cause of liver mass is secondaries.
- Poor general condition of the patient.

Any differential diagnosis in your mind?

Yes sir, though I think on the basis of clinical features, it is a hepatic mass due to secondaries but I will keep in mind other causes of hepatic mass like.
- Hepatocellular carcinoma (hanging type)
  (Other types of HCC are pushing and infiltrating)
- Hepatocellular carcinoma with cirrhosis
- Hydatid cyst
- Hemangioma liver
- Lever adenoma, etc.

Salient Features

1. Hepatocellular Carcinoma
- Middle aged man
- Associated with chronic liver disease particularly with HBV and HCV
- May be presented with symptoms of chronic liver disease (malaise, weakness, jaundice, ascites, variceal bleed, encephalopathy) ill defined upper abdominal pain, hepatic mass
- Serum AFP increases > 4 time (normal value 200 ng/ml).

2. Hydatid Cyst
- Common condition in countries around the Mediterranean
- Very slow growing mass grow 1-2 cm per year
- Usually smooth surface, firm in consistency but it becomes hard while it is calcified
- Cyst is usually quite large (> 5 cm) when symptoms do occur
- Symptomatic patients commonly present right upper quadrant pain or dyspepsia
- Firm hepatic mass can often be palpable
- Ultrasound detects approximately 90% of hydatid cyst in liver
- Serum immunoelectrophoresis is currently the most reliable procedure. 90% sensitivity, if individuals infected with *E. granulosus*.
- ELISA for *Echinococcus* IgE.

3. Hemangioma
- Most common liver lesion
- Female are five times more commonly affected
- Most common presentation is asymptomatic abdominal mass may be with dull aching pain or GI symptoms
- Gaint hemangioma (> 4 cm in size) may cause obstructive jaundice, biliary colic, gastric outlet obstruction, etc.
- On examination, the mass is usually located in the epigastrium or left upper quadrant
- Compressibility of tumor is diagnostic
- USG shows hyperechoic lesion with finely indented circular border
- NCCT – Hypodense lesion

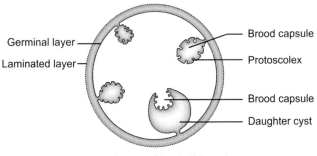

Anatomy of hydatid cyst

- CECT: Peripheral enhancements initially. Within 3 minutes complete opacity appears.

  ↓

  3-30 minutes—Isodense
  ↓ Thereafter
  Again hypodense
- In MRI the term used is **'lights up' lesion**
- **In case of any doubt do USG, CECT and MRI. Among the three if any two suggestive of hemangioma then it is to be treated as hemangioma.**

How will you proceed in this case?

I will confirm my diagnosis first by doing ultrasound abdomen.

It shows—The organ of origin:
- Nature of the mass
- Displacement/ pressure effects on surrounding structures
- It picks up the characteristics lesions like-hemangioma hyperechoic lesion
- Multiple nodular lesions in secondaries, etc.
- Lymphadenopathy, ascites, etc.
  Others:
  i. Primary site is identified by gastroscopy, colonoscopy, contrast X-ray, CT scan, etc.
  ii. I will do LFT, tumor markers like CEA
  iii. Liver biopsy if primary is not identified
  iv. CECT abdomen to detect primary site and to stage the disease and
  v. All baseline investigations to make the patient fit for anesthesia if surgery is planned.

Suppose it is secondaries in liver how will you manage the case?

I will look for primary sites. If it is from colon or kidney, surgery has got a definite role.

Palliative hemicolectomy should be offered, if primary is in the colon, along with solitary secondary in the liver, can be resected.

If secondaries in a single segment or lobe, segmentectomy or lobectomy can be done.

Otherwise chemotherapy is the treatment of choice.

How will you plan chemotherapy?

Depending upon the primary, I will choose the drugs. Example:

Carcinoma stomach – mitomycin, cisplatin and 5FU
Carcinoma colon – cisplatin or folfox regimen, oxaliplatin, 5FU, etc.

What's all other methods to ablate the tumor locally in secondaries in liver?

The other modalities of treatment are:
- Microwave therapy
- Radiofrequency ablation (single lesion <4 cm in size)
- Laser therapy
- Ultrasound or electrolyte therapy
- Ethanol injection, etc.

What's all the common primary sites often give rise to metastasis in liver?

Most common sites are:
- Carcinoma colon: 65%
- Carcinoma pancreas: 63%
- Carcinoma breast: 61%
Others:
- Carcinoma ovary: 52%
- Carcinoma rectum: 47%
- Carcinoma stomach: 45%
From:
- Carcinoma lung: 36%
- Carcinoma kidney: 27%

What are the routes of hepatic metastasis?

Metastasis reach the liver by four routes:
i. Direct invasion [Stomach, colon, bile duct, gallbladder (50-70% cases)].
ii. Lymphatics [Breast, lung via mediastinal nodes].
iii. Hepatic artery (lung, melanoma).
iv. Portal vein (carcinoid, other GI malignancies).

The portal vein by far the most common route.

Can you tell me the treatment protocol in a case of carcinoma in liver?

How will you follow-up the patient postoperatively?

Follow-up after hepatic resection should include frequent visits (initially 3 months) with intensive evaluation of any abnormality.

Postoperative abdominal CT scan and plasma CEA level should be obtained to establish the recurrence.

10 -20% patients may develop a re-resectable recurrence.

Overall prognosis of liver secondaries is poor. Patients die of malignant cachexia, infection, liver failure, etc.

Algorithm of treatment of hepatic tumor

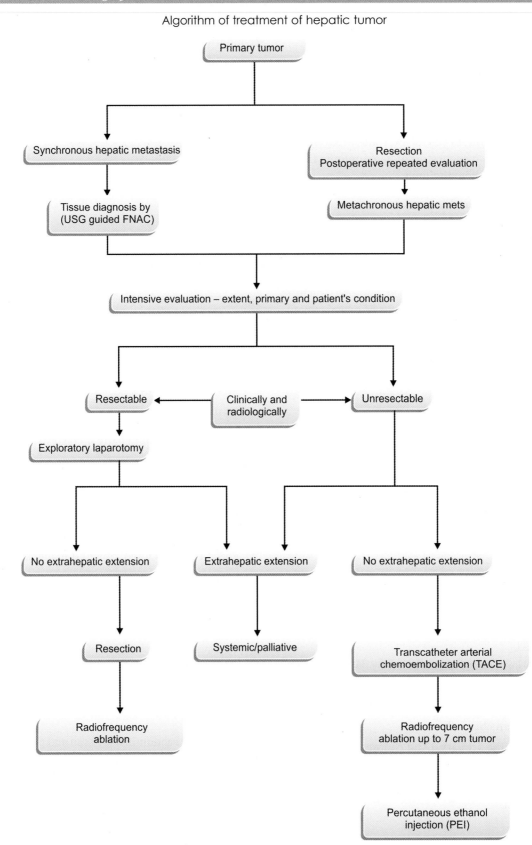

SHORT NOTES ON HEPATOCELLULAR CANCER

Hepatocellular concer (HCC) is the most common solid organ cancer worldwide and causes more than 1 million deaths annually. The disease is most commonly related to liver injury and is prevalent in south and Southeast Asia and China where the incidence of HBV infection is high. The tumor commonly presents late and is usually advanced, beyond scope of useful therapy at presentation due to the superb regenerative capability of the liver.

Etiology

HBV and HCV

The geographic distribution of HCC mirrors the incidence of HBV infection and is common in China, Taiwan, and Singapore, Malasia, Indonasia and countries of tropical Africa. Areas with high HCV infection like Japan and Italy are also affected commonly.

Cirrhosis of Liver, Previous Adenoma

Toxins

The most common toxin implicated is aflatoxin from fungal infestation of groundnuts and grains. The implicated toxin is aflatoxin B2. Other chemicals like alcohol, nitrites, hydrocarbons, organochlorine pesticides and thorotrast are implicated in the causation of HCC.

Genetic

Genetic loading is an important issue in HBV related HCC. In addition some metabolic diseases like hemochromatosis, Wilson's disease, glycogen storage disease, tyrosinemias are also related to the development of HCC.

Pathology

The outcome of the cancer is more related to the resectability than the histologic differentiation of the lesion. Three major macroscopic types: hanging, pushing and infiltrative types, the former two being easily amenable to resection.

The fibrolamellar variant is an unsusal form seen in young patients with a high resectability and usually not associated with HBV raised AFP or cirrhosis.

HCC may also be seen along with cholangiocarcinoma and this differentiation is associated with poor differentiation.

Clinical Presentation

The lesions commonly present with insidious symptoms of ill health, weight loss, ill defined upper abdominal pain, dyspepsia or a large hepatic mass. It may be the first presentation of cirrhosis. Other presentations include jaundice, hepatic failure, portal hypertension, variceal bleed and occasionally the dramatic tumor rupture.

A few patients < 5% may have paraneoplastic syndrome fever, porphyria, carcinoid syndrome, polycythemia hyperthyroidism, etc.

Confirm extent of disease; determine hepatic remnant function and biologic determinants of prognosis.

It is not absolutely necessary for histology when dealing with a mass lesion which is resectable as resection alone is the single most important prognostic indicator.

Confirm the Diagnosis

A combination of clinical findings, imaging and AFP level > 500 ng/ml is fairly confirmatory of the diagnosis. Presence of HBsAg/anti HCV is further confirmatory. FNAC is not mandatory due to the risks of bleed and seeding unless the plan is to start on a nonsurgical therapy for the patient. The accuracy of FNAC in diagnosis in the absence of a raised AFP is to the tune of 70%.

Define Extent of Disease

The common metastatic sites of HCC are bone, liver, adrenal, and lungs which need to be appropriately imaged to ascertain and rule out metastatic disease. Extent of disease in the liver particularly the growth pattern, proximity and involvement of hepatic and portal veins and intraparenchymal mets define the resectability of the disease. Further information on the vascular anatomy and its relation to the lesion can be obtained by USG, Doppler, angiography and three-dimensional CT.

Of late advances in technology have made it possible to calculate the remnant hepatic volume and also define the relationship of the tumor to the intrahepatic venous and biliary anatomy with software called Hepavision.

Determine Hepatic Remnant Function

The next important factor defining the possibility of resection is the function of the hepatic remnant. It is well known that the liver has an excellent regenerative capacity but most livers with HCC are cirrhotic or functionally compromised due to the causative disease HBV/HCV infection or the metabolic derangement. *In essence HCC is a tumor in a compromised **cirrhotic** HBV/HCV infected liver as outcomes are dependent on recurrences and cirrhotic decompensation.*

Liver function tests derangements, which are commonly observed, are serum albumin and alkaline phosphatase levels derangements. Serum bilirubin elevation is suggestive of deranged remnant and/or biliary obstruction. The most useful clinical system is the Child Pugh score (given below) with a grading of B or C carrying a worse outcome. In general Child C patients are offered only supportive care as they do not tolerate any modality of therapy.

Dynamic function of the liver is commonly done with Indocyanine glue (ICG) clearance, BSP clearance, C aminopurine clearance. ICG clearance is the commonly done assay which assesses the residual lCG (Indocyanine glue) at 15 minutes and a value of <15 is indicative of a lower risk for surgery.

Biologic determinants of prognosis.

These parameters are available following the resection and include presence of cirrhosis, angioinvasion, degree of differentiation, satellite nodules, nodal metastasis and other molecular markers of poor prognosis.

Treatment

The treatment modalities with possibility of cure are liver resection and liver transplantation. All other modalities of therapy like chemoembolization, ethanol injection, cryosurgery, radiofrequency ablation and systemic chemotherapy and hormonal therapy do not confer any improvement in survival though there is an improvement in quality of life.

Hepatic Resection

Advances in the understanding of the lobar anatomy of the liver, improvements in anesthesia, introduction of equipment like the harmonic scalpel and the CUSA dissector have made liver resections safe procedure. It is possible in noncirrhotic patients to excise up to 70% of the liver with hope of regenerative compensation by the remnant. The limits for patients with damaged liver are however much lower and the maximal resection tolerable in well compensated patients would be a hemihepatectomy. It is rarely possible to resect more than 20-25% of the functioning parenchyma in a cirrhotic patient. Patients with cirrhosis are also compromised with the presence of hypoalbuminemia, coagulopathy, altered anatomy, portal hypertension and poor regenerative capability.

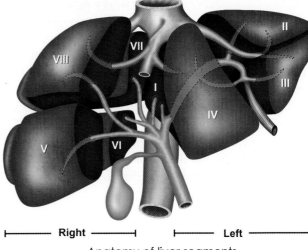

Anatomy of liver segments

Mortality of surgery is less than 5% and survival following surgical resection is 30-35% at 5 years, prognostic factors affecting survival are:

Hepatic and portal venous invasion	*Satellite lesions*
Nodal metastasis	Poor differentiation
Cirrhosis	
Nomenclature of surgical procedure	
Right hemihepatectomy	Segments 5, 6, 7, 8
Left hemihepatectomy	Segments 1, 2, 3, 4
Left lateral segment excision	Segments 2, 3
Isolated caudate lobe excision	Segment 1
Wedge excision	Nonanatomic
	Excision of involved liver with clear margin
Central hepatectomy	Segments 4, parts of 5 and 8

Surgical technique involves complete mobilization of the liver, intermittent inflow occlusion and careful dissection with CUSA or ultrasonic scalpel. The smallest resection that will remove all the tumor is the preferred procedure which is decided on table along with the available investigations.

Present studies have confirmed that surgery does add to survival even in patients with multiple tumors, adjacent organ invasion and obstructive jaundice. The only finding suggestive of poor survival is the presence of hepatic and portal venous invasion. Though the lesion may be technically resectable few would proceed to long-term survival.

Neoadjuvant Therapy

The aim of the therapy is to reduce the size of a large lesion for an attempt at Ro resection which would have not been possible otherwise. Numerous agents such as adriamycin and gemcitabine have been used in the recent years. The other modalities have been hepatic arterial embolization of chemotherapeutic agents, radiocolloids and immuno-therapeutic agents (OK 432). Though studies have shown improvements in survival and resectability the results are not uniform and no benefit has been unequivocally demonstrable.

An alternative approach to the problem of resectability is to occlude the portal venous supply by portal vein embolization to the affected segment and allow for a hypertrophy of the remnant which will allow for a safer resection.

Adjuvant Therapy

The majority (2/3rd) will recur with disease locally or systemically due to the nature of the liver, nature of the disease and both. Modalities attempted include chemoembolization and systemic chemotherapy. No randomized control trial has demonstrated a benefit of chemotherapy in any form in preventing or delaying recurrence and improving survival. This is largely due the fact that the tumor is not amenable to chemotherapy due to the multidrug resistant (MDR) gene hyperexpression in hepatic tumors.

Chemoprevention studies have shown some benefit of polyprenoic acid in the adjuvant selling iodine 131 labeled lipiodol has also shown to have a benefit in the adjuvant setting but problems of dosimetry and availability limit wide usage of the product.

Size <5 cm

Well differentiated tumors

No vascular invasion

No nodal metastasis with all above modalities of therapy the survival is to the tune of 30-35% in various studies. With careful selection and aggressive postoperative care the mortality is around 5%. Factors which predict a better survival in univariate analysis are:

No satellite lesions

Noncirrhotic.

Hepatic Transplantation

Transplantation as an option for HCC arises from the following facts.

The cirrhotics who underwent transplantation and were found to have nodules which were cancer experienced survivals no different from the patients without HCC, i.e. in the range of around 60% at 5 years which is superior to the best resection results. HCC is a disease in a diseased liver which is prone to develop tumors. It would be naive to leave behind a liver which has once proven to form cancer and hoping for no recurrence. It is also the only option for a patient with a small HCC, poor liver function and no metastasis.

The major obstacle for HCC is the availability of organs. HCC patients are low in the MELD score which governs the allocation of organs to waiting end stage liver disease (ESLD) patients. In addition patients with lesions larger than 5 cm are currently not candidates for receiving an organ. Use of live related donors for the same is also subject to ethical debate due to the issues of recurrence.

Nonsurgical Ablative Therapies
Percutaneous Ethanol Injection (PEI)

The method was first described by Suguira in 1983. Lesions can be injected at surgery, laparoscopically or percutaneously. The limiting factor is the size which should be be <3 cm and less than 3 in number for a single sitting. Nonrandomized and randomized small studies have shown that the procedure can lead to survivals comparable to resection and chemoembolization.

PEI is recommended indicates for poor risk patients with multiple small tumors where resection is not possible.

Radiofrequency Ablation

Radiofrequency ablation (RFA) is a increasingly popular modality for small HCC and recurrences in operated patients who are not for surgery now. RFA is cheaper equipment compared to the cryosurgery probe and easier to use. Limitations of size number are similar to PEI.

Transcatheter Arterial Embolization (TACE)

The liver has a dual blood supply and it has been noted that the tumors are selectively supplied by the artery. Hence, selectively embolizing the feeding artery has a potential to destroy the tumor. Liodol has affinity to escape into the perivascular space in tumor tissue and coat the endothelium preventing diffusion of nutrients. Addition of chemotherapeutic agents like adriamycin and mitomycin increases the local availability of the drug and overcomes the p glycoprotein efflux pump hence adding on to the cell destruction.

The treatment results in improvement of quality of life parameter with no objective survival improvement. This is possibly the only therapy possible in multicentric HCC and large painful lesions. Head-to-head comparisons with other forms of therapy and variations in the mode and materials of embolization have been difficult and difficult to interprete also.

Radiotherapy

The tolerance of the liver to RT is low. Whole liver RT has shown no efficacy which may be marginally improved with addition of cisplatin. I 131 labeled oil has been used for embolization but no survival difference has been noted. The problems of dosimetry, toxicity and availability have been alluded to before.

Chemotherapy

The role of systemic chemotherapy is limited due to the inherent chemo refractoriness of the tumor secondary to the multi drug registant (MDR) gene and the p-glycoprotein. The most commonly used agents are doxorubicin and gemcitabine. No agent has shown to have any survival benefit and response are partial and ill sustained.

Immunotherapy and Hormonal Therapy

Interferon alfa or beta interferon in a dose of 18-50 mU/m^2 has shown better response than and marginal improvements in survival compared to chemotherapy.

The tumors express estrogen and androgenic receptors. Trials with the use of antiestrogens and antiandrogens have shown no improvement in survival.

Summary of treatment options:

Assess tumor anatomy and extent

Assess hepatic reserve.

If the above is amenable to resection proceed for surgery.

If not, attempt TACE, PEI or RFA.

If a candidate is fit for transplant and organ is available go for transplant.

Metastatic disease symptomatic care or palliative chemotherapy.

Summary of management

Initial assessment

Clinical examination

CT abdomen and chest

MRI/Doppler for vasculature

LFT, prothrombin time

General fitness assessment for surgery

Grade risk by child Pugh score A, B, C

Assessment will divide patients to 4 groups

Small tumor <5 cm with child A or correctable B operate

Small tumor < 5 cm with child B or C

RFA/PEI/TACE

Chemo- or immunotherapy based on performance status

Large tumor > 5 cm with child A or correctable B operate

Large tumor > 5 cm with poor liver function TACE or supportive care

Multicentric tumor	TACE
Metastatic tumor	Treat lesion in the liver as for symptom Systemic chemotherapy/ immunotherapy if good performance status.

Child Pugh's grading of hepatic reserve

Measurements	1 point	2 points	3 points
Bilirubin mg/dl	< 2	2-3	> 3
Prothrombin time	1-3 sec	4-6 sec	> 6 sec
Prolongation INR	< 1.7	1.7 – 2.3	> 2.3
Albumin g/dl	> 3.5	2.8 – 3.4	< 2.8
Ascites	None	Mild	Severe
Encephalopathy	None	Grade 1-2	Grade 3-4

A = 5-6 points   B = 7-9 points   C= 10-15 points.

CASE 8 — Carcinoma Gallbladder

My patient, Kela Devi, a 60-year-old female, resident of Meerut, UP, admitted to this hospital with complaints of:

- Pain right upper abdomen for last 5 months
- Itching all over the body for last 1 month
- Yellowish discoloration of urine and eyes for last 20 days.

History of present illness: My patient was apparently asymptomatic 5 months back since when she started having pain in her right upper abdomen.

Initially it was off and on.

Presently it is dull aching, continuous pain, not radiating to any site. No relieving or aggravating factors noticed as such.

For last 1 month she has been having itching sensation all over the body which is gradually progressing.

With some medication, after getting admitted in this hospital, the itching is slightly reduced for last ten days.

History of yellowish discoloration of eyes and urine for last 20 days which is gradually progressive but there is no history of clay color stool till date.

But history of unquantified weight loss, anorexia present.

But there is no history of:

- Fever, chills and rigor, vomiting, hematemesis or malena. No history of chest pain.

Hemoptysis, jaundice or bone pain, etc. (features suggestive of distant metastasis).

Past history: Not a known case of HTN, DM, TB or a gallstone disease. No history of previous operation.

Personal history: Postmenopausal women. She has got a history of smoking and tobacco chewing since childhood.

Family history: Not contributory.

On examination: (General survey).

Patient is looking ill but cooperative.

Average built, and nourished.

P-68/min, BP 116/70 mm Hg

Pallor+, icterus++, no edema or generalized lymph adenopathy noticed.

Scratch marks all over the body. No features of chronic hepatic insufficiency, (like confusion, spider telangiectasia palmar erythema, tremor, etc.).

Systemic Examination

Abdomen

Inspection:

- Scaphoid in shape but there is an obvious bulge in right upper quadrant, noticed
- Umbilicus central
- All quadrants move with respiration
- No visible veins, visible peristalsis or pulsation
- No scar marks
- Flanks not full
- Hernial sites and external genitalia appear normal.

Palpation: Temperature not raised, nontender.

There is a lump measured 10 × 6 cm, at right hypochondrium extending towards right lumbar region. Firm/hard in consistency.

- Irregular surface
- Pyriform in shape
- Well defined lower, medial and lateral margins
- Upper margin could not be palpable
- Moves with respiration
- Side-to-side mobility is there.

Fingers cannot be insinuated between right costal margin and the lump.

Liver is palpable 2 cm on midclavicular line. Smooth, nontender, hepatic dullness on 5th intercostal space. No other organomegaly.

No supraclavicular lymphadenopathy.

Digital per rectal examination and pervaginal examination show no 'Blumer shelf'.

- Respiratory system:
    - Bilateral air entry equal, no adventitious sound heard. Others

– Systemic examination including CNS, CVS.

– Musculoskeletal systems are essentially normal.

Summary of the Cases

My patient, a 60-year-old female, presented with right hypochondrial pain for last 5 months, itching all over the body for last 1 month and yellowish discoloration of urine and eyes for last 20 days.

There is a history of unquantified weight loss and loss of appetite.

On general examination there is pallor, icterus and scratch maks present all over the body on systemic examination there is a 10 × 6 cm pyriform shaped intra-abdominal lump which firm/hard in consistency, upper margin marged with liver, moves with respiration and side-to-side mobility is there. Liver is enlarged 2 cm on right midclavicular line.

So this is a case of most probably carcinoma gallbladder.

DIFFERENTIAL DIAGNOSIS

GB mass probably malignant:
CBD malignancy, i.e. cholangiocarcinoma.
Hepatocellular carcinoma.
Portal lymphadenopathy.

How will you proceed in this case?

I will confirm my diagnosis first.

I will do ultrasound abdomen to assess the lesion in gallbladder.

I will see
- Extension of GB mass
- Involvement of liver
- Lymph nodes involvement
- The status of CBD, pancreas, etc.
  [USG guided FNAC to get the tissue diagnosis for palliative chemotherapy in a case of inoperable tumor].

Next I will do the CECT abdomen
- To confirm the USG findings
- To see the extent of the mass
- To stage the disease
- To assess the extent of lymphadenopathy.
- Ascites if any, etc.

The characteristics of GB mass in CT scan are:
- Mass replacing GB or protruding into the GB or filling the gallbladder. The mass may be infiltrating type,

exophytic type or there may be only irregular abnormal thickening of GB wall.
- Gallbladder mass may extend into the liver.
- Loss of fat plane in GB fossa.
- Irregular mucosal thickening of GB. Usually mucosal thickening > 4 mm is more suggestive of malignancy.

Next I will do liver function test to exclude hepatic involvement.

Tumor markers CEA, CA 19-9 which can be elevated in carcinoma gallbladder. (These are not specific markers for carcinoma GB as these markers are elevated in other GI malignancies also.

How will you to differentiate between carcinoma, GB and chronic cholecystitis in CECT?

In CECT carcinoma, GB will show enhancement of tumor mass and/or irregular thickening of GB wall whereas in chronic cholecystitis there will be nonenhancing regular thickening of fibrotic GB wall.

What will you do next?

If the patient is operable I will do all baseline investigations to make the patient fit for anesthesia. Then I will offer definite surgery.

What is the role of MRCP in this case?

In this case there is a role of MRCP, as the patient has got jaundice we can consider MRCP. It has got good delineation for biliary tree. It shows the site and nature of obstruction.

The indications of MRCP are:
i. When stenting is not contemplated
ii. When bilirubin level is ≤ 15 mg%
iii. As a noninvasive procedure to a contrast sensitive patient and debilitated patients who are not suitable for CECT or any invasive surgical procedure.

What are the indications of ERCP in this case?

ERCP is only indicated when bilirubin is >15 mg% and preoperative stenting is contemplated. Otherwise in a case of carcinoma GB without jaundice ERCP is not indicated. Some surgeons prefer pre of stenting of CBD if serum bilirubin is >15 mg%.

How will you treat the patient?

I will assess the operability of this patient from clinical and radiological examination.

If the patient is operable I will make him fit for anesthesia and do radical cholecystectomy.

What do you mean by radical cholecystectomy?

1. Resection of 2 cm wedge of liver at GB bed along with whole GB mass.
2. Station I and Station II lymph nodes dissections.

What do you mean by station I and station II lymph nodes in a case of carcinoma GB?

Station I lymph nodes are:
- Cystic, pericholedochal, periportal lymph nodes. Station II lymph nodes are:
- Celiac, retroduodenal and peripancreatic nodes, etc.

What does extended radical cholecystectomy mean?

In extended radical cholecystectomy along with 2 cm wedge resection of liver and clearance of stations I and II, LNS, CBD is excised along with resection of invaded duodenum or colon. Only CBD excision does not come in extended radical cholecystectomy as because many surgeons like to excise CBD for better clearance of lymph nodes in the procedure of extended cholecystectomy.

How will you assess the patient of carcinoma GB as an inoperable case?

I will consider two things to group the patient as inoperable.
No. 1 Patient factors
- *Age:* elderly patient cannot tolerate extensive surgical procedure
- Poor general condition
- Uncontrolled comorbid conditions
- Presence of infection, etc.

No. 2 Tumor factors
- Distant metastases like involvement of peritoneum or extra-abdominal distant metastases like supraclavicular lymph nodes involvement
- Invasion to main portal vein
- Invasion to hepatic artery both lobes of liver
- Invasion to surrounding structures, etc.
  Note: Metastasis confine to one lobe of liver or invasion to duodenum or pancreas or colon without liver mets may be considered for extended resection.

What are the palliative procedures for unresectable tumor?

i. Simple cholecystectomy—if possible may prevent development of acute cholecystitis.
ii. Choledochojejunostomy with Roux en Y limb of jejunum as a by pass procedure to relieve jaundice.
iii. Gastrojejunostomy is the procedure to relieve gastric outlet obstruction.
iv. To relieve pain, celiac ganglion is blocked with alcohol injection.
v. ERCP and stenting of CBD and PTBD where ERCP not possible. Both the procedures are done to palliate jaundice and pruritus in inoperable cases.

What is the role of chemotherapy in carcinoma GB?

The role of chemotherapy is not significant in a case of carcinoma GB.

Any how, Cisplatin, 5 Fu are used as palliative procedure. Nowadays Gemcitabine is commonly used.

Is there any role of radiotherapy in carcinoma-gallbladder?

Radiotherapy has got very little role in carcinoma-gall bladder. Some radiotherapists like to use radiotherapy as adjuvant therapy. But different studies show no survival benefit as such. To tell the truth, in this case it is like something is better than nothing.

What is TNM staging in a case of carcinoma gallbladder?

Tis—Carcinoma *in situ*
T_1a—Tumor invades mucosa
T_1b—Tumor invades muscularis
T_2—Tumor invades serosa
T_3—Tumor invades 2 cm of liver or only one adjacent organ.
T_4 tumor invades 2 cm of liver or two or more adjacent organs involvement.

Nodal Status

N_0 – No evidence of nodal involvement.
N_1 Metastasis to regional lymph nodes (Nowadays station I and station II are considered a single station).
Metastasis:
M_0 No distant metastasis
M_1 Distant metastasis.

Why carcinoma gallbladder spreads so rapidly?

As GB has got
i. No submucosal layer
ii. Muscle layer is very thin
iii. Veins from GB directly drain into hepatic veins.

What are the risk factors of developing carcinoma gallbladder?

- Porcelain gallbladder
- Gallbladder polyp >1 cm/multiple GB polyps

- Long standing gallstone (commonly larger stone > 2 cm)
- Adenomyomatosis of gallbladder
- Choledochal cyst
- Anomalous pancreaticobiliary duct junction (APBDJ) 17%
- Chronic typhoid carriers
- Carcinogen like nitrosamines exposure, etc.
- Family history of carcinoma gallbladder.

[Remember, 93% of carcinoma gallbladder patients show gallstone in gallbladder but only 3% gallstone causes carcinoma gallbladder].

A patient undergoes cholecystectomy due to gallstone disease. HPE report shows the tumor invades muscularis. What will be the next step of management?

Tumors invade muscularis means it is T_{1b}.

Initially it was thought that simple cholecystectomy was enough for T_{1b} lesion. But nowadays, radical cholecystectomy in the treatment of choice in T_{1b} lesion of gallbladder.

So, if cholecystectomy specimen shows T_{1b} lesion completion radical re-section so my has loobe done.

If tumor is confined in mucosa only simple cholecystectomy is enough for the patient.

What is Nevin's staging of carcinoma gallbladder?

Stage	Depth of tumor
I	Mucosa
II	Muscularis
III	Serosa
IV	Liver invasion
V	Adjacent organs or distant metastasis

SHORT NOTE ON CARCINOMA GALLBLADDER

Gallbladder carcinoma is a relatively rare cancer often diagnosed in an advanced stage due to nonspecific symptomatology. Though associated with a dismal prognosis until recently, recent advances in imaging and surgical techniques along with emerging options in palliative chemotherapy have improved the outlook in these cancers. While complete surgical resection remains the only hope of cure in these cancers. Palliative biliary decompression and chemotherapy can result in substantial improvement in quality of life.

Incidence varies throughout the world, with maximum incidence and highest mortality occurring in northern India and north-eastern Europe. The ratio of affected women to men is variable according to region, ranging between 1.5:1 and 6:1. Risk increases with age, with the maximum incidence occurring in the 7th decade.

PATHOLOGY

Most gallbladder cancers (99%) are adenocarcinomas. Infrequently, tumors of the gallbladder can be of mesenchymal origin – leiomyosarcoma, rhabdomyosarcoma, or, more rarely, carcinosarcoma, small cell carcinoma, carcinoid tumor, lymphoma, or melanoma. Because of the proximity of the gallbladder to segments IVb and V of the liver, direct invasion by tumor occurs often. Cancer typically spreads around the bile duct, to the cystic and pericholedochal nodes. Direct invasion of the adjacent structures such as duodenum, colon, anterior abdominal wall and common hepatic ducts is extremely common. Distant metastases to the lung and brain have been observed.

DIAGNOSTIC EVALUATION

Imaging studies guide preoperative diagnosis, determine stage, and helps to assess resectability. Multiple discontinuous liver metastasis, ascites, peritoneal metastasis, distant metastasis, extensive involvement of the hepatoduodenal ligament, encasement or occlusion of major vessels, biliary involvement not amenable to reconstruction, and poor performance status are indications of unresectable disease. Direct involvement of duodenum, liver or colon is not a contraindication to surgery.

Laparoscopic staging should be considered prior to laparotomy in potentially resectable disease because of high rate of occult metastatic disease. If the patient has radiologically unresectable disease, pathological diagnosis can be obtained by needle biopsy to proceed with palliative therapy.

Ultrasonography is the most common radiologic study used to asess gallbladder diseases. Findings suggestive of allbladder cancer are discontinuous gallbladder mucosa, mural thickening, mural calcifications, a mass protruding into the lumen, a fixed mass in the gallbladder, and its fossa, loss of interface between the gallbladder and its fossa, polyps larger than 1 cm, sessile polyps and those with eroded mucosa are suspicious for carcinoma and should be resected. Ultrasound-guided fine needle aspiration is safe and effective in providing a definitive diagnosis of gallbladder and biliary tract carcinomas.

COMPUTED TOMOGRAPHY (CT) SCAN

Computed tomography (CT) scans are more useful in determining resectability by better assessing the extent of disease. Helical CT scans can predict resectability with 93.3% accuracy. CT scanning however is a poor modality for detection of omental spread.

OTHER DIAGNOSTIC TOOLS

Endoscopic retrograde cholangiopancreatography (ERCP) and percutaneous transhepatic cholangiography (PTC) are often used as therapeutic measures to relieve biliary obstruction by placement of a stent. Bile sampling through ERCP can establish the diagnosis of carcinoma gallbladder up to 40% cases. Noninvasive procedures such as magnetic resonance imaging (MRI) and magnetic resonance cholangiopancreatography (MRCP) have generally replaced these procedures, as they better define resectability. MRI with MRCP is effective in preoperative evaluation of gallbladder carcinoma. The sensitivity of MRI and MRCP in studies has ranged from 67 to 100% for direct liver invasion and 56 to 92% for lymph node metastasis. Elevated carcinoembryonic antigen (CEA) and CA19-9 in the presence of biliary obstruction and nonspecific symptoms raises the suspicion of gallbladder cancer, but the sensitivity of CEA is only 50% and that of CA 19-9 is approximately 80%.

SURGICAL MANAGEMENT

The only potentially curative therapy for gallbladder cancer is complete surgical resection. Historical data on the results of curative surgical resections have been disappointing until the last decade. In the past decade however, better understanding of the patterns of tumor spread and progress in preoperative radiologic evaluation have led to better patient selection and an appreciation of the need for aggressive surgical resection for cure. Complete resection must include removal of the cancerous gallbladder any adjacent organ invaded by tumor, and any potentially involved lymph nodes.

GUIDELINES BY TUMOR STAGE

T_1 tumors are typically diagnosed incidentally after simple cholecystectomy for presumed gallstones. If a T_1 tumor is discovered intraoperatively, the cystic lymph node should be excised and the portal lymph nodes carefully evaluated, although they are unlikely to be involved. If a T_1 tumor is identified pathologically after conclusion of the operation, no further surgery is warranted.

Simple cholecystectomy is inadequate surgery for T_{1b} and T_2 lesions. The standard subserosal plane for surgical excision during routine cholecystectomy often violates a T_2 tumor. Furthermore, lymph node metastases are found accompanying 33% of T_2 tumors. Appropriate surgical care for a T_2 tumor is radical cholecystectomy, which involves removal of the gallbladder with at least 2 cm of the surrounding liver (segments IVB and V), and en bloc lymphadenectomy of the hepatoduodenal ligament lymph nodes, with or without bile duct excision. Radical re-resection for a pathologic T_2 lesion discovered after a simple cholecystectomy significantly improves survival. In some studies, the survival benefit is limited to tumors associated with cancer cells within 5 mm of the excised margin at the initial cholecystectomy. Radical resection for T_3 and T_4 gallbladder disease- especially in the absence of nodal metastasis-has gathered support in recent years, with data confirming 5 years survival rates of 15 to 67% and 7 to 33% for T_3 and T_4 tumors, respectively.

Lymph Node Involvement

For patients with N1 disease, regional lymphadenectomy may cure metastasis to cystic, portal, and portocaval lymph nodes. Five-year survival rates ranging from 45 to 60% have been reported for patients with regional NI disease after radical resection. Radical lymphadenectomy for N2 disease, which involves removal of retropancreatic, periduodenal, periportal, superior mesenteric, aortocaval, or celiac lymph nodes, has been advocated by few investigators. Surgery includes a hepatopancreaticoduodenectomy in addition to radical cholecystectomy. However, this approach has been associated with high morbidity and mortality rates. Therefore, radical resection should be reserved for patients with stages I to III disease, i.e. tumor invasion up to T_3, with nodal involvement confined to the hepatoduodenal ligament, posterosuperior pancreaticoduodenal region, and along the common hepatic artery.

The present NCCN guidelines distinguish between patients: (1) in whom cancer is found incidental surgery or on pathologic review and (2) those who exhibit a mass on ultrasound or present with jaundice. Within these groups the algorithm differentiates between those with resectable disease and those with unresectable disease. Patients who present with an incidental finding of cancer at surgery may be treated with cholecystectomy and resection of gallbladder fossa and lymphadenectomy with or without partial hepatic resection and with or without bile duct excision. A similar approach is appropriate for patients who present with a mass on ultrasound or with jaundice, for whom surgery is considered after more extensive evaluation, including staging laparoscopy, CT or MRI, liver function tests, chest radiograph and surgical consultation.

Among patients in whom gallbladder cancer is diagnosed as an incidental finding on pathologic review, those with T_1 lesions may be observed. Patients with T2 or greater lesions should be considered for surgery, after CT/MRI confirms the absence of metastatic disease. In addition, for those who undergo laparoscopic operations, resection of port sites with or without bile duct excision should be considered because of the risk of local recurrence at these sites.

Adjuvant therapy for resectable patients, except those with T_1, NO disease, should include adjuvant 5-fluorouracil (5-FU)-based chemotherapy and radiation.

Palliative Treatment of Advanced Disease

Patients with unresectable tumor but without jaundice and who do not have obvious metastatic disease may benefit from a regimen of 5-FU-based and gemcitabine chemotherapy and radiation similar to the regimen used adjuvantly. However, overall survival *of* such patients remains poor. Because there is no definitive treatment with proven survival benefit, be supportive care or enrollment in a clinical trial are considered appropriate options for patients with unresectable disease. *For jaundiced patients whose disease is considered unresectable after preoperative evaluation, a biopsy should, be performed to confirm the diagnosis. In such patients biliary decompression would be an appropriate palliative procedure. Best supportive care or consideration of gemcitabine and/or 5-FU- based chemotherapy or best supportive care is also appropriate.*

Follow-up

Follow-up consists of imaging studies every 6 months for 2 years. If the patient's disease progresses. The initial workup guidelines should be followed again.

CASE 9

Renal Lump

RENAL CELL CARCINOMA

My patient, Ramanand a 60-year-old male resident of Punjab/Rajasthan (Renal/vesical calculus more common) presented to this hospital with complain of:

Pain at the left flank off and on for last 6 months.
Passage of blood in urine twice within last 4 months.
Lump left side of mid abdomen for last 2 months.

History of Present Illness

My patient was apparently asymptomatic 6 months back since when he has been having pain off and on in his left side of mid abdomen.

Pain is insidious in onset.
Dull aching.
Continuing for few minutes to hours.
Nonradiating (usually subcostal to towards umbilicus).
No relieving or aggravating factor as such.

He has got a history of passage of blood in urine twice within 2 months.

1st episode—2 months back—sudden onset with obstruction in the passage of urine.

2nd episode—9 days back, sudden onset with difficulty in passing urine on catheterization clot was coming out painlessly—irrigation done. He was relieved after that and no further episode is these till date.

He also noticed a lump in his left side of mid abdomen which is gradually progressive in nature, painless, approximately 6 × 4 cm. He has also got a history of anorexia and weight loss for last 2 to 3 months.

There is no history of any other urinary disturbance like retention of urine or sudden increase of urine volume (malignant obstruction/hydronephrosis).

No history of fever, fatigue, giddiness, headache (paraneoplastic syndrome).

Or vomiting, alteration of bowel habit (exclusion of growth in descending colon).

No history of chest pain, hemoptysis (75%), bone pain (20%), jaundice (18%), etc. (exclusion of distant metastasis).

Past History

No history of hypertension, diabetes, tuberculosis.
No history of any past allergic reaction.
No history of any significant operation in the past.
(*NB*—Renal transplant causes up to 80% risk of developing RCC).

Personal History

Farmer by occupation. (Exposure to heavy metals, petroleum products increases the risk of development of carcinoma).

Smoker, 10-15 bidi per day for last 15 years.

Cigarette 5-10 per day for last 5 years (smoking increases two folds risk).

Family History

Not contributory.

On General Examination

The patient is cooperative, anxious looking average built and nourished. BP-160/88 mm Hg in right arm supine.

Pulse- 80/min, regular, normal in volume.

Condition of the arterial wall is normal. No radioradial or radiofemoral delay. All peripheral pulses are palpable. Pallor +. No icterus, no edema or generalized lymphadenopathy.

Systemic Examinations

Abdomen
On inspection
- Scaphoid/protruded with obvious bulge on left side of mid abdomen

- Umbilicus center
- All quadrants move with respiration
- No visible veins, scar marks
  Flanks are not full
- Renal angle appears normal—not full
- Hernial sites and external genitalia appear normal—varicocele noticed in the left.

On palpation
- Some of the inspectory findings are confirmed
- Local temperature not raised, nontender
- Abdomen soft
- There is a 6 × 4 cm retroperitoneal lump at left lumbar region extending towards left hypochondrium- reniform shaped, firm in consistency, moves slightly with respiration, well defined lateral, medial and lower margins- rounded – irregular- variegated – ballotable and bimanually palpable. It does not cross midline; fingers can be insinuated between left costal margin and the lump. (Most of the time upper margin is not easily palpable)
- Left renal angle nontender. No fullness palpable
- No other swelling palpable in the abdomen
- No hepatosplenomegaly
- No free fluid in abdomen
- No supraclavicular lymphadenopathy
- Hernial sites appear normal
- No varicocele noticed.

Percussion
- Dull /tympanic over the lump [usually resonant as colon is lying over but in case of large lump colon is displaced and dull node can be heard].
- Renal angle dull on percussion.

Auscultation
  No renal bruit.
  Normal peristaltic sound heard.
Per rectal examination
  No 'Blumers self' found.
  Grade II prostate palpable.

Other systemic examinations
Respiratory system: Bilateral air entry equal, no adventitious sound heard.
  CVS: S1 S2 normal, no murmur.
  Other systemic examinations are within normal limits.

Summary of the Case

My patient, a 60-year-old male chronic smoker, presented with complaint of pain in left flank intermittently over last 6 months, two episodes of hematuria and a lump in left lumbar region of the abdomen for last two months. He has got the history of unquantified weight loss and anorexia without any history suggestive of metastasis.

On examination: Patient is slightly anemic.

There is a 6 × 4 cm, well defined, smooth, ballotable, retroperitoneal lump at left lumbar region which is bimanually palpable and moves with respiration and does not cross the midline.

Fingers can be insinuated between the costal margin and the lump.

So this is a case of left renal lump most probably malignant.

Differential Diagnosis

- Carcinoma descending colon. (In case of right sided lump carcinoma ascending colon).
- Retroperitoneal lymphadenopathy/mesenteric lymphadenopathy.
- Soft tissue sarcoma.
- Splenic mass (In case of left renal mass only).

How to proceed in this case?

First to confirm the diagnosis, USG of abdomen is the investigation of choice. It can detect:
- Anatomy and organ of origin.
- Type of the mass – solid /cystic.
- Lymph node involvement.
- Any fluid in abdomen.
- Liver metastasis.
- Extrarenal extension of tumor.
- Involvement of adrenal gland, etc.
- <2 mm parenchymal thickness suggestive of dysfunction of kidney.

Contrast Enhanced CT Scan of Abdomen:
- Procedure for confirming USG finding
- Can detect the extent of the lesion, infiltration of the adjacent viscera
- To detect retroperitoneal lymph nodes involvement and liver metastasis
- To stage the disease
- To see the functional status of opposite kidney which is very important to plan the surgery
- Any thrombus in renal vein or IVC.

Color Doppler Flow Imaging (CDFI)

To detect thrombus inside the vessel or involvement of the vessel wall.

MRI

Indications

- Involvement of the bilateral kidney
- Solitary kidney involvement
- Where nephrons sparing surgery in the kidney is essential (82-96% sensitivity, suitable for renal failure and pregnant mother).

Other Metastatic Workup

- Liver function test
- Coagulation profile.
- Chest X-ray PA view (to exclude any lung metastasis)
- Bone scan:
  - In case of any bone pain
  - Increase level of alkaline phosphatase.

  All other basic investigations to be done for anesthetic fitness.

What is the role of IVU in RCC?

When CECT scan is not available IVU is done to see the kidney function. Nowadays a CECT is available almost every where so IVU is not routinely used.

What is the role of bone scan in RCC?

Bone scan is not done routinely. It is indicated when there is a bone pain or increased blood alkaline phosphatase.

Why this is a renal lump?

- Anatomical position
- Reniform shaped
- Ballotable
- Bimanually palpable
- Lump does not cross the midline
- Fingers can be insinuated between the lump and the costal margin
- Moves with respiration (though retroperitoneal)
- There is a band of colonic resonance anteriorly and dull on percussion posteriorly.

Why you think it is a malignant tumor?

- Elderly patient
- Painless lump at the loin
- Painless intermittent hematuria
- Weight loss, anorexia
- Lump is firm in consistency with irregular surface
- Renal angle is dull

- Moderate degree of varicocele on left side.
  All these features suggestive of malignancy.

Do you consider a FNAC in this case for diagnosis?

FNAC can breach the capsule of kidney which may cause shedling of tumor cell along the niddle track. So there will be change of staging of the tumor. So FNAC should not be done in a case of RCC.

How to diagnose the case?

Usually renal malignancy is diagnosed on clinical ground and radiological basis. CECT abdomen is playing a very important role to diagnose malignancy in kidney.

What is the role of renal angiography in renal tumor?

A good CECT play an important role in necessary aspects. So renal angiography is not done routinely. It is indicated.

- In bilateral renal carcinoma, solitary kidney affected by tumors where nephron sparing surgery is very essential
- It shows involvement and extend of tumor in the vessels, i.e. renal vein, IVC, etc.
- It also shows the neovascularization of the tumor.

What is the classical triad in RCC?

Classical triads are:
- Flank pain
- Hematuria
- Flank mass.
  This is found only in 10% cases.
Pain is due to:
- Rapid growth pressing the surrounding structures and infiltration into the surrounding tissues
- Hemorrhage in the tumor
- Involvement of retroperitoneal nerve plexus.
  Hematuria occurs when the tumor extents up to renal pelvis and invade the vessels.
  Palpable mass in the flank or abdomen is seen in 25% of cases only.
  This triad of symptoms indicate advance disease.

What is Stauffer syndrome?

Stauffer describes a reversible syndrome of hepatic dysfunction in the absence of hepatic metastasis associated with the RCC (3-20%). Stauffer syndrome tends to occur in association with fever, fatigue and weight loss and it is typically resolved after nephrectomy. This symptom is due to overproduction of granulocyte macrophage colony stimulating (GM-CSF) factors by the tumor.

STRUCTURES OF KIDNEY

What are the common sites of origin of kidney tumors?

Clear cells of proximal renal tubule is the most common site of origin. Clear cells are nothing but the epithelial cells. Tumor arising from the collecting duct is most aggressive among the other tumors of kidney.

What is standard surgery for carcinoma kidney?

Radical nephrectomy is the surgery of choice. It includes en bloc resection of kidney along with the tumor with or without same sided adrenal gland, surrounding Gerota's fascia. Proximal ½ of the ureter and lymph nodes form the Crus of diaphragm to aortic bifurcation.

What are the indications of radical nephrectomy with ureterectomy?

- Transitional cell carcinoma of kidney (involving pelvis, calyces or ureter)
- Grade V vasicoureteric reflux with nonfunctioning kidney (benign condition).

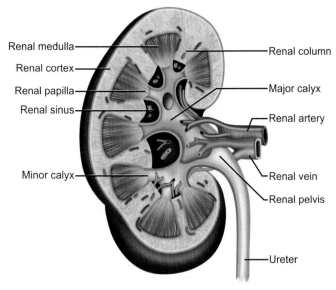

What are the approaches for kidney tumor?

1. Flank/loin/lumbar incision is the most common approach.
   Transcostal, extrapleural, extraperitoneal.
   Indications:
   i. Nephrectomy
   ii. Pyelolithotomy
   iii. Open drainage of perinephric abscess.

Advantage: Direct access to kidney.

Disadvantages: Space limited above by 12 rib, below iliac a crest. So it is not suitable for very large tumor.

2. *Subcostal approach:* Through the bed of 12 rib. Indicated in upper pole kidney tumor.
3. *Midline:* Transperitoneal approach
   Indications—Renal trauma
   Bilateral kidney tumor.
   Renal cell carcinoma (RCC)
   When costal angle is narrow.
4. Roof top/ Extended subcostal incision:
   Indications—bilateral kidney tumor.
   Wide costal angle.
5. Thoracoabdominal incision through XIth intercostals space.
   Indication: 1. Big tumor
                    2. Upper pole tumor.
6. *Lumbotomy:* It is done in prone position by giving posterior vertical incision (Gilvernet approach) it is non-muscle cutting approach.
7. *Others:* Laparoscopic or retroperitoneoscopic approach.

What will be the approach when tumor is extended into renal vein/ IVC/right atrium?

a. **Involvement of renal vein:** Ligation of the renal vein is to be done proximal to the site of tumor extension.
b. **IVC involvement:** In this case IVC is to be dissected with proximal control of IVC is essential. Long venotomy may be done to remove tumor thrombus.
c. **Involvement of right atrium:** It invites CTVS surgeons help. Tumor extension form the IVC and right atrium is to be removed under cardiopulmonary bypass.

What is therapeutic embolization?

Indications:
1. For a large tumor it is done aiming to regress the size of the tumor and to reduce the vascularity which is very much helpful during surgery.
2. For palliative procedure in case of a locally advanced inoperable case. Surgery to be done within 72 hours of therapeutic embolization.

What is the indication of nephron sparing surgery in RCC?

The indications of nephron sparing surgery are:
1. Bilateral renal tumor.
2. Renal tumor in a solitary kidney.

What are the differential diagnosis of renal lump?

1. *Splenic mass:* Typical characteristic of splenic lump (already discussed in general guideline of abdominal lump).
2. *Colonic lump:* Mobility more in side-to-side, restricted vertically, more GI symptoms.
3. *Retroperitoneal lymphadenopathy:* Nonmobile.
4. *Mesenteric lymphadenopathy:* Side-to-side mobile, restricted along the axis of the mesentery.

What is the treatment of metastatic RCC?

1. *Palliative nephrectomy:* It is done to alleviate symptoms like pain, hemorrhage, hypertension, hypercalcemia, erythrocytosis, etc.
2. *Immunotherapy:* Interferon therapy, IL2 therapy.

What is the role of radiotherapy and chemotherapy in RCC?

Renal cell carcinoma (RCC) is refractory to most of the chemotherapeutic agents. Only 5FU has a response rate of 10%, along with interferon response rate is increased up to 19%. Radiotherapy is primary therapy for palliation like painful osseous lesions or brain metastasis.

What is angioinfarction?

In case of very large and highly large vascular tumor a selective renal arteriogram is done through transfemoral route and artery is blocked by gel, foam, autologous blood clot, metal coils, muscle, etc. As a result of infarction of kidney mass occurs. It has got other advantages like reduced vascularity, reduced size of the tumor mass which are beneficial during the surgery. Angioinfarction is also done as a palliative measure in case of locally advanced inoperable cases.

SHORT NOTES ON RENAL CELL CARCINOMA

INTRODUCTION

Renal cell carcinoma (RCC) is the most common neoplasm arising from kidney and constitutes approximately 85-90% of all primary malignant renal tumor. It has got special characteristics like:

- Lack of early warning sign.
- Various clinical manifestations.
- Resistant to chemo as well as radiotherapy.

Multiple terms has been used to describe renal adenocarcinoma like hypernephroma, Grawitz tumor, clear cell carcinoma, alveolar carcinoma, etc.

Epidemiology

Renal cell carcinoma (RCC) accounts approximately 3% of all adult malignancies.

Male-female ratio is 2:1.

Age of incidence is usually between 4 and 6th decade.

Etiology

The real cause of RCC is unknown. A number of cellular, genetic, hormonal and environmental factors have some factors play possible role to develop RCC.

- Cigarette smoking increases two fold risks in smokers.
- Exposures to asbestos, solvents, and cadmium are also associated with increased incidence.
- Renal transplantation itself and with its associated immunosuppressive drugs increases 80 folds risk.
- *Hereditary:* Two hereditary forms of RCC describe having incidence up to 70%.
  a. *Von Hippel-Lindau disease:* 35-40% patient develop RCC, mostly bilateral and aggressive.
     NB: Von Hipple-Lindau disease is an autosomal dominant disease associated with inactivating mutation of VHL tumor suppression gene of chromosome no 3.
     Components of VHL syndromes are:
     - RCC up to 70%
     - Pheochromocytoma 10-20%
     - CNS and retinal hemangioblastoma
     - Pancreatic islet cell tumor
     - Endolymphatic tumors
     - Cystic lesions- like renal pancreatic and epididymal cysts.

  b. *Hereditary papillary renal cell carcinoma:* It is characterized by a predisposition to develop bilateral multiple renal tumor with a papillary histologic appearance. In compare to VHL patients, the major neoplastic manifestations, appear to be confined to the kidney.

Other factors are:
1. Obesity, urban living
2. Hypertension
3. Unopposed estrogen therapy
4. Abuse of phenacetin containing analgesic
5. Renal dialysis
6. Cystic kidney disease associated with chronic renal insufficiency.

Pathology

Renal cell carcinoma (RCC) originates from the proximal renal tubular epithelium. These tumors occur with equal frequency in either kidney. RCC originate in the cortex and tend to grow out in the perinephric tissue which causes bulge of the tumor and mass effect.

1. **Adenocarcinoma:** It is most common of all renal cancers in adults. They are typically round and have a pseudocapsule of condensed parenchyma and connective tissue.

   Bilateral tumor occurs in 2% of sporadic cases. The histological subtype include:

   a. *Clear cell most common (75%):* Arises from the proximal tubule—growth pattern is acinar or sarcomatoid.

   b. *Chromophilic (15%):* Bilateral and multimodal- site is proximal tubule—growth pattern is papillary and sarcomatoid.

   c. *Chromophobic (5%):* Course is indolent-arises from cortical collecting duct—growth pattern is solid, tubular or sarcomatoid.

   d. *Collecting duct:* Very aggressive—arises form medullary collecting duct—growth pattern is papillary or sarcomatoid.

   This tumor invades local structures and frequently extents into renal vein. Metastasis occurs through lymphatic and bloodstream. Most common sites are lung (75%), soft tissues (35%), and bones (20%), including small bones like fingertips (2%), liver (18%), and brain (8%).

2. **Transitional cell carcinoma:** Arises from renal pelvis uncommon tumor-affects multiple sites of urothelial mucosa- low grade tumor—usually detected late.

   They spread sheet like in the retroperitoneum, encasing vessels and producing urinary tract obstruction.

3. **Others:** Renal tumors, although rare, include lymphoma, sarcoma, juxtaglomerular tumor, hemangiopericytoma. Benign tumors like angiomyolipoma, adenoma, etc. and metastatic tumors like lung, overy, colon, breast, etc. are also there.

   [Natural history of adenocarcinoma- more unpredictable tumor with a variable growth pattern and may remain localized for many years. Metastatic foci may remain indolent and undetected for many years after removal of primary].

DIAGNOSIS

1. Clinical
2. Radiological
3. Laboratory investigations.

Clinical

Renal cell carcinoma (RCC) patients remain asymptomatic for most of its course. The classical triad of symptoms are:

a. Flank pain.
b. Flank hematuria.
c. Flank mass.

Usually this triad is uncommon and occurs only in 10% cases in advance case of the disease. Anyway most common presentation is:

a. *Hematuria (40%):* Painless vermifrom (uniform clot), throughout the stream of urine.
b. *Flank pain (40%):* Palpable mass at flank or in the abdomen found in 25% of cases.

Constitutional symptoms are weight loss (30%), fever (20%), night sweat, malaise, etc.

Signs are:

Hypertension (25%)

Hypercalcemia (5%)

Varicocele –usually left sided and this is due to obstruction of testicular vein found in 2% cases of male patients.

Paraneoplastic syndrome- occurs in 10-40% cases in RCC and it includes:

Symptoms	Signs
Cachexia	Anemia
Weight loss	Hypertension
Headache	Polyneuromyopathy
	Dermatomyositis

Stauffer syndrome –nonmetastatic hepatic dysfunction

Amyloidosis

Raised ESR

Erythrocytosis

Hypercalcemia

A paraneoplastic syndrome present at the time of diagnosis does not confer poor prognosis but the patient whose paraneoplastic metabolic disturbances fails to normalize after nephrectomy suggest the presence of clinically undetectable metastatic disease and have very poor prognosis.

Other Presentations

Approximately 30% of the patients present with metastatic disease—painful enlargement of the long bone, pathological fracture, persistent cough, hemoptysis, etc.

Occasionally persistent pyrexia is the only symptom of the disease.

Radiological

A fare number of patients are diagnosed with RCC have small tumors discovered incidentally on imaging studies.

- *Plain X-ray abdomen:* Cases of focus of renal calcification- seen in 5-10% of cases. Central calcification is found approximately 85% of cases.
- *IVU:* Nowadays it is not routinely used in the initial evaluation of renal masses because of its low sensitivity and specificity. CECT abdomen is far better imaging modality than IVU. IVU even may not detect small to medium size tumor.
- USG—Providing excellent initial imaging [described previously].
- CECT abdomen—The imaging procedure of choice described previously.
- Renal angiography—Described earlier.
- MRI—Currently the preferred imaging technique providing a three-dimensional picture of the tumor with an accuracy of 82-90%.
- Vascular involvement is the best demonstrated with MRI.
- Especially valuable where, contrast is contraindicated for allergic patients.
- Patients of renal failure.
- Pregnant patients.
- Metastatic workup.
  1. Chest X-ray—essential to detect lung secondaries. Characteristic 'Cannon Ball' appearance is shown in RCC.
  2. Bone scan—as described before.

3. FNAC—for cytological diagnosis is controversial. But logically it may be used for patients with indeterminate masses where inflammatory lesion, abscess and where metastases are suspected. The relatively low diagnostic yield, suboptimal accuracy and risks of tumors seeding are the reasons for controversy.

STAGING

In common clinical practice the Robson modification of Flocks and Kadesky system is used as it is very simple and useful.

The Robson staging system is as follows:

Stage I: Tumor confined within the capsule of kidney.

Stage II: Tumor invades perinephric fat but it is within the fascia of gerota and or invades ipsilateral adrenal.

Stage III:

a. Tumor invades the renal vein or IVC.
b. Tumor invades regional lymph nodes.
c. Both a and b.
d. Tumor invades adjacent viscera (excluding ipsilateral adrenal) or distant metastasis.

TNM Classification: (AJCC, 2002)

The major advantage of the TNM system is that it is clearly differentiate individuals from tumor thrombi from those with local nodal disease.

TNM classification system is as follows:

- Primary tumor (T).
- Tx—Primary tumor cannot be assessed.
- T0—No evidence of primary tumor.
- T1—Tumor 7 cm or less in greatest dimensions limited to the kidney.
  1. T1 a—Tumor 4 cm or less in greatest dimensions.
  2. T1 b—Tumor more than 4 cm in greatest dimension but less than 7 cm in dimension.
- T2—Tumor more than 7 cm in greatest dimension but limited to kidney.
- T3—Tumor extends into major veins or directly invades adrenal glands or perinephric tissues but not beyond the fascia of gerota.
  1. T3 a—Tumor invades adrenal glands or perinephric tissues but not beyond the fascia of gerota.
  2. T3 b—Tumor grossly extends into renal vein or IVC below the diaphragm.
  3. T3 c—Tumor grossly extends into inferior vena cava above the diaphragm.
  4. Tumor directly invades the fascia of gerota.

N-Regional Lymph Nodes

- Nx—Regional lymph nodes cannot be assessed.
- N1—No regional lymph node metastasis.
- N2—Metastasis in single regional lymph nodes.
- N3—Metastasis in more than one regional lymph nodes.

Distant Metastasis

Mx—Distant mets cannot be assessed.

M0—No distant metastasis.

M1—Distant metastasis.

Stage Grouping

Stage I—T1, N0, M0.

Stage II—T2, N0, M0.

Stage III—T1-2, N1, M0 or T3 a-c, N0-1, M0.

Stage IV—T4 or any T, N2 M0 or any T, any N, M1.

Management

Surgical resection remains the mainstay of treatment in localized renal cell carcinoma and it is also done for palliation in metastatic disease.

1. *Incidental renal tumors:* usually small in size. Surgical exploration-> frozen section-> the total/partial nephrectomy is the treatment of choice.

2. *Localized RCC:* Radical nephrectomy is the standard procedure for localized RCC. This entails early ligation of renal artery – followed by renal vein.

   En bloc removal of gerota fascia and its contents including resection of kidney perirenal fat, proximal half of ureter with or without ipsilateral adrenal gland with ipsilateral regional lymph nodes dissection. 20-30% patients of clinically localized diseases develop metastatic disease after nephrectomy.

   Recent evidence suggests that the adrenal gland should not be removed because of low probability of ipsilateral adrenal metastasis and more morbidity associated with adrenalectomy.

   Indications of adrenalectomy are:

   i. Involvement of adrenal in preoperative CT scan.

   ii. Gross extension of tumor into the gland in scan intra-operatively.

   iii. Tumors > 5 cm and located in the upper pole.

3. Lymphadenectomy—removal of all nodes between Crus of diaphragm above and bifurcation of aorta below advantages:

   i. Gives pathological staging.

   ii. Removal of micrometastasis.

   iii. Relieves pain and backache.

   iv. Prevents nodal relapse. 5 years survival improving only about 10%.

   v. Prognosis of the disease.

4. In case of extension of tumor thrombus in major veins in 5% patients tumor invades in renal vein or IVC.

   If IVC is involved vascular control to be obtained both below and above the tumor thrombus.

   Tumor thrombus to be resected intact through venotomy with subsequent closure of IVC.

   If the tumor thrombus reaches at right atrium. Cardio- pulmonary bypass procedure to be adopted to remove the tumor thrombus.

5. Role of nephron sparing surgery:

   Only incase of bilateral RCC—synchronous or RCC in a solitary kidney.

   Role of nephron sparing surgery in patient with unilateral RCC is controversial where the contralateral kidney is normal.

   Nephron sparing surgery usually limited to tumor <4 cm in size local relapse –occurs in 2% cases and it - can be salvaged with radical nephrectomy but still radical nephrectomy is the procedure of choice.

   Favoring points for radical nephrectomy are:

   - Low risk (1-2%) of development of metachronous tumor in the opposite normal kidney.
   - Low risk of opposite normal kidney dysfunction.
   - Presence of multifocal tumors.
   - Nephron sparing surgery technically more demanding and carries high risk of morbidity.

6. Laparoscopic nephrectomy has got all the advantage of minimal invasing surgery like- short recovery period, less morbidity, less blood loss, etc.

   But the main disadvantages are spillage, limited experience and technical difficulties in defining surgical margins but it may be tried for removal of small volume renal cell carcinomas usually which have been termed as incidental renal tumors.

7. Treatment of metastatic RCC: At the time of diagnosis approximately 20-30% patients have metastatic disease. The question whether it is solitary mets or disseminated.

   In solitary mets (usually 5% loses) surgical resection is recommended in selected patients with metastatic RCC. The procedure may not be curative in all patients but may produce some long-term survival. The incidence of increase survival have been studied after resection of primary tumor and isolated mets excision.

Disseminated Mets

Treatment—palliative nephrectomy to relieve the symptoms like pain, hemorrhage malaise, hypercalcemia, hypertension. Various reports suggest regression of metastatic RCC.

Cytoreductive nephrectomy is performed to decrease tumor burden and thereby symptoms.

Immunotherapy

Interferon alfa—affects the tumor growth by its antiproliferative and immunomodularity properties. Interleukin 2 affects the tumor growth by activating lymph node cells.

Role of chemoradiotherapy – already discussed.

Prognosis

5-year survival rate approximately:

T1 RCC—95%

T2 RCC—85%

T3—60%

T4—20%

Patient with regional lymph node involvement or extra-capsular extension have a survival rate of 10-25%. Although renal vein involvement does not have negative effect on prognosis.

Follow-up

Stages I and II disease- every 6 months for 2 years physical exam, chest X-ray, KFT, LFT, calcium to be checked up.

For stage III RCC same tests to be done every 3 or 4 months for first 2 years and every 6 months for next 3 years.

Abdominal CT scan should be ideally performed 6 months for first 2 years, then yearly up to 5 years and thereafter as indicated.

My patient, Hamid, a 40-year-old male, farmer in occupation, resident of Rajasthan, presented to this hospital with chief complaints of:

- Pain in left loin for last 9 months.
- Swelling in the left loin for last 6 months. [Other presentations– DIETL's crisis (described below), dysurea, frequency, urgency of urination, retention of urine, features of chronic kidney disease, etc.].

History of Present Illness

My patient was apparently asymptomatic 9 months back since when he developed pain in left loin. The pain is insidious in onset, dull aching in nature, lasting for half to 1 hour, radiating sometimes towards the thigh, relived by passage of urine or with some analgesic. He noticed swelling in the left loin for last 6 months which is gradually increasing in size. There is a history of sudden attack of pain and increase size of the swelling. The pain is reduced following the passage of large volume of urine, swelling is also reduced thereafter.

There is no history of hematuria, difficulty in passing urine, burning micturition, features of renal dysfunction, etc.

Past History

No history of hypertension, diabetes, tuberculosis.
No history of any past allergic reaction.
No history of any significant operation in the past.
(NB—Renal transplant causes up to 80% risk of developing RCC).

Personal History

Farmer by occupation. (Exposure to heavy metals, petroleum products increases the risk of development of carcinoma).
Smoker, 10-15 bidi per day for last 15 years.
Cigarette 5-10 per day for last 5 years (smoking increases two folds risk).

Family History

Not contributory.

On General Examination

The patient is cooperative, anxious looking average built and nourished. BP-160/88 mm Hg in right arm supine.
Pulse- 80/min, regular, normal in volume.
Condition of the arterial wall is normal. No radioradial or radiofemoral delay. All peripheral pulses are palpable. Pallor +. No icterus, no edema or generalized lymphadenopathy.

SYSTEMIC EXAMINATION

Abdomen

Mostly similar to RCC. Specific points of hydronephrosis are described below.

There is a retroperitoneal lump in the left loin, 12 × 8 cm in size, reniform shaped, tense cystic in nature, smooth surface with well defined margin, rounded; move up and down with respiration, ballotable and bimanually palpable, fingers can be insinuated in between the swelling and the left costal margin. Rest of the examinations are as described in RCC.

Summary of the Case

A 40-year-old male presented with complaint of pain in the left loin for last 9 months and swelling at the same side for last 6 months without any history of hematuria, burning micturition.

On examination—general survey is essentially normal, systemic examination of abdomen reveals 12 × 8 cm retroperitoneal tense cystic lump with smooth surface, well defined margins, ballotable and bimanually palpable. The lump moves with respiration. There is band of resonance in front of the swelling.

PROVOSIONAL DIAGNOSIS

Most probably this is case of left sided hydronephrosis.

Differential Diagnoses

1. *A simple cyst of kidney:* Rare and usually painless. There is no history of reduction of size with passage of urine.
2. *Polycystic kidney disease:* Early age of onset, bilateral disease, (but one sided cystic lesion may be more prominent and palpable than the other) may be associated with hematuria, UTI, hypertension, uremia, chronic kidney disease, etc.
3. *Hydatid cyst of kidney:* Very rare incidence (5-7% of all hydatid disease), very slow growing – 1 cm /year, associated with urticaria.

How will you proceed in this case?

Sir, first I will confirm my diagnosis. The ultrasonography of abdomen is the investigation of choice. It can detect:
1. Cystic or cystic components of solid mass.
2. Degree of dilatation of pelvic calyceal system.
3. Condition of ureter whether it is dilated or not.
4. Any calculus in kidney or ureter.
5. Assessment of cortical tissue of kidney to predict the degree of dysfunction of the affected kidney.
6. Assessment of contralateral kidney.

What is the next step?

The next step is intravenous urogram (IVU):
- To see cause of hydronephrosis and the site of obstruction.
- To assess the kidney function both affected and contralateral kidney.
- To see the changes in the pelvic calyceal system, i.e. the grade the hydronephrosis.

What are the types of hydronephrosis?

Hydronephrosis can be grossly divided into:
1. *Obstructive:* Where definite obstruction causes hydronephrosis.
2. *Nonobstructive:* Where there is no obvious obstruction but pelvic calyceal system is dilated.

What are the causes of obstructive hydronephrosis?

Unilateral Hydronephrosis

Intraluminal:
1. Calculus in pelvis or ureter
2. Sloughed papilla in papillary necrosis.

Intramural:
2. Congenital stenosis of ureter.
3. Congenital narrowing of pelvic ureteric junction.
4. Ureterocele or congenital small ureteric orifice.
5. Neoplasm of ureter or bladder which blocks ureteric orifice.

Extramural:
1. Idiopathic retroperitoneal fibrosis (Ormond's disease).
2. Tumor arising from adherent structures like carcinoma cervix, carcinoma prostate, carcinoma cecum, colon or rectum.

Bilateral Hydronephrosis

Congenital Causes

1. Congenital strictures or pin hole meatus.
2. Phimosis.
3. Posterior urethral valve in male urethra.
4. Congenital contracture of bladder neck.

Acquired

1. Benign prostatic hyperplasia.
2. Carcinoma prostate.
3. Postoperative bladder neck contracture.
4. Post-traumatic/ inflammatory urethral stricture.
5. Secondary phimosis.

Note: Congenital PUJ obstruction is the most common cause of hydronephrosis.

What are the causes of nonobstructive hydronephrosis?

1. **Residual hydronephrosis:** Obstruction relieved but HDN persisting.
2. **In pregnancy:** As a result of high level of circulating progesterone on the ureteric smooth muscle causing dilatation of renal pelvis and ureter. It is considered normal in pregnancy. Normal size of ureter and pelvis returned back within 12 weeks after delivery.
3. **In diabetes insipidus.**
4. **Vesicoureteric reflux grades IV and V.**
5. **Extrarenal pelvis:** The dilatation first effect the pelvis alone-pelvic hydronephrosis.

How will you differentiate between obstructive and nonobstructive hydronephrosis?

5. **Diethylenetriamine pentaacetic acid (DTPA)** isotope renogram (if available) [DTPA given IV- not absorbed by the tubules of kidney- filtered by glomeruli-frusemide

increases the filtration, thereby it gives dynamic representation of kidney function.

NB—Tc^{99m} scan is particularly useful to prove that the hydronephrosis is due to obstruction.

If DTPA scan is not available Whitaker test is to be done.

Process

A percutaneous puncture, through loin of the kidney is made- normal saline is infused at a constant rate (usually 10 ml/min) with monitoring intrapelvic pressure. Normal pressure ≤ 15 mm Hg.

16-22 mm Hg is equivocal, >22 mm Hg indicates obvious obstruction.

What is the role of retrograde pyelography in the diagnosis?

Usually IVU is enough to see the site of obstruction. But if IVU shows the affected kidney is nonfunctioning and the site of obstruction is not obvious or doubtful, in such case retrograde pyelography may take care to locate the site of obstruction.

Process

Urograffin is injected through ureteric catheter which is to be put through by cystoscope prior to putting urograffin. It will show ureter, pelvis and thereby site of obstruction.

How do you grade hydronephrosis?

Grade I: Mild blunting of calyceal fornix.
Grade II: Obvious blunting of calyx, intruding papillary shadow.

Grade II: Rounding of calyx, No papillary shadow seen.
Grade IV: Ballooning of calyx.

How to manage the case?

After confirming the diagnosis baseline investigations like complete blood count, sugar, LFT, KFT, chest X-ray, PA view, ECG, routine urine examination to be done and Anesthetic clearance is to be taken. For the surgical correction.

What is the preferred surgery in PUJ obstruction?

Anderson-Hynes pyeloplasty, where a reasonable thickness of functioning parenchyma is present.

What is endoscopic pyelolysis?

Endoscopic pyelolysis usually done in case of idiopathic PUJ obstruction. But the long-term benefit of this procedure is doubtful.

Process

Under radiological control a specially designed balloon which is passed through ureter disrupt the PUJ.

What is Dietl's crisis?

In case of intermittent hydronephrosis patient experience an acute attack of renal pain and thereafter swelling appears in the loin.

Some hours later, following the passage of large volume of urine the pain subsided and the swelling disappears.

[**NB:** Dielt was professor of pathology, Karkan, Poland.]

SHORT NOTE ON HYDRONEPHROSIS

1. *Definition:* Hydronephrosis is an aseptic dilatation of pelvic calyceal system due to partial and /or intermittent obstruction to the outflow of urine. [Remember—complete obstruction leads to renal atrophy].
2. *Etiology:* Described male female ratio 2:1
3. *Pathology:* As a result of some kind of obstruction, either partial or intermittent, the calyces become progressively dilated though initial pressure can be sustained by pelvis, later calyces and renal parenchyma

↓

Gradually the renal parenchyma progressively thinned out and destroyed by the pressure atrophy

↓

Leading to compromised secretary function

↓

≤ 2 mm parenchymal thickness suggests renal dysfunction

↓

In bilateral obstruction after this, the patient will develop renal failure.

A kidney; destroyed by long standing hydronephrosis, is a thin walled loculated sac containing pale fluid.

4. Clinical features as described.
5. Complications of hydronephrosis are:
   • Pyonephrosis
   • Perinephric abscess
   • Renal failure in bilateral cases.
6. Investigations- as described earlier.
7. Treatment-
   Pyeloplasty in described below.

PYELOPLASTY FOR SYMPTOMATIC PUJ OBSTRUCTIONS

Indications for surgery are:
1. Recurrent attack of renal pain.
2. Increasing hydronephrosis
3. Evidence of parenchymal damage.
4. Infection, etc.

Types

I. Dismembered pyeloplasty.
II. Flap pyeloplasty- so called membered pyeloplasty.

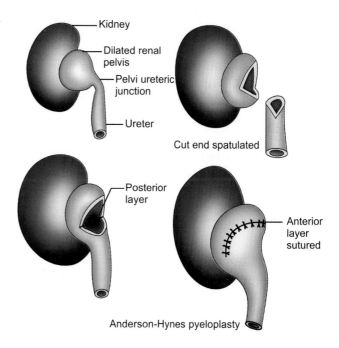

Anderson-Hynes pyeloplasty

Dismembered Pyeloplasty

Like Anderson-Hynes-currently most urologists rely on a variation of a dismembered pyeloplasty for the majority of their patients, because this procedure is almost universally applicable for repair of PUJ obstruction.

It can be used regardless of whether the ureteral insertion is high in the pelvis or already dependent.

It also allows reduction of redundant pelvis, where necessary or straightening of a lengthy or tortuous proximal ureter.

In addition, anterior and posterior transposition of PUJ obstruction can be accomplished when the obstruction is associated with accessory or aberrant lower pole vessels.

Finally, in compare to all flap techniques, only a dismembered pyeloplasty allows complete excision of the anatomically and functionally abnormal PUJ.

Relative contraindications, i.e. it is not suitable for:
  i. Lengthy or multiple proximal ureteric strictures.
  ii. PUJ with small and relatively inaccessible intrarenal pelvis.

Exposure to the PUJ: It is accomplished by first identifying the proximal ureter in the retroperitoneum. The ureter is dissected cephalad for the renal pelvis to preserve ureteral blood supply leaving behind a large amount of periureteral tissue.

Flap Procedure

i. *Foley's Y-V plasty* was originally designed for reconstruction of a PUJ obstruction associated with high ureteral insertion. But it is supplanted by Anderson- Hynes pyeloplasty.

   Contraindications- when transposition of lower vessels is required.

   Also lower value when significant reduction of renal pelvic size required.

ii. *Culp-DeWeerd spiral flap:* Best suited to large, readily accessible extrarenal pelvis in which the ureteral insertion is already in a dependent oblique position. Although most such patients are generally also good cases for dismembered pyeloplasty.

   Spiral flap may be of particular value when the PUJ obstruction is associated with a relatively long segment of proximal ureteral narrowing or stricture.

iii. *Scardino-Prince vertical flap:* Limited application today.

   It is suitable when dependent PUJ situated at the medial margin of a large square (box shaped) extrarenal pelvis.

   But mostly supplanted by a standard dismembered pyeloplasty.

Intubated ureterotomy: It is rarely used today. Primary role was for repair of lengthy or multiple ureteral strictures. If the stricture is associated with PUJ obstruction the intubated ureterotomy may be combined with any of the standard pyeloplasty techniques.

Note: If all of the above method fails—Ureterocalycestomy is the answer.

My patient, Raghuvir, a 58-year-old man, resident of Calcutta, West Bengal, presented with chief complaints of:

- Alteration of bowel habit for last 10 months.
- Bleeding per rectum along with passage of mucous with stool for last 7 months.
- Lump at left side of his mid abdomen and flank along with pain off and on for last 4/5 months.

My patient was apparently asymptomatic 10 months back since when he has developed alteration of bowel habit, i.e. he used to pass motion once or twice in a day but for last 10 months he noticed increasing constipation and passing motion once in 3/4 days and he noticed also alternating constipation followed by diarrhea for last 10 months.

- He has also got a history of passage of fresh blood per rectum, particularly during defecation at a regular interval. Nowadays, he has also noticed there is a passage of mucous with stool frequently.
- Since, last 4/5 months he developed a lump in his left mid abdomen and flank along with dull aching pain at the site of lump off and on. Pain is slightly relieved by defecation.
- There are history of unquantified weight loss and loss of appetite for last 4/5 months.

   There is a history of intestinal obstruction one month back, managed conservatively.

   There is no history of any urinary symptoms like hematuria, flank pain, retention of urine, etc. (to exclude renal lump).

- No history back pain, compressive features like venous compression causing varicose vein, swelling leg or discomfort/pain loin (compression on ureter causing hydronephrosis, etc.).

   (To exclude retroperitoneal soft tissue sarcoma).

- No history of chest pain, hemoptysis, bone pain, jaundice, etc. (To exclude distant metastasis).

Past History

He is not a known case of HTN, DM or TB or any heart disease (to exclude co-morbidity).

- No past history of any significant operation in past (operation for ulcerative colitis or Crohn's disease; adenomatous polyp, etc. are important).

Personal History

He used to have red meat and fatty food regularly (Red meat and saturated fat increases the incidence of colonic cancer).

- He is a smoker for last 20-25 years used to smoke 8-10 cigarettes per day.
- He is a known alcoholic also for last 10/15 years, 2/3 pegs/day minimum.

Family History

No history of any similar complaints or death of any family member due to similar complaints. [To exclude **familial adenomatous polyposis (FAP)**].

General Examination

Patient is cooperative, anxious looking, average built, averagely nourished. **Mild pallor** is there but there is no icterus, edema or generalized lymphadenopathy P-86/min, Temperature not raised BP 110/76 mm Hg, right arm supine respiration 16/min.

Systemic Examination

GIT: Inspection

- Abdomen is scaphoid
- Umbilicus is center
- There is a obvious bulging in left lumbar region
- All quadrants move with respiration
- No visible peristalsis or pulsation seen
- There is no visible vein, dilated vein or scar mark
- There is a obvious bulge in left lumbar region, flanks are not full
- Hernial sites, external genitalia appear normal.

On palpation: Abdomen soft, temperature normal, nontender, there is a 8 × 6 cm spherical. Retroperitoneal lump at left lumbar region extending above towards left hypochondrium below towards left iliac fossa and medially towards umbilicus. Surface smooth, firm in consistency, margins are palpable rounded but indistinct. There is slight side-to-side mobility of the lump but mobility is totally restricted craniocaudally. It does not move with respiration.

There is no hepatosplenomegaly, no other palpable mass, no free fluid in abdomen.

External genitalia, hernial sites are normal.
Supraclavicular lymph nodes not palpable.

Digital Rectal Exam (DRE)

* Rectum–no evidence of any growth, no 'Blumer self' palpable at rectovasical pouch but fingers are smeared with blood.

Other Systemic Examinations

Respiratory—Bilateral air entry equal. No adventitious sound heard.

CVS— S_1S_{11} (Normal) No murmur heard.
Others are essentially normal.

SUMMARY OF THE CASE

My patient, a 58-year-old man presented with complaint of alternation of bowel habit for last 10 months. Bleeding per rectum along with passage of mucous with stool for last 7 months.

Lump left mid abdomen and flank along with dull aching pain off and on for last 4/5 months with weight loss and loss of appetite.

On examination patient is mild anemic. There is a 8 × 6 cm retroperitoneal firm lump at left iliac fossa extending towards left hypochondrium above and left iliac fossa below, smooth surface, margins are palpable but in distinct. There is no mobility up and down but it is slightly mobile side-to-side, does not move with respiration.

So my provisional clinical diagnosis is:
Carcinoma descending colon without any clinical evidence of distal metastases.

Why are you considering this as a colonic carcinoma?
Sir,
* Elderly male, known smoker, alcoholic and red meat eater.

* Presented with alteration of bowel habit, bleeding per rectum along with mucous with stool, lump left side of abdomen along with dull ache and colicky pain off and on.
* History of weight loss, loss of appetite are there.
* On examination patient is anemic.

There is a retroperitoneal lump in left lumbar region moves side-to-side; not up and down, margins are palpable but not distinct, firm in consistency, nontender.

Whats are the other possibilities?
Other possibilities are:
  i. Tuberculosis in discending colon
 ii. Left sided renal lump
iii. Retroperitoneal soft tissue tumor
 iv. Lymphoma

  i. **Features of TB colon:**
    * It mimics carcinoma colon.
    * Patient presents with tenesmus, diarrhea or discharge from the painful fistula or recurrent subacute obstruction.
    * Few patients present with lump abdomen.
    * Features of evening rise of temperature, weight loss, etc.
 ii. **Renal Lump**
    * Presents with hematuria, flank pain, mass abdomen.
    * Reniform shaped mass.
    * Renal lump though retroperitoneal, but moves with respiration.
    * Does not cross the midline.
    * Ballotable, bimanually palpable.
    * Fingers can be insinuated between the lump and costal margins.
    * Band of colonic resonance over the lump.
iii. **Retroperitoneal soft tissue tumor**
    * Elderly people.
    * Retroperitoneal central mass.
    * Painless progressive mass.
    * Smooth surface.
    * Crossing midline.
    * No urinary, GI symptoms.
    * Fixed.
    * Does not move with respiration.
    * All margins are not distinctly palpable except lower margin.
 iv. **Lymphoma**
    * More common in male.
    * Bimodal presentation 20-30 years and 50 years.
    * Cervical lymph nodes involvement is the most common, abdominal lymphadenopathy less common.

- 'B' symptoms like weight loss (>10% in 6 months), fever, pruritus. Bone pain, etc. 'A' is absence of these symptoms.
- Splenomegaly is very common.

(Details are written in concerned chapters).

Ok, how will you proceed in this case?

Sir,

I will confirm my diagnosis first.

I will do

i. **Colonoscopy (160 cm long, flexible):** The investigation of choice in suspected colonic malignancy provided the patient is fit enough to undergo the bowel preparation by enema.

Advantages: It picks up primary lesion, any synchronous polyp or even multiple carcinomas (occur in 5% of cases).

- Biopsy is taken for histological diagnosis.

Disadvantages: There is a small chance of perforation, failure to get to the cecum in 10% of cases.

ii. *Double contrast barium enema:* It is a second line investigation and usually used when colonoscopy is contraindicated.

It shows:

- Cancer of the colon
- Irregular filling defects
- Synchronous lesions, etc.

(Truly it is rarely done nowadays as CECT abdomen is the investigation of choice after colonoscopy).

Disadvantages

- It should not be done in case of intestinal obstruction.
- False positive occurs 1-2% of cases and false negative in 7-9% of cases. (In impending colonic obstruction– a study with water soluble contrast may be done).

Suppose histopathology came as adenocarcinoma colon then how will you stage the disease?

I will do:

- Chest X-ray PA view to roule out pulmonary mets.
- Liver function test to see the level of alkaline phosphatase (ALP), SGOT, SGPT level. Markedly elevated levels suggest liver metastasis.
- **USG abdomen** used as a screening investigation for liver metastases over the size of 1.5 cm.
  - To see the lymph nodes involvement
  - Ascites, etc.

- **CECT abdomen**
  - To determine the local invasion
  - Extent of the disease.
  - Intra-abdominal metastases
  - Lymph nodes involvement.

Anything more will you like to do?

I will also assess blood carcinoembryonic antigen (CEA) level. Normal value 2.5–5 ng/ml.

Elevated level favors the diagnosis of carcinoma in case any doubt and it has got a good prognostic value in serial follow-up.

A rising CEA level in follow-up period may suggest recurrence before the clinical disease becomes apparent. CEA is a glycoprotein tissue and in colorectal cancers but it is absent in normal colorectal mucosa.

Note: CEA is not a specific marker for colorectal cancer It may be elevated in so many conditions like.

Malignant: Carcinoma stomach, pancreas, lung, breast, etc.

Benign: Cirrhosis of lever, pancreatitis, ulcerative colitis, renal failure, smokers, etc.).

What is the role of spiral CT in carcinoma colon?

It is very useful in elderly patients where colonoscopy as well as contrast enema both are contraindicated or where both the procedures are not diagnostic.

In some centers, it is the standard procedure above the age of 80 years.

What is virtual colonoscopy?

It is also called **CT colonography.** The technology uses helical CT and three-dimensional reconstruction to detect intraluminal colonic lesions.

Bowel preparation, oral and rectal contrast and colonic insufflations are used to maximize sensitivity. It is a non-invasive procedure and very good imaging for colorectal cancer and in future it may replace colonoscopy.

Whats are the contraindications for surgery in case of carcinoma colon?

- Moribund patient, not fit for surgery
- Multiple metastases and
- Where chance of survival is less.

Suppose patient is operable what will you do?

Sir, I will do all baseline investigations.

- CBC platelets count
- Sugar- both fasting (F) and postprandial (PP)

- KFT
  - Urine {RE
            ME
  - Stool { Re
           Occult blood
  - ECG, etc.

I will send to patient to anesthetist for preanesthetic check up. If patient is fit for surgery I will plan for left hemicolectomy.

How will you prepare the patent for surgery?

I will
i.   Build up patient's nutrition
ii. Correct patients anemia
iii. I will prepare the gut before operation.

How will prepare the gut?

- Low residue diet 48 hours before surgery
- I will start liquid diet 24 hours before surgery
- Gut irrigation with polyethylene glycol (so called peg lac) – a balanced salt solution

100 gm of peglec is dissolved in 2 liter of water on previous day and has to be taken over 2 hours (9 -11 am). It's enough to clear the motion.

- Tab. Metoclopramide or domperidone (10 mg) is given to reduce nausea
- ORS water 1 L may be given day before evening and early morning of up day
- A rectal washout may be necessary
- Antibiotic preparation – aim is to sterilize the gut. Luminal antibiotics like erythromycin base 1 gm + Tinidazole 1 gm or 11 am, 1 pm and 11 pm on the day before operation at 1 pm, 3 pm and 11 pm. When surgery is planned at 9 am next day.
- Systemic antibiotics are also administered usually third generation cephalosporin, metronidazole and aminogly-coside at the start of surgery, repeat doses to be given after 6 hours and 16 hours in postoperative period.

(Bowel preparation before colorectal surgery is still controversial but present literature suggests that no bowel preparation is safe for right sided colonic surgery.)

What is your plan in this case?

Sir,
If patient is operable I will do left **hemicolectomy**.
I will remove:
- Left one-third of transverse colon
- Splenic flexure
- Descending colon
- Proximal sigmoid colon

- A long with part of transverse mesocolon and sigmoid mesocolon and to remove locoregional lymph nodes.

What is extended left hemicolectomy?

In extended left hemicolectomy inferior mesenteric artery, at the level of aortic origin is ligated and distal transverse colon, descending colon, sigmoid colon and upper rectum are removed along with removal of locoregional lymph nodes (mesenteric and pericolic lymph nodes).

(However, there have been no prospective studies demonstrating a benefit from extended left hemicolectomy).

What are the tests for operability, i.e. how will you assess the resectability?

When the abdomen is opened and the tumor is assessed for resectability
i.   **Assessment of liver:** Liver is looked for any secondary deposits. Though liver secondary is not necessarily a contraindication for surgery because in colonic carcinoma the best palliative treatment is removal of the tumor.
ii. **Peritoneum:** Particularly the pelvic peritoneum is looked for small white seed like neoplastic implantation which may be found in omentum also. These deposits suggests advanced carcinoma and palliative resection is advisable.
iii. **Lymph nodes assessment:** Enlargement of different groups of lymph nodes may not be always involved, they may be inflammatory. Fixed metastatic lymph nodes indicate inoperability but palliative resection to be performed if possible. If resection is not possible proximal colostomy is the answer.
iv. **Fixity of growth:** Local fixity does not always imply local invasion, it may be due to extensive local inflammatory response. So, fixity of tumor does not always mean inoperability.

Suppose an elderly patient presents to you with acute intestinal obstruction along with left sided colonic mass what should be your approach?

In such case I will do initial colostomy to relieve the obstruction
↓
After 4-6 weeks curative/palliative resection to be done
↓
Colostomy clouse, i.e. restoration of gut to be done after 8 weeks (average 6-12 weeks)

If the growth is stenosing in nature (which is most common varity in left side) can cause close loop obstruction because of the competent ileocecal vulve.

As a result pressure increases in the cecum (As per laplace rule), eventually it may lead to perforation. Perforation may occur at the site of tumor also.

In such a case emergency cecostomy or colostomy to be done.

Resection and anastomosis of the segment at the time depends on the patient general condition, Hb% level and serum albumin status. Resection of growth can be done in emergency but primary restoration of continuity should not be done and it is always better to do an end colostomy after resection.

Usually it is not done in emergency. It is done after 3-6 weeks after making the patient surgically fit.

Is there any alternate procedure is there for left sided colonic growth with acute intestinal obstruction?

In such a case, transanal self-expanding metal stent can be used instead of de functioning colostomy.

What will you do if a solitary liver secondary is found during resection of colonic tumor?

In such case, I will do metastectomy even for multiple secondaries, segmental resection, lobectomy also recommended.

What is 'second look operation' in carcinoma colon?

Second look operation is most often helpful in carcinoma colon to resect residual or recurrent tumors.

It was proposed by Owen Wangensteen so it is called 'Owen Wangensteen's second look surgery.

Do you know what is Turnbull's no touch technique?

In a case of colonic carcinoma, during the process of resection early division of blood vessels and ligated at their origins, before handling the tumor to prevent dissemination of the tumor cells by blood stream.

This is called *Turnball's no touch technique*.

Suppose after opening the abdomen you find the left colonic tumor is unresectable what will you do next?

Sir, I will do a transverse colostomy as a palliative procedure and I will plan for adjuvant chemotherapy. Nowadays the commonly used regime is called FOLFOX containing 5 FU, leucoverin and Oxalpiatin. Other regimes are FLOX containing 5FU and Oxalpiatin.

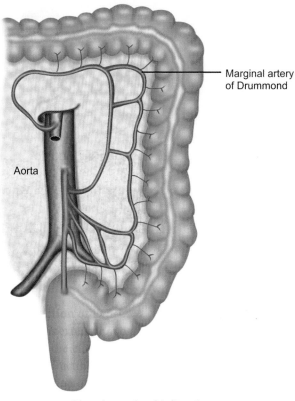

Blood supply of left colon

What chemotherapy you will prefer for colonic carcinoma?

As a adjuvant therapy Inj. 5FU+ Levamisole or Inj 5Fu+ leucovorin has shown to have beneficial effect in terms of long-term survival. Minimum 6 cycles chemotherapy to be given 4 weeks interval.

What are the indications for chemotherapy in carcinoma colon?

The indications are:
- T_3, T_4 lesions
- Lymph nodes involvement
- Poorly differentiated carcinoma
- Lymphovascular invasion
- Signet cell colonic carcinoma.

What is the role of laparoscopic surgery in colonic carcinoma?

Laparoscopic colonic resection is coming up though it is still controversial started in 1991. Principles are same like an open operation. It requires skill in advanced laparoscopy.

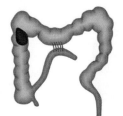 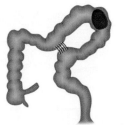

Ileocolic anastomosis　　　Colocolic anastomosis

Bypass procedures in colonic carcinomas

What is the follow-up procedure in an operated carcinoma colon?

- Follow-up at an interval of 3 months for initial 2 years as 70% of recurrent disease appears in 2 years.
- There after, every 6 months review is required up to 5 years.
- Next yearly review.

What all will you do in follow-up?

- Clinical examination
- Fecal occult blood test
- Liver function test
- CEA level assessment
- Chest X-ray PA view
- Colonoscopy every 6 months for first 2 years and next every yearly for 5 years.

A raise level of CEA is an indication of colonoscopic examination or CT scan abdomen.

What can be the functional effects of left and right hemicolectomy?

Left hemicolectomy results increase frequency of motions. Whereas in right hemicolectomy stool will be loose (as absorption of water is less in absence of right colon and volume will be more around 600-700 ml (Normal volume is 250 ml).

Why obstructive features are common in left sided colonic growth?

There are two reasons for this:
- i. Left sided growth is usually stenosing in nature.
- ii. Stool is formed and solid in colon.

What is right hemicolectomy?

Right hemicolectomy includes:
- Resection of cecum, appendix, ascending colon, right 1/3rd of transverse colon and 10 cm of terminal ileum.
- Removal of locoregional lymph nodes, i.e. epicolic, paracolic, intermediate groups of lymph nodes. Here ileo-transverse anastomosis is to be done.

What is extended right hemicolectomy?

- In extended hemicolectomy, all structures are removed like right hemicolectomy but right 2/3rd transverse colon is to be removed instead of right 1/3rd.
- Here trunk of middle colic artery is tied whereas in right hemicolectomy right branch of middle colic artery is tied.

How lymphatic spread occurs in colonic carcinoma?

Lymph spread in carcinoma colon is sequential to different groups of lymph nodes.
- i. Epicolic lymph nodes lying on the colonic wall.
- ii. Pericolic lymph nodes lying on the immediate vicinity of the colonic wall along the marginal artery.
- iii. Intermediate lymph nodes lying along the main arterial branches like – ileocolic, right colic, middle colic, left colic, sigmoid arteries.
- iv. Mian/principle lymph nodes are lying along the inferior or superior mesenteric vessels.

What is spurious diarrhea?

There is increase frequency of motion but stool contains only mucosa and blood specially in the early morning. Patient usually passes 10-12 motions per day.

Why in colonic growth alternate constipation and diarrhea occur?

Constipation occurs as stool gets obstructed by the growth as the stool in colon is hard. Gradually the colonized bacteria start fermenting the stool and stool liquefies and passes, so called diarrhea occurs.

What is tenesmus?

The Greek word tenesmus means ineffective and painful straining of stools. Its an urge to pass motion, may be intermittent or constant and usually accompanied by pain despite of straining efforts; little or nothing is passed.

How will you identify rectosigmoid junction?

- The position from peritoneal reflection, i.e. 4 cm above the lower margin of upper rectal reflection of peritoneum.
- At the level of sacral promontory
- The distance of 15 cm from the anal verge.
- The most useful practical approach to identify the recto-sigmoid junction is the confluence of the taenia coli.

What is 'Laplace' law in close loop obstruction?

Laplace rule T (wall tension) = P (pressure in the wall)

$$\frac{R \text{ (radius of the luman)}}{W \text{ (wall thickness)}}$$

$\uparrow$ Pressure = $\uparrow$ radius of the close loop

$\Downarrow$

$\downarrow$ wall thickness

$\Downarrow$

Rupture of close loop

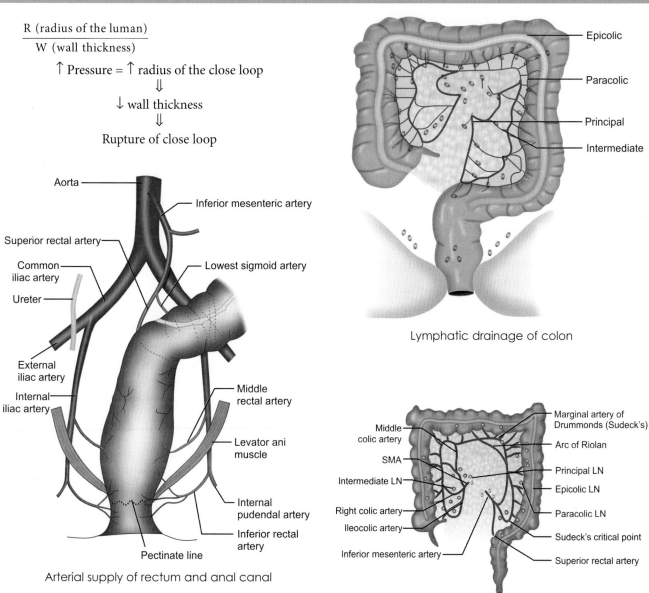

Arterial supply of rectum and anal canal

Lymphatic drainage of colon

Arterial supply and lymphatic drainage of colon

A classic form of closed loop obstruction seen in the presence of a tight carcinomatous stricture of the colon with a patent ileocecal valve.

The inability of the distended colon to decompress itself into the small bowel results in an increase in intraluminal pressure, greatest at the cecum.

Ok, one thing can you tell me on X-ray how will you identify obstructed small bowel from obstructed large bowel?

Small bowel: Jejunum–valvulae conniventes which completely pass across the width of the bowel. These are regularly placed giving a concertina or ladder effect.

- Ileum – featureless
- Cecum–distended cecum looks like a rounded gas shadow in right iliac fossa.

Large bowel: Hustral (folds are placed irregularly and the indentations are not placed opposite to one another).

SHORT NOTE ON CARCINOMA COLON

- Adenocarcinoma most common variety of colonic carcinoma
- Genetics

Normal colonic mucosa → Dysplastic aberrant crypt foci → early adenoma → intermediate adenoma → DCC → Late adenoma → Carcinoma

- Etiology:
  - Intake of excessive dietary animal fat like red meat increases the risk
  - Smoking, alcohol increase the risk
  - Even after cholecystectomy—increased secretion of bile acid may increase the risk
  - Irritable bowel disease, ulcerative colitis, Crohn's disease increase the risk of malignancy.
  - Hereditary nonpolyposis colonic cancer (HNPCC).
- **Premalignant conditions of colonic carcinoma**
  i. Neoplastic
     a. Familial adenomatous polyposis (FAP)
     b. Turcot's syndrome
     c. Lymphomatous polyposis
     d. Leukemic polyposis
  ii. Inflammatory
     a. Ulcerative colitis
     b. Crohn's disease
     c. Granulomatous polyposis
  iii. Juvenile polyposis
     a. Peutz Jeghers syndrome
     b. Neurofibromatous polyposis
     c. Lipomatous polyposis
     d. Cronkhite Canada syndrome
  iv. Unclassified
     a. Metaplastic polyps
     b. Pneumatosis cystoids intestinalis.

- *Types of neoplastic polyps are:*
  i. Adenotubular 80%
  ii. Tubulovillous
  iii. Villous
  - Type of colonic cancer
    Macroscopically there are four type of carcinoma colon:
    i. Annular or constricting type commonly seen in left side and gives rise to obstructive symptoms
    ii. Tubular ⎫
    iii. Ulcerative ⎬ all three varieties present
    iv. Cauliflower ⎭ commonly with bleeding
- The sites of distribution of colonic cancer in Fig. 10.6
- **Clinical Features:**
  Left sided tumors: Left sided tumors two times more common than right, though the present days incidence of carcinoma colon is being shifted left to right.

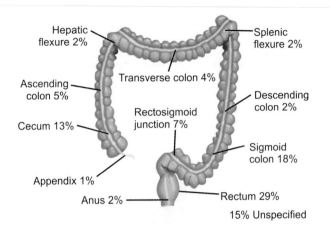

Sites of distribution of colonic cancer

Clinical features are: common symptoms are usually associated with increasing intestinal obstruction.

- Pain: Colicky in nature, referred to suprapubic area, constant pain may suggest an advanced tumor
- *Alternation of bowel habit:* It means change of bowel habits from regular like once or twice a day to on, i.e. in three days or more. There may be a difficulty to get the bowel move

  It may be habits of having constipation followed by diarrhea other way
- *Distention of abdomen:* Usually lower abdominal distention along with pain and which is relived by passing flatus or motion
- *Palpable lump:* Carcinoma colon is a slow growing malignancy. Lump may be palpable per abdomen, per rectal or by manual palpation. Rectal bleeding, tenesmus are the other features.

  Special features of carcinoma sigmoid, sense of incomplete evacuation, tenesmus accompanied by passage of mucous and blood, bladder symptoms may be there.
- *Right sided colonic carcinoma:* Right sided colonic carcinoma, patients usually present with: (i) Iron deficiency anemia and (ii) Abdominal mass.

  In both the case if there is metastases jaundice, ascites, hepatomegaly may be associated features.
- *Investigations:* Investigations for colonic carcinoma as described early.
- **TNM classification of colonic cancer**
  AJCC TNM staging system.

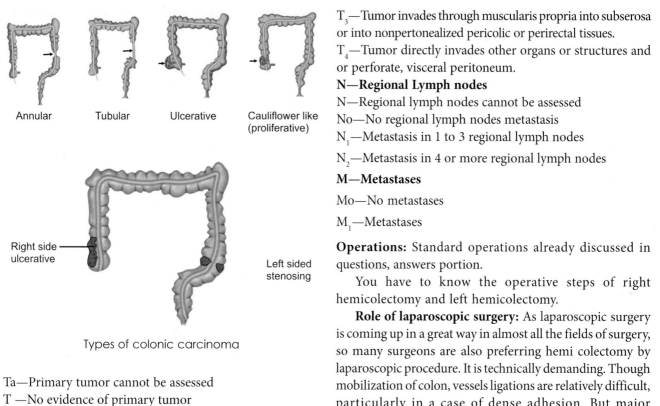

Annular   Tubular   Ulcerative   Cauliflower like
(proliferative)

Right side
ulcerative

Left sided
stenosing

Types of colonic carcinoma

Ta—Primary tumor cannot be assessed

T —No evidence of primary tumor

T—Carcinoma *in situ* intraepithelial or invasion of lamina propria

T_1—Tumor invades submucosa

T_2—Tumor invades muscularis propria,

T_3—Tumor invades through muscularis propria into subserosa or into nonpertonealized pericolic or perirectal tissues.

T_4—Tumor directly invades other organs or structures and or perforate, visceral peritoneum.

N—Regional Lymph nodes

N—Regional lymph nodes cannot be assessed

No—No regional lymph nodes metastasis

N_1—Metastasis in 1 to 3 regional lymph nodes

N_2—Metastasis in 4 or more regional lymph nodes

M—Metastases

Mo—No metastases

M_1—Metastases

Operations: Standard operations already discussed in questions, answers portion.

You have to know the operative steps of right hemicolectomy and left hemicolectomy.

Role of laparoscopic surgery: As laparoscopic surgery is coming up in a great way in almost all the fields of surgery, so many surgeons are also preferring hemi colectomy by laparoscopic procedure. It is technically demanding. Though mobilization of colon, vessels ligations are relatively difficult, particularly in a case of dense adhesion. But major laparotomy is avoided this way and in laparoscopic procedure postoperative recovery is faster and patient compliance is more as there is minimal amount of pain.

Specimen retrieval is via a small incision.

Carcinoma Stomach—The Captain of Men's Death

My patient, Amir Khan a 56-year-old man, resident of Tirupatti, Chennai, presented to this hospital with complaint of:

- Pain upper abdomen for last 8 months.
- Sensation of fullness after meal with regular vomiting for last 6 months.
- Weakness, weight loss and loss of appetite for last 4 months.
- My patient was apparently asymptomatic 8 months back since when he started having upper abdominal pain off and on. The pain is dull aching insidious in set, continuous, aggravated after having meal, non-radiating and subsides sometime automatically, sometimes on medication.
- Sensation of bloating and fullness after meal with regular vomiting for last 6 months.
- Initially vomiting occurred almost daily but gradually vomiting has become less for last 2 months (As the stomach is being distended gradually and capable to contain more food material) once or twice in a week.
- Vomiting is projectile in nature contains food material taken more than 12 hours before which is nonbilious.
- He has got a feeling of rolling mass in abdomen from left to right, feeling of fullness is more often.
- My patient has got history of loss of appetite and unquantified weight loss for last 4 months.
- But there is no history of peptic ulcer disease in the past (which may lead to gastric outlet obstruction).
- There is no history of hematemesis and melena (to exclude upper GI hemorrhage).
- There is no history of alteration of bowel habits, distention of lower abdomen (to exclude carcinoma transverse colon).
- There is no history of hemoptysis, cough, chest pain, jaundice, etc. (to exclude metastases).

Past History

- No history of diabetes but he is hypertensive for last 4/5 years and on regular medication.
- No history suggestive of acid peptic disease.
- No significant operative history in the past.

Personal History

- Nonvegetarian.
- Used to have high salt diet, smoked fishes regularly.
- He is a chronic smoker, smokes 20 bidi/day for last 15 years, occasional alcoholic also.

Family History

- His father also died of carcinoma stomach. Family history of gastric carcinoma is there.

General Survey

- Patient is cooperative, average built, but poorly nourished. Pallor present but there is no icterus, edema or generalized lymphadenopathy. Patient is dehydrated.
- **System examination:**
- **Inspection:** Abdomen scaphoid, there is no obvious bulge in abdomen, umbilicus in center position, all quadrants move with respiration.
- There is visible peristalsis moving left to right side of abdomen (occasionally found) but there is no visible veins, pulsation, scar marks, etc. Flanks are not full. Hernial sites and external genitalia appear normal.
- **On palpation:** Abdomen soft, temperature is normal, nontender.
- This is a large, palpable intra-abdominal spherical mass extending from left hypochondrium towards epigastrium and the umbilical region.

- The mass is pushed inwards and seems to be disappeared by examining finger.
- There is a intra-abdominal globular firm mass 4.3 cm, uneven surface, margins are palpable irregular, moves up and down with respiration. The lump is mobile from side to side.
- No other lump palpable, no hepatosplenomegaly.
- There is no free fluid in the abdomen bowel sounds audible. Succusion splash is present (Ausculto percussion reveals a distended stomach and greater curvature lying below umbilicus).
- **There is no supraclavicular lymph node palpable**.
- Digital rectal examination. There is no 'Blumer shelf' palpable. Only grade II prostate palpable.
- **Other systemic examination:**
- **Respiratory system:** Bilateral air entry equal. No adventitious sound present.
- **CVS:** $S_1 S_{II}$ (Normal) no murmur.
- Others systemic examinations are essentially normal.

SUMMARY OF THE CASE

My patient, a 56-year-old male from Chennai, smoked fish eater and smoker, presented with upper abdominal pain and discomfort for 8 months, feeling of fullness of abdomen and regular vomiting for 6 months, weight loss, anorexia for last 4 months.

On examination: Poorly nourished patient, anemic and dehydrated.

Systemic examination reveals: Stomach is distended along with features of gastric outlet obstruction and there is a 4 × 3 cm spherical mass at epigastrium which is firm in consistency, uneven surface, irregular margins, mobile from side-to-side. Succusssion splash is present (Ausculto percussion reveals the distended stomach with greater curvature lying below the umbilicus).

So, my provisional diagnosis is—this is a case of carcinoma stomach with gastric outlet obstruction.

Any other diagnosis in your mind other than carcinoma stomach?

Sir, from history and clinical examination I feel it is a case of carcinoma stomach but I will definitely exclude carcinoma transverse colon as because of the position of the tumor along with anemia and lassitude.

How will you proceed in this case?

Sir, first I will confirm my diagnosis by doing:

   I. **USG abdomen** to see the:
   - Organ of origin
   - Nature of the swelling solid and cystic or both
   - Any free fluid abdomen
   - Status of liver
   - Lymphadenopathy, etc.

   Remember USG is poor imaging modality to evaluate the growth (carcinoma) of the stomach but we are used to do it as it is first, easily available and gives a gross idea about the lesion.

   II. **Barium meal which may show**
   - Irregular filling defect
   - Loss of rugosity
   - Delayed emptying
   - Dilated stomach in carcinoma pylorus.

   III. **Upper GI endoscopy and biopsy** to confirm the diagnosis and it is the investigation of choice. Diagnostic accuracy is 95%. Multiple biopsies are recommended for more accuracy.

   IV. **CECT abdomen**
   - To stage the disease, i.e. extension of the disease
   - Infiltration into the surrounding structures depth of invasion in stomach wall
   - Secondaries
   - Lymph nodes involvement
   - Operability, etc.

   CT chest-to exclude pulmonary metastasis, in an advanced disease.

Any other investigations you would like to do?

Sir, I will do Hb%, LFT and all baseline investigations for preanesthetic checkup.

Suppose this patient is operable how will you treat the patient?

Sir, if the growth is in pylorus, I will do distal gastrectomy with proximal 5 cm clearance along with the removal of greater omentum, lesser omentum and D2 lymph nodes and I will do gastrojejunostomy.

What kind of gastrojejunostomy will you do?

Sir, I will do anterior gastrojejunostomy.

Why anterior gastrojejunostomy?

Sir, as there is a maximum chance of recurrence in gastric bed. So better to avoid usual posterior gastrojejunostomy.

What is the main drawback at anterior gastrojejunostomy?

Sir, due to nondependent drainage regargitant vomiting and nausea, retching may be the irritating problems.

What do you mean by D2 lymph nodes dissection?

D2 lymph node dissections mean removal of D1 group and D2 group of lymph nodes.

What are the different groups of lymph nodes related with carcinoma stomach.

There are four groups of lymph nodes called D1, D2, D3 and D4.

(D means Dissection)

D1 lymph nodes are 1-6:

1. Right cardiac nodes
2. Left cardiac nodes
3. Lymph nodes along the lesser curvature
4. Lymph nodes along the greater curvature
   a. Along the short gastric vessels
   b. Along the left gastroepiploic vessels
   c. Along the right gastroepiploic vessels
5. Suprapyloric nodes
6. Subpyloric nodes.

D2 lymph nodes include 7-11 group:

7. Nodes along the left gastric artery
8. Lymph nodes along the common hepatic artery
9. Lymph nodes along the celiac axis
10. Lymph nodes along the splenic hilum
11. Lymph nodes along the splenic artery.

D3 lymph nodes include 12-16 groups:

12. Lymph nodes at the hepatoduodenal ligament
13. Retroduodenal lymph nodes
14. Lymph nodes at the root of mesentery
15. Lymph nodes around the middle colic artery
16. Para-aortic lymph nodes.

D4 lymph nodes include 17-18 group [only it is dealt in proximal carcinoma stomach]:

17. Lymph nodes around lower esophagus
18. Supradiaphragmatic lymph nodes.

Suppose the growth is in the body or more proximal what will you do?

Sir, in such a case I will do total radical gastrectomy, D2 lymph nodes dissection with Roux en Y esophagojejunal anastomosis.

Other questions are:

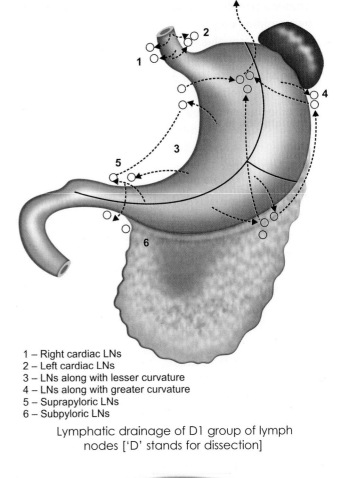

1 – Right cardiac LNs
2 – Left cardiac LNs
3 – LNs along with lesser curvature
4 – LNs along with greater curvature
5 – Suprapyloric LNs
6 – Subpyloric LNs

Lymphatic drainage of D1 group of lymph nodes ['D' stands for dissection]

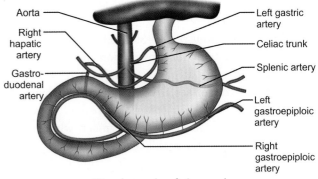

Blood supply of stomach

During endoscopic biopsy what all are essential to remember?

i. Multiple biopsies to be taken to have a diagnostic. Accuracy more than 95%.

ii. Gastric carcinoma may be difficult to distinguish from gastric lymphomas, because of submucosal location of lymphoid neoplasma. So it is important to obtain biopsy specimen in an adequate depth.

What are the palliative procedures in a case of in operable carcinoma stomach?

- If growth is not resectable palliative gastrojejunostomy can be done.
- If the growth causing recurrent bleeding and obstruction palliative gastric resection is the way.
- Stenting or recanalization with laser may be helpful for in operable gastroesophageal junction growth.
- Palliative chemotherapy also helps in improving survival.

What is the role of neoadjuvant chemotherapy in carcinoma stomach?

In a case of locally advanced carcinoma stomach a combine preoperative chemotherapy is given to down stage the disease.

It is proved that neoadjuvant chemotherapy renders locally advanced inoperable case, operable.

What are the chemotherapeutic agents, commonly used in carcinoma stomach?

A combination of epirubicin, cisplatin and 5 FU is very effective.

Recently thiotepa, floxuridine, nitrosoureas, mitomycin, anthracyclines and cisplatin in different combinations are being used effectively.

What is the role of adjuvant chemotherapy?

In early gastric cancer surgery alone has excellent cure rate. But in advanced gastric cancer, risk of tumor recurrence increases as the stage increases, so adjuvant chemotherapy has gained importance in recent years though it gives only modest benefit in gastric cancer.

What about radiotherapy in carcinoma stomach?

In a word, radiotherapy is not much effective in gastric cancer. But trials going on this issue.

However, radiotherapy has been used in combination with chemotherapy as an intraoperative modality and also as palliative modality different studies suggest that patients receiving adjuvant chemoradiation (5FU + Leucovorin + 45 Gy of radiation) are not likely to become the standard of care for the patients with stages II, III A and III B gastric carcinoma.

Radiotherapy is very useful for painful bony metastasis.

What is the recent best modality of treatment for a case of operable gastric cancer?

The recent evidence suggests that total (radical) gastrectomy, combined with D2 lymphadenectomy, appears to be the procedure of choice irrespective of sites.

A combined modality treatment also holds promise.

Tell me the conditions where abdominal pain aggravates after having meal?

The conditions are carcinoma stomach:
- Gastric ulcer
- Chronic pancreatitis
- Carcinoma pancreas
- Chronic mesenteric ischemia.

Is there any tumor marker in gastric carcinoma?

There are many tumor markers related to gastric cancer like CEA, CA 19-9, CA 125, CA 72 are important tumor markers to assess recurrence and prognosis of carcinoma stomach.

Most important tumor marker is T2-4 which disappears after surgery and re-appears with regional or distant recurrence.

Do you know the CT staging of carcinoma stomach?

Yes sir,

Stage I: Intramural growth only without wall thickening
Stage II: Wall thickening > 1 cm
Stage III: Involvement of adjacent structures
Stage IV: Metastases to liver, lymph nodes or distant sites like lung, bone, etc.

What are the other causes of gastric outlet obstruction?

The causes of gastric outlet obstruction are:
- Consequence of chronic duodenal ulcer
- Gastrointestinal stromal tumor (GIST) involving stomach
- Extrinsic compression by enlarged lymph nodes
- Gastric lymphoma
- Carcinoma head of pancreas
- Adult hypertrophic pyloric stenosis
- Bezoar, etc.

What are the effect of gastric outlet obstruction?

- *Anatomical effect:* Because of obstruction there will be hyperperistalsis in the stomach to overcome the obstruction.
- Hypertrophy of stomach musculature as a result.
  Later on there will be a huge dilation of the stomach.
- *Metabolic effect:* Metabolic effect as a result of gastric outlet obstruction is hypochloremic, hypokalemic metabolic alkalosis as a result of loss of H^+, Cl^- and K^+ due to repeated vomiting.
- *Mechanism:* In initial stage vomiting causes loss of H^+ and Cl^- leading to hypochloremic alkalosis.
  Na^+ level may be normal and loss of K^+ may not be manifested.

Kidney tries to compensate this alkalosis by excreting low chloride and more bicarbonate.

In late stage—If vomiting persists

↓ more dehydration

↓ hyponatremia develops

To conserve circulatory volume kidney reabsorbs water and Na^+ (due to aldosterone effect)

↓

Na^+ ions retained by distal renal tubules by exchange of H^+, K^+ ions in urine as a result kidney passes acidic urine leading to paradoxical aciduria and hypokalemia.

Ultimately there will be hypochloremic, hypokalemic metabolic alkalosis with paradoxical aciduria.

How will you manage the case of metabolic alkalosis?

Sir, I will start

- 1N to 2N HCl which is effective to correct severe metabolic alkalosis. 1-2 liters of solution to be transfused over 24 hours. Monitor of pH, $PaCO_2$ and Na^+, K^+, and serum Ca^+ every 4 hourly is mandatory.
- Ammonium chloride can be used to correct the alkalosis effectively but very carefully as it more prone to develop ammonia toxieity.
- IV potassiumo .5-1 meg/kg body weight.
- Correction of dehydration and underlying cause is essential.

What is gastric tetany?

As a result of severe vomiting. Seum levels of Na^+, Cl^-, K^+, Mg drop leading to metabolic alkalosis and alkalosis can lead hypocalcemia causing tetany which is called gastric tetany.

What is Mary Joseph's nodule?

Mary Joseph's – a nursing superintendent of St Mary's Hospital, USA noticed the presence of an umbilical nodule in many patients of advance gastric cancer. By her name this umbilical nodule is called Mary Joseph's nodule. (The secondary spreads through ligamentum of teres).

How will you assess in operability in carcinoma stomach?

Patient is considered to be in operable if:

i. Patient has hematogenous metastases like involvement of liver, lung, etc.

ii. Involvement of distant peritoneum.

iii. N4 nodal (more than 18 regional nodes) disease and beyond.

iv. Fixation to structures that cannot be removed.

What is the role of laparoscopy in carcinoma stomach?

Laparoscopy is very sensitive for staging of metastatic disease. Especially in identifying tumors deposits which cannot be detected by conventional imaging.

What does early and advanced gastric cancer mean?

Early gastric cancer is defined as the cancer that remains limited to the mucosa or the submucosa regardless of the presence or absence of nodal metastasis (T1, any N).

Whereas advanced gastric cancer involves the muscularis and beyond.

What is Troisier's sign?

In advanced carcinoma stomach lymph nodes of left supraclavicular region are involved. These lymph nodes are called Virchow's lymph nodes and this sign is called Troiser's sign.

Q. 30. Tell me the TNM staging of carcinoma stomach.

T – Primary tumor

T_0—No evidence of primary tumor

T_1S—Carcinoma *in situ*

T_1—Tumor involves lamina propria or submucosa

T_2—Tumor involves muscularis or subserosa

T_3—Tumor involves serosa

T_4—Tumor invades adjacent structures

N —Lymph nodal status

N_0—No lymph nodes involvement

N_1—Involvement of 1-6 regional lymph nodes

N_2—Involvement of 7-15 regional lymph nodes

N_3—Involvement of > 15 regional lymph nodes

M—Metastasis

M_0—No distant metastasis

M_1—Distant metastasis

How can you manage early gastric cancer?

Present day's concept for management of early gastric cancer is endoscopic submucosal resection where it is possible.

CARCINOMA STOMACH—SHORT NOTE

- **Carcinoma Stomach**
  - Called captain of men's death
  - Second most common cancer in the world
  - More common in male
  - In India it is common in **South India.**

- **Etiology**

  A multifactorial disease. The risk factors are diet:
  - Excessive salt take
  - Deficiency of antioxidant
  - Food with more nitrosamines increases the risk
  - Smoked salmon fish

  Risk factors for proximal gastric cancer
  - Obesity young age
  - High socioeconomic status
  - Genetic factors.

  Risk factors for distal gastric cancer:
  - Old age
  - *Helicobactor pylori* responsible for body and distal stomach carcinoma
  - Low socioeconomic group
  - In Asian countries it is common in distal stomach.

- **Other important risk factors are:**
  - 10% familal
  - Blood group 'A' is more susceptible for carcinogens
  - Pernicious anemia
  - Gastric polyp, adenomatous polyp > 2 cm
  - Familial adenomatous polyposis
  - Chronic gastritis, gastric dysplasia
  - Smoking, alcohol
  - Giant hyperplasia gastric mucosal folds (Mènètrier's disease).

- **Classification:**

  I. Borrmann classification:
     - Single polyploid carcinoma (Exophytic growth)
     - Ulcerative carcinoma with clear margin (vlcerative growth)
     - Infiltrating
     - Diffuse carcinoma linitis plastica

  II. Japanese classification: Early gastric cancer
      i. Protruded
      ii. a. Elevated
          b. Flat
          c. Depressed
      iii. Excavated.

  III. Lauren classification:
     - *Intestinal gastric cancer:* In this variety the tumor resembles a carcinoma else where in the tubular gastrointestinal tract and forms polypoid tumors or ulcers.
     - *Diffuse gastric cancer:* It infiltrates deeply into the stomach without forming obvious mass lesions but spreads widely in the stomach wall.

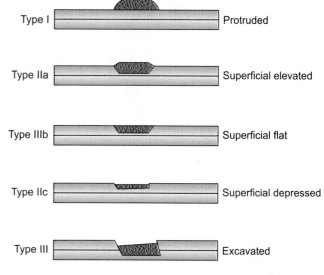

Japanese classification for Early Gastric Cancer

IV. Who classification of carcinoma stomach on pathological varieties:
    i. Adenocarcinoma
       a. Intestinal type
       b. Diffuse type
    ii. Papillary adenocarcinoma
    iii. Tubular adenocarcinoma
    iv. Mucinous adenocarcinoma
    v. Signet ring cell carcinoma
    vi. Adenosquamous carcinoma
    vii. Squamous cell carcinoma
    viii. Undifferentiated carcinoma
    ix. Unclassified carcinoma

V. Ming's classification:
   i. Expanding
   ii. Infiltrating

Common Sites of Gastric Cancer

i. Most common site is prepyloric and pyloric region 65%.
ii. Body 25%.
iii. Fundus and gastroesophageal junction (GE junction) 10%.

- **Microscopically**
  - Adenocarcinoma most common
  - Adenosquamous or squamous cells carcinoma rare it occus usually near GE junction.

- **Clinical features:**
  - Typical features of gastric cancer are anorexia with marked weight loss, upper abdominal discomfort or

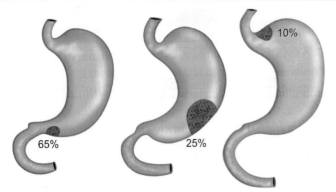

Precent of cancers stomach at different sites

pain and a sense of fatigue but unfortunately these features appear in advanced gastric cancer

- Early gastric cancer may often be confused with benign peptic ulcer disease
- I advanced carcinoma early satiety bloating, distention vomiting along with abdominal pain or discomfort features of gastric outlet obstruction (GOO).
- 3 'A' are the most common features
- A—anorexia
- A—anemia
- A—asthenia
- Malena is more common than hematemesis
- Dysphagia with mass in upper abdomen.
- **On physical exam:** Mass in pylorus lies just above the umbilicus, mass arising form the body lies more proximal at epigastrium
  - Ascites+ve , Troisier's sign (involvement of left supra-clavicular nodes)
  - +ve Trousseau's sign, i.e. migrating thrombophlebitis present.
  - Anemia, cachexia
  - Multiple nodular mass may be palpable on DRE called Blumer shelf at rectovesical pouch in male and pouch of Dougla in female.
  - Krukenberg tumor may be palpable
  - Sister Mary Joseph's nodule at umbilicus
  - Along with jaundice, liver may be palpable with secondaries.
- **Investigations** – already discussed
- **Treatment** – already written in questions answers portion.
- **Know the steps of gastrectomy phase**
- **Notes on gastrointestinat stromal tumors (GISTs)**
- **What is GISTs?**

- Gastrointestinal stromal tumors are the most common mesenchymal tumors of GI tract and are most frequently arise from the stomach.
  Leiomyoma and leiomyosarcomas are grouped as GIST
- **Sites:** Most common site is stomach 60-70%.
  - 30-40% other sites of GI tract.
- **Histological origin:** Histologically GIST originate from the cells of Cajal, autonomic nerve related GI pacemaker cells that regulate intestinal motility.
- **Presentations:** After 4th decade, mean age 60 at diagnosis
  - Most common presentations are GI bleeding.
  - Patients may presents with lump abdomen hematemesis, malena once the tumor ulcerate.
  - Nonspecific presentations are anorexia, weight loss, anemia, etc.
  - Abdominal mass with features of gastric outlet obstruction, etc.
- **Investigations**
  i. Endoscopic biopsy is diagnostic in approximately 50% of case. As by endoscopy mucosa appears normal there by biopsy may be inconclusive. The lesion starts usually in mesenchyma, therefore involvement of mucosa is unlikely.
  ii. Barium meal X-ray may help in diagnosis.
- **Biological Behavior**
  - Biological behavior of GIST is peculiar. Small tumor behave like benign and large tumor like malignant
  - 70 -80% GISTs are positive for CD34 a hematopoietic progenitor cell antigen.
  - A subset of GISTs lack C-kit mutations C-kit is a transmembrane tyrosine kinase receptor which is responsible for cells growth.
- **Treatment:**
  Surgery is the mainstay of treatment. The goal of surgery is a margin negative resection to include en bloc resection of adjacent organs if involved by direct extension.
- **Small tumor:** Wedge resection of stomach may be curative.
- **Large tumor:** Partial gastrectomy to be done.
- **Recurrent disease:**
  Salvage surgery to resect recurrent disease has not been demonstrated to improve survival.
- **CT/RT** has not been proven to be effective.
- **Prognosis:**
  - Over all 5 years survival for gastric GISTs is up to 48% (19-56%).
  - After complete resection over all 5 years survival is up to 63% (32-63%).

- USG guided FNAC can be performed carefully to diagnose GISTs.
- **Follow-up:** Most recurrence occur usually in the first 2 years, presenting as a local disease most often, it is associated with liver metastases.
- **Imatinib mesylate** a competitive inhibitor of certain tyrosine kinases dose 400-600 mg daily for 2 years to prevent recurrence.
  Imatinib mesylate is approved for use in CD 117 positive unresectable and/or metastatic GISTs.

Gastric Lymphoma

- Gastric lymphoma is an interesting disease commonly occurs in 6th decade.
- Type
  A. *Primary:* When it is localized to the stomach it accounts for approximately 5% of all gastric neoplasm. Primary gastric lymphoma arises from 'B' cell and from Mucosa Associated Lymphoid Tissue (Maltoma).
  B. *Secondary:* Stomach is involved secondary to generalized lymphadenopathy. This is more common. Most commonly found in the cardia or body of the stomach as opposed to the antrum.
- **Pathology**
  - Primary gastric lymphoma remains in the stomach for a long period before involving the lymph nodes
  - In an early stage, the disease takes the form of a diffuse mucosal thickening which may ulcerate and lymph nodes involvement is late.
  - Lymphocytes are usually not found in normal gastric mucosa but have been found in association with *H. pylori* infection.
  - Most common lymphoma is diffuse large B cell lymphoma (55%) next common is Maltoma 4% .
- **Clinical features:**
  i. 3 'A'—Anorexia
     — Anemia
     — Asthenia
  ii. Lump abdomen with or without gastric outlet obstruction
  iii. Hematemesis, malena.
- **Diagnosis:**
  i. Endoscopy generally reveals nonspecific gastritis or gastric ulcerations with mass lesions being unusual.
     Occasionally a submucosal growth pattern will render endoscopic biopsies nondiagnostic.
  ii. CECT abdomen and chest to detect lymphadenopathy

An enlarge lymph nodes should be biopsied. *H. pylori* testing should be performed by histology if negative confirmed by serology.
  iii. Complete blood count, bone marrow aspirations are required.

- **Criteria for diagnosis primary gastric lymphoma:**
  - Lymphoma localized to stomach only
  - No other lymphadenopathy like superficial mediastinal detected.
  - Bone morrow, CBC, liver, spleen are normal.

In secondary gastric lymphoma lymphocytosis is common feature bone marrow may be involved–lymphadenopathies to other sites.

Treatment

Primary gastric lymphoma controversial but it seems most appropriate treatment is surgery alone.

Lesions in fundus or proximal stomach which is more common site total gastrectomy is the answer lesion in antrum or distal part—Distal gastrectomy.

Some other groups claim that primary gastric lymphoma may be treated by chemotherapy alone. But logically C$^+$ alone may be appropriate for the patients with systemic disease only.

Gastric involvement with diffuse lymphoma like in non-Hodgkin's lymphoma is to be treated usually with chemotherapy alone.

For complications like perforations or bleeding, gastrectomy is the ultimate answer.

The chemotherapeutic agents are:
MOPP
M—Mechlorethamine
O—Oncovin (vincristine)
P—Procarbazine
P—Prednisolone
CHOP
C —Cyclophosphamide
H—Hydroxydaunomycin
O —Oncovin
P—Prednisolone
CVP
C—Cyclophosphamide
V—Vincristine
P—Prednisolone
Presently monoclonal antibody like rituximab approved as a single agent or combination with CHOP in treatment of both low grade follicular NHL and diffuse high grade lymphoma.

Dose – 375 mg/m^2 slow infusion every 3-4 weekly.

My patient, Hari Ram, a 60-year-old farmer resident of Gujarat, presented with:
- Heaviness and lump in the central part of left mid abdomen for last 1 year.
- Backache along with it for same duration.

History of Present Illness

My patient was apparently asymptomatic 1 year back since when he developed heaviness in the central part of the abdomen and feeling of a lump at the same site. The size is gradually progressive, and painless. He also complains of backache almost with the same duration intermittently with no relieving or aggravating factor, non-radiating, relieved automatically or by analgesics.

There is a history of unquantified weight loss and loss of appetite for last 6 months. There is no history of abdominal trauma (precipitating factor), fever, and night sweats, pruritus (lymphoma).

No history suggestive of obstruction in either urinary or GI tract (obstructive symptoms).

No history of tingling, numbness but low back pain is there (compression in the lumbar nerve).

No history of chest pain, bone pain or weakness, malaise jaundice (exclude metastases).

Past History

No history of hypertension, diabetes, radiation exposure (radiation increases 50 times risk of STS), chemical exposure (exposure to phenoxy acetic acid, chloramphenicol, vinyl chloride, arsenic).

Operative History

No history of previous operation (long standing scar may develop STS).

Drug History

No history of intake of drugs like methysergide, hydralazine, alpha methyldopa.

No history of exposure to gadolinium dye.

Family History

Not suggestive.

Personal History

Farmer by occupation. No history of smoking 10-15 bidies per day. No history of alcohol. Off and on exposure to insecticides.

General Survey

Patient is cooperative.
    Lying comfortably on bed.
    Average built, and nourished.
    Pulse 80 per min.
    BP 112/70 mm Hg right arm supine. Temp (N) Resporatory 16/min
    No pallor, jaundice, edema, generalized lymphadenopathy or any other suggestive signs are there.

Systemic Examinations

Upper GI tract is within normal limit.

Abdomen

Inspection: Abdomen is scaphoid in shape but there is an obvious bulge around umbilicus, all quadrants moving with respiration, no visible vein, peristalsis or scar marks, noticed. External genitalia appears normal (testicular tumor may sometimes cause abdominal lymphadenopathy).

Palpation

Temperature not raised, nontender, flanks are not full, umbilicus central, there is obvious bulging at umbilical left lumbar, hypogastrium and partly at left iliac fossa. All quadrants move equally with respiration.

Deep palpation: There is a about 10 × 8 cm spherical retroperitoneal lump (as in knee elbow position it does not fall forward) the lump is around at left lumbar region, extending to umbilical partly region, left hypogastric and left iliac fossa).

Nonmobile, not moving with respiration, smooth surface, firm inconsistency, deeply placed, so all margins are not distinctly palpable except lower margin.

Percussion

Tympanitic (for bowel loop over it) on percussion.
Auscultation: Normal bowel sounds are heart, no bruit.
Other systems are within normal limit.

SUMMARY

My patient, 60-year-old farmer, presented with heaviness with painless progressive central mid abdominal lump along with low backache for last 1 year without any trauma or obstructive features. General examination is essentially normal. There is a 10 × 8 cm spherical retroperitoneal lump, fixed, smooth surface, ill-defined margin and does not move with respiration.

So my provisional diagnosis is retroperitoneal soft tissue sarcoma.

Points in Favor

Elderly man, retroperitoneal central mass, painless, smooth surface, crossing midline, no urinary or GI symptoms.

Points against: No risk factors, 1 year history without vascular or urinary tract involvement.

Other Possibilities

1. Retroperitoneal lymph node enlargement.
   Points in favor: Elderly patients, deeply placed, large retroperitoneal mass, firm, variegated consistency, mostly smooth.
   Points in against: No primary malignancy noted. Any B symptoms like fever, weight loss, fever, etc. are not there.
2. Renal lump.
3. Adrenal lump.

QUESTIONS AND ANSWERS

How will you proceed in this case?
I will confirm my diagnosis first.
  I will do **IUSG abdomen**.
  It has got a diagnostic role. It shows:
  i. Organ of origin.
  ii. Solid mass or complex mass where cystic component is there along with solid.
  iii. Involvement of lymph nodes.
  iv. It is useful adjoining to MRI/CT when findings are indeterminate and for delineating adjacent vascular structures.
  II CECT abdomen—(Most preferred for retroperitoneal tumor).

To see the extent of soft tissue tumor burden and proximity of the tumor to the vital structures.

CT can provide a detailed survey of abdomen and pelvis and delicate adjacent organs and vascular structures.

[Remember for extremity sarcomas, MRI is better than CT scan].

MRI perfectly delineates muscle groups and it distinguishes bone, vascular structures, nerves and tumors and relation with tumor. A base line image is usually obtained 3 months after surgery.

III Biopsy—either FNAC or tru Cut.
FNAC—Diagnostic accuracy 60-90%.

It is indicated for primary diagnosis of soft tissue sarcoma provided the experienced cytopathologist is present at that center.

But FNAC cannot grade the tumor.

It is used mainly to sample deep seated tissue and to diagnose metastasis and recurrence.

Tru Cut Biopsy

It is safe, accurate and economical to diagnose STS.

The tissue is sufficient for several diagnostic tests, i.e. histological typing and grading of sarcoma, accuracy > 95%.

Incisional Biopsy

It is a reliable diagnostic method for definitive and specific histologic identification.

Indicated (i) when FNAC or tru cut biopsy is not sufficient or inconclusive, (ii) Deep or superficial tumor >3 cm.

Excision Biopsy

Usually done when the tumor size is < 3 cm and the tumor is easily accessible.

What is the role of CECT chest in case of a soft tissue sarcoma?

In all cases of STS, CECT is not required.

CECT chest to be done to exclude pulmonary metastasis.

i. In case of high grade tumor or intermediate tumor and tumor > 5 cm.

ii. Soft tussue tumor, which have more predilection for lymph nodes metastasis like synovial cell sarcoma, clear cell sarcoma, angiosarcoma, rhabdomyosarcoma (Remember SCAR).

How will you treat a case of soft tissue sarcoma?

Extremity sarcoma

In past two decades, a multimodality treatment approach has improved survival and quality of life for patients with extremity sarcoma.

But the mainstay of treatment is wide local excision, i.e. the tumor is to excised with a 2 cm margin of surrounding normal soft tissue.

- In T1 N0 M0—postoperative eratively neither CT nor RT are recommended.
- But in T2 N0 M0 lesions—wide local excision and adjuvant CT and/ or RT recommended.
- For stages II, III disease – Neoadjuvant CT and /or RT-> Surgery-> Adjuvant CT and /or RT recommended.
- If the primary is unresectable or marginally resectable at presentation.

Preoperative CT and /or RT

↓Assess

Resectable   Unresectable

↓   ↓

Surgery   Palliative CT/RT

(WLE) Symptomatic palliative resection, ablation, etc. + CT and/or RT

- In metastatic disease:

If mets is detected at the time of diagnosis, the primary tumor can be managed as follows:

Metastasectomy may be considered if single organ or limited metastasis

↓

With neoadjuvant and or adjuvant CT/ RT or both.

↓

Radiofrequency ablation if mets is less than 3 cm can be done up to 7 cm tumor maximum.

Alternative option is chemoembolization for controlling the metastasis.

Treatment for retroperitoneal sarcoma is:

Complete surgical resection is the treatment of choice for both primary and recurrent retroperitoneal sarcomas with minimum 1 cm margin (2 cm is better).

[Usually retroperitoneal sarcoma involves vital structures so the margins are often compromised because of anatomical constraints. However, complete resection still possible in 40-60% of cases].

Chemotherapy has got very limited role in retroperitoneal sarcoma.

Preoperative CT/RT still to be determined regarding their roles in treating retroperitoneal sarcomas.

SMALL NOTES ON STS

Soft tissue can be defined as nonepithelial, extraskeletal tissue including voluntary muscles fat, fibrous tissue along with vessels and nerve supplying these tissues.

It excludes reticuloendothelial system, glia, supporting tissue of various parenchymal organs, i.e. tissue of mesodermal origin.

Soft tissue comprises almost 50% of total body weight.

Malignant tumors of soft tissue are called sarcoma and characterized by:

- Locally aggressive growth.
- Invading surrounding structures.

- Recurrence.
- Distant metastasis.

Previous radiation therapy, exposure to chemicals immunodeficiency, long standing scars, chronic irritation and genetic cancer syndromes like Gardner's syndrome, von-Recklinghausen's disease are responsible to develop soft tissue sarcoma.

The lower extremities are the most common site approxmately 40%, trunk-19%, upper extremities 13% and retroperitoneum 12-13%, head neck 9% and other sites 1% only. Gastrointestinal stromal tumor is one of the variants of STS.

On the basis of its aggressiveness and morphology sarcomas are graded as low, intermediate and high grade.

Systemic spread at the presentation is relatively uncommon 7-25% only.

The most common site of metastasis is lung and bones.

Common variants of soft tissue sarcomas are:

- Malignant fibrous histiocytoma (most common worldwide).
- Liposarcoma (most common in our country).
- Fibrosarcoma
- Leiomyosarcoma
- GIST
- Synovial sarcoma
- Rhabdomyosarcoma- most common in childhood
- Malignant mesenchymal tumor
- Malignant peripheral nerve sheath tumor
- Clear cell sarcoma.

Tumor Grades

Gx—Grade cannot be assessed   Low grade
G1—Well differentiated   Low grade
G2—Moderately differentiated   Low grade
G3—Poorly differentiated   High grade
G4—Undifferentiated.   High grade

TNM staging:
T1—The tumor is < 5 cm.
T2—The tumor is 5-10 cm.
T3—The tumor is 10-15 cm.
T4—The tumor is > 15 cm.
Each stage is divided into:
a. Superficial tumor.
b. Deep tumor.

[Superficial tumor means the tumor is located superficial to superficials fascia without invading the fascia.

Deep tumor is located beneath the superficial fascia or the tumor invading superficial fascia.

Most of the tumors are usually deep tumors.

Regional lymph nodes (N)

Nx—Regional lymph nodes cannot be assessed.
N0—No regional lymph node metastasis.
N1—Regional lymph node metastasis.

Distant metastasis

Mx—Distant metastasis cannot be assessed.
M0—No distant metastasis.
M1—Distant metastasis.

SHORT NOTE ON LIMB SALVAGE SURGERY

Limb salvage surgery is the standard care of most extremity sarcomas.

Neoadjuvant chemotherapy and or radiotherapy and availability of improved prosthesis may facilitate limb salvage surgery.

Isolated Regional Perfusion

Isolated regional perfusion is an investigational approach for treating extremity sarcomas. It is mainly as a limb sparing alternative for locally advanced soft tissue sarcomas or as a palliative treatment to achieve local control for the patients of distant metastatic disease.

Both artery and vein can be used for limb perfusion.
External iliac vessels are used for thigh tumors.
Femoral /popliteal vessels are used for calf tumors.
Axillary vessels for upper limbs tumors.

Gastrointestinal Stromal Tumor (GIST)

Surgery remains the mainstay of treatment for both localized and locally advanced GIST. Complete resection with negative margins improve the survival.

Systemic chemotherapy not effective for GIST.

Imatinib (C-Kit inhibitor) is the only effective systemic therapy for metastatic or locally advanced GIST.

Dose-400-600 mg daily for 2 years.

[C-Kit – It is a transmembrane glycoprotein receptor with tyrosine kinase activity. It is related to regulation of cell growth and survival].

Chemotherapeutic drugs commonly used in sarcomas are: Doxorubicin.

Dacarbazine and Ifosfamide.

Prognosis

Overall 5 years survival of all stages of STS is 50-60%.
80% patients of metastatic disease die within 2-3 years.

HIGHLIGHT ON RETROPERITONEAL SPACE AND ITS DISEASES

Anatomy

The retroperitoneal space is bounded:
  i. Anteriorly by posterior parietal peritoneum.
 ii. Posteriorly by vertebral column, iliopsoas muscle, quadratus lumborum muscle and tendinous part of the transverse abdominis muscle.
iii. Superiorly by diaphragm and 12th rib.
 iv. Inferiorly by levator ani muscle and pelvic diaphragm.

Abnormalities in Retroperitoneal Space

a. Diseases of the specific retroperitoneal organs like adrenal, kidney, vascular diseases, etc.
b. Retroperitoneal tumors
   Benign—   Lipoma
                Neurofibroma
                Fibroma.
   Malignant:
        Liposarcoma
        Malignant fibrous histiocytoma.
        Lymphoma (most commonly with NHL)
        Secondaries to retroperitoneal lymph nodes.

Characteristics of Retroperitoneal Mass

- Large, firm to hard mass.
- Nonmobile, usually surface is smooth but in lymphoma it is nodular.
- Margins not well defined.
- Nontender.
- Not moving with respiration.
- Does not fall forward on knee elbow position.
- Resonant or percussion (as intestine in the front).

Features of Soft Tissue Sarcoma

- Mass felt per abdomen.
- All features of retroperitoneal mass.

- Presenting features:
  - Back pain.
  - Mass abdomen.
  - Compressive features line venous compression causing varicose vein compression of ureter causing hydronephrosis.
  - Gastric outlet obstruction, intes final obstruction.

Investigations

To confirm the diagnosis first.
1. USG abdomen:
   - To see the retroperitoneal mass.
   - Compressive features like hydronephrosis.
   - LN involvement, etc.
   - USG guided FNAC- sensitivity 60-93%.
   - Tru cut biopsy- sensitivity 90%.
2. CECT abdomen:
   - Confirm the USG findings.
   - To see the vascular involvement, celiac trunk, Superior mesenteric artery (SMA), IVC.
3. MRI: Accurately delineates the muscle group.
   - Distinguishes among bone, vessels and nerve and soft tissue involvement.
4. To exclude metastasis
   Chest X-ray to exclude pulmonary metastosis initially.
   CECT chest – to be considered when the tumor size is >5 cm to exclude pulmonary metastasis.

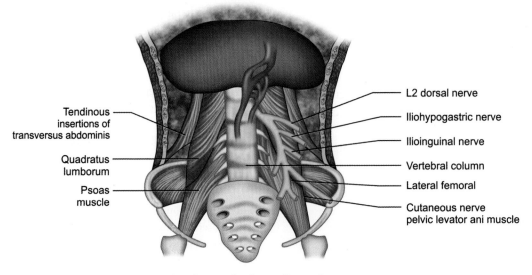

Anatomy of retroperitoneal space

Treatment of STS

- *Neoadjuvant therapy:* Role of preoperative CT/RT still under evaluation.
- *Surgery:* Wide local excision with 2 cm margin of surrounding normal soft tissue. It usually involves the adjuvcant organs often.
- Palliative debulking surgery may be undertaken when the tumor is inoperable.

- Postoperative radiotherapy—either brachytherapy or external beam radiotherapy- effective.
  Dose—60-70 Gy is enough for postoperative treatment.
- Chemotherapy- not much more effective for retroperitoneal STS. The chemotherapeutics agents used are: Doxorubicin, Dacarbazine and Ifosfamide.
- In recurrent disease surgery again is the mainstay of treatment.

My patient, Omvati, a 40-year-old lady, resident of Mathura from very low socioeconomic status, presented with complain of:

- Pain left upper abdomen for last 2 years.
- Passage of black stool for last 6 months.

My patient was apparently asymptomatic 2 years back since when she has been having pain in his left upper abdomen which is insidious onset, continuous, dull aching, nonradiating, aggravated on exertion, relieved after medication but sometimes the pain is very embarrassing.

Sudden onset at the left flank.

History of—passage of black stool one episode 6 months back. Stayed for 2-3 days.

History of unquantified weight loss and anorexia are also there but there is no history of:

- Fever with chill and rigor.
- Hematemesis, vomiting.
- Jaundice in recent past.
- Petechial spots in the body.
- No urinary disturbance or GI symptoms.
- No history suggestive of any chronic hepatic insufficiency.
- Bowel, bladder habits are normal.

Past History

- No past history of HTN, DM, IHD, etc.
- No history of blood transfusion in past.
- No history of any regular injection intake.
- No significant history of operation in past.
- No history of drug allergy.
- No history of injections, being given to the patient.

Personal History

Housewife, from low socioeconomic background.
Nonalcoholic.
She is premenopausal lady.
Family history: Not contributory.

General Examination:

Patient is cooperative, anxious looking average built and nourished.

    P- 80/min, BP-130/80 mm Hg, Pallor +, Icterus +.

    No edema or generalized lymphadenopathy noticed.

Abdomen:

On inspection:

- Abdomen is scaphoid.
- Umbilicus center.
- All quadrants moving with respiration.
- There is an obvious bulge at left hypochondrium and left lumbar region.
- No visible veins around umbilicus and in the flank.
- No scar marks.
- Flanks are not full.
- Hernial sites and external genitalia appear normal.

On palpation:

- Temperature not raised.
- Nontender.
- There is a 15 cm intra-abdominal mass occupying left hypochondrium, left lumbar and umbilical region.
- Crossing midline 2 cm.
- All margins palpable except upper margin which is merged within costal margin.
- At anterior border one notch is felt.
- Smooth surface.
- Moves with respiration.
- Nonballotable.
- So most probably it is splenomegaly.
- No hepatomegaly but free fluid is there on shifting dullness.
- Hernial sites and external genitalia are normal.
- No supraclavicular LN palpable.
- Digital rectal examination (DRE): NAD.

Other Systemic Examination

Respiratory system: Bilateral air entry equal, no adventitious sound heard.

CVS- S1, S2 (N), No murmur.

Others are essentially normal.

Summary

My patient, a 40-year-old lady presented with history of pain in left upper abdomen off and on for last 2 years and one episode of passage of black stool 6 months back without any history of fever, hematemesis or urinary symptoms.

On examination: Patient is anemic and mild icteric.

There is a 15 cm splenomegaly without hepatomegaly or ascites.

My provisional diagnosis is:

This is a case of portal hypertension, most probably due to noncirrhotic portal fibrosis or idiopathic cirrhosis.

Why do you say so?

- Female patient, aged 40 years.
- There is persistent splenomegaly with anemia.
- Ascites is there.
- No history of remarkable fever in the past.

Why the portal hypertension (PHT) here is not due to extrahepatic portal vein obstruction?

As the patient is 40-year-old. By the age either the disease outgrows or the patient would have been died till this time due to massive hemorrhage. Sometimes, patient may survive a long only when patient is under active treatment.

What are the differential diagnosis?

Differential diagnosis:

1. Tropical splenomegaly:
   - Hyperendemic area of malaria, kala-azar.
   - Common in female.
   - History of fever which is not seen in PHT.
   - Both spleno- and hepatomegaly.
2. Chronic myeloid leukemia (CML):
   - Average age 55 years.
   - Patient asymptomatic 11% cases.
   - Splenomegaly 90% cases.
   - Massive splenomegaly 10% cases.
3. Left sided isolated portal hypertension (Sinistral PHT) seen in chronic pancreatitis.

What is the clinical triad of portal hypertension?

- Splenomegaly
- Ascites
- Hematemesis/melana.

Suppose this is a case of portal hypertension-how will you proceed in this case?

I will confirm my diagnosis first.

I will do

i. Complete hemogram to rule out hypersplenism [Hyper-splenism manifested by leukopenia (WBC<4000 /cumm) and thrombocytopenia (platelet count <100000) has been reported in 33% cases].

ii. Pancytopenia owing to destruction of blood cells in the spleen.

iii. LFT- to differentiate cirrhotic from noncirrhotic portal hypertension (in cirrhosis total protein and serum albumin will be decreased).

To rule out—Active parenchymal disease (where SGOT, SGPT increased) which is contraindicated for surgery.

i. Coagulation profile:
   a. Prothrombin time (PT)
   b. Partial thromboplastin time (PTTK)
   c. Bleeding time (BT)
   d. Clotting time (CT)
   e. INR will be prolonged due to reduced PT and PTTK. [In cirrhosis PT is raised which is unresponsive to vit K].

ii. *Viral markers:* Hepatitis B surface antigen. HCV antibodies – to be done in all patients with suspected liver parenchymal disease.

USG Abdomen with Color Doppler

To establish the diagnosis to see the collaterals, **Varices at splenic hilum and stomach is diagnostic of PHT.**

It shows bright echo texture, nodular surface of liver in cirrhosis, periportal fibrosis in NCPF and normal liver in Extrahepatic portal vein obstruction (EHPVO). It also shows portal cavernoma (multiple small venous channel replacing thrombosed portal vein).

It may differentiate EHPVO from intrahepatic PHT by showing patency or thrombosis in portal vein.

In EHPVO—it shows extent of thrombus in portal vein, superior mesenteric vein, splenic vein, and left renal vein.

Diameter of portal vein and splenic vein and renal vein before shunt surgery.

Along with color Doppler it helps to detect direction of blood flow.

- Hepatopetal—to the liver.
- Hepatofugal—away from the liver.

To see the obstruction in hepatic veins or IVC in Budd-Chiari syndrome.

Upper GI Endoscopy

- To exclude esophagogastric varices and to grade the varices.
- To rule out other causes of hematemesis like gastric ulcer, duodenal ulcer, erosions, etc.
- To exclude nonvariceal cause of PHT, i.e. gastropathy.
- To exclude fundal varices. (It is found in left sided portal hypertension).

Liver Biopsy

- It is indicated to establish the etiology of PHT particularly in the doubtful cases.
- It is indicated in chronic Budd-Chiari syndrome to rule out secondary cirrhosis which may change the plan of management.

(Liver biopsy is contraindicated in presence of ascites and in deranged INR).

Spiral CT Angiography

- It gives a good picture of portal venous system.
- Gives all information before contemplating shunt surgery.
- It is useful to establish ectopic varices.
- It replaced the conventional venography.

Disadvantages

- Costly as restricted availability.
- It does not give any information about portal venous pressure.

MR Angiography

Has greater sensitivity than CT angio but more costly but it is most useful in Budd-Chiari syndrome.

How will you manage a case of bleeding esophageal varices?

I will do
i. Blood transfusion-after proper grouping and cross-matching.

ii. I will correct coagulopathy by giving injection vit K and by transfusing FFP.
iii. Depending on the availability of endoscopy:

If ndoscopy is available, endoscopic variceal ligation (EVL) or sclerotherapy to be done.

If it is not available, pharmacotherapy is the choice (as described below).

i. Esophageal balloon tamponade (Sengstaken-Blackemore tube).
ii. Pharmacotherapy – injection vasopressin/Octreotide/Somatostatin.
iii. Endoscopic sclerotherapy or banding.
iv. Assessment of portal vein patency by Doppler ultra-sound or CT.
v. TIPSS—Transjugular intrahepatic porta systemic stent shunts- to reduce portal venous pressure – resulting in reduction of variceal bleeding but this is not a permanent solution. It is used as a temporary measure till permanent treatment is offered like liver transplantation in cirrhotic patient.
vi. Surgical options:
   a. Portal decompressive procedures- portosystemic shunts.
   b. Nondecompressive procedure called Sigura and Fatagua operation consisting of:
      - Esophageal transection
      - Splenectomy
      - Gastric devascularization.
   c. Last option—Liver transplantation.

What is hypersplenism?

Hypersplenism is characterized by:
- Pancytopenia (anemia, leukopenia and thrombocytopenia).
- Splenomegaly.
- Reactive bone marrow hyperplasia.
- All are reversed by splenectomy.

Symptomatic hypersplenism-manifested by:
- Recurrent sepsis.
- Epistaxis
- Spontaneous petechiae, platelet count <50000/ cumm, WBC< 2000/cumm
- Low Hb in absence of GI bleeding. Thereby repeated blood transfusion, even twice in a week, is required which demands surgical intervention.

What are the indications of splenectomy in portal hypertension?

i. Prophylactic splenectomy is indicated to prevent traumatic splenic rupture which may endanger the life. Usually it is carried out with esophagogastric devascularization.

ii. Left sided portal hypertension (sinistral portal hypertension) in a patient with isolated splenic vein thrombosis, usually as a sequelae of chronic pancreatitis.

iii. Symptomatic hypersplenism—where platelet count <50,000/cumm; WBC<2000/cumm and low Hb where repeated blood transfusion is required.

In active bleeding varices what is procedure of choice sclerotherapy or banding?

In active bleeding varices sclerotherapy is the procedure of choice. Banding will be a very difficult procedure because of active bleeding; the point of bleeding for banding is not properly visible in active bleeding.

When will you consider pharmacotherapy?

The indications of pharmacotherapy are:
- For primary prophylaxis and to prevent recurrent variceal bleeding.
- Control of active (acute) variceal bleeding.
- To control the bleeding from portal hypertensive gastropathy.

  Prophylactic beta-blocker to be given in all cases of PHT.

  In massive GI bleeding due to PHT, pharmacotherapy should be started immediately while patient is being shifted for endoscopy.

What is the role of beta-blockers in PHT?

Beta-blockers block beta-adrenergic receptors
↓
Thereby allow increased alpha-adrenergic activity
↓
Leading to splanchnic arteriolar vasoconstriction.
↓
Decrease portal venous pressure
Beta-blockers also decrease heart rate and cardiac output
↓
Tending to decrease portal venous inflow
↓
So reduces the risk of variceal bleeding

[Dose of beta-blockers to be adjusted to achieve 20-25% reduction of resting heart rate (absolute heart rate 55-60/min) usual dose of propranolol is 40 mg once or twice daily].

How do you grade the varices in upper GI endoscopy?

Grade I   Varices visible on Valsalva's maneuver only.

Grade II   Varices occupy <25% of the circumference of the esophageal lumen.

Grade III Varices occupy 25-50%, of the circumference of the esophageal lumen.

Grade IV   Varices obliterating the lumen of esophagus.

Which type of varices are more prone to develop for active bleeding?

- Varices upon the varices.
- Presence of cherry red spots on varices.
- Grade IV varices.

What are the surgical procedures for portal decompression?

There are two types of portal systemic shunts:
a. *Selective:*
   - Warren—Distal splenorenal shunt.
   - Inokuchi—Left gastric – caval shunt (coronocaval shunt).
b. *Nonselective:*
   - Whipple—Portocaval shunt.
   - Linton—Proximal splenorenal shunt.
   - Drapanas—Interposition mesocaval shunt.
   - Cooley—Side to side splenorenal shunt with spleen preservation.

What are the types of porta systemic shunts?

There are three types of porta systemic shunts:
i. Porta caval—(End to side/ side to side)
   - Selective—distal splenorenal shunt (DSRS splenorenal shunt).
   - Partial shunts—small diameter porta caval shunt (Sarfeh shunt).
ii. Central splenorenal:
   - Proximal (side to side)—coronocaval shunt (Inokuchi).
iii. Mesocaval:
   - Cavomesenteric
   - Mesocaval 'H' graft.

Whats all are the indications for elective surgery as the primary modality of treatment for PHT?

The indications are:
i. Left sided portal hypertension also called sinistral portal hypertension. Splenectomy is the curative surgery for this situation.
ii. Symptomatic hypersplenism surgery is indicated for correction of hypersplenism.

iii. Bleeding from ectopic varices which are not amenable to endotherapy.
iv. Massive splenomegaly which is more prone to rupture on trivial trauma.
v. Continue growth retardation.
vi. Portal biliopathy- to decompress portal cavernoma.
vii. A rare blood group patient, patient is in remote area and where advanced medical facility is not available.
viii. Patient's choice.
    Elective surgery as rescue therapy
    • Failure of endoscopic sclerotherapy [EST]
    • Significant rebleed in defaulters.

What are the indications for TIPSS?

i. To control acute esophageal gastric variceal bleeding after failure of pharmacotherapy and endoscopic treatment.
ii. Repeated variceal bleeding despite of adequate endoscopic treatment.
iii. Refractory ascites in patient with cirrhosis.
iv. Hepatorenal syndrome.
v. Budd-Chiari syndrome- to treat PHT as well as fluid retention.

Why the patient of PHT may present with obstructive jaundice?

Obstructive jaundice may be due to extensive pressure on the bile duct by periportal and pericholedochal varices.

What is the present concept of the variceal grades?

Presently varices are divided into two:
i. Large varices diameter > 5 mm
ii. Small varices diameter < 5 mm.

Do you know the grades of encephalopathy?

Encephalopathy is a sign of hepatic decompression.

Grade I: Euphoria, mild confusion slurring of speech, disorder in sleep rhythm.

Grade II: Drowsy, but responds to simple commands, inappropriate behavior.

Grade III: Sleeps most of the time but arousable, marked confusion, in coherent speech.

Grade IV: Unarousable. May respond to noxious stimuli.

SHORT NOTE ON PORTAL HYPERTENSION

Normal portal venous pressure is 5-8 mm Hg.
A portal venous pressure is > 10 mm Hg.
(>14 cm of water) is called portal hypertension.
Patient becomes symptomatic usually when the portal venous pressure is > 12 mm Hg.

Anatomy

Portal vein is formed by joining of splenic vein and superior mesenteric vein at the level of L2 vertebra behind the neck of pancreas.

Inferior mesenteric vein opens into splenic vein.
The main tributaries of portal veins are:
• Splenic vein
• Superior mesenteric vein
• Left gastric vein.
• Right gastric vein.
• Cystic veins.
• Right gastroepiploic vein.

Sites of porta systemic anastomoses:
i. At the lower third of esophagus:

Portal—The esophageal branches of left gastric vein.
Systemic—Esophageal veins draining the middle third of esophagus into azygos vein.

ii. Anorectal junction:
   • Portal—Superior hemorrhoidal vein-inferior mesenteric vein-splenic vein-portal vein.
   • Systemic—Middle and inferior hemorrhoidal veins-internal iliac-common iliac-IVC.

iii. Around umbilicus:
   Portal—Paraumbilical veins travel in the falciform ligament and accompany the ligamentum teres-left branch of portals vein.
   Systemic—Superficial veins of anterior abdominal wall (superior and inferior epigastric)-external iliac-IVC.

iv. Retroperitoneal space:
   Portal, veins of ascending colon, descending colon, pancreas.
   Systemic—Renal, lumbar and phrenic veins.

v. Bare area of liver:
   Portal—Veins of liver
   Systemic—Diaphragmatic veins.

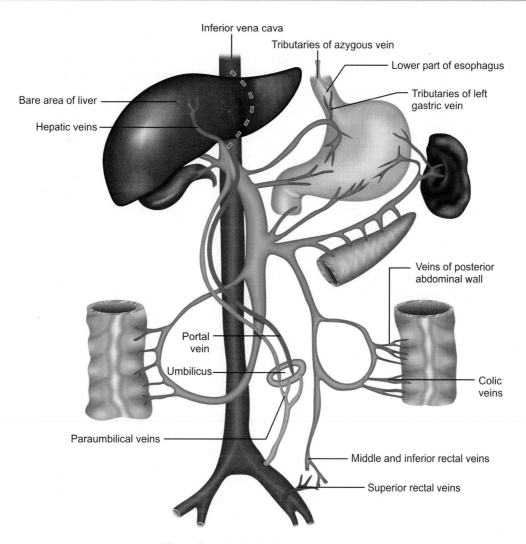

Inferior vena cava

Tributaries of azygous vein

Lower part of esophagus

Tributaries of left gastric vein

Bare area of liver

Hepatic veins

Veins of posterior abdominal wall

Portal vein

Umbilicus

Colic veins

Paraumbilical veins

Middle and inferior rectal veins

Superior rectal veins

Sites of porta Systemic Anastomoses

Natural porto systemic shunt:

i. Gastro adrenorenal veins.

ii. Linorenal veins.

It is developed significantly more in Extra-hepatic portal venous obstruction (EHPVO).

Classification of PHT

According to the site of obstruction

1. Prehepatic: Presinusoidal
   - Splenic vein thrombosis.
   - Splenic arteriovenous fistula.
   - Splenomegaly.
2. Intrahepatic:

Presinusoidal:
- Noncirrhotic portal fibrosis (NCPF)
- Schistosomiasis.
- Idiopathic portal fibrosis.
- Congenital hepatic fibrosis.
- Chronic active hepatitis.
- Primary biliary cirrhosis.

Sinusoidal:
- Cirrhosis.
- Alcoholic hepatitis.

Postsinusoidal:
- Vascular occlusive disease.
- Alcoholic terminal hyaline sclerosis.

3. Posthepatic:
  • Budd-Chiari syndrome
  • Inferior venous congestion.

Portal Hypertension Incidence

India	Western country
i. Cirrhosis <50%	> 80%
ii. NCPF 10-25%	3-5%
iii. EHPVO 30-40%	5%
iv. Budd-Chiari syndrome 8-25%	<1%

Natural History of PHT

Natural history depends on the etiology of PHT:

In both cirrhosis and NCPF—the obstruction is intrahepatic there by the venous flow is hepatofugal, i.e. away from the liver.

The loss of portal perfusion occurs much slowly in NCPF.

Different effects of PHT in paitent of cirrhocis and NCPF

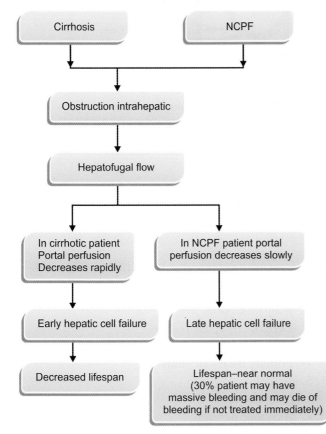

Development of liver cell failure occurs much later in comparison to cirrhotic portal hypertension. Non-nodular variety of NCPF patients have near normal lifespan but nodular variety behaves like cirrhotic patients; have deterioration of liver functions by 20 years.

In **EHPVO [Extrahepatic portal venous obstruction]**
Portal cavernoma maintains hepatopetal flow, i.e. flow
Towards the liver
↓
Adequate hepatic portal perfusion
↓
Preservation of hepatocytes functions
↓
Lifespan-normal

Few line on NCPF [Non-cirrhotic portal fibrosis]

Etiology still not established but it is believed that NCPF is due to perisinusoidal fibrosis
  ↓ causing obliteration of peripheral portal vein
   Leading to PHT
  Age group affected 30-50 years.
  Female predominant and from low socioeconomic background.
  Highest in northern and eastern parts in India.
  Imaging study- normal sized liver – peripheral cut off of terminal portal venous radicals ('Cut off' sign).
  Main intrahepatic portal vein remains-normal.

Few Lines of Extrahepatic Portal Venous Obstruction (EHPVO)

Common in developing countries. In India incidence rate is 40% among all cases of PHT.
  Seen in both adults and children.
  EHPVO occurs in children 75% of PHT among children.

The most common causes are:
• Neonatal peritonitis
• Dehydration due to diarrhea.
• Umbilical sepsis leading to portal pyemia.
• Congenital abnormalities- atresia/ stenosis of portal vein.

Adults and children:
• Hypercoaguable states.
• Polycythemia rubra vera.
• Protein C,S, antithrombin III deficiency.
• Neurofibrosis.

Adults:
- Iatrogenic trauma to portal vein.
- Chronic pancreatitis, pancreatic carcinoma.
- Abdominal trauma.

Left sided PHT:
- Also called sinistral PHT.
- Seen in patients with isolated splenic vein thrombosis.
- It causes isolated varices in gastric fundus.
- Splenectomy- curative.

Cirrhotic PHT

Causes
- Alcohol.
- Post necrotic (Hepatitis B and C virus)
- Primary biliary cirrhosis.
- Primary sclerosing cholangitis.

Budd-Chiari syndrome:
- Incidence in India—10-25%.
- Due to hepatic venous outflow obstruction.
- Three types:
  Type I—Major hepatic vein obstruction. IVC patient.
  Type II—IVC obstruction above the level of hepatic vein obstruction.
  In India – pregnancy related hypercoagulability.
  - Infections
  - IVC web/ membrane.
  - Idiopathic.

Treatment:
  TIPSS
  Portocaval shunt- nonspecific.
  Mesocaval/mesoatrial shunt-specific.

CLINICAL PRESENTATION OF PHT

i. GI bleeding is the most common manifestation of portal hypertension [hematemesis, melena]. Almost 75% patients rebleed.
ii. Patients may present with hematemesis and melena or hematochezia. Hematemesis is spontaneous, painless, and profuse.
iii. Patient may present with anemia with splenomegaly often seen in NCPF and EHPVO.
iv. Patient may present with the features of hypersplenism.
v. Others are: ascites, jaundice, growth retardation, etc.

Mechanism of Variceal Bleeding

1. Hepatic venous pressure gradient (HVPG) = WHVP – FHVP (Wedge hepatic venous pressure- free hepatic venous pressure).

   HVPG reflects portal pressure, WHVP reflects sinusoidal pressure and FHVP reflects hepatic venous pressure.

2. Stress in the wall of the varix: (remember TPR)
   Lap lace law
   $T = p \times r/w$
   T = wall tension, P = pressure in varix
   R = radius of varix and w = wall thickness.

$$\downarrow \text{Pressure} = \downarrow \text{Radius of varix}$$
$$\downarrow$$
$$\downarrow \text{Wall thickness}$$
$$\downarrow$$
$$\text{Rupture of varices}$$
$$\downarrow$$
$$\text{Bleeding}$$

How to measure portal pressure?

The liver receives 2/3rd of its blood supply from portal vein. Portal vein wedge hepatic venous gradient (WHVP) = Wedge hepatic venous pressure (WHVP)–Free hepatic venous pressure (FHVP).

   Normal pressure gradient is 5-6 mm Hg.

   A gradient of 12 mm Hg or more develops bleeding varices.

   Hepatic venous pressure gradient reflects portal venous pressure. WHVP reflects sinusoidal pressure.

   FHVP reflects hepatic venous pressure.

PHARMACOTHERAPY IN PHT

1. Splanchnic vasoconstrictors > decrease portal blood flow > low PHT.

Drugs used are:
i. Beta blockers-nonselective (Propranolol, nadolol, carvedilol) propranolol is the most commonly used beta blocker.

   Mechanism of action: These drugs (i) causing splanchnic arteriolar vasoconstriction leading to decrease portal venous inflow, (ii) decreasing heart rate and cardiac output, also reduces portal venous infow.

Dose to be adjusted to achieve 25% reduction in resting heart rate. Dose of propranolol initially 10 mg thrice daily.

ii. Vasopressin and its analogous- Glypressin, Terlipressin, ornipressin.

Hormones- somatostatin

Somatostatin analogue, octreotide, vapreotide.

2. Vasodilators:

Mechanism of action: Reduce intrahepatic vascular resistance.

Drugs are:

i. **Nitates**
- Short acting- NTG.
- Long acting – Isosorbide mononitrate.
Isosorbide dinitrate.

iii. Alpha-adrenergic antagonist- Prazosin.

3. Miscellaneous agents:

Metoclopramide.

Calcium channel blockers.

ACE inhibitors – Losartan.

Vasopressin-mechanism of action- causing splanchnic arteriolar vasoconstriction leading to decrease portal venous inflow.

Dose: 20 units in 200 ml of crystalloid solution over 20 minutes IV infusion.

Commonly used in acute variceal bleeding.

Adverse effect:

Myocardial and mesenteric ischemia 25% cases.

- **Somatostatin:**

Mechanism of action- splanchnic arteriolar vasoconstriction

↓

Low portal inflow

↓

Low PHT

Dose: IV bolus dose 250 mgm followed by continuous IV infusion 250 mgm/hr.

Adverse effect: Hyperglycemia.

- **Octreotide:**

Mechanism of action: Significantly low azygos blood flow

Low wedge hepatic pressure gradient (WHPG)

↓

↓ PHT

Dose: 50 mgm IV followed by infusion 50 mgm/hr continuous.

Usually it is used in conjunction with endotherapy to control acute variceal bleeding.

- Endoscopic therapy:

(Sclerotherapy and Banding)

Sclerotherapy: It is highly practiced to control both acute variceal bleeding and long-term control.

Sclerosants used are:

Synthetic products: 1.5% sodium tetradecyl sulfates
                                          0.5-1% polidocanol.

Fatty acid derivatives: 5% sodium morrhuate
                                          5% ethanolamine oleate.

Other agents: Absolute alcohol
                                 3% phenol in water.
                                 5% phenol in oil.

Among all 3% phenol has been reported highly effective safe, economical and easily available sclerosant.

Schedule of injection: Varices are usually injected at weekly interval till obliteration of varices.

Few centers recommended 3 days interval injections initially for first 3 times followed by monthly injections till obliteration.

Follow-up:

- Endoscopy has to be repeated at 3 months interval for 1st year, then every 6 months interval for 2nd year and then yearly is sufficient.

Techniques of EST	Advantages	Disadvantages
i. Intravariceal	Less risk of ulceration and perforation and stricture formation	Injection site bleeding
ii. Paravariceal	No risk of bleeding from injected site. Less risk of systemic complications.	Take long-time to obliterate the varices, stricture. formation, can cause bleeding from eroded varix.
iii. Combination technique	Has advantages of both intravariceal and paravariceal techniques.	Risk of perforation, stricture formation due to paravariceal technique.

- Chance of recurrent bleeding is up to 70% in their lifetime. So long-term management is essential to prevent recurrent bleeding.

Efficacy: EST is effective in controlling acute variceal bleeding in 80-90% of patients. Over all mortality is < 2%.

VARICEAL LIGATION

Varices are ligated with elastic band. Application is started just above GE junction. 2-3 bands are applied to each varix ascending fashion.

To control acute variceal bleeding endoscopic variceal ligation (EVL) is equally effective as EST. But technically EVL is more difficult than EST in presence of massive bleeding as the field of vision is obstructed.

Disadvantages

Endoscopic variceal ligation (EVL)
Recurrence rate higher as para esophageal varices are not obliterated.
Not suitable for small varices (Grades I, II).
Very expensive (Approx 5000/ sitting).

COMMONLY USED PORTA SYSTEMIC SURGERIES

Porta caval shunt: (a) End to side (b) Side to side.
a. *End to side*: Portal vein devided and end of portal vein is anastomosed with the side of IVC.

Indication in emergency control of variceal bleeding where medical management has failed, the end to side porta caval shunt is the surgery of choice as it effectively decompreses the portal venous system and can be rapidly constructed.
b. *Side to side*: It maintains the continuity of portal vein; so it decreases sinusoidal pressure.

It is more effective in relieving ascites and prevents recurrent variceal hemorrhage too.
Indications: Budd-Chiari syndrome – as the portal vein serves as a major efferent conduit in relieving ascitis and as well portal hypertension.

Disadvantages of Porta Caval Shunt

i. Loss of portal perfusion
↓
Deterioration of liver functions.
ii. Hepatic encephalopathy- mostly in cirrhotic patients (40-50%) and in NCPF (20-40%).

Proximal Splenorenal Shunt (Linton)

Requires minimum 8 mm diameter of splenic vein and 10 mm of left renal vein.

Splenectomy to be done and hilar end of splenic vein is anastomosed to renal vein.

This shunt is a central shunt and functionally similar to porta caval shunt.

This is very popular in India as because it deals with:
i. Symptomatic splenomegaly and hypersplenism.
ii. Patients with EHPVO without any risk of developing encephalopathy.

Disadvantages: It is a nonselective shunt; there is a risk of encephalopathy even in patients with NCPF.

So it is not recommended in NCPF and cirrhotic patients.

Mesocaval Shunt

a. Interposition 'H' grafts- nonselective shunt. There is a interposition of autologous vein graft/synthetic graft between SMV and IVC.
b. Cavomesenteric shunt- in this infrarenal IVC is sutured and proximal end of IVC is anastomosed to side of SMV.

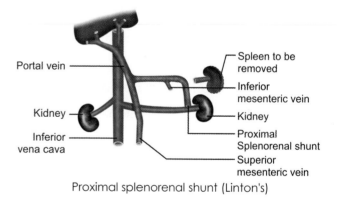

Proximal splenorenal shunt (Linton's)

It is a shunt of choice in children with EHPVO where splenic vein is not patent.

It is not suitable in adults as it may cause high incidence of pedal edema.

Indications of mesocaval shunt
i. Ectopic variceal bleeds.
ii. Budd-Chiari syndrome.
iii. Alternative to proximal splenorenal shunt where splenic vein is not patent.

Advantages

As the porta dissection is not done, it does not interfere with future liver transplant and hence this shunt is used as a long-

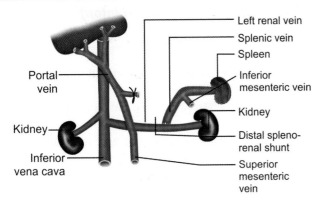

Distal spleno-renal shunt (Warren's DSRS) selective

term bridge to liver transplantation as a definitive surgical procedure, thereby in patients with failed TIPS.

Side to Side Splenorenal Shunt (Cooley Shunt)

It is a total lienorenal shunt with splenic preservation.

Indications
  i. Small diameter of splenic vein.
  ii. In porta biliopathy or ectopic varices.
  Advantage of the shunt: It relieves hypersplenism and decrease splenic size.

Distal Lienorenal Shunt (Warren Shunt)

Here distal end of splenic vein is anastomosed with the side of the left renal vein.

  Portal perfusion is maintained via mesenteric supply. It reduces the risk of postoperative hepatic encephalopathy. It also decreases hypersplenism.

Disadvantages
• Complex surgery, chance of shunt thrombosis is higher.

• Problem of early rebleed because of incomplete decompression in the initial phase prior to dilatation of short gastric veins.
• Not suitable for the patient with extensive thrombosis.
• Not suitable for intractable ascites, massive splenomegaly and emergency situation.

Coronocaval Shunt (Inokuchi Shunt)

Here left gastric vein anastomosed with IVC. Technically, it is very demanding but difficult.

NONSHUNT SURGERY

  i. Transthoracic extensive devascularization of lower esophagus.
  ii. Transabdominal devascularization of upper half of lesser curvature of stomach.
  iii. Splenectomy
  iv. Vagotomy.
  v. Pyloroplasty.

LIVER TRANSPLANTATION

In cirrhotic patient liver transplant cures liver cell failure and thus eliminates resistance to portal blood flow.

ELECTIVE LONG-TERM MANAGEMENT OF PHT

• Endoscopic sclerotherapy is the procedure of choice in the management of PHT irrespective of the etiology but it needs lifelong follow-up.
• The choice of surgery depends on the etiology, sites of bleeding, hypersplenism, portal biliopathy, etc.
• Thorough knowledge of hemodynamics of portal blood flow, anatomy of portal venous system is essential before shunt surgery.

CASE 15

Pelvic Mass

My patient, Mrs Kalawati, a 42-year-old female, who is a resident of Delhi, housewife by occupation, gravida 3, para 2, living 2, abortion 1, presented with the chief complaints of:

Pain in lower abdomen for 3 months.

Lump lower abdomen for 2 months.

The patient was apparently well 3 months back, since when she has pain lower abdomen. The pain is in the right iliac fossa, of moderate intensity, non-radiating, dull-aching, relieved by medication, not related to food intake or bowel motion. Pain not aggravated during menses, no history of dyspareunia (endometriosis, infected or twisted ovarian cyst).

The lump abdomen is in right lower abdomen which was noticed 2 months back when it was the size of a lemon and has gradually increased to the present size. It is not associated with bladder or bowel symptoms.

No history of fever, discharge per vaginum (to look for evidence of abdominal tuberculosis/pelvic inflammatory disease).

No history of, weight loss (tuberculosis/ovarian malignancy).

No history of bowel or bladder complaint (urinary tract infection, dysentery, pressure symptoms of ovarian mass).

Menstrual history: Menarche – 13 years of age, since then cycle is regular 4-5days/ 28-30 days duration, associated with mild dysmenorrhea. LMP was 2 weeks back, no history of preceding amenorrhea (to rule out pregnancy related complications, e.g. ectopic pregnancy, threatened abortion).

Obstetric history: 2 full term normal vaginal deliveries, 1 MTP was done at 2 months amenorrhea, 12 years back followed by bilateral tubal ligation.

Personal history: Vegetarian, non-smoker, non-alcoholic.

Medical and surgical history: No history of TB, DM, HT, epilepsy, bronchial asthma, blood transfusion, thyroid disorder. No history of previous surgery.

Family history: No history of TB/DM/HT/ovarian or colonic carcinoma in the family.

On Physical Examination

General Examination

Patient is conscious, cooperative and well oriented to time, place and person. She is of average built and nutritional status. Her height is 160 cm and weight is 64 kg, making her BMI–25 kg/m^2. She is afebrile to touch; her radial pulse is 84/min, good volume, synchronous, all peripheral pulses palpable, no radiofemoral delay, and vessel wall not palpable.

Her RR is 14/min thoracoabdominal.

Her blood pressure is 130/80 mm Hg in right brachial artery supine position.

There is mild pallor (clinically 9 gm%), no lymphadenopathy (may be present in case of tuberculosis or ovarian malignancy [supraclavicular lymph nodes]), no thyromegaly.

CVS examination: S1S2 normal, no adventitious sounds heard.

Respiratory system examination: Bilateral bronchovesicular breadth sounds are heard.

CNS system examination: Motor and sensory system is normal on examination.

Gynecological Exam:

Abdominal Exam

On **inspection** abdomen is scaphoid, umbilicus is central inverted, all quadrants moving well with respiration, no visible veins, lump or scar marks. Flanks are not full, all hernial sites appear normal.

On **palpation**, a spherical, firm, non-tender mass 4 × 4 cm is palpated above the pubic symphysis in the right iliac fossa. The mass has restricted side-to-side mobility, smooth surface and its lower limit cannot be reached. The skin overlying the mass is healthy.

On **percussion**, No evidence of free fluid in abdomen. On **auscultation**, bowel sounds are present.

Per speculum examination: no abnormality detected, pap smear taken.

Per vaginum examination: Same mass is felt in the right fornix, 8 × 10 cm smooth walled, cystic, with restricted mobility, tender on deep palpation, cervical motion not transmitted to the mass, mass felt separate from the uterus, groove sign felt between the mass and the uterus (the mass is probably, ovarian in origin, i.e. it is separate from the uterus).

Uterus: Anteverted multiparous size, nontender and deviated to the left.

What is your provisional diagnosis?

A 42-year-old para-2, live-2, abortion 1 with pelvoabdominal mass with pain abdomen.

What is the difference between abdominopelvic mass and pelvoabdominal mass? Why do you say this mass is pelvoabdominal?

A mass that arises from the pelvis and grows in size and thus reaches the abdomen is a pelvoabdominal mass. The mass is palpable per abdomen but on examination one cannot get below the mass. On the other hand an abdominopelvic mass originates in the abdomen and with further increase in its size it dips into the pelvis. However, the lower limit of such a mass is usually reached on per abdomen examination.

What is your differential diagnosis?

The mass could be:
a. Uterine origin: Pregnancy, fibroid
b. Ovarian origin: Ovarian cyst (functional, benign, malignant), endometriotic cyst, hydrosalpinx, para-ovarian cyst.
c. Urinary bladder mass.
d. Encysted fluid collection.

　　Also this patient has presented with pain lower abdomen, I would like to rule out any torsion which is especially possible with a large ovarian cyst or a subserous fibroid. However, torsion is seen in patients presenting with pain of acute onset.

What are fibroids or leiomyomas? What is their incidence and how do they commonly present?

Leiomyomas are most common tumors of the uterus. They are seen in over 25% of women aged 35 years and above and

are benign. They are well circumscribed, encapsulated solid tumors of the uterus. They contain fibrous tissue and muscle tissue in interlacing bundles. Most leiomyomas are asymptomatic, small and clinically inconsequential. They are diagnosed an ultrasonography scans. Symptoms vary depending upon the size and location of the fibroids and include menstrual disturbances like menorrhagia, polymenorrhea, pain, infertility, recurrent miscarriages, abdominal masses and pressure symptoms of bladder, kidneys and bowel.

How will you differentiate an ovarian mass from fibroid uterus?

Fibroid uterus may be uniformly smooth or nodular and regular in outline, nontender and firm to feel. Uterus is not felt separately. They can be palpated as irregular asymmetric enlargements of uterus. Cervical motion gets transmitted to the mass.

　　Ovarian cysts / tumors, are cystic, firm mass felt separate from uterus on bimanual palpation (the mass is felt separate from the uterus elicited by a groove sign) the cervical motion is not transmitted to the ovarian mass. However, it is sometimes difficult to differentiate pedunculated subserous fibroid and broad ligament fibroid from an ovarian mass by clinical examination.

How will you confirm your diagnosis?

I would first do an ultrasound (preferably a transvaginal ultrasound) to determine the site of origin of the mass, the nature of the mass (solid, cystic or of mixed echogenicity, hemorrhagic or endometriotic).

　　Please note following important USG findings/ appearances of the cysts:

Functional cyst: Unilocular, isoechoic cyst with smooth margins.

Chocolate cyst: Homogeneous ground glass with speckled appearance.

Dermoid cyst: Shows mixed echogenicity, with some solid (hyperechoic areas) and some isoechoic areas (fluid). It may also show areas of calcification (teeth/bone).

Hydrosalpinx: Sausage shaped complex cystic structure with reduced resistive index (RI) in the adnexal region.

What features on ultrasound go in favor of a benign or malignant mass?

Following features go in favor of benign or malignant features:

Benign features	Malignant features
Thin walled cyst	Thick walled
Simple or anechoic cyst	Solid tumor/solid areas in the cyst
No loculations	Multilocular
No septations	Thick septations
Unilateral	Bilaterality
No free fluid/ ascites	Presence of free fluid/ ascites
Smaller size	Larger size

What are the various gynecological causes of pelvic mass by approx frequency and age group?

Infancy: Functional cyst, germ cell tumor.

Prepubertal: Functional cyst, germ cell tumor.

Adolescent: Functional cyst, pregnancy, dermoid /other germ cell tumors, obstructing vaginal or uterine anomalies, epithelial ovarian tumor.

Reproductive: Functional cyst, pregnancy, uterus fibroids, epithelial ovarian tumor.

Perimenopausal: Fibroids, epithelial ovarian tumor, functional cyst.

Postmenopausal: Ovarian tumor, functional cyst, secondaries of gynecological origin in the bowel.

Whats are the characteristic features that suggest the provisional diagnosis of encysted tubercular peritonitis?

The patient usually above the age of puberty
Presents as a loculated mass abdomen,
There will be history of TB or features suggestive of TB.

What are the nongynecological causes of pelvic mass?

Arteriovenous malformation, diverticulosis, complicated appendicitis, bowel tumor, lymphadenopathy, gastro-intestinal masses like appendiceal abscess, appendiceal tumor, diverticular abscess, colonic tumor, genitourinary-Pelvic kidney, retroperitoneal-hematoma, lymphocyst, lymphoma, sarcoma.

What is an adnexal mass?

A lump in tissue near the uterus, usually in the ovary or fallopian tube. Adnexal masses include ovarian cysts, ectopic (tubal) pregnancies, paraovarian cysts, subserous or broad ligament fibroid.

Why this is not an ectopic on the basis of history? How will you definitely rule out an ectopic?

This 42-year-old lady is tubectomized and her last menstrual period is just 2 weeks back with normal flow. I will however rule it out for sure by doing a urine pregnancy test.

In this lady who is 42 years old what other investigations specific to this adnexal mass would you do?

I would do all routine investigations as this patient has a 10 cm cystic mass which would most probably require a surgical intervention of some form. These investigations include Hb, TLC, DLC, platelet count, blood urea, serum creatinine, Random blood sugar, X-ray chest and ECG for preanesthetic evaluation.

Secondly, I would do investigations specific to tuberculosis including ESR, Mantoux test, ELISA for TB.

Thirdly, in this perimenopausal age group it is important to rule out malignancy and I would do tumor markers and Doppler ultrasonography in this patient.

What are the tumor markers specific to ovarian malignancy?

CA-125 is a tumor marker specific to epithelial ovarian tumors. The CA-125 is also elevated in other cancers including endometrial, pancreatic, lung, breast, and colon cancer, and in menstruation, pregnancy, endometriosis, and other gynecologic and nongyne-cologic conditions.

The other tumor markers include AFP, LDH, hCG and CEA and PLAP.

What is the importance of various tumor markers?

Tumor markers can be used for one of four purposes: (1) screening a healthy population or a high risk population for the presence of cancer; (2) making a diagnosis of cancer or of a specific type of cancer; (3) determining the prognosis in a patient; (4) monitoring the course in a patient in remission or while receiving surgery, radiation, or chemotherapy.

What is the importance of Doppler ultrasonography?

Doppler ultrasonography is to measure the blood flow into a tumor. Malignancy is characterized by high vascularity which is seen as low resistance flow on Doppler. The resistance index is < 0.4 in malignant tumors.

How will you manage this case if the features on the above investigations are suggestive of benign ovarian mass?

A diagnostic laparoscopy followed by operative laparoscopy/laparotomy under general anesthesia can be planned after preanesthetic check up.

Laparoscopic ovarian cystectomy with a frozen section where facilities are available can also be done.

How will you manage this case if the features on the above investigations are suggestive of malignant ovarian mass?

If all investigations done point towards malignancy then the patient should be taken up for staging laparotomy and panhysterectomy total with infracolic omentectomy and if facilities of frozen section are available they should be asked for.

What are the steps of staging laparotomy?

Staging laparotomy is begun with a planned midline vertical incision and the abdomen is opened in layers. Any ascitic fluid or free fluid is sampled and then peritoneal washings are taken from prevesical space, pouch of Douglas, both paracolic gutters, and both subdiaphragmatic spaces. Then all peritoneal structures are palpated to look for intraperitoneal disease. Therafter removal of the entire mass along with abdominal total hysterectomy with bilateral salpingo-oophorectomy is done.

What are functional ovarian cysts? How are they managed?

Functional cysts are seen in women in childbearing years. On USG they appear as clear cysts. They do not occur in women an oral contraceptive pills. Their management includes observation and conservative approach if the cyst is <6 cm. They are then reassesed after 3-4 months. If the mass resolves, no further action is to be taken. If on the other hand, they persist or grow, laparoscopy is indicated. However, even a functional cyst can pose a problem when their size is >6 cm. They turn and undergo torsion which presents with pain of acute onset and thus needs to be surgically tackled immediately.

What is a dermoid cyst? How will you diagnose and treat it?

Dermoid cyst is the most common benign ovarian neoplasm. Its peak incidence is between 20 and 40 years. It originates from primordial germ cells, composed of well-differentiated derivatives of all the 3 germ layers—ectoderm, mesoderm and endoderm. It is generally benign, but rarely may undergo malignant transformation in 0.5-2% of cases. Most common carcinoma associated with dermoid cyst is squamous cell carcinoma. On gross examination it appears round or oval with smooth glistening gray white surface. It is bilateral in 8-15% of cases. It is the most common ovarian tumor to be B/L and undergo torsion. Torsion is a frequent complication because they are relatively buoyant and mobile. On USG it may be either unilocular or multilocular. On X-ray abdomen calcification may be seen secondary to osseous differentiation or teeth in the pelvis. Treatment in young patients involves doing an ovarian cystectomy with preservation of normal ovarian tissue and close inspection of contralateral ovary.

What is torsion ovarian cyst? How will you diagnose and treat it?

A torsioned ovarian cyst occurs when the cyst twists on its' vascular stalk, disrupting its blood supply. The cyst and ovary (and often a portion of the fallopian tube) die and necrose. Patients with this problem present with severe unilateral pain with signs of peritonitis (rebound tenderness, rigidity). This problem is often indistinguishable clinically from a pelvic abscess or appendicitis, although an ultrasound scan can be helpful. Treatment is surgery to remove the necrotic adnexa. If surgery is unavailable, then bedrest, IV fluids and pain medication may result in a satisfactory, though prolonged, recovery. In this suboptimal, non-surgical setting, metabolic acidosis resulting from the tissue necrosis may be the most serious threat. Mortality rates from this condition (without surgery) are in the range of 20%. Other surgical conditions which may resemble a twisted ovarian cyst (such as appendicitis or ectopic pregnancy) may not have a good outcome if surgery is delayed. For this reason, patients thought to have a torsioned ovarian cyst should be moved to a definitive care setting where surgery is available.

What is endometriosis? What are the common sites affected by this disease?

Endometriosis is a condition in which implants of normal appearing endometrial glands and stroma are found outside their normal location in the uterine cavity. The most common sites of endometriosis are the ovaries, the uterosacral ligaments and the peritoneum of the cul-de-sac and bladder. It is common in the nulliparous women and in the 2nd to 4th decades of their life.

How is chocolate cyst formed?

In patents with endometriosis when the ovary is involved, they become enlarged, cystic and a collection of dark chocolate colored fluid accumulates within an ovarian cyst. They usually do not exceed 12 cm in diameter, and are often difficult to differentiate clinically from ovarian neoplasm. Ovary is often adhered and may have restricted mobility on clinical examination. Nodularity and tenderness of the uterosacrals (Nodularity of the uterosacrals/ POD may also be present due to metastatic deposits from the primary in the ovaries or other sites, e.g. GIT) and other structures may help in the differential diagnosis. Most common symptom is chronic pelvic pain, other symptoms are dyspareunia, infertility.

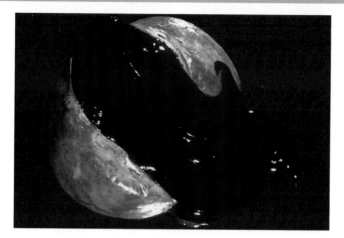

Chocolate cyst

What are paraovarian cysts?

A cystic mass in the adnexal region may be neither ovarian nor tubal in origin but caused instead by remnants of embryologic structures. The paraovarium, located within the portion of the broad ligament containing the fallopian tube, consists of vestigial remnants of the Wolffian duct. Paraovarian cysts are found as distal remnants of the Wolffian duct system. They are located between the fallopian tube and the ovary and when enlarged, fallopian tube is often found stretched over the cyst. They are unilocular and are filled with clear yellow fluid. They often persist into the postmenopausal period and are diagnosed incidently on ultrasound or other imaging studies done for other complaints. The ovaries can usually be identified separate from these cysts on USG.

What is hydrosalpinx? How does it commonly present? What are the complications associated with it?

Hydrosalpinx is collection of mucus secretion into the fallopian tube. It is usually due to repeated attacks of mild endosalpingitis by pyogenic organisms of low virulence but highly irritant, e.g. *Staphylococcus, E.coli, Gonococcus, Chlamydia trachomatis, Mycobacterium tuberculosis*, etc.

It is commonly asymptomatic but may also present with chronic pelvic pain, infertility or rarely, in severe cases as adnexal mass. It may be unilateral or bilateral. On USG a sausage shaped complex cystic structure with reduced resistance index (RI) in the adnexal region is suggestive of the diagnosis. The tube is retort shaped. The wall is shiny and smooth, and contains clear fluid which is usually sterile. Depending on the tubal diameter, hydrosalpinx may be **Mild** <15 mm; **moderate** 15-30 mm; **severe** >30 mm. The complications associated with it include formation of tubo-ovarian cyst, torsion, infection from the gut and rupture.

Why is hydrosalpinx retort shaped?

During initial infection, the fimbriae are edematous and indrawn with the serous surface adhere together to produce closure of the abdominal ostium. The uterine ostium gets closed by congestion. The secretion is pent up to make the tube distended. The distention is marked in the ampullary region than the more rigid isthmus. As the mesosalpinx is fixed, the resultant distention makes the tube curled and looks retort shaped.

How do you ovarian stage malignancy?

Ovarian neoplasms may be primarily cystic, solid, or mixed. Some are benign, some are malignant. The TNM and FIGO staging are given in Table 14.4.

How do you classify ovarian tumors on histopathology?

There are three main types of ovarian tumors based on histopathology: Epithelial, germ cell and sex cord tumors.

Epithelial ovarian tumors are derived from the cells on the surface of the ovary. This is the most common form of ovarian cancer and occurs primarily in adults. It includes serous tumor, endometrioid tumor, mucinous cystadenocarcinoma, Brenner's tumor.

Germ cell ovarian tumors are derived from the egg producing cells within the body of the ovary. This occurs primarily in children and teens and is rare by comparison to epithelial ovarian tumors. Germ cell tumor accounts for approximately 30% of ovarian tumors but only 5% of ovarian

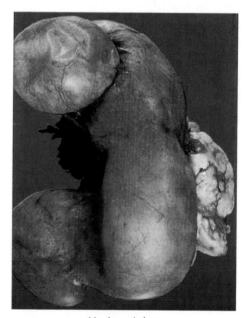

Hydrosalpinx

TNM	FIGO	Description
Tx		Primary tumor cannot be assessed
T0		No evidence of primary ovarian tumor
T1	**Stage I**	**Tumor limited to ovary (ies)**
T1a	Ia	Tumor limited to 1 ovary; capsule intact, no tumor on ovarian surface. No malignant cells in ascites or peritoneal washings.
T1b	Ib	Tumor limited to both ovaries; capsules intact, no tumor on ovarian surface. No malignant cells in ascites or peritoneal washings.
T1c	Ic	Tumor limited to 1 or both ovaries with any of the following: capsule ruptured, tumor on ovarian surface, malignant cells in ascites or peritoneal washings.
T2	**Stage II**	**Tumor limited to pelvis**
T2a	IIa	Extension and/or implants on the uterus and/or fallopian tubes. No malignant cells in ascites or peritoneal washings.
T2b	IIb	Extension to and/or implants on other pelvic tissues. No malignant cells in ascites or peritoneal washings.
T2c	IIc	Pelvic extension and/or implants (stage IIA or stage IIB) with malignant cells in ascites or peritoneal washings.
T3	**Stage III**	**Tumor limited to the abdominal cavity**
T3a	IIIa	Microscopic peritoneal metastasis beyond pelvis (no macroscopic tumor).
T3b	IIIb	Macroscopic peritoneal metastasis beyond pelvis <=2 cm at largest diameter
T3c	IIIc	Peritoneal metastasis beyond pelvis >2 cm at largest diameter and/or
or N1	-pet IIIc-g	Regional lymph node metastasis.
M1	**Stage IV**	**Remote metastases**
		Tumor involving 1 or both ovaries with distant metastasis.
		If pleural effusion is present, positive cytological test results must exist to designate a stage IV case. Parenchymal liver metastasis is equivalent to stage IV.

cancers; because most germ cell tumors are teratomas and most teratomas are benign. Germ cell tumor tends to occur in young women and girls. The prognosis depends on the specific histology of germ cell tumor, but overall is favorable.

Sex cord stromal ovarian tumors are also rare in comparison to epithelial tumors and this class of tumors often produces steroid hormones. These include estrogen-producing granulosa cell tumor and **virilizing** Sertoli-Leydig cell tumor or arrhenoblastoma and account for 8% of ovarian cancers.

Mixed tumors, containing elements of more than one of the above classes of tumor histology.

Cancers derived from other organs can also spread to the ovaries (**Metastatic cancers**).

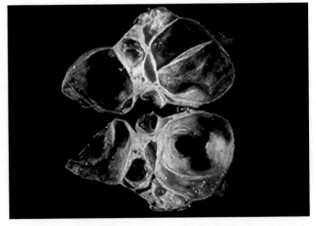

Papillary serous cystadenoma

SUMMARY

Gynecological causes of pelvic mass by approx. frequency and age group

Infancy
- Functional cyst
- Germ cell tumor

Prepubertal
- Functional cyst
- Germ cell tumor

Adolescent
- Functional cyst
- Pregnancy
- Dermoid /other germ cell tumors.
- Obstructing vaginal or uterine anomalies
- Epithelial ovarian tumor

Reproductive
- Functional cyst
- Pregnancy
- Uterus fibroids
- Epithelical ovarian tumor

Perimenopausal
- Fibroids
- Epithelical ovarian tumor
- Functional cyst

Postmenopausal
- Ovarian tumor
- Functional cyst
- Bowel-malignant tumor or inflammatory or metastasis.

Non-Gynecological Causes of Pelvic Mass

Arteriovenous malformation
Diverticulosis
Complicated appendicitis
Bowel tumor
Lymphadenopathy

Gastrointestinal
- Appendiceal abscess
- Appendiceal tumor
- Diverticular abscess
- Colonic tumor

Genitourinary
- Pelvic kidney

Retroperitoneal
- Hematoma
- Lymphocyst
- Lymphoma
- Sarcoma

CASE 16 — Carcinoma Oral Cavity

My patient, CR Bomber, a 65-year-old male, resident of Rajasthan, presented with complain of ulcerative swelling in right side of his mouth cavity for last 1 year.

My patient was apparently asymptomatic 1 year back since when he noticed a small sizeeulcer at inner side of his right cheek.

The ulcer is gradually progressive and not responding to usual treatment. It was painless initially. Nowadays, there is a burning sensation over it, particularly on taking food.

For last 3-4 months a swelling appeared around the ulcer and attained its present size approx 3 × 2.5 cm.

But there is no history of regular pain or pain referring to ear.

No history of dyspnea, cough (chronic smoker or tobacco chewer have COPD).

No history of bleeding from ulcer or no history of growth in the other subsets of oral cavity.

No history of restricted mouth opening, difficulty in protruding of tongue, chewing food, halitosis (unpleasant smell).

No history of voice change, difficulty in breathing (dyspnea), difficulty in swallowing (dysphagia), defective speech (to exclude synchronous lesion or infiltration to the surroundings).

No swelling in the neck (Neck nodes).

Past history: No history of HTN, DM, exposure to radiotherapy, etc.

Personal history: Chronic smoker- 2 bundle (40) bidi/ day for last 15-20 years.

Tobacco chewer for last 15 years. He used to keep the tobacco at right lower part of his oral vavity.

He is nonalcoholic.

Family history: Family history is not contributory.

General survey: Patient is cooperative, anxious looking average built, averagely nourished.

P- 80/min, BP- 118/80 mm Hg. Temp (N) Refp. 18/min

No pallor, icterus, edema or generalized lymphadenopathy noticed.

LOCAL EXAMINATION

Externally

The face appears normal, no asymmetry, deformity or growth or skin involvement over the cheek noticed.

No neck swelling noticed.

Internally

Oral hygiene poor.
Teeth not broken around the site of the lesion.

Inspection

There is 3 × 2.5 cm ulceroproliferative growth at right lower gingivobuccal sulcus extending posteriorly over external gingiva from lower 2nd premolar to 1st molar tooth approx 1.5 cm in length.

- Oval shaped lesion, margin irregular, edge thickened and everted.
- Floor- uneven, pale and whitish patches over the floor.
- There is no active discharge and the surrounding area is healthy.
- No surrounding edema.
- All other subsets look normal.

Palpation

- Inspectory findings are confirmed.
- Ulceroproliferative growth is tender and bleeds on touch.
- Base of the ulcer is indurated, but not fixed to underlying bone.
- Other subsets are normal.
- No palpable lymph nodes in the neck.

Systemic Examination

Respiratory System:
- Trachea is central
- Bilateral air entry is equal and no adventitious sound heard
- CVS: S1, S2 normal. No murmur heard
- Others systems are essentially normal.

SUMMARY

My patient, a 65-year-old male, chronic smoker and tobacco chewer, presented with ulceroproliferative growth at right side of his oral cavity, inner aspect of cheek for the last one year, which is gradually progressive, initially painless, but now he is having pain over it while chewing food.

But there is no difficulty in chewing food or in mouth opening and there is no lymphadenopathy in the neck.

On examination general survey is essentially normal.

On local examination there is 3 × 2.5 cm ulcero-proliferative growth in right lower gingivobuccal sulcus extending posteriorly over gingiva from lower 2nd premolar to 1st molar.

Oval shaped, irregular margin, edge everted.

Floor- uneven, pale looking and whitish patches over the floor.

So my provisional diagnosis is carcinoma right lower gingivobuccal sulcus.

Clinically T2 N0 M0.

Questions

Why do you think it is carcinoma?
- Elderly patient
- Chronic smoker
- Tobacco chewer
- Having painless progressive ulceroproliferative disease
- Everted edge
- Bleeding on touch.

All point towards carcinoma.

Why he is having pain now?

As the ulcerative lesion progresses gradually and floor of the ulcer exposing more and more, the nerve endings are exposed. So pain sensation is there on exposure to any kind of irritation like after taking food.

How will you proceed in this case?

Sir, I will confirm my diagnosis first

- I will do incisional biopsy (wedge biopsy) from the margin of the lesion.
- Next I will do orthopan tomogram: Oblique and occlusion views of the mandible or CT scan oral cavity to demonstrate involvement of the bone.

If CT scan is available – orthopantomogram is not required as CECT scan is better. It can show the involvement of mandible, extension of the lesion – infratemporal fossa, base of skull, masticator space, tonsillar fossa are involved or not which are indicative of inoperability.

Involvement of surrounding muscles, soft tissue, skin, etc.

Involvement of cervical lymph nodes.

Indirect laryngoscopy is required to rule out the synchronous lesions.

What is the role of MRI in oral carcinoma?

MRI, when available, is the investigation of choice for oral and oropharyngeal cancer. Its great advantage over CT is that the image is not degraded by the presence of metallic dental restorations. It's a very good in imaging soft tissue infiltration. It is very useful in assessing cancers arising in tongue and floor of mouth. Its specificity and sensitivity in diagnosing cervical lymph nodes metastasis is similar to that of CT.

Can you tell me the TNM staging of oral cancer?

Yes Sir,

T stage depends on the size of the primary lesion:

T1 <2 cm.
T2 2-4 cm
T3 >4 cm
T4 involvement of skin, muscle or bone.

a. Involvement of skin of cheek, deep muscles of tongue (genioglossus, hyoglossus, palatoglossus and styloglossus) and cortical bone of mandible.

b. Tumor invades the masticator space, pterygoid plates, and base of skull or encases internal carotid artery.

N refers to disease in lymph nodes:

N0 No palpable lymph node
N1 Single node <3 cm
N2a Single ipsilateral node 3-6 cm in size.
N2b Multiple ipsilateral nodes <6 cm.
N2c Bilateral or contralateral node <6 cm.
N3 Nodes >6 cm.
M0- No systemic metastasis.
M1- Systemic metastasis.

Stage grouping:

Stage I	T1, N0, M0
Stage II	T2, N0, M0
Stage III	T3, N0, M0, T1-3, N1, M0
Stage IV	T4, N0-3, T1-4, N2-3, M0 and M1 diseases.

What s about your case – it is early or late stage?

Sir, clinically my patient is T2 N0 M0, i.e. it is an early lesion.

What treatment modalities you can offer to this patient?

In early lesion, i.e. T1, T2 disease, surgery and radiotherapy give equally good results.

But as a surgeon I will definitely offer surgery if the patient is willing and he is fit enough for the surgery.

In present days laser excision is also a good alternative option.

What surgery will you offer for this case?

I will do
   i.   Wide local excision of the lesion. Ideally 2 cm of healthy mucosal surface to be obtained.
   ii. Segmental resection of the mandible to obtain wide margins to facilitate reconstruction.
   iii. Raw area is covered with split skin graft.
   iv. If necessary, a flap of mucosa from floor of mouth and adjacent tongue can be raised to cover small defect suited in the posterior part of cheek.

   Today, the most popular flap is pectoralis major myocutaneous flap. The island of skin is obtained form skin below and medial to the nipple.

Suppose this was a case of T3/ T4 lesion. How would you do the reconstruction after wide local excision with hemimandibulectomy?

The defect to be reconstructed in four layers:
   i.   Defect in the mucosal layer.
   ii. Deficiency in the mandible.
   iii. Loss of soft tissue.
   iv. Loss of skin.
   The reconstruction has to be done layer by layer:
   i.   Raw area of mucosa is covered with a split skin graft.
   ii. Small defects (T1 lesions) may be closed primarily. If necessary, a flap of mucosa from floor of mouth or adjacent tongue can be raised to close the defect.
   For women, myofacial flap (pectoralis fascia and pectoralis major) is preferred to reduce the bulkyness.

Advantages:

Soft tissue defect is also adequately compensated by pectoralis major myacuteneous flap (PMMC flap). Other flap like forehead flap, flap from palate may also be used.
   iii. Repair of bone defect:
       The defect may be bridged by:
       1. Titanium implant
       2. A piece of autogenous rib or iliac crest.
       3. An osteomyocutaneous flap, e.g. rib with a PMMC flap.
       4. Free flap with microvascular anastomosis which is considered the best.
   iv. *Loss of soft tissue:* Soft tissue defect may be managed adequately by PMMC flap or palate flap if it is relatively smaller.
       Pectoralis major myocutaneous (PMMC) flap is most commonly used flap – supplied by pectoral branch of acromiothoracic artery- which is arising from axillary artery.
   v.   *Skin defect:* A small defect can be managed with PMMC flap itself as the island of skin is obtained from the skin below and medial to the nipple.
       Large defect is best managed by deltopectoral flap which is supplied by perforators of internal mammary artery.

What is the policy of neck nodes management in carcinoma oral cavity?

1. *For N0 neck:* The policy is to do supraomohyoid dissection involving removal of I to III level neck nodes.
   • Specimen is submitted for frozen section.
   • If metastasis positive completion of neck dissection to be done otherwise not required.
   • If frozen section facility not available and nodes show metastases of histopathological examination-completion of neck dissection to be done at the earliest in the same hospital stay.
       For N0 neck only elective neck dissection is done when the neck is entered for an excision of primary, i.e. hemimandibulectomy.

2. *For operable positive neck nodes:* Complete removal of level I to V neck nodes is mandatory. To remove all these nodes, usually sternocleidomastoid and internal jugular veins are removed. Every attempt is made to preserve the spinal accessory nerve (Type I MRND).

What are the types of mandibulectomy you know?

1. Marginal mandibulectomy—where the alveolar part is removed, preserving the lower border.

   Teeth loss is there but minimum cosmetic deformity.

   Marginal mandibulectomy is a good operation for the lesions of floor of mouth.

2. Segmental mandibulectomy

   Indications:
   - Clinical or radiological invasion of mandible, i.e. of course an indication for segmental resection of bone.
   - To obtain wide margins.
   - To facilitate reconstruction.
   - In lesions involving full thickness of cheek.

3. Arch preserving mandibulectomy: To preserve the arch of mandible. It prevents the pouting of lower lip and there by preventing continuous drooling of saliva (the deformity is known as "Andy Gump deformity").

4. Hemimandibulectomy.

What are the criteria for nonrespectability in carcinoma oral cavity?

Extensive disease

   i. Involving tonsil, soft palate, hard palate.
   ii. Involvement of pterygoid muscle, infratemporal fossa, premasticator spaces, base of skull, involvement of internal carotid artery.
   iii. Extensive fungative growth of skin.
   iv. Fixed lymph node metastasis at neck.

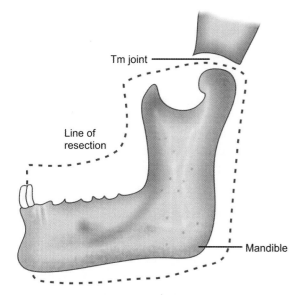

Doted line shows the area of haemimandibulectomy

   v. Perineural spread and direct invasion of regional structures.
   vi. Poor general condition along with uncontrolled co-morbid condition.

What are the indications of adjuvant treatment?

The indications of adjuvant therapy (Radiotherapy or chemotherapy) are:
- The resection is less than required and either gross or minimal disease has been left behind.
- Margin positive of the resected specimen.
- Multiple lymph nodes involvement and or extranodal spread of disease.
- Tumor invades infratemporal fossa.
- High grade tumor.

What is the standard adjuvant therapy and when and how to start?

The standard adjuvant therapy is postoperative radio-therapy.

It should be started usually 4 to 6 weeks after operation.

   Dose is about 50-60 gray and it is delivered over a period of 6 weeks.

   [Side effects are osteoradionecrosis of the jaw, teeth problems, dryness of mouth and delayed trismus due to post-radiation fibrosis].

Is there any role of neoadjuvant (preoperative) radiotherapy in a case of carcinoma oral cavity?

Initially preoperative radiation was the standard treatment. It was the idea that preoperative radiotherapy to the tumor with intact blood supply would be more effective. But there is considerable morbidity due to delayed wound healing, skin flap necrosis. Secondary fatal hemorrhage from the carotid vessels.

   But despite of all this few surgeons like to offer pre-operative radiotherapy in case of extensive disease, particularey when the disease involves skin of cheek, for better locoregional control prior to surgery.

   However, over the years, postoperative radiotherapy has become the standard treatment in headneck cancer.

What is the role of chemotherapy in head-neck cancer?

In head and neck cancer, preoperative chemotherapy produces dramatic regression, but it has not improved the over all survival.

Postoperative chemotherapy is alternative to radiotherapy.

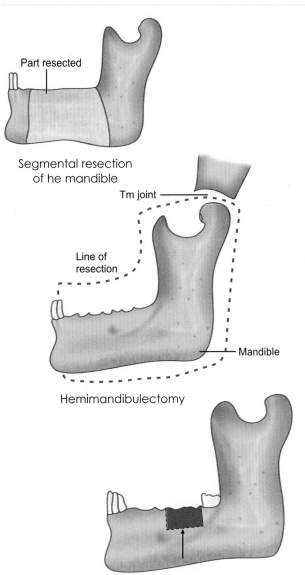

Segmental resection
of he mandible

Hemimandibulectomy

Marginal mandibulectomy

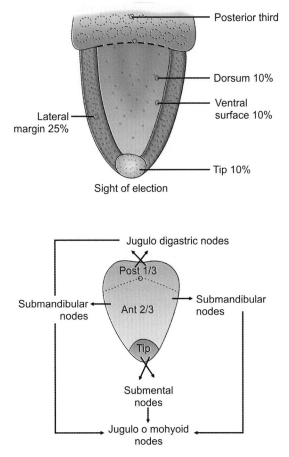

Sight of election

Lymphatic drainage from different parts of tongue

Tell me the precancerous lesions in oral cavity?

1. Lesions of definite risk of malignancy are:
   - Leukoplakia
   - Erythroplakia
   - Chronic hyperplastic candidiasis.
2. Lesions carry more risk of malignancy are:
   - Submucous fibrosis.
   - Syphilitic glossitis.
   - Sideropenic dysphagia (Plummer Vinson syndrome/ Paterson-Kelly syndrome).
3. Lesions may be associated with malignancy:
   - Oral lichen planus.
   - Discoid lupus erythematosus.
   - Dyskeratosis congenita.

What are the subsets of oral cavity?

The subsets are:
  i. Lips
 ii. Tongue
iii. Palate
 iv. Gingivobuccal sulcus with gingiva (gums)
  v. Floor of mouth
 vi. Buccal mucosa (inner side of cheek).

Most common site of oral cancer is tongue at middle third of the lateral margins. Second most common site is floor of mouth.

Have you heard the term field cancerization?

Yes Sir, Slaughter is the man who coined the term 'field cancerization'.

In this theory it is said that chance of involvement of malignancy in other subsets is 4% every year if the patient has developed cancer in any subset of oral cavity.

Tell me something about leukoplakia?

WHO defined leukoplakia as 'any white patch or plaque that cannot be characterized clinically or pathologically as any other disease'.

Chance of malignant transformation rate is 2.4% at 10 years which increased to 4 5 at 20 years. Tobacco smoking and chewing is undoubtedly an important etiological factor.

The pathological changes are:

- Hyperkeratosis—parakeratosis > dyskeratosis > Acanthosis > Carcinoma *in situ*.

Can you tell me which types of leukoplakia are more prone to develop malignancy?

- Speckled or nodular leukoplakia.
- Leukoplakia of elderly patient who continues tobacco chewing and/or alcohol consumption.

- Leukoplakia of long duration.
- Leukoplakia in floor of mouth and lateral margin of tongue.

How will you manage the patient of leukoplakia?

i. I will ask the patient to stop smoking /chewing of tobacco or alcohol intake.

ii. If there is any sharp tooth I will extract the tooth.

iii. Biopsy can be taken if the lesion is indurated associated with fissure or surface ulceration.

iv. Otherwise I will excise the lesion if there is severe dysplasia or any suspicion of malignant changes.

v. Excision can be surgical or by laser (carbon dioxide laser).

IMPORTANT SHORT NOTE ON CARCINOMA ORAL CAVITY

INTRODUCTION

In Asia oral/oropharyngeal cancer is the most common malignant tumor. India and Sri Lanka where chewing tobacco is used with betel nuts and reverse smoking is practiced, there is a very high incidence of oral cancer and account for as many as 50% of all cancer.

The incidence is greater in man than women. It is predominantly a disease of the elderly, 60 years and above.

The single greatest risk factor is tobacco.

RISK FACTORS

All forms of tobacco have been implicated as causative agents including cigarette, cigar and pipe tobacco as well as chewing tobacco.

In West cigarette smoking along with alcohol abuse, the risk of both in combination being greater than the summation of the risk of each individually (>15 times greater risk).

In Asia and far East, chewing 'pan' betel nut and reverse smoking (burning end inside the mouth) are the major etiological factors.

Heavy alcohol usage is an additional causative factor.

In lip carcinoma, which included in statistics for oral cancer, is more similar to skin cancers. Sun exposure and pipe smoking are also the important factors.

Age is frequently named as a risk factor for oral cancer.

Biological factors include viruses and fungi, have been found in association with oral cancers.

Human papilloma particularly HPV 16 and HPV18 have been implicated in some oral cancers.

Different subsets and premalignant lesions are described in questions and answers part of this chapter.

Clinical Presentation

- Patient usually presents with persistent oral ulcer.
- Any sore or discolored area in oral cavity which persists for more than 2 weeks should be a suspicious lesion.
- Symptoms like a mass in oral cavity or neck which is painlessly progressive.
- Other symptoms are difficulty in chewing, swallowing, excess salivation, hoarsness of voice, etc.

Diagnosis as Described Earlier

Choice of Treatment

The principle treatments for primary tumors are still surgery and radiotherapy.

If radical radiotherapy is chosen as treatment of choice, surgery is reserved for 'salvage', i.e. for recurrent or residual disease.

If surgery is chosen as treatment of choice, radiotherapy is used as adjuvant therapy either preoperative or post-operative period.

But fundamentally the operation remains the definitive curative procedure.

However, the treatment of choice depends on the following factors:
a. Tumor factors.
b. Patient factors.
c. Resources factors.

Tumor Factors

1. *Site of origin:* Treatment of choice depends on the part of oral cavity in which the tumor arises.
   Example: Surgery is preferable for the tumor arising involving alveolar processes.
   For other sites surgery and radiotherapy are alternatives.
2. Stage of the disease:
   In early stage, i.e. T1, T2 disease surgery and radiotherapy are equally effective.
   But in advanced disease, surgery followed by radiotherapy is the preferable option.
   Where there is involvement of cervical lymph nodes, the primary and nodes, both are normally treated surgically.
3. Tumors arising from previously irradiated tissue is to be preferably treated by surgery.
4. Field change when multiple primary tumors are present or there is extensive premalignant change, surgery is the treatment of choice.
5. *Histology:* Adenocarcinoma, melanoma are usually treated surgically as these tumors are relatively radio- resistant.

Patient Factors

Age is a very important factor. Radiotherapy given to a young patient may induce malignancy in years to come.

Elderly patient tends to be poor surgical risks, but on other hand, they also tend to do badly with radiotherapy which causes different adverse effects along with debility and poor nutritional status.
   i. Co-morbidity rehabilitation potential and patient wishes are also considered important factors.
   ii. *Resources factors:* Availability of well trained surgeon or radiotherapist with the facility of radiotherapy and ability of patient to bear the cost of treatment, etc.

Surgery for Oral Cancers in Different Subsets

Lip: Lip is usually considered separately from cancers of other oral cancer as it behaves more like skin cancers.

TNM staging is also slightly different from cancer oral cavity.

T4a- in Lip Ca: Tumor invades through cortical bone, inferior alveolar nerve, floor of mouth or skin (chin, nose)

T4b- same as oral Ca.

T1, T2 lesions are cured by wedge resection and primary closure. Usually up to 1/3rd of the lip can be removed with V or W shaped excision with primary closure.

T3 and T4 lesions require resection of involved tissues, bilateral supraomohyoid neck dissection with reconstruction in three layers, mucosa, muscles and skin.

Tongue: Small lesions can be excised; keeping 1 cm healthy margin, the defect left will granulate, as in less than one-third of tongue excision formal reconstruction is not necessary.

Tongue lesion around 2 cm requires partial glossectomy and lesion more than 2 cm requires hemiglossectomy.

Tongue lesions infiltrating styloglossus muscle, floor of mouth and alveolus- major resection and mandibulectomy is done via a lip split incision and there by reconstruction is mandatory.

Neck dissection: Tongue cancer with no nodal status minimum supraomohyoid neck dissection to be done.

Lesion in the midline or one sided lesion crossing midline – Bilateral supraomohjoid dissection (SOHD) is required.

In clinically palpable nodes, MRND same sided is mandatory.

Floor of mouth: Second common subsite for oral cancers. This cancer usually extends to involve the tongue and/or mandible.

Thereby, composite resection of mandible along with wide local excision of the tumor, keeping at least 1 cm healthy margin, and neck dissection to be done.

The neck dissection status is as Ca tongue.

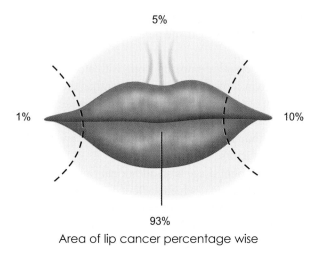

Area of lip cancer percentage wise

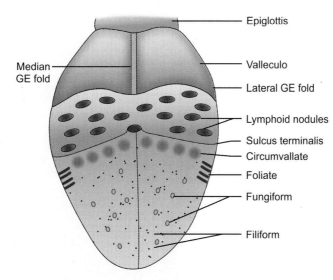

Anatomy of the tongue showing parts and papillae

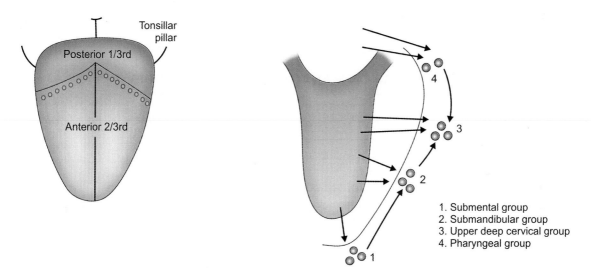

1. Submental group
2. Submandibular group
3. Upper deep cervical group
4. Pharyngeal group

Anatomy and lymphatic drainage of tongue

Reconstruction is done in layer, mucosal layer covered with split skin graft (SSG).

Deficiency in mandible is reconstructed by titanium plate/ ribs/ iliac crest/ ribs with PMMC flap/ free flap with microvascular anastomosis.

Loss of soft tissue and skin – reconstructed by PMMC and deltopectoral flap respectively.

Ca Buccal Mucosa

For T1, T2 buccal mucosal cancer surgery or radiotherapy give equally good results.

Surgery- wide local excision with SOHD in N0 neck.

In oral defects up to 3 × 5 cm, buccal fat pad is useful as a local flap for reconstruction.

The forehead flap, an axial flap based on the superficial temporal artery is also used.

T3, T4 lesion—WLE with segmental or hemi-mandibulectomy with MRND are required. Mandibular reconstruction is best done in the forms of various free flaps like radial free fore arm flap (RFFAF), fibular free flap (FFF).

Soft tissue defect is covered with PMMC flap and skin defect by deltopectoral flap.

Retromolar Trigone (RMT)

15% of oral cancer occurs in RMT.

RMT lesion is very difficult to treat as it has got inherent tendency to involve deeper structures such as ramus of mandible, pterygoid muscles, the masticator space and base of skull.

Another mode of spread is through foramen of inferior alveolar nerve into the ramus of mandible.

Often lip split and segmental resection of mandible and excision of part of pharynx are required.

Small defects can often be reconstructed with a masseter or temporalis muscle flap. Larger defects are best reconstructed with a free radial fore arm flap.

Hard palate and upper alveolus:

A tumor confined to the hard palate upper alveolus and floor of antrum can be resected by partial maxillectomy. For more extensive tumor confined to the infrastructure of maxilla requires total maxillectomy.

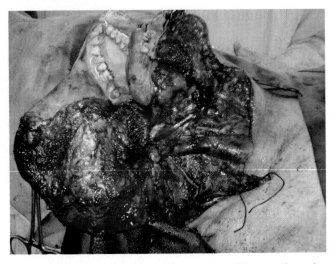

Carcinoma oral cavity—wide local excision and neck dissection

SHORT NOTE ON MANAGEMENT OF NECK NODES

SURGICAL ANATOMY

The cervical lymph nodes are arranged anatomically as follows:

a. **The outer circle of superficial nodes:** These include submental, submandibular, facial, preauricular, post-auricular and anterior cervical nodes.

b. **The inner circle surrounding larynx, trachea, and pharynx:** These include-pretracheal, paratracheal and retropharyngeal nodes.

c. **The deep cervical nodes** surrounding internal jugular vein (IJV) lies in between the outer and inner circles, and drain them. These are grouped into antero-inferior, postero superior and postero-inferior (jugulo – omohyoid, supraclavicular) nodes.

The clinically useful description (originally proposed by MSKCC) divides the nodes into the following lymph node levels:

I   Submental, submandibular
II   Upper jugular
III   Middle jugular
IV   Lower jugular
V   Posterior triangle (Upper, middle, lower)
VI   Central compartment
VII   Superior mediastinal

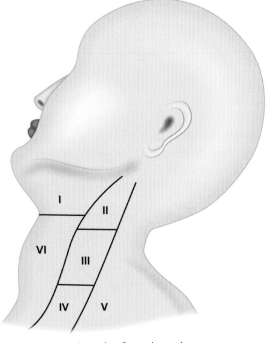

Levels of neck nodes

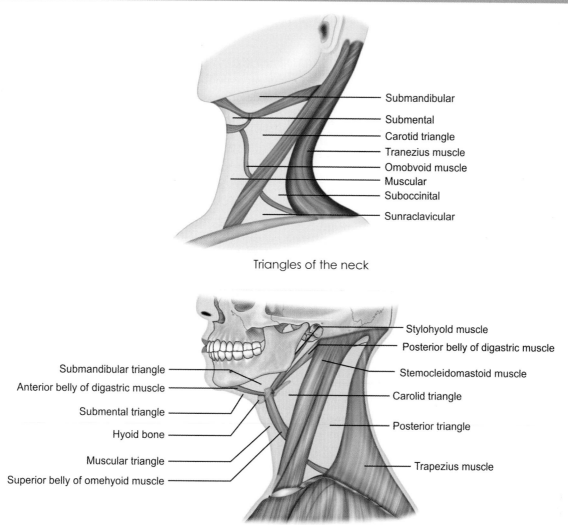

Triangles of the neck

Triangles of neck

The clinical landmarks for differentiating between levels II and III, II and IV are:
a. Hyoid bone
b. Cricoid cartilage.

The surgical landmarks for the same are:
a. Carotid artery bifurcation
b. Omohyoid muscle crossing the internal jugular vein.

ONCOLOGIC RELEVANCE OF LYMPH NODE LEVELS

The patterns of lymph node metastases, as determined by Lindberg (1972) and Jatin Shah (1990) are predictable: These patterns are as follows:

Level I : Oral Cavity, anterior part of nose, mid-face, maxillary sinus.

Level II : Oral cavity, nasal cavity, nasopharynx, oropharynx, hypopharynx, larynx, parotid

Level III : Oral cavity, nasopharynx, oropharynx, hypopharynx, larynx

Level IV : Hypopharynx, larynx, cervical esophagus

Level V : Nasopharynx, oropharynx

Level VI : Thyroid, larynx (Glottis, subglottis), cervical esophagus.

Thus, the first draining lymph nodes of various sites are:

- Oral cavity   : I, II, III
- Larynx, pharynx : II, III, IV
- Thyroid   : VI, VII, IV
- Parotid   : Parotid, preauricular, II, III, V (upper)

EVOLUTION OF NECK DISSECTION

Radical neck dissection (RND) was first described by *Crile (1906)*, a hundred years ago. He described the procedure for removing the lymphatics of the neck along with removal of the sternocleidomastoid muscle (SCM), internal jugular vein (IJV) and spinal accessory nerve (SAN). *Hayes Martin (1951)* advocated the RND as standard of care for cervical metastases. *Bocca and Pignataro (1967)* introduced the concept of conservative (*Functional*) neck dissection, sparing the non-lymphatic structures, interestingly in both No and N+ necks.

In the 1970s and 1980s, modified RND was proposed for reducing the morbidity of RND by preserving SAN/ IJV/ SCM, *Spiro et al (1985)* and *Shah (1990)* validated selective neck dissections especially supra omohyoid neck dissection (SOHND) for oral cavity lesions and Lateral neck dissections lesions of the hypopharynx and larynx.

STANDARDIZING NECK DISSECTION TERMINOLOGY

The terminology for describing neck dissections was standardized by the American Academy of Otolaryngology, Head and Neck Surgery (1991, 2000). The classification is as follows:

Comprehensive Neck Dissection

- Radical Neck Dissection (RND)
- Modified RND
- Extended RND

Selective Neck Dissection

- Supraomohyoid neck dissection (SOHND)
- Extended SOHND
- Lateral ND
- Posterolateral ND
- Central sompartment ND.

Comprehensive neck dissection: Removes all lymph node groups that would be included in a classic RND, SAN/IJV/ SCM may or may not be preserved.

Radical neck dissection: Lymph node levels I to V are removed. SAN, IJV, SCM are removed.

Extended RND: Extended to include removal of one or more additional lymph node groups nonlymphatic structures or both. These may include parotid nodes, levels VI, VII nodes,

hypoglossal nerve, digastric muscle, skin, external carotid artery.

Modified RND: All lymph node groups (I to V) are removed. One or more nonlymphatic structures are preserved. Some authors describe various types as follows:

Type I   : Preserves SAN
Type II   : Preserves SAN and SCM
              IJV Sacrifices (Jatin Shah's cancer of head and neck)
           : Preserves SAN, IJV (Stell and Maran's head and neck surgery; 4th Edn)
              Eugene M Myers' Cancer of Head and Neck, 4th Edn
Type III   : Preserves SAN, SCM, IJV.

In view of the confusion, it is desirable that the preserved structure should be named, e.g.: modified RND with preservation of SAN.

[Remember type 1, preserve 1(SAN) type 2, preserve 2 (SAN and IJV) type 3, preserve 3 (SAN, IJV and SCM)]

Selective ND: One or more lymph node groups, which are removed in RND, are preserved. The SAN, IJV and SCM are routinely preserved. These were originally recommended for N0 neck. However, they are also being advocated for N+ neck by some workers.

a. *Supraomohyoid neck dissection:* Lymph node levels I, II, III are removed.
b. *Extended SOHND:* Level IV is also removed. This is recommended for oral tongue lesions for 'skip metastases' (Byers et al, 1997), but has not accepted by some others.
c. *Lateral neck dissection (Jugular neck dissection):* Lymph node levels II, III, IV are removed. This is recommended for lesions of hypopharynx and larynx.
d. *Anterolateral neck dissection:* Lymph node levels I, II, III, IV, V are removed. This is recommended for oropharyngeal lesions when surgery is used for treatment of the primary.
e. *Posterolateral neck dissection:* Lymph node levels II, III, IV, and V are removed. This is recommended for posterior scalp lesions.
f. *Central compartment neck dissection:* Lymph node level VI is removed (i.e. lymphatics from hyoid to suprasternal notch and laterally up to carotid arteries). Recommended in differentiated Ca thyroid.
g. *Functional neck dissection:* Pignataro introduced the concept of conservative neck dissection in which all non-

lymphatic structures are spared. Only lymph nodes are removed, interestingly in both NO and N+ neck nodes.

It is claimed that this type of neck dissection is equally effective in controlling regional metastasis.

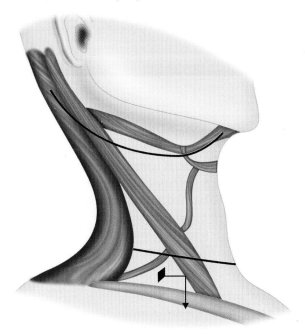

McFee incision for modified radical neck dissection

EVALUATION OF THE NECK

Presurgical staging of the neck is done by clinical palpation, but imaging adds to the sensitivity and specificity.

CT and MR imaging can be used. This criteria for indicating metastasis involvement are size [>15 mm (jugulo-digastric), >12 mm (submandibular), >10 mm (other nodes)], central necrosis, ring-enhancement and extranodal invasion.

USG is useful, but is operator dependant. It is often used for guided fine needle aspiration cytology studies.

Positron emission tomography (PET) localizes regions of increased glucose metabolism and can be used to evaluate patients clinically staged as N0. The sensitivity of PET can also be combined with the anatomic detail of CT. At present most centers use it only in case of suspected recurrent/residual disease.

STAGING OF CERVICAL NODAL METASTASES

The AJCC staging has universal acceptance.
• N refers to disease in lymph nodes.

N0 No palpable lymph node
N1 Single node <3 cm
N2a Single ipsilateral node 3-6 cm in size.
N2b multiple ipsilateral nodes <6 cm.
N2c Bilateral or contralateral node <6 cm.
N3 Nodes >6 cm.

MANAGEMENT OF THE N0 NECK

The approach to management of the clinically N0 neck is sometimes controversial, as there is no firm data to suggest improved survival with elective treatment as compared to close observation. It is considered that elective treatment is recommended in patients with more than 20-25% risk of occult metastases. Elective neck dissection and elective irradiation have both been shown to be equally effective (90% control rates). When the neck is entered for resection of the primary tumor or for reconstruction, elective neck dissection is preferred to irradiation.

Selective neck dissections are ideally suited for the elective setting. Super selective neck dissections (e.g. levels I, II) have also been advocated by some workers as being oncologically safe with reduced morbidity.

SELECTION OF SURGICAL PROCEDURE

An algorithm for selection of neck dissection is given below:-

Sentinel node mapping, though the standard of care in N0 neck in cutaneous melanomas of the heads and neck, is still under evaluation for squamous cell carcinomas. Intra-operative radiolympho-scintigraphy is used to detect uptake in nodes which are then dissected out.

ROLE OF RADIOTHERAPY

Elective radiation, where indicated, is as effective as neck dissection in the N0 neck. In the N+ neck surgery may be combined with postoperative radiotherapy (RT) to reduce local failure rates. The indications for post operative RT are bulky nodal disease (N2, N3), extranodal extension and multiple level involvements.

The National Comprehensive Cancer Network gives detailed Clinical Practice Guidelines in Oncology, which are updated regularly (www.nccn, org).

My patient, Sarukh khan, a 30-year-old male, resident of Nepal, Soldier in Indian Army, presented with chief complains of:

- Pain left leg while walking for last 1½ years
- Blackish discoloration of left great toe for last 1 month
- *HOPI:* My patient having the history of pain in his left leg while he starts walking for a distance (Intermittent claudication). Initially the pain was started after half a kilometer still he could able to manage walking but for last 6 months he is unable to walk more than 300 meters. He has to stand for few minutes than only he can start walking again.
- Nowadays, during rest at night he also experiences pain in his left leg, get relieved on hanging the leg from the bed.
- Since, last one month along with pain he also noticed blackish discoloration of his great toe following a minor trivial trauma.
- The black discoloration of left greatoe is gradually progressive along with pain.
- But there is no history of chest pain, breathlessness and syncope (to exclude cardiac disease/pulmonary embolism]
- No history suggestive of superficial thrombophlebitis (Redness along with the superficial vein).
- No history of pain, pallor of toes and or finger on exposure to cold (to exclude Raynaud's disease)
- No history of impotence, claudication of hip, gluteal region (different level of arterial occlusion).
- No joints pain, difficulty in movement, etc. (to exclude rheumatoid arthritis, SLE, etc.).

Past history: No history of diabetes, hypertension, hyperlipidemia, no past history of vascular disease. No history of previous surgery.

Personal history: He is a chronic smoker. Smokes 20-30 bidi per day. Occasional alcoholic.

Family history: No family history of peripheral vessels disease, atherosclerosis, etc.

General Survey: Patient is cooperative, anxious looking On average built, averagely nourished. No pallor, icterus, edema and generalized lymphadenopathy. Pulse 76/ minute radial, BP 128/78 mm Hg right arm supine. Temperature normal. Respiration 16/min.

Local Examination:

- Right lower limb appears normal (Normal limb first).

Left lower limb

- Attitude—standing comfortably
- Deformity muscle wasting, thigh, calf
- Buerger's angle: leg appears pale at 30° (But in black complexion it is very difficult to observe)
- Guttering of vein (bluish discoloration along the venous line)
- Signs of peripheral ischemia
- Affected area here left great toe, blackish great toe left, dry, no edema and signs of progression noticed. (Describe ulcer if any).

On Palpation:

- *Temperature:* Left lower limb is colder than the right
- *Affected part:* Blackish discoloration of left great toe, No gangrene as such (If gangrenous change describe that)
  - Peripheral pulses

–	Right lower limb	Left lower limb
Femoral	++	++
Popliteal	++	+
Anterior tibial artery	++	–
Posterior tibial artery	++	–
Artery dorsalis pedis	++	–

- Capillary filling > 3 seconds (suggestive of ischemia)
- Venous filling > 20 seconds (suggestive of ischemia)
- Cross leg test positive (Oscillatory movement of the leg) suggestive of absent poplitealartery pulsation.
- Buerger's test (Vascular angle) < 30°
- Test for DVT—Homan's sign negative.

Next examine
- The muscle wasting
- Movement of joints, neuropathy
- Inguinal lymph nodes.

On Auscultation
No bruit heard over femoral, aortic, carotid arteries.

Systemic Examination
CVS S1 S11 (N) No murmur heard. Others systemic examination is essentially normal.

Summary of the Case
My patient is a 30-year-old male, chronic smoker, presented with complain of intermittent claudication which is gradually progressive for last 1½ years and blackish discoloration of his left great toe for last 1 month without any history of cardiovascular events.

On examination: general survey is essentially normal.

Left lower limb is colder; Buerger's angle is less than 30°. Peripheral pulses are absent in left anterior tibial artery, posterior tibial artery and artery dorsalis pedis.

There is blackish discoloration in left great toe which is not on progression and no gangrenous changesnaticed.

So this is a case of peripheral artery occlusive disease affecting the left lower limb with ischemic changes at left great toe most probably due to Buerger's disease.

What is Buerger's disease?
It is a nonatherosclerotic segmental inflammatory disease that most commonly affects small and medium sized arteries, veins and nerves of the arms and legs.

This is also termed as thromboangiitis obliterans.

Why you thinking this PAOD patient having Buerger's disease?
- 30-years-old young male
- Chronic smoker
- History of intermittent claudication
- Infrapopliteal arterial occlusions and signs of ischemic changes
- In this patient atherosclerosis is unlikely
- Pregangrenous changes are there in left great toe.

What do you mean by intermittent claudication?
Sir, 'claudio' means 'I limp'. There is a crampy pain in the muscle during walking. Three characteristic features of intermittent cludications are:
  i. Pain starts after some walking distance
  ii. Pain disappears on rest
  iii. Again it appears on walking or during exercise.

What are the grades of intermittent claudication?
Grade I: Pain starts after the 'claudication distance' but patient continues to walk (as on exercise muscle blood flow increases and P substances swept away).

Grade II: Claudication is there but patient can still manage to walk with effort.

Grade III: Here after the claudication distance, the patient has to stop walking or exercise, i.e. patient has to take rest.

This is known as **Boyd's classification**.

What do you mean by claudication distance?
Claudication distance is a walking distance when the patient starts having pain.

How will you differentiate between vascular and neurogenic claudication?
i.   In vascular claudication patient usually experiences pain after a certain distance or exercise.
      Neurologic pain usually starts after a few steps.

ii.   In vascular claudication pain is usually relieved on rest but in neurogenic claudication pain is usually relieved on adaptation of certain posture.

iii. In vascular claudication usually the pain radiates from below upwards but in neurogenic claudication pain radiates from above downwards.

iv.   In vascular claudication peripheral pulsation may not be felt or weak. In neurogenic claudication peripheral pulses are not affected.

What is rest pain?
In peripheral vascular disease the term 'rest pain' is used which is continuous and aching in nature and patient experience, the pain even on the rest. The pain is worse at night, gets aggravated on elevation of the effected limb.

The pain is due to ischemic changes in the somatic nerves so called **'cry of the dying nerves'**.

Why the pain is worse at night?

At night, particularly, during rest, the heart rate as well as the blood pressure is decreased. Thereby further hypoperfusion may aggravate the ischemic pain.

Patient concentration, at night goes more towards the pain so; psychologically patient feels more pain at night.

How one can assess the claudication distance of an indoor patient?

Simple by a 'Treadmill Test' and claudication distance is measured observing the point of time at which patient starts having pain.

You were telling the word 'pregangrenous' changes in the left great toe? What do you mean by that?

Pregangrene is characterized by:
- Rest pain
- Color changes
- Edema
- Hyperesthesia
  With or without ischemic ulceration.

How will you confirm your diagnosis?

Sir, I will do angiography which may show:
- Involvement of small and medium sized vessels such as tibial, peroneal, plantar, etc.
- Segmental occlusive lesions (diseased arteries interspersed with normal appearing arteries).
- Distally more severe disease and normal proximal arteries
- No evidence of atherosclerosis.
- Collateralization around areas of occlusion called corkscrew collaterals.

Angiography is not essential for Buerger's disease as the disease involves small medium size vessels and surgery is not feasible. Moreover the disease is best diagnosed clinically.

What is the role of color Doppler study in this case?

- In Buerger's disease if the vessel is partially occluded there will be audible turbulence. In complete blockage no signal will be audible
- Segmental pressures' as well as, ankle brachial pressure index (ABPI) by applying cuff, can be measured.
- Pulse wave tracing analysis may helpful to assess occlusive arterial disease.

How ABPI is significant in artery occlusive disease?

From the value of ABPI we can assess the severity of PAOD
- Normal ABPI is 1

- ABPI 0.9 indicate some degree of arterial occlusion and patient present with claudication
- ABPI < 0.3 indicates critical ischemia and incipient necrosis.

How will you manage a case of Buerger's disease?

Aim-to prevent the progression of disease only. Thereby, prevention of amputation.

So first and foremost thing I will do encourage the patient to discontinue smoking and tobacco completely tell him. "Opt either cigarette or limb, but not both please"

Second regular graded exercise

In acute phase
- Inj Iloprost (prostaglandin analog) which is effective in improving symptoms.

Other drugs for Buerger's disease are:
- Antiplatelet like aspirin, clopidogrel
- Vasodilator like nifedipine
- Rheological agents like pentoxifylline 400 mg twice daily and cilostazol 100 mg twice daily.
- Analgesic, etc.

What is the role of surgery in Buerger's disease?

Due to diffuse segmental involvement and distal nature of disease. Surgical revascularization is next to impossible.

But the following surgery can be considered on specific demands like.

i. *Bypass surgery:* If the patient has severe ischemia and there is a distal target vessel, bypass surgery with the use of autologous vein can be considered.

ii. *Sympathectomy:* It is proven in treating pain and helps in healing of superficial ischemic ulceration; and this is most commonly performed surgery for Buerger's disease to relieve the rest pain mainly.

iii. *Omental transfer:* Surgical use of omental transfer has been reported to produce promising results.

iv. *Ilizarov technique:* Inflicted fracture of the affected limb leading to neoangiogenesis.

v. *Profundoplasty* done for blockadge of profunda femoris so as to open more collaterals.

vi. *Amputation* is and should be the last choice. It is performed when there is obvious gangrene with line of demarcation is found.

What is the newer developing therapy for Buerger's diseases?

Sir, recently the gene, vascular endothelial growth factor (VEGF) therapy in patients with Buerger's disease is promising.

What is chemical sympathectomy?

Lumbar sympathetic trunk can be blocked by injecting phenol/alcohol into the lumbar sympathetic ganglion under fluoroscopic control.

5 ml of phenol in water (1:15) is injected into the lumbar sympathetic trunk besides the bodies of 2nd, 3rd, 4th lumbar vertebra.

Which sympathetic ganglia will you remove in lumbar sympathectomy?

In unilateral sympathectomy L1, L2, L3, and L4 ganglia to be removed.

But in bilateral sympathectomy L1 ganglion is to be preserved to avoid developing impotence.

Removal of which ganglion is more effective preganglionic or postganglionic?

Removal of preganglionic fiber is more effective as preganglionic fibers are related with anterior aspect of thigh.

How will you judge whether the sympathectomy has been done accurately or not?

If the sympathectomy is done properly:
- The skin temperature will increase
- The limbs become warm
- Rest pain will be reduced or disappeared immediate post of period.

Do you know the Fontaine classification in chronic limb ischemia?

Yes sir,

Stage I	Asymptomatic
Stage II	Intermittent claudication, limiting lifestyle
	(a) well compensated
	(b) poorly compensated
Stage III	Rest pain due to ischemia
Stage IV	Ulceration or gangrene due to ischemia.

What is Buerger's exercise?

Buerger's exercise is meant to relieve rest pain. The process is alternate elevation depression of the affected lower limb from the bed level.

What is Leriche's syndrome?

When the block is in the common iliac or aortoiliac segment causing intermittent claudication in the buttock and often associated with impotence. This is called *Leriche's syndrome.*

What is Peacock's regimen?

For originally the Peacock's regimen is Reserpine + T3 (Triiodothyronine) 25 mg TDS for 2 weeks.

Presently immunotherapy with Azothiaprime + Steroid is given in uncontrolled cases.

What do you know about chronic critical limb ischemia?

Chronic critical limb ischemia is characterized by:
- Recurrence of ischemic rest pain for 2 weeks or more.
- Ulceration /gangrene of toes/foot
- Ankle systolic pressure < 50 mm Hg
- Ankle brachial pressure index (ABPI).

Know perfectly
- Capillary filling test.
  How to perform the test: press tip of nail or pulp of great toe for few seconds and release. Look how much time is taken for the blanched area to turn pink after the pressure is released. Normal filling time is 3 seconds, in ischemic limb it takes >5 sec
- Venous filling test
  How to perform the test: Keep both of your index finger over a vein, keeping asteady pressure on the vein move the heart side finger proximally. The distal finger is now released and observe venous refilling. Normal time is up to 10 seconds more than 15 seconds is suggestive of ischemia.
- Palpation of all peripheral pulses against bones
- Artery palpate against
- Superficial temporal artery zygomatic bone
- Carotid artery the spine of C6 vertebra called Chassaigne tubercle.
- Subclavian artery against mid clavicular point
- Axillary artery against head of humerous at lateral axillary border
- Brachial artery at medial condyle of humerous
- Radial artery at lower end of radius
- Ulnar artery at styloid process of ulna
- Femoral artery at neck of femur in between ASIS and pubic tubercle
- Popliteal artery at prone position-lower end of femur and in supine position against tibial condyle
  (To palpate the popliteal artery use bimanual technique both thumb at tibial tuberosity anteriorly.
- And all fingers are placed between two head of gastrocnemius. Compress posterior aspect of tibia below knee and palpate the artery.

- Anterior tibial artery at lower end of tibia, lateral to extensor hallucis tendon. Ask the patient to extend the great toe, the tendon will be prominent
- Posterior tibial artery against calcaneum, just behind the medial malleolus
- Dorsalis pedis artery against middle cuneiform bone, lateral to extensor hallucis longus
- Cross leg test (Fuchsig's test): Ask the patient to sit on a chair with legs crossed and look for oscillatory movement of upper leg. If the oscillatory movement present, it means popliteal artery is pulsatile.
- Buerger's postural test: Ask the patient to raise the legs, keeping the knee straight. In normal individual the leg will remain normal color even at 90 degrees angle but in ischemic limb elevation to a certain degree will cause marked color changes, i.e. pallor. A vascular angle less than 30 degrees indicates severe ischemia.
  (Guttering of veins: In case of severe ischemia on raising the limb even 10-15 degrees pale blue gutter appears along the course of veins. This is called guttering of veins.)
- Test for DVT: Homan's sign, Moses sign, and Neuhof's sign.
- Homan's test: Forcible dorsiflexion of the foot which stretches the calf muscles will cause pain. But it is only 30% sensitive.
- Moses sign: Gentle sgueezing of calf from one side to other side is painful.
- Neuhof's sign: Thickening and deep tenderness of calf muscle.

Collateral Pathway in Chronic Aortic Occlusion

1. Superior mesenteric artery to distal inferior mesenteric artery-39% via superior hemorrhoidal artery to medial and inferior hemorrhoidal artery to internal iliac artery.
2. Lumbar arteries to posterior gluteal artery–37% to internal iliac artery.
3. Lumbar arteries to lateral and deep circumflex iliac artery–12% to common femoral artery.
4. Winslow's pathway–12%. Subclavian to superior epigastric to inferior epigastric to external iliac artery at the groin.

SHORT NOTES ON PAOD (BUERGER'S DISEASE)

Buerger's disease also called thromboangiitis obliterans (TAO).

The disease is exclusively seen in males of younger age group. Not seen in female due to some genetic reason. Seen only in smokers and tobacco users. Commonly India, Korea, Japan, Israel, Turkey.

Always lower limbs one side affected first, upper limbs are involved only after limbs involvement of lower.

Etiology

- To tell the truth, the cause of Buerger's disease in unknown
- But it is fact that there is an extremely strong association between the heavy use of tobacco
- There is an extremely high prevalence of TAO among people of low socioeconomic class who smokes bidis.

Pathogenesis

- Smoking → Hyperchromocysteinemia
  Raised lipoprotein
  ↓
  Impaired endothelium dependant vasorelaxation
  ↓
  Vasospasm and hyperplasia of intima
  ↓
  Pan arteritis involving small, medium arteries
  segmental involvement
  ↓
  Once blockage occurs, collateral open up and blood supply is maintained to ischemic area called *compensatory PAOD*
  ↓
  Eventually artery, vein, nerve all are involved
  ↓
  Smoking continues
  Disease progress into collaterals, blocking them leading to severe ischemia called *decompensatory PAOD*
  ↓
  Critical limb ischemia
  ↓
  Rest pain, ulceration and gangrene

Stages

i. *Acute:* An occlusive, highly cellular, inflammatory thrombus with less inflammation in the walls of the blood vessels.
ii. *Subacute:* The progressive organization of the thrombus in the walls of blood vessels.
iii. *Chronic stage:* Organized thrombus and fibrosis of blood vessels.

Clinical Features

- Typically occurs in young male (20-45 years) smoker
- Claudication of the limb, rest pain, ulceration and gangrene
- Gangrene may occur spontaneously or following trauma
- Gangrene is digital but may spread giving rise to 'mummified foot'
- Recurrent migratory superficial thrombophlebitis.

CHRONIC AND CRITICAL LIMB ISCHEMIA

Etiology of chronic limb ischemia.

Chronic limb ischemia is common in males

M: F = 1.5: 1

Peak age of incidence is 70-80 years. Up to 50% of patients with CLI have severe multiocclusive disease. The patients have high risk of major amputation and death (> 10% every year).

Although understanding of artery occlusion is very important to manage the case accurately.

The important causes of lower limb arterial occlusions are:
- Atherosclerosis
- Thromboangiitis obliterans (TAO)
- Arterial trauma
- Popliteal artery entrapment
- Cystic adventitial disease of the popliteal artery

The major risk factors include:
- Smoking – single most important risk factor
- Hyperlipidemia
- Hypertension
- Diabetes mellitus.

Diagnostic Criteria

- History of smoking
- Young male 20-45 years
- Infrapopliteal arterial occlusions
- Superficial migratory thrombophlebitis
- The presence of diabetes mellitus rule out the diagnosis TAO.

Investigations

i. Arterial Doppler and Duplex scan to see:
- The site of occlusion
- Extend of occlusion
- Occlusions of collaterals
- Distal run off through collaterals.

ii. Angiogram shows the:
- Blockage and extension
- Cork screw appearance of the vessels collaterals
- Distal run off.

iii. Ultrasound abdomen to exclude:
- Blockage of aorta
- Aneurysm if any.

iv. ESR, blood sugar, lipid, etc. autoantibody, CRP, RA factor antinuclear antibody (ANA), etc.

Best Advice for the patient is stop smoking, 'opt for either cigarette or limb, but not both.

Pathophysiology of CLI is still not cleared. But it appears that atherosclerosis is a dynamic and hematological disturbance. Although atherosclerotic changes in the large vessels leading to occlusion or stenosis which causing chronic as well as critical limb ischemia.

Microvascular changes also play an important role to develop CLI.

The atheromatous plaque may be progressive and cause more deterioration of limb ischemia or it may heel or regress. As a result of obstruction survival of the affected limb will depend on the followings:

Macrocirculation: The fundamental process in the pathogenesis of CLI is atherosclerosis. Atherosclerosis plaques may develop in three stages:

i. Early fatty streak in the intima

ii. Fibrous plaques formation

iii. Complicated plaques like calcification, extensive necrosis, etc.

Microcirculation: Microcirculation is composed of arterioles, capillaries, venules, interstitial spaces as well as lymphatic channels.

↓

In chronic ischemia perfusion pressure seems to be reduced

↓

Increase plasma viscosity

↓

Leading to clumping of RBC's and release of ABP-promotes platelet aggregation

↓

Neutrophils are activated and release injurious substance like collagenase elastase and gelatinase damaging endothelium

↓

Damaged endothelium becomes swollen and permeable

↓

Increase permeability further reduces tissue nutrition.

↓

149

Classification of chronic limb ischemia
  i. Functional ischemia
  ii. Critical ischemia.

Functional limb ischemia: Occurs when blood flow is normal in the resting extremity but cannot be increased in response to exercise. Clinically, claudication is the manifestation.

Critical limb ischemia: Critical limb ischemia is basically due to reduction of peripheral perfusion to the extent that the basal metabolic needs of the tissue are not met as per demand.

- Recurrence of rest pain for more than two weeks
- Persists ulcer or gangrene in the toes/foot
- ABPI ≤ 3

The chronic critical limb ischemia has got the following two criterias:

  i. Recurring ischemia, rest pain persists for more than two weeks and requires regular analgesic with an ankle systolic pressure of 50 mm Hg or less or both.
  ii. Ulceration or gangrene toes/foot with similar hemodynamic parameters.

A clear distinction of functional and critical limb ischemia is not always possible.

One thing to be cleared that disorders that may cause leg pain include diabetic neuropathy nerve root compression, reflex sympathetic dystrophy, whereas ulceration may be induced by venous disease, diabetic neuropathy, etc.

Management of Chronic Limb Ischemia

Aortoiliac occlusive disease: A wide range of therapeutic options are available for the management of aortoiliac occlusive disease and they are broadly categorized as:

1. Anatomic repair or direct reconstructive surgical procedure on the aortoiliac vessels.
2. Extra anatomic repair or indirect bypass procedures that avoid normal anatomic pathways.
1. Direct anatomic surgical reconstruction may be:
    a. Aortoiliac end arterectomy
    b. Aortofemoral bypass – gold standard for widespread intra abdominal disease and multilevel disease.

2. Extra anatomic or indirect bypass—usually effective for the patients who are less likely to tolerate major abdominal operations and it is done usually in subcutaneous pathways.
3. Catheter based interventions or endovascular intervention.

Indications for endovascular aortoiliac interventions are:
  i. Percutaneous transluminal angioplasty for focal stenosis of the aorta or iliac arteries
  ii. Dissection and residual stenosis after percutaneous transluminal angioplasty (PTA) are adequately treated with stent placement.
  iii. Focal stenosis at aortic bifurcation.
  iv. Patients with multilevel disease (Hybrid procedures).
  v. Long-term patency of angioplasty or stenting is almost equal to surgery.

Infrainguinal Occlusive Disease

- Femoral—popliteal tibial artery occlusive disease.
- Superficial femoral artery is the most common infra-inguinal artery affected.
- If proximal popliteal artery is patent, bypass from the common femoral artery proximally to popliteal artery distally is the procedure of choice.
- If the popliteal artery below the knee is patent, bypass is done to this segment using reversed saphenous vein.
    - Thromboendarterectomy is a viable alternative but the procedure of choice
    - Profundoplasty currently used in difficult and extreme cases.

Endovascular procedures: Angioplasy and stenting of infra inguinal arterial segment is not as good as for iliac vessels partly because of the long segment involvement, however in selective patients with short segment stenosis with good distant run off, endovascular techniques may be tried.

Infrapopliteal occlusive disease:
- Bypass procedure is better when distal segment is patent.
- Angioplasty
- Percutaneous transluminal angioplasty (PTA) but out come is less favorable than bypass procedure.

CASE 18 — Varicose Vein

My patient is Ram Krishna, 40-year-old, traffic police resident of Gaya, Bihar, presented with complaint of:

- Swelling along the vein in his right lower limb for last 4 years
- Pain in the right limb for last 1 year
- And ulcer at lower part of leg for last six months.

My patient was apparently asymptomatic 4 years back since when he started developing swelling along the vein of his right lower limb.

Swelling is insidious in onset, slowly progressive and attained its present prominency.

- For last 2 years he has been having pain in his right lower limb. Pain appears when he stands for a long time during his duty, Pain is dull aching in nature. At the end of day he feels crumpy pain over the swelling. The pain is relieved on lying down. i.e. when he takes rest and on elevation of the limb.
- For last 6 months he has developed an ulcer at lower leg just above the medial malleolus. The ulcer is surrounded by a pigmentary skin changes with mild pain over the ulcer site along with itching. There is no active discharge or edema around the ulcer.

    But there is no history of tauma, intermittent claudication, rest pain or gangrene (to exclude arterial disease (as along with the arterial disease healing will be hampered\delayed).
- No history of any lump lower abdomen or constipated bowel habit (abdominal lump and loading colon lead to varicose vein).
- No History of pain and swelling in the calf with fever ever (to exclude DVT).

Past history: No history of HTN, DM, and No history of prolong immobilization or DVT (in case of female take history of long term intake of OCP). No history of any abdominal operation in past.

Personal History

- Traffic police in occupation Job demands long standing.
- He is also a known smoker.
- Smoke 5-6 bidi/day for last 10 years.

Family history: His father was a Riksha puller and had varicose vein (Varicose vein is familial)

General Examination

- Patient is cooperative looking comfortable; average built, well nourished.
- No Pallor, icterus, edema, lymphadenopathy noticed Pulse 72/min, BP 126/78 mm Hg right arm supine, Temperature not raised, Respiration 16/min.

Last Examination

The patient has been examined both standing and lying position.

- *On inspection:* Left lower limb appears normal (Normal limb inspection first).
- *Attitude:* Patient stands comfortably (In arterial disease patient likes to hang his leg down form bed to get relieved from pain).
- *Deformity:* There is a varicose vein at the medial aspect of right lower, leg great saphenous vein territory is involved, extends just above medial malleolus to thigh but limb lengthening, pulsatile vein (seen in *Kippel Trenaunay syndrome*) or superficial thrombophlebitis not noticed.

    Skin of leg
    - (look for chronic veinous insufficiency)
    - Loss of hairs
    - Shiny skin—thin skin, etc.)
- No signs of chronic venous insufficiency.
- No history of hemorrhage, pigmentation, eczematous lesion, equinus deformity (complications of varicose vein). There is an ulcer approximately 3 × 2 cm above the medial malleolus, shallow, oval shaped, sloping edge,

healing margin, purple blue in colors, but no active discharge from the ulcer, floor is covered with pink gramulotion tissue
- No cough impulse visible at saphenous opening.

On Palpation
- Temperature in both lower limbs is equal
- Course of long saphenous vein is thickened but nontender
- No cough impulse felt at saphenofemoral junction (Morrissey's cough impulse test)
- **Brodie-Trendelenburg test:** To see incompetency of the saphenofemoral valve and incompetency of the communicating veins.

  How to perform the test: Ask the patient to lie down and empty the saphenous vein by elevating and milking the veins. Saphenofemoral junction is to compress with thumb or to apply a tourniquet just below the saphenofemoral junction and ask the patient stand up.

  First method- the pressure is realeased, if the varices fill rapidly from above; it indicates the incompetency of the sapheno femoral valve.

  Second method—Same procedure is repeated upto milking of vein. Pressure is now not released and look. If the veins are being filled up gradually, it suggests incompetency of communicating veins.

  If any of the above two is found, the Trendelenburg's test is said to be positive.

Why it is called Brodie-Trendelenburg test?

Brodie had started doing the test but it had been popularized by Trendelenburg.
- **Tourniquet test:** It is a variant of Trendelenburg test. Multiple tourniquets are tied round the thigh and at leg at different levels which can determine the position of the incompetent communicating veins. (Minimum 4 tourniquets to be applied).

  How to perform the test: After emptying of veins as above first tourniquet is tied below the saphenous opening. Second one is below the adductor canal perforators. Third one is tied just below the knee perforators. Fourth one is placed just below the 15 cm above ankle perforators. Now the patient is asked to stand and see which part of superficial veins is being filled up that can determine the position of the incompetent communicating vein.
- **Modified Perthes test:** To exclude deep vein thrombosis. (How to perform the test: a tourniquet is tied just below the saphenous opening without emptying the vein and asks

the patient to walk fast for few minutes. if the communicating and deep veins are normal the varicose veins will shrink and if these are blocked, the varicose veins will be more distended and patient will have crampy pain.

What is original Perthes' test then?

Here the affected limb is wrapped with elastic bandage. And ask the patient walk around or exercise. the patient will have bursting pain in the leg.)
- **Schwartz test:** In long standing case feeling of impulse of tapping in both directions.

  How to perform the test: Make a tap at the lower part of the varicose vein and feel the impulse at the saphenous opening with a finger of other hand. Feeling of impulse indicates this is a long standing case.
- Fegan's method to indicate the sites of perforators.

  How to perform the test: Ask the patient to stand and mark the excessive bulges of varicosities and ask the patient to lie down. The limb is elevated to empty the veins. Now at the markings palpate the deep fascia. Gaps or pits in the deep fascia can be felt which indicate the sites of incompetent perforators.

Palpation of Ulcer
- Inspectory findings confirmed base of the ulcer is indurated, nontender.
- No active bleding on touch
- Peripheral arterial pulses—Femoral, popliteal, anterior tibial, posterior tibial, artery dorsalis pedis are normal (++).
- No inguinal lymphadenopathy palpable.
- Auscultation—No bruit is heard over the veins - (External iliac, femoral)

Systemic Examination
  GIT—Abdomen:
  0- Soft
  - Bowel sound +
  No lump palpable
  No hepato splenomegaly
  CVS - SII SII (Normal), No murmur.
  Other examinations are essentially normal.

Summary of the Case
- My patient is a 40-year-old traffic Police and chronic Smoker, presented with varicosity along the right long saphenous vein for last 4 years, dull aching and crumping pain at the same site for last 1 year and ulcer at lower

part of leg for last 6 months. Without any history of intermittent claudication, DVT of any abdominal lump.

- General survey is essentially normal.
- **On local examination:** There is varicose vein of long saphenous vein without any complication except a venous ulcer at the lower part of leg. The edge of the ulcer is slopping and it is on the process of healing.
- Trendelenburg test shows -sapheno femoral incomptency without incompetency of the communicating veins.
- Modified Perthe's test sugests no deep vein thrombosis.
- All peripheral plsation are normal. So this is a case of Right sited varicose vein at great saphenous territory with saphenofemoral incompetence.

How will you proceed in this case?

Sir, I will confirm my clinical findings first.
I will do
i. CDFI (Color Doppler flow imaging)
    I will see
    - The patency of deep vein
    - Saphenofemoral Junction—competent or not.
    - Venous reflux at the site of perforators in competence.
    - To exclude any associated artery disease.
    - see the venous flow, venous patency etc.
      Duplex Scan of this ultra sound Doppler imaging will reveal, along with direct visualization veins gives the functional and anatomical status and patency of deep veins, perforators incompetence, etc. very accurately.
ii. USG abdomen to exclude any intra-abdomey lump pressing major vessels.
iii. From venous ulcer, discharge to be sent for culture, sensitivity and biopsy to be taken from ulcer edge to rule out Marjolin's ulcer.
iv. X-ray of the area to exclude periostitis.

What is the role of venography in this case?

Sir, ascending venography was very common investigation done before color Doppler. It is good investigation to rule out DVT.

Wht is descending venography then?

Sir, descending venography is done when ascending venography is not possible. It is good investigation to see imcompentent veins.

Why deep vein thrombosis is very important thing to see in a case of varicose vein?

Sir, if DVT is present along with varicose vein both surgery and sclerotherapy are contraindicated.

Why DVT is contraindicated for surgery?

Sir, though superficial veins usually drain 10% of lower limb blood from skin, subcutaneous tissues but when the deep veins are thrombosed \diseased, superficial veins are the only channel of draining blood. So surgery is contraindicated for varicose vein. Same way sclerotherapy to superficial vein will lead to completely nonfunctional superficial veins which is not deserved in presence of DVT.

In this case what will you do?

Sir, I will make the patient fit for surgery by doing baseline investigations and preanesthetic checkup.
    If the saphenofemoral junction is incompetent.
    I will do
a. Trendelenburg operation which consists of:
    i. Juxtafemoral flush ligation of long saphenous vein (i.e. flush with femoral vein).
    ii. Ligation of superficial circumflex, superficial external pudendal, superficial epigastric vein and unnamed tributaries.
        (All tributaries to be ligated otherwise recurrence will be the fate).
b. Stripping of vein - Myers stripper is used to strip off the vein. (Stripping from below upward is technically easier, immediate application of crepe bandage reduces the chance of bleeding and hematoma formation).

OK, how much vein will you do the stripping?

Sir, I will do the stripping from thigh to just below knee or the reverse which is better, because in the leg long saphenous vein and sapheous nerven run side by side. Injury to saphenous nerve causing saphenous neuralgia.

If perforators are incompetents along with varicose vein what will you do?

I will mark the perforators by Fegan's method before surgery and I will ligate the perforators' deep to deep fascia through incisions in antero medial side of the leg. I can also do it through Linton's vertical approach.

What is SEPS?

Sir,
    SEPS is Subfascial Endoscopic Perforator Ligation Surgery. It is cosmetically very demanding procedure. SEPS is ideal when whole leg is pigmented or full of eczematous lesion or lipodermatosclerosis due to complications of varicose vein.

Have you heard TRIVEX method?

Yes Sir,

It is a very old method, hardly follow now a days hereby subcutaneous illumination, a large quantity of fluid is injected percuteneously to identify the superficial veins and identified superficial veins are removed using suction. It may cause bruising, grooves, skin changes etc.

What is most recent method for vericose veins ablation?

Sir,

Endoluminal laser ablation of varicose veins is the most modern method for varicose veins ablation.

Ok, how will you manage this ulcer in your patient?

Sir,

Usually in patient with varicose ulcer due to superficial vericosity, the ulcer heals well after varicose veins surgery.

But conservative treatment like regular dressing, control of infection, elastic stockinette, etc. are required for quick healing.

How stockinette or compression bandage help in healing ulcer?

A pressure of 30-45 mm Hg has to be applied at the ulcer site which makes the venous pressure tends to which altimately hastens the healing.

What are the complications of vericose vein surgery?

The complications of varicose vein surgery are:
- Infection —10%
- Haematoma formation
- DVT 1%
- Saphenous nerve injury leading to saphenous neuralgia
- Recurrence

Ok, tell me one thing before patient is anesthetized or morning of surgery will you do something?

Sir,

In the morning after patient takes bath I will mark main trunk of varicose vein along with the communication veins and the sites of perforators in competence with gentian violet. In a word it's to be done prior to anesthesia for easy identification during surgery.

How will you manage the r~~esidual vericosities?

Residual vericosities to be managed either by compression bandage or by injection sclerotherapy.

(Examiner will say -very good.

You say -thank you very much sir).

When do you plan for injection sclerotherapy in varicosity?

Usually sclerotherapy is indicated in:
- Minor vericosities where main trunks of long and short saphenous veins are normal.
- Residual vericosities following surgery.

What are the sclerosant agents commonly used and how?

The common sclerosant agents are:
- Sodium tetradecyl sulphate
- Polydocanol and
- Phenol in olive or almond oil.

Varicose vein is maked 23 gauge or 25 gauge needle is introduced into vein when patient lying. The limb is elevated to empty the vein. A small volume, say .5ml (1/2cc) of sclerogent agent to be injected in to the empty vein.

Immediately the vein is to be compressed with finger first then a farm pressure bandage to apply aiming that the walls of the vein will be remained in contact. Compression bandage to be applied for 4-6 weeks till the veins are transform in to fibrouscords.

How does sclerotherapy help in varicose vein?

Injected sclerosant agent destroys the endothelial lining and results in fibrous cord formation within 4-6 weeks. The compression bandage put such way so that to walls of vein remain in contact, no chance of thrombus formation within the vein and ultimately there is sclerotic and fibrotice occlusion of the vein so that no recanalisation occurs anyway.

What is microsclerotherapy?

Microsclerotherapy is applied to very small veins like venous stars, reticular veins in the skin.

Small amount sclerosant agent (0.1ml) is injected through 30 gauge needle. Compression to be applied for stars.

What are the probable complication of sclerotherapy?

The usual complications are:
- Skin pigmentation
- Superficial thrombophlebitis
- Skin ulceration if injected in extravenous space.

How does venous ulcer develop?

- Valves of superficial and deep veins incompetency.
- Reverse flow of blood from superficial to deep veins.
- This is more marked during standing or walking.

⇓ Result in

Ambulatory venous hypertension

1. Fibrin cuff theory:
   i. Defective macro circulation:
   - Increased pressure in the capillaries.
   - Extravasation of blood elements from capillaries.
   - A perivascular cuff is formed consisting of fibrin collagen and fibronectin.
   - The fibrin cuff acts as a barrier to diffusion, nutrient exchange, and anoxia.
   - Resulting in tissue damage.
   - Ulceration this is called 'fibrin cuff' theory.
2. Leukocyte trapping hypothesis:
   - Ambulatory venous hypertension causes leukocyte migration and sequestration in the capillaries.
   - Activated leukocyte release proteolytic enzymes and oxyzen free radicals.
   - Causing damage of capillary endothelium and thrombosis of microcirculation.
   - Tissue damage.
   - Skin ulceration.

Where is the common site for venous ulcer and why?

This is just above and ground the medical malleoli because of large number of perforators which transmit pressure changes directly into superficial system.

This area is called *Gaiter's zone* (Gaiter: is the covering for the lower part of leg used by the hoarse rider).

How will you treat venous ulcer?

1. Bisgaard regimens
   - Elevation of limb
   - Massage of the indurated area and whole calf
   - Active and passive exercise.
   Above the measures are required to reduce edemas increase venous drainage which promote healing.
- Apply pressure bandage
- Cleaning of ulcer with H_2O_2, normal saline and providone iodine
- Dress with EUSOL (Edinburgh University Solution of lime containing boric acid, sodium hypochlorite, calcium hyperoxide)
- Four layers bandage (Remember—WCEC)
  - First layers—wool
  - Second layers—crepe bandage
  - Third layers—elastic
  - Fourth layer—coban
  To achive high compression pressure which maintains the venous pressure tends to Ommlg which promotes healing.
- Antibiotics depending on culture sensitivity of the discharge.

- Splitskin graft (SSG)—when there is heathy granulation tissue at ulcer bed.
2. Specific treatments for varicose veins are:-
   - Trendelenburg operation
   - Stripping of veins, ligation of perforators
   - Venous valve repair (Kistner's valvuloplasty) or valve transplantation and drugs like stanozolol, reduce fibrosis. Resulting in increasing oxygenetion of tissue and ulcer heal.

What is venous claudication?

This is nothing but an acute bursting pain on ambulation as a result of chronic venous insufficiency.

What is Saphena varix?

The dilated terminal end of long saphenous vein is called saphena varix.

Here thrill and cough impulse may be palpable.

What are the difrent types of varices?

1. Thread veins or layer—the varicose of the smaller dermalvessels; 5 to 1 mm in maximum diameter appearing as red or purple spots, usually around ankle.
2. Reticular varicose smaller veins located in subcuteneous regions varices of 1-3 mm diameter
3. Small varicose vein < 3 mm in diameter
   Large varicose vein > 3 mm in diameter.

How pigmentation occurs in venous ulcer?

As a result of:
- Incompetence of venous valves
- Long standing stasis of blood chronic ambulatory venous hypertension
- RBC diffuses into tissue planes
- Lysis of RBC's
- Release of hemosiderin
- Pigmentation.

What is MRV?

It is a noninvasive procedure and MRV is magnetic resonant venography. It has excellent delineation for the veins.
- It gives functional and anatomical informations of the varicose vein like competency of SF junction.
- Patency of deep vein, perforators incompetence, etc.
- It also reveals the relationship of vein with surrounding structures, i.e. artery, nerve, etc.
  Only drawback of this imaging study is it is very costly thereby not available every where.

What are the indications for varicose vein surgery?

1. Cosmetic purpose
2. Symptoms of heaviness and triedness
3. Symptoms of itching and thickening of skin
4. Bleeding from varicose vein
5. Phlebitis
6. Eczema, lipodermatosclerosis
7. Ulceration etc.

What is venous closure method?

In this method an ablation catheter is passed into long/ short saphenous vein at SF/SP junction under ultrasound guidance. The catheter is to be withdrawn slowly to destroy the varicose vein hematoma and pain is less in this method.

What are the drugs can be used for varicos veins?

1. Calcium dobesilate-500 mg BD
2. Diosmin 450 mg BD or diosmin 450 mg+hesperidin 50 mg (DAFLON 500 mg)
3. Toxerutin 500 mg BD to TDS benefits of all these drugs are still are on doubt.

What is echosclerotheapy?

When the sclerotherapy is done under duplex ultra sound image guidance, then the sclerotherapy is termed as echosclerotherapy.

What is ian-aird test?

On standing proximal segment of long saphenous vein is emptied with two fingers. Pressure from proximal finger is released to see the rapid feeling from above which confirms saphenofemoral incompetence.

How will you differentiate between saphena varix and femoral hernia?

Saphena varix is enlarged terminal part of long saphenous vein, usually along with varicose vein.

It is soft, disappears with lying, fluid thrill, impulse on coughing, venous hum present.

Whereas femoral hernia usually an oval swelling at or just below the groin crease and a tight swelling, usually it does not disappear on lying, fluid thrill, venous hum not present.

SHORT NOTE ON VARICOSE VEIN

---

1. Varicose veins are dilated, tortuous and elongated veins where the blood flow is reversed through its faulty valves.
2. Types of varicose veins
    A. Congenital
    B. Primary varicosities
    C. Secondary varicosities
   A. *Congenital:* Absence of valves in external iliac veins.
   B. *Primary varicosities:* The causes are idiopathic but most probably due to:
    • Congenital incompetence or absence of valves
    • Weak venous wall may permit dilatation causing incompetence of valves.
    • Weakness or wasting of muscles
    • Stretching of deep fascia, etc.
   C. Secondary varicosities causes are:
    • *Occupational:* Where job demands standing for long hours (traffic police, guards, rikshaw puller, etc.)
    • Recurrent thromfbphlebitis
    • Obstruction to venous outflow-like gravid uterus, abdominal lump, retroperitoneal fibrosis, fibroid, pelvic tumor ovarian cyst, etc.

• Pregnancy due to hormonal effects of estrogen causing relaxation of vein wall smooth muscle, and compression of pelvic veins.
• Destruction of valve-due to deep vein thrombosis.
• High pressure flow-like in A-V malformation either longenital or acquired.
   Iliac vein thrombosis etc.

Common sites of varicosities

1. Lower limblong and short saphenous varicosities.
2. Pampiniform plexusvaricocele
3. Vulva
4. Sites of Porto systemic anastomosis like—esophageal varices in rectum piles, etc.
1. *Physiology of venous dinage in lower limb:* Blood flows into the leg because it is pumped by the heart through the arteries. By the time, the blood emerges from the capillary the pressure is about 20 mm Hg but by this pressure blood can return towards heart.

   In addition to this, pumping action of muscles help blood to flow towards the heart.

There is also a foot pump, due to pressure in the plantr veins during walking, which helps in propelling the blood upwards.

On exercise, the calf and thigh muscle contract, compressing the veins and ejecting blood towards the heart. The direct ion of venous blood flow is controlled by the venous valve. The pressure within the calf compartment rises to 200-300 mm Hg during walking and this is more than enough to propel the blood in the direction of the heart.

During the phase of muscle relaxation the pressure within the calf falls to a low level and blood from superficial veins flow through the perforating veins into the deep veins.

Consequence of this is that the pressure in the superficial veinsfalls during walking. Normally the pressure in the superficial veins of the foot and ankle falls from a resting level 80-100 to 20 mm Hg.

3. *Effect of deep and superficial venous incompetence on the vascular physiology of the leg:* Incompetence of deep veins usually has a more severe effect on the venous physiology than the superficial venous incompetence as the deep veins are much larger than the superficial veins. The effect of reverse flow in the deep or superficial veins is to prevent the superficial venous pressure from falling during exercise as a result there will be persistently raised venous pressure. Called *'ambulatory venous hypertension'* which is the main cause of venous leg ulceration.

4. System of veins in lower limb there are:
   - Deep venous system
   - Superficial venous system
   - Communicating veins
   - Perforating veins.

Deep Venous System

This accompanies the main arteries and is well supported by powerful muscle which compresses the vein as a result blood returns to the heart.

The deep venous system comprises the fermoral, popliteal veins, veins or venae.

Comitantes accompanying the anterior tibial, posterior tibial and peroneal arteries and the valveless veins draining the calf muscle (solealvenous sinus) these deep veins are also provided with veins.

The high pressure deep venous system communicates with the low pressure superficial venous system at the following sites:

Short saphenous vein: Saphenopopliteal junction 2 cm below the knee to 15 cm above the knee.

Long saphenous vein: Saphenofemoral junction constant larges.
- Adductor canal by inconstant perforators (Hunterian) at mid thigh.
- Short saphenopopliteal junction-constant.
- Perforators below the knee (Dodd's perforator).
- Posteromedial aspect of the leg by constant perforators, 5, 10, 15 cm above medical malleolus (Cockett and Boyd's perforators).
- Posterolateral aspect of the leg by inconstant perforators.
- Remember CBD-H (heapticartery) from below upwards.
- Perforators at the level of ankel (May or kuster perforators).

Superficial Venous System

Long saphenous vein is the largest vein in the body. It commences from medial side of the dorsal venous arch of the foot and courses infront of the medial malleolus and ascends to the posteromedical side of the knee. Than the vein inclines laterally and forward in the thigh towards the saphenous opening which is 4 cm below and lateral to the public tubercle. It pierces the cribriform fascia and passes deeply to enter the femoral vein, the vein contains more than 12 valves, the saphenous nerve accompanies the vein in the leg.

Short saphenous vein commences from lateral side of the dorsal venous arch and passes behind the lateral malleolus and then ascends obliquely backward towards the middle of popliteal fossa, where it pierces the deep fascia to enter the popliteal vein in most cases. The sural nerve accompanies the vein in the lower third of the leg.

Communicating veins: These are superficial veins lying superficial to the deep fascia communicating between great (long) and short saphenous veins.

Perforating Veins

These veins connect between superficial venous system to deep venous system. Perforators are:

Direct and Indirect

Direct perforators: These perforators communicate directly between the superficial and deep veins.

Indirect perforators: These perforating veins from the superficial vein communicates the venous plexus in the muscle another perforating veins drains into the deep veins thereby indirectly connecting the superficial and deep veins.

Aetiology of Congenital Varicose Veins

Theory 1: There is no valve in IVC and common iliac veins but about 80 percent of people have valves in external iliac veins which save, SF junction from high pressure.

Those who are not having (20% people) the valves congenitally, develop venous hypertension crossing SF junction leading to varicosities at SF junction and down below.

This occurs mostly in young people whose family history is positive.

Theory 2: Thrombus at soleal sinuses extends to one of the calf perforators-leading to incompetent perforator.

- Develops venous hypertension transmitted to deep to superficial venous system. Distention of the superficial veins.
- Varicose veins.

5 CEAP Classification of Venous Disease

- C clinical
- Grade 0-6 A asymptomatic S symptomatic.
- Grade O no visible or palpable signs of venous disease.
- Grade 1 telangiectasia or reticular veins.
- Grade 2 varicose veins.
- Grade 3 edema along with varicose vein.
- Grade 4 skin changes ascribed to venous disease (pigmentation, lipodermatosclerosis etc.)
- Grade 5 skin changes with healed ulcer.
- Grade 6 skin changes with active ulceration.
  - E etiological.
  - Congenital-
  - Primary-
  - Secondary
  - A Anatomical — Deep venous disease and
    — Perforators incompetence

  P- Pathological ⎡— Reflux
                     ⎢— Obstruction
                     ⎣— Reflux and obstruction

Cavaliers sign: It is the sign demonstrating in competentcy of sapheno femoral valve.

Here thumb is kept at saphena varix and the patient is asked to cough. A tremor is felt like a jet of water intering into it and filling it.

Klippel-Trenaunay syndrome:

The syndrome is a triad of
- Pulsatile varicose vein
- Haemangioma and
- Lengthening of limb.

Clinic Feature

- Leg fatigue, pain, saccular dilated veins, nocturnal muscle cramps.
- Along with varicose vein, pigmentation on the medial or lateral aspects of the ankle, dermatosclerosis atrophy of skin eczematous dermatitis, etc.
- Venous claudication
- Venous ulceration
- Cosmetically look ugly.

Complications of Varicose Vein

i. Hemorrhage -may occur from minor trauma.
ii. Phlebitis—it occurs spontaneously or secondary to minor trauma
iii. Ulceration—as a result of ambulatory venous hypertension.
iv. Pigmentation—due to hemosiderin formation as a result of lysis of RBC.
v. Eczematous dermatitis.
vi. Lipodermatosclerosis—skin becomes thickened, fibrosed and pigmented. This is due to high venous pressure which causes fibrin accumulation around the capillary.
vii. Calcification of vein.
viii. Periostitis in a case of long standing ulcer over the tibia.
ix. Equinus deformity-this occurs as a result of long standing ulcer when the patients find relieve of pain on walking on toes. With the passage of time if the patient continues to walk on toes, tendoachilles tendon becomes shorter and stiffer to cause the equinus deformity.

MEDICAL MANAGEMENT OF CHRONIC VENOUS DISEASE (CVI)

The phlebotropic agent—calcium dobesilate.

And flavonoids have shown symptomatic improvement in CVI.

Flavonoids: Are effective in releving CVI associated pain night cramps also in controlling lower extremity edema.

Mechanism of action: It reduces leukocyte adhesion to endothelium and limits the consequences of noxious stimuli of inflammatory response.

Calcium dobesilate 500 mg BD: Increases lymphatic flow and macrophage related proteolysis it is also a nitric oxide donor. Studies have shown in improving subjective symptoms of CVI.

Diosmin 450 mg BD: Therapy increases the venous tone actually in early CVI, phlebotropic drugs along with compression stockings are the first line of treatment. Stanazol is very promising drug for healing of ulcers.

May Husni procedure: In patients who have obstruction of the superficial femoral vein, the long saphenous vein may be connected to the popliteal vein in the same limb, allowing the blood flow along the superficial veins more easily. However, in the majority of patients with chronic superficial femoral vein obstruction the blood flows along the long saphenous vein to reach the end, therefore this operation is not required.

Palma operation: In case of iliofemoral thrombosis, common femoral vein lower the block is communicated to opposite femoral vein through opposite long saphenous vein. Practice the following test repeatedly phase.

i.   Brodie-Trendelenburg test: Why it is called so?
      As it was invented by sir Benjamin Brodie but it was popularized by friedrich Trendelenburg).
ii.   Multiple tourniquet test.
iii. Parthes' and modified Parthes' test
iv.   Fegans test
v.   Pratt's test
vi.   Schwartz test
vii. Morrissey's cough impulse test.

Short saphenous vein: Varicosity neglected enity in a case of short saphenous incompetence application of the venous tourniquet to the upper thigh has paradoxical effect of increasing the strength of reflux as shown by faster filling time the sign is pathognomonic of short saphenous vein.

   (The saphenopopliteal junction is lying 2 cm below to 15 cm above the knee).

   Marked with pen with the patient standing the short saphenous vein is emptied by elevation of the leg, firm thumb pressure to be applied to the ink mark the patient is aked to pressure is released if saphenopopliteal junction is incompetent; the vein will be filled immediately.

   Practical purposes—there is no other incompetent perforating vein in the short saphenous system.

Surgery:

Flash ligation of saphenopopliteal junction.

- Stripping of short saphenous vein is more beneficial than just a ligation at saphenopoplited junction It is to be from above downwards using a rigid stripper to avoid injury to sural nerve.

Trendelenburg: Name is related to:

i.   Trendelenburg test for varicose vein.
ii.   Trendelenburg position head low and leg up position.
iii. Trendelenburg gait—a waddling gait due to hip instability suggesting weak abduction at hip.
iv.   Trendelenburg sign—seen in congenital dislocation of hip.
v.   Trendelenburg operation—for varicose vein.

DEEP VEIN THROMBOSIS (DVT)

Pathophysiology

Vchow's triad	Stasis
	Hypercgulability
	Vein wall injury

Causes/Risk factors.

General

- Elderly age, obesity
- Immobilization longer than 3 days
- Pregnancy and postpartum period
- Major surgery in previous 4 weeks
- Long car/Plane trips more than 4 hours -**called economy class syndrome.**

Medical

- Postoperative—Most common cause
- Cancer debilitating illness
- Previous DVT
- Stroke
- Acute myocardial infraction.
- Sepsis
- Nephrotic syndrome
- Ulcerative colitis.

Trauma to ankle, thigh, pelvis
- Muscular violence.

Hematologic

- Polycythemia rubra vera
- Thrombocytosis

- Inherited disorders of coagulation/fibrinolysis
- Antithrombin III deficiency
- Protein C deficiency
- Factor V Leiden
- Dysfibrinogenemias and disorders of plasminogen activation
- Drugs/ Medications
- Oral contraceptives
- Estrogens
- Heparin induced thrombocytopenia.

Travelers Thrombosis

- Thrombosis of travelers who travel air or car for a long duration > 4 hours.

Thrombosis: Thrombosis can occur in individuals, who sit with computer for a long time.

Postoperative Thrombosis: This is the most common cause of thrombosis. Common after the age of 40 years incidence following surgeries is 30%. Both legs are affected in 30% case.

Most commonly seen after:
- Prostate surgery
- Hip surgery
- Major abdominal surgery
- Gynecological surgery
- Cancer surgery, etc.

Bed ridden more than 3 days in postoperative period increases the risk of DVT.

Sites

1. Pelvic veins—common
2. Leg veins—common in femoral and popliteal veins (common in left side)
3. Upper limb veins like axillary vein thrombosis
   - Neuhof's sign: Thickening and deep tenderness on palpation of deeper part of calf muscles.
   - Unfortunately, most often DVT patients are asymptomatic and present suddenly with features of pulmonary embolism, i.e. breathelessness, chest pain, hemoptysis.

Different diagonosis of DVT:
i. Ruptured Baker's cyst
ii. Ruptures plantaris tendon
iii. Calf muscle hematoma
iv. Cellulitis leg
v. Superficial thrombophlebitis.

Investigations

- Venous Doppler |
- Duplex scanning | already described
- Venogram |

Others
- MRI: MRI is investigation of choice for suspected iliac vein of inferior vena caval thrombosis
- In second or third trimester pregnancy, MRI is more accurate than Duplex ultrasonography because of gravid uterus which alters Doppler venous flow characteristics

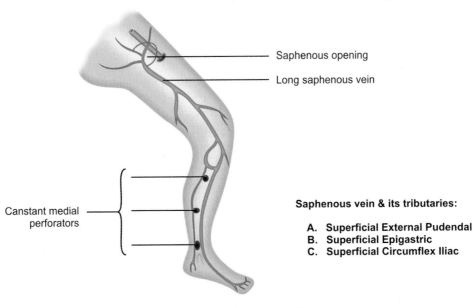

Saphenous opening

Long saphenous vein

Canstant medial perforators

Saphenous vein & its tributaries:

A. Superficial External Pudendal
B. Superficial Epigastric
C. Superficial Circumflex Iliac

Long saphenous Vein and its Tributaries

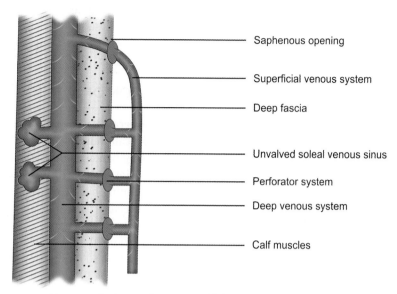

Venous drainage from superficial to deep in lower limb

- In suspected calf vein thrombosis, MRI is more sensitive than any other noninvasive study.

  When directly compared, duplex ultrasonography has superior sensitivity and specificity.
- **Phlegmasia alba dolens**: Major drainose veins the lower limb DVT, like DVT femoral vein, commonly in deep femoral vein causing painful congestion and edema of leg with lymphangitis which further increases the edema and worsens the condition, loosely called whiteleg. Pulse may be palpable in these patients.
- **Phlegmasia cerulea dolens**: Involves not only major drainage ileofermoral massive venous obstruction but also it involves their collaterals by thrombosis causing cyanotic leg. The leg is usually marked by edematous, painful and cyanotic petechiae are often present and edema is so massive that ankle pulses may not be palpable

  If it is not treated urgently, it may lead to venous gangrene where the increasing edema occludes the arteries and produces limb ischemia.

Clinical Features

- Commonly—it is asymptomatic.
- Fever early symptom—most common
- Pain and swelling in the calf and thigh. Pain is so severe that patient may not move the leg
- Features of pulmonary embolism—dyspnea, chest pain, hemoptysis.

On Examination

- Leg is tender, warm, pale or bluish with shiny skin
- Homan's sign—Passive forceful dorsiflexion of the foot with extended knee will cause pain in the calf
- Moses sign—Gentle squeezing of lower part of the calf from side-to-side is painfull. Careful gentle squeezing is important—otherwise if may dislodge the thrombous to form an embolus

Fribrinolysis: Streptokinase 6 lakhs to start with and later one lakh hourly. Urokninase, tissues plasminogen activator may also be used to dissolve thrombus. It is to be avoided when patient is on heparin.

Venous thrombectomy is done using Fogatity venous balloon catheter.

IVC filter prevents thromboemboli to reach the heart. Kimray Greenfield filter, M- Uddin umbrella filters are used.

Palma Operation

In iliofemoral thrombosis, common femoral vein below the block is communicate to opposite femoral vein through opposite long saphenous vein.

Palma Operation for iliofemoral block using opposite saphenous vein femoral vein is connected to otherfemoral vein.

May-Husni operation: When blockage is in popliteal vein, popliteal vein below the block is anastomosed to long saphenous vein so as to bypass the blood across the popliteal block.

Lab Studies

- D- dimer assays have low specificity for DVT; therefore, they should only be used to rule out DVT, not to confirm the diagnosis.
- A new rapid ELISA assay has high sensitivity for plasma measurement of D-dimer patients with low to moderate risk.
- A positive D-dimer assasy—all patients with a moderate to high risk of DVT, require a diagnosis study.
- Protein S, protein C, antithrombin III, factor V Leiden.

Treatment

i.   Advice: Rest, elevation of limb bandaging the entire limb with crepe bandage
ii. Anticoagulants - Heparin, warfarin, phenidone
iii. For fixed thrombus - Initially high dose of heparin of 25,000 units/day for 7 days is given.
     - Then warfarin for 6 months
     - Low molecular heparin can be used
     - Dose to be adjusted by assessment of APTT, INR (APTT—Activated partial thromboplastin time)

iv. For fire thrombus
     - Fibrinolysis
     - Thrombectomy using Fogarty catheter
     - IVC filter

PREVENTION OF DVT

i.   **Postoperative patient:** Positioning of legs with pressure on the calf muscles.
ii. Pressure bandage to be applied to the legs after major surgeries, elevation of leg, early ambulation, maintaining hydration are very important aspects.
iii. In suspected cases, after major surgeries patient can be put 5000 units' heparin/ day for minimum 5-7 days.
iv. IV Dextran 70 during surgery 500 ml to be transfused and another 500 ml postoperatively can prevent DVT
v.   Smoking, OCP, oestrogens to be stopped 6-8 weeks prior to elective surgery.

Complication of DVT

- Pulmonary embolism
- Infection
- Venous gangrene
- Recurrent DVT
- Proximal propagation of thrombus 20-30%
- Partial recanalization post phlebitic syndrome
- Chronic venous hypertension at ankle region causing venous ulceration.

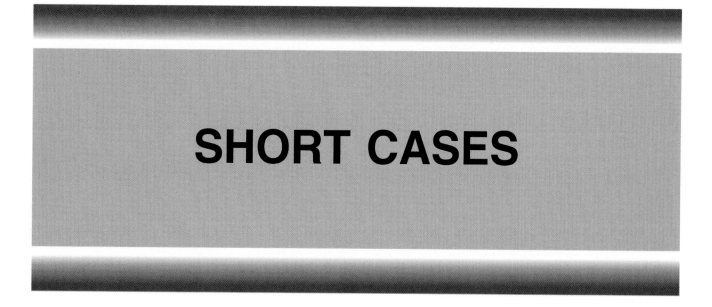

SHORT CASES

Short cases almost equally as important as a long case. Time allotted is 15 Minutes each. Usually 3 short cases are given.

In a short case- History should be only minimal relevant, Avoid negative history except very important one. Only mention the positive points from general survey and local examinations.

In this book I have presented short cases slightly extra for learning purpose. Practically you have to make it short as per above guide line please.

Lastly I will say, ultimately in examination your attitude, way of presentation and the impression you create that matters to make you through the 'Gateway' to Surgery. Never try to fool the examiner by giving smart wrong answers or giving many ir-relevant points in answer etc ie quality is alway preferable not quantity.

CASE 19 — Carcinoma Breast

My Patient Suman, a 43 years old, premenopausal lady, resident of Pathan Kot, Punjab, presented with a lump in her left breast for last 1 year.

My patient was apparently asymptomatic 1 year back when she noticed a lump in her upper outer part of left breast incidently while she had a feeling or stretching sensation during taking bath at the area.

The lump is
- Gradually progressive
- Painless
- Attained its present size approximately 3 × 3 cm from its initial size of a peanut.

But there is no history of
- Trauma, nipple discharge, retraction and crack in the nipple
- No other swelling noticed in the same breast and opposite breast or no swelling in both the axilla
- No skin changes over the breast
- No swelling in the left arm.

No history of (as per following sequence)
- Bone pain
- Cough, hemoptysis, chest pain
- Weight loss malaise anorexia, jaundice. Or
  (To exclude seizure, metastases in bone, lung, liver and brain respectively.)

Past History

- Not a known case of HTN, DM, TB
- No past history of HRT (Hormone Replacement therapy) or long-term OCP intake
- No history of operation in past
- No history of radiation exposure also in past.

Personal History

- Housewife, married at 24 years of age
- 1st childbirth- 3 years after marriage
- Both children were breast fed
- She is not an alcoholic
- Menstruation- regular. Menarche at the age of 11 years. Cycle stays for 3-4 days at 28 ± 2 days interval.

Family History

- No family history of same incidence of lump breast in her first or second degree relations.

On Examination

- She is cooperative, looking anxious, average built, well nourished.
  Pulse- 80/min, BP- 110/70 mm of Hg right arm supine. Temperature (N), RR-16/min there is no pallor, icterus, edema or generalized lymphadenopathy.

Local Examination

- Patient has been examined in sitting, sitting with hand raised, supine, recumbent and bending forward positions.
- On inspection both the breasts appear normal except left sided nipple is retracted.
- There is no venous engorgement, no skin changes like ulcer, no peau d' orange.
- No swelling noticed in both the breasts.
- Nipple areola complex appears normal. No fissure or eczematous lesion noticed.

On Palpation

- In the right breast (normal breast first) and axilla- no lump is palpable.
- Local temperature not raised, nontender.

In the left breast
- There is a 3 × 3 cm spherical lump
- At left upper outer quadrant of the breast
- No local rise of temperature

- Nontender
- Firm in consistency
- Well defined, irregular margin
- Uneven surface
- Mobile
- Not fixed to the underlying structure or overlying skin. No other swelling palpable in the breast.
- No axillary Lymph nodes palpable in the same site of axilla or opposite axilla.
- Supra clavicular lymphnodes are not palpable.

Systemic Examinations

- **Musculoskeletal system**- no spine or any bony tenderness (as bone mets are common and involvement of bone is earliest).
- **Chest** - Bilateral air entry equal, no adventitious sound heard.

Abdomen

- Soft
- No hepatosplenomegaly
- No free fluid
- CVS and CNS: Essentially normal
  I would also like to do per rectal and per vaginal examination.

Summary of the Case

My patient, a 43 years old perimenopausal lady presented with a lump at upper and outer part of her left breast which is painlessly progressive for last 1 year.

General survey is essentially normal.

- *On local examination* there is a 3 × 3 cm firm, mobile, well defined lump in the upper and outer quadrant of her left breast which is not fixed to underlying structure or overlying skin but there is an obvious retraction in the left nipple without any other changes of nipple areola complex. There is no evidence of involvement of axillary lymph nodes or distant metastasis clinically.

So, my provisional diagnosis is- this is a case of carcinoma left breast, clinically T2 N0 M0.

Why do you consider it is carcinoma breast?

This is a case of Carcinoma breast because
- Premenopausal lady
- Rapidly progressive lump, painless
- Lump is firm with well defined irregular margin and uneven surface

- Nipple is retracted in the same side of the lump.
  [If axillary lymph node is involved or if there is skin involvement/chest wall involvement/nipple retraction, these points will also go in favor of carcinoma breast].

What are the other possibilities?

The other possibilities may be

Fibroadenoma breast. [If it is large- cystosarcoma phyllodes also called serocystic disease of brodie].

How will you proceed in this case?

I will confirm my diagnosis first. I will do mammography of both breast then FNAC for tissue diagnosis.

What will you do first-mammography or FNAC?

Sir, I will do mammography first as because FNAC may distort the breast architecture and it may mimic like carcinoma breast.

What will all you see in mammography?

In malignancy I will look for
- Distortion of breast architecture
- Micro calcification <.5 mm)
- Stippled calcification is important characteristics
- Dilatation of ducts
- Soft tissue mass dense, stellate, irregular margins and spiky projections
- Nipple retraction etc.
  Mammography shows malignant lesion and micro-calcification.

Do you know BIRADS classification of mammography findings?

Yes sir, BIRADS means Breast imaging reporting and data System.

In BIRADS

Category 0-
- Used for screening purpose if negative and additional investigation /imaging evaluation is required.

Category I-

Negative.
- .05% chance of malignancy. Annual screening recommended for >45 years women.

Category II-

Benign findings. May be cyst or fibroadenoma. Follow-up yearly is recommended.

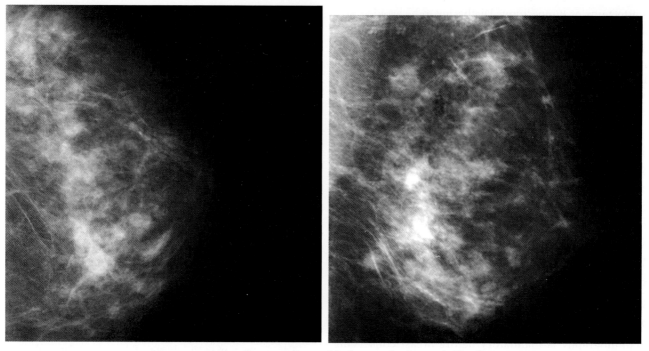

Mammography show malignant lesion and microcalcification

Category III-

Probably benign findings- short interval follow-up is suggested (6 months interval). Chance of cancer < 2%.

Category IV-
- Suspicious abnormality.
- FNAC / true cut to be considered.
- Chance of malignancy 25-50%.

Category V-
- Highly suggestive of malignancy (75-99%)
- FNAC / Biopsy suggested for tissue diagnosis.

Category VI
FNAC proven carcinoma breast.

How will you do FNAC?

I will aspirate the tissue form the tumor under negative pressure.

Procedure:

Clean the area with antiseptic solution
↓
Fix the lump
↓
Take 22/23 gauge needle attached to a 10 ml syringe and put it inside the tumor

↓
Create negative pressure
↓
Move the needle in different direction
↓
Take it off and make slides.

What is the predictive value of FNAC?

- Sensitivity is up to 95%
- Specificity is almost 100%
- False negative is 2-10%.

Suppose your FNAC result come negative. What will you do next?

I will do repeat FNAC. If it comes negative I will do true cut biopsy.

Or I can do directly true cut biopsy.

Tissue also is used for hormone receptors study.

What are the indications of incisional biopsy?

When repeat FNAC is inconclusive.

True cut biopsy inconclusive or true cut middle not available.

When the breast mass is more than 4 cm.

[Note- while taking incision for biopsy it should be planned to be inside the subsequent incisional area for mastectomy or lumpectomy. Diathermy to be avoided as it may damage the histological picture of the tumor and may destroy the hormonal receptors status.]

What is the role of frozen section biopsy in suspected carcinoma breast?

In suspected Ca breast when the repeated FNAC is inconclusive- some surgeons like to do still frozen section biopsy to see the nature of the growth. If it shows malignancy MRM/ lumpectomy with axillary clearance is to be considered.

The drawbacks of frozen section biopsy are-
- It is difficult to differentiate an invasive carcinoma from severe atypia or carcinoma *in situ*.
- Experienced pathologist is required to give the proper opinion on which surgical option is fully depended.

Why mammography is mandatory before the planning for breast conserving surgery?

Mammography is mandatory before breast conserving surgery because it can show whether the CA breast is multicentric or multifocal.

If it is multicentric - BCS is contraindicated.

[Multi centric- multicentricity refers to the occurrence of a second breast cancer outside the breast quadrant of the primary cancer.

Multifocal- multifocality refers to the occurrence of a second cancer within the same breast quadrant as the primary cancer.]

How will you stage the early Ca breast?

Early CA breast means
- T1, T2, N1 M0 Or T3, N0, M0 disease
- Where chance of distant mets, bone mets are relatively less
- So, I will do the following investigations to stage the disease
- LFT to exclude liver involvement
- Chest X-ray PA view- to exclude lung involvement
- USG abdomen- to exclude liver mets- lymphadenopathy, ascites etc.

Do you know perfectly the TNM classification of carcinoma breast?

Yes sir.
- Tx- Primary tumor cannot be assessed
- T0- No evidence of primary tumour
- Tis- Carcinoma *in situ*

[Tis (DCIS)- Ductal Carcinoma *in situ*
Tis (LCIS) - Lobular carcinoma *in situ*
Tis (Paget's) Paget's disease of the nipple without tumor].
- T1- tumor 2 cm or less in greatest dimension
- T1 mic-micro invasion 0.1 cm or less in greatest dimension
- T1a- Tumor more than .1 cm but not more than .5 cm in greatest dimension
- T1b- Tumor more than .5 cm but not more than 1 cm in greatest dimension
- T1c- Tumor more than 1 cm but not more than 2 cm in greatest dimension
- T2- Tumor more than 2 cm but not more than 5 cm in greatest dimension
- T3- Tumor more than 5 cm in greatest dimension
- T4- tumor any size with direct extension to
  a. Chest wall or
  b. Skin involvement or
  c. Both chest wall or skin involvement or
  d. Inflammatory breast carcinoma.
- T4a- Extension to the chest wall (intercostal muscles, ribs and anterior fibers of serratus anterior not pectorals major)
- T4b- Skin- Oedema, including Peau d'sorange or ulceration or satellite nodules confided to the same breast.
- T4c- Both T4a and T4b
- T4d- Inflammatory breast carcinoma.

Regional lymph nodes- clinical N.
- Nx- Regional lymph node can not be assessed.
- N0- No regional lymph node involvement.
- N1- Metastasis to ipsilateral axillary lymph nodes.
- N2- Metastasis in ipsilateral axillary lymph node fixed or matted or in clinically apparent ipsilateral internal mammary nodes in the absence of clinically evident axillary lymph node metastasis.
- N2a- Metastasis in ipsilateral axillary lymph node fixed to one another (matted) to other structure.
- N2b- Metastasis only in clinically apparent ipsilateral internal mammary nodes and in the absence of clinically evident axillary lymph nodes metastasis.
- N3a- Metastasis in ipsilateral infraclavicular lymph node(s).
- N3b- Metastasis in ipsilateral internal mammary lymph node(s) and axillary lymph node(s).

Distant metastasis (M)-
- Mx- Distant metastasis cannot be assessed.
- M0- No distant metastasis.
- M1- Distant metastasis.

What do you mean by early CA breast and locally advanced Carcinoma breast?

- Early CA breast is T1, T2, N0/ N1, Mo or T3 N0 M0.
- Locally advanced CA breast is T3, T4 and any N, M0 or any T, N2, N3, M0.
  [Metastatic Ca breast any T, any N, M1]

How will you manage the case of early Ca breast?

After confirmation and staging of Ca breast I will do all base line investigations to make the patient fit for anesthesia.

I will plan for breast conserving surgery in this case.

What do you mean by breast conserving surgery?

Breast conserving surgery consisting of
  i. Lumpectomy, i.e. wide local excision of the lump with 1 cm margin.
  ii. Axillary clearance and
 iii. Postoperative padiotherapy - which is an integral part of BCS, called Breast conserving therapy (BCT)
    [Postoperative radiotherapy can be avoided in a) elderly patient >70 years b) where all dissected lymph nodes are negative and c) in ER, PR positive status.]

What are all you look before you proceed for BCS, i.e. what are all the contraindications of BCS?

Breast conservation, nowaday, to be considered for all patients because of the important cosmetic advantages but relative contraindications to breast conservation therapy include

- Prior radiation therapy to the breast or chest wall.
- Multicentric disease.
- Involved surgical margin or unknown margin status following re-excision.
- Scleroderma or other connective tissue disorders.

What all will you consider before breast conserving surgery?

Sir,
- I will assess the stage of Ca breast; I will prefer to do BCS in early Ca breast.
- I will take patient consent for BCS and give importance to patient choice.
- I will inform the negative aspects of BCS like chance of recurrence is 10%. Patient has to receive postoperative radiotherapy which takes usually 6 weeks.
- Breast should be adequate size to allow uniform dosage of radiation.
- And of course I will confirm whether radiotherapy facility available/affordable or not.

When will you consider mastectomy in early Ca breast?

  i. Recurrence after BCS.
  ii. Margin positive after lumpectomy.
 iii. Multicentric carcinoma breast.
  iv. Poorly differentiated carcinoma breast, and
   v. Of course, patient choice is very important.

Why axillary clearance is essential in a case of Ca breast?

Axillary lymph node involvement is no
  i. Important prognostic factor of the disease.
  ii. LN involvement is a deciding factor for adjuvant therapy.
 iii. And it stages the disease.

What are the prognostic factors for a patient of Ca breast?

Prognostic factors of Ca breast is divided into
a. Tumor factors.
b. Host factors.

a. Tumor factors are:
   - Nodal status.
   - Tumor size.
   - Histologic/nuclear grade.
   - Pathological stage.
   - Hormone receptors status.
   - DNA content (Ploidy, PHASE fraction).
   - Extensive intraductal component.
b. Host factors:
   - Age.
   - Menopausal status.
   - Family history.
   - Previous breast cancer.
   - Immunosuppression.
   - Nutrition.
   - Prior chemotherapy.
   - Prior radiotherapy.

What are the indications of simple mastectomy?

Indications of simple mastectomy are
- Recurrence of BCS/margin positive after lumpectomy.
- Extensive DCIS.
- Cystosarcoma phyllodes
- In the form of palliative toilet mastectomy.
- Atypical hyperplasia of the breast.

What are the types of modified radical mastectomy?

i. Patey's MRM- it consists of en block resection of breast and axillary lymph nodes.

ii. Here, the pectoralis minor muscle is removed for adequate axillary dissection, i.e. to clear the level ii and iii axillary lymph nodes.

iii. All levels of Axillary lymph nodes.

Scanlon's procedure—where the pectoralis minor is divided for adequate clearance of axillary nodes level III. (Remember Sub Division. Here, S-scanlon and D-divition)

Auchincloss—where the pectoralis minor is retracted for giving clearance of level III axillary lymph nodes.

What are the adjuvant therapy after BCS?

Adjuvant therapy in the form of:

a. Radiotherapy - which is an integral part of breast conserving surgery.

b. Chemotherapy.

c. Radiotherapy- part and parcel of BCS - 50 gy is the dose for whole breast and lymph nodal field with 100 gy boost to the local site of tumor.

d. Chemotherapy- tumor >1 cm is considered as systemic disease and chemotherapy is essential irrespective of lymph nodal status.

The common chemotherapeutic regimes used are

i. CAF- Cyclophosphamide 500 mg/sqm body surface area.
   • Adriamycin- 50 mg/sqm body surface area.
   • 5 Fluorouracil - 500 mg/sqm body surface area.
   • Chemotherapy to be repeated every 21 days for 6 such cycle. Blood counts and kidney function test (urea, creatinine) are mandatory before each cycle of chemotherapy.

ii. CEF-
   • C- Cyclophosphamide.
   • E- Epirubicin.
   • F- 5- Fluorouracil.

iii. CMF- Cyclophosphamide.
   • Methotrexate.
   • 5 fluorouracil.

Side effects of these chemotherapeutic drugs are:
• Nausea.
• Vomiting.
• Alopecia.
• Myelosuppression.
• Cardiac toxicity (with Adriamycin).
• Premature menopause, etc.

What all will you expect from the pathologist while you sending the specimen?

I will ask

i. Type of tumor histopathologically.

ii. Comments on margin of the specimen whether the margin is free of tumor or not resection margin, skin involvement, etc.

iii. Grading of tumor - type of cell differentiation.

iv. Hormone receptor status - ER/ PR.
   • HER2 receptors status.

v. Axillary lymph nodal status—very important to stage the disease and for prognostic factor and of course for the treatment plan.

What is the role of hormone therapy in this case?

• Tamoxifen is very much effective in both pre- and post-menopausal patients with +ve ER/ PR status, in most of the cases except ER -ve premenopausal lady.

• Aim to prevent recurrence as well as to prevent development of opposite breast cancer.

• Mechanism of action:
   – Tamoxifen blocks the uptake of estrogen by estrogen receptors of the breast tissue

• Dose- 20 mg tab/day for 5 years.

• Why to give this hormone therapy? - It reduces the incidence of contralateral breast cancer.

• Side effects are- hot flushes as it initiates early menopause.

• Vaginal bleeding.

• Bone pain.

• Irregular menses.

• Increase the risk of carcinoma endometrial carcinoma 2-3 folds.

• May increase thromboembolic events.

• Fluid electrolytes imbalance.

• Transient hypercalcemia.

What are the indications of radiotherapy in early Ca breast?

The indications of radiotherapy in early Ca breast are:

i. As an integral part of breast conserving surgery.

ii. Larger tumor size > 5 cm - depends on surgeon's preference.

iii. Lymphnode involvement more than four out of 10 lymph nodes.

What others hormonal therapy is used in Ca breast?

i. Oral aromatase inhibitors like Anastrazole, 1 mg, Letrozole 2 mg once a day—specifically effective in post menopausal women.
   Mechanism of action—Aromatase inhibitors blockage the synthesis of estrogen by the adrenal gland.

ii. LHRH—agonist like goserelin.

Different Incisions in Breast Lump

i. 'Webster' - excision through a circumareolar incision.
ii. Galliard Thomas incision. Excision through sub-mammary incision.
iii. Stewart incision Horizontal incision for mastectomy.

Study Thoroughly

- Anatomy breast
- Blood supply
- Lymphatic drainages
- Level of axillary's lymph nodes

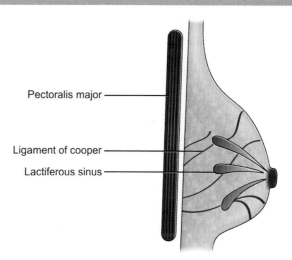

Anatomy of the breast

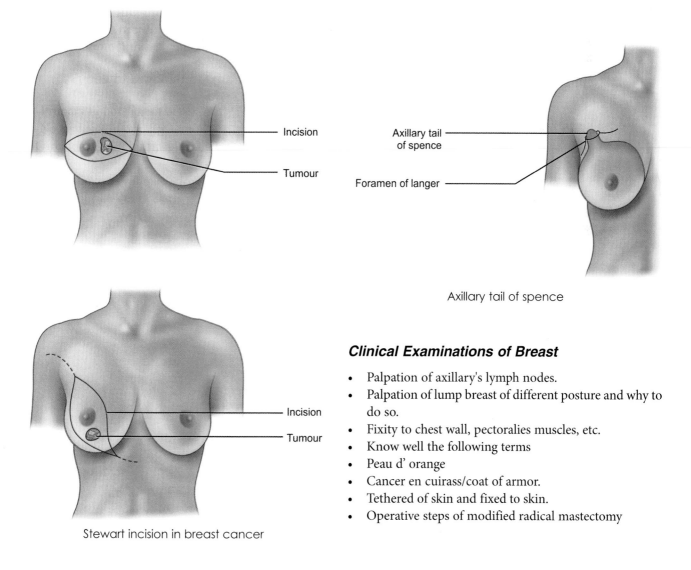

Incision

Tumour

Axillary tail of spence

Foramen of langer

Incision

Tumour

Axillary tail of spence

Stewart incision in breast cancer

Clinical Examinations of Breast

- Palpation of axillary's lymph nodes.
- Palpation of lump breast of different posture and why to do so.
- Fixity to chest wall, pectoralies muscles, etc.
- Know well the following terms
- Peau d' orange
- Cancer en cuirass/coat of armor.
- Tethered of skin and fixed to skin.
- Operative steps of modified radical mastectomy

LOCALLY ADVANCED CA BREAST

Case to be presented as before. The case summary of LABC is like this-

My patient Anita, a 55-years-old postmenopausal lady presented with a lump in her left breast for last 1 and ½ years. The lump is painlessly progressive and attained its present size approx 6 × 4 cm from its initial size of a marbel approximately 2 × 1.5 cm.

She also noticed a lump in her left axilla for last 1 year which is gradually increasing in size.

But there is no history of any other lump in opposite breast or axilla. No history of chest pain, coughs, haemoptysis or bone pain.

General survey is essentially normal.

On Examination

- Right breast appears normal. The left breast is drawn upwards, the lump is visible at upper outer quadrant, and the nipple areolar complex is slightly inverted. The Peau'd' orange appearance in the skin over the lump. The lump is 6 × 4 cm, fixed to the chest wall and the skin over the lump. Firm in consistency margins are well defined, irregular, surface is uneven.
- In axilla one lymphnode is palpable at left axilla which is fixed.
- No lymphoedema in the left arm or no supra clavicular lymphadenopathy noticed.
- Systemic examination is normal. So, this is a case of locally advanced carcinoma breast.
- Clinically T4c N2 Mx.

what do you mean by locally advanced carcinoma breast?

Locally advanced means
   T3, T4 any N, M0.
   Or any T, N2/N3, M0 (stage IIIA and IIIB).

How will you investigate the patient?

- I will confirm my diagnosis first [as written in early Ca breast.
- All investigations are same like early Ca breast.
- Extra investigations- to be done is whole body bone scan to exclude skeletal metastasis.
- CECT chest to exclude pulmonary mets.

How will you treat the patient?

- I will assess the patient whether she is operable or not.
- In this patient the lump is fixed to the chest wall and axillary lymphnode also fixed.

- So, this is apparently inoperable. I will offer neoadjuvant chemotherapy (3-6 cycles), aim is to make the patient operable (the tumor will be free from chest wall).
- Then I can do modified radical mastectomy.
- If the tumor is still fixed to the chest wall I can offer only treatment like (i) palliative simple mastectomy: Fdan, ulcer or fungative lesion persist (ii) CT/RT (iii) Hormonal therapy.

Which locally advanced carcinomas are inoperable?

   i. Very large tumor i.e high tumor breast ratio.
   ii. Fixed to the chest wall even after neoadjuvant chemotherapy.
   iii. Extensive involvement of skin, fungating mass, ulcerative growth.
   iv. Large and fixed axillary lymphnode excludes the possibility of axillary clearance.

Can breast conserving surgery play any role in LABC?

In present days, BCS is surgery of choice in carcinoma breast even in LABC. But the condition is to make the tumor operable and/or to downgrade the tumor by giving neoadjuvant chemotherapy.

If the tumor has good response to chemotherapy BCS can be offered.

Postoperative radiotherapy and remaining cycles of chemotherapy to be given.

There after hormonal therapy as per ER/ PR and menopausal status.

What are the indications of radiotherapy in a case of Carcinoma breast?

Indications are
- Positive margins.
- Involvement of skin and muscle.
- Residual disease.
- TX and PT3 lesion. [P stands for pathological lesion]
- More than three nodes positive.
- Perinodal involvement.
- Vascular or lymphatic involvement.
- More than 25% nodes positive. If the number of removed nodes less than 5.
- Part of BCS, the therapy is called BCT.
- N2 disease.

Postaxillary boost to be given if more than 10 nodes positive.

What is the ideal time for radiotherapy?

Preferable time to give radiotherapy within 14-16 weeks after surgery.

What is the prognosis of locally advanced carcinoma breast?

- 5 years survival is 45-50%.
- 10 years survival is 25-30%.

Do you know 'Pragmatic' classification of breast cancer?

Group	Approximate 5 years survival rate	Example	Treatment
Very low risk primary breast	>90%	Screen detected DCIS,	Local

contd...

contd...

cancer		tubular or special types	
low risk primary breast cancer	70-90%	Node negative with favourable histology	Locoregional with or Without systemtic
High primary breast cancer	<70%	Node positive with unfavourable histology	Locoregional with systemic
Localy advanced primary breast cancer	<30%	Large primary or inflammatory	Primary systemic
Metastatic breast cancer	_____	_____	Primary systemic

CARCINOMA BREAST WITH DISTANT METASTASES

How will you investigate a case of Ca breast with distant mets?

All the investigations are like in LABC (locally advanced breast cancer):

- FNAC.
- Chest X-ray - PA.
- LFT.
- USG/ CT abdomen.
- Whole body bone scans.
- Other specific investigation like CECT brain/skeletal survey/CT chest etc depends on the site of metastasis.

How will you treat the patients of metastatic Ca breast?

Treatment of this patient, are to relieve symptomatically and to provide palliation by giving - chemotherapy, hormonal therapy, radiotherapy and limited surgery.

[Chemotherapy- first line drugs CAF- Cyclophosphamide. Adriyamycin and 5 Fu (Anthracyclin base).

Newer drugs- taxanes- paclitaxel and docetaxel, more effective as a single agent or as a combined chemotherapy.

Pamidronate to prevent osteoporosis.

Hormonal therapy- Tamoxifen in ER positive patient.

In premenopausal patient - 1st line treatment is tamoxifen or ovarian ablation.

2nd line ovarian ablation after tamoxifen.

In postmenopausal patient - anti estrogen (Tamoxifen)

2nd line treatment - aromatase inhibitors like anastrozole, letrozole.

(In postmenopausal lady, the source of estrogen is extra ovarian, i.e. adrenal gland. So aromatase inhibitors which prevent the synthesis of estrogen are very effective in postmenopausal women.).

Radiotherapy- palliative radiotherapy to breast, lymphnodal fields, bone mets to relieve pain, brain mets, to decompress the spinal cord mets. To some extent it may be given to liver mets also to provide effective palliation of symptoms.

Surgery- for providing palliation
- Simple or toilet mastectomy.
- Extended simple mastectomy when axillary lymphnode, also removed for palliation along with breast lump.
- Solitary lung mets, hepatic mets, brain mets may have some benefit.
- Ovarian ablation in premenopausal women (LHRH analogue may bring about reversible chemical castration).

What is sporadic, familial and hereditary breast cancer?

Sporadic- where there is no family history of breast cancer in two generation. Incidence- 65-75%.

Familial- where there is family history of breast cancer in either first or second degree relatives. There is no definite mode of inheritance. Incidence- 20-30%.

Hereditary- there is a family history of breast cancer in 1st or 2nd degree relatives where mode of inheritance is autosomal dominant.

History of related ovarian (70%) or colonic cancer in the family. Incidence- 5-10%.

How obesity and alcoholism are related to carcinoma breast?

Obesity- the major source of estrogen in postmenopausal women is the conversion of androstenedione to estrone by adipose tissue, obesity is associated with long-term increase in estrogen exposure.

- **Alcoholism**- Alcohol consumption is known to increase serum level of estradiol, the evidence suggests that chronic consumption of fatty foods contributes to an increased risk of breast cancer by increasing serum estrogen levels.

BRCA Mutation:
- BRCA1 and BRCA 2 which are inherited in an autosomal dominant.
- BRCA 1 is located on chromosome 17 q.

- BRCA 2 is located on chromosome 13 q.
- BRCA1 associated breast cancer are invasive ductal carcinoma poorly differentiated.

The distinguishing clinical features of BRCA1 are:
- Early age of onset, compared with sporadic cases.
- Higher prevalence of bilateral breast cancer.
- Associated cancers in some affected individuals, specifically ovarian cancer and possibly colon and prostate cancers.

BRCA2- estimated breast cancer risk is 62.

Representing a, l00-fold increase over the general male population risk.

Associated with invasive ductal carcinomas more likely to be well differentiated.

Distinguishing clinical features -
- Early age of onset, compared with sporadic cases.
- Higher prevalence of bilateral breast cancers.
- Presence of associated cancers in some affected individuals, especially ovarian, colon, prostate, pancreas, gall bladder, bile duct, stomach cancers, as well as melanoma.

IMPORTANT NOTES ON CA BREAST

Incidence

The incidence of cancer breast is slightly increasing, coming very close to that of Ca cervix, which is the common cancer in women. It is the most common cause of mortality in woman aged 40 to 55. Incidence increases with age, peaking in the sixth decade.

Predisposing factors

There is a large number of predisposing factors or risk factors which increase the possibility of getting Ca breast. However, only ten percent of patients have any of these factors. Hereditary, genetic predisposition, hormonal factors and diet etc are few of these risk factors.

Strong family history of Ca breast in mother, sister and maternal aunt, presence of mutation of BRCA 1 and BRCA 2 gene, early menarche, nulliparity, late menopause, excessive use of estrogens, increase the risk. Atypical hyperplasia increases the risk too.

Late menarche, first child at or before 18 years of age, early menopause, and oophorectomy before 35 years, decrease the risk.

There is an increase risk in American women and ladies of the upper socioeconomic class. Excessive use of fat, alcohol, cholesterol rich diet and exposure to radiation may increase risk too.

Past history of Ca Breast in the opposite side is the biggest risk factor.

Pathology

Carcinoma breast generally arises from Terminal duct lobular unit (TDLU) more than 95% cancers are adenocarcinomas, being ductal or lobular, each of these can be invasive or *in situ*. Invasive ductal carcinoma (IDC) is most common, found in over 80% cases, the most common variety of IDC is not other vice specified (NOS), found in over 80% cases of IDC, other types of IDC are tubular, papillary, comado, medullary and colloid. DCIS, LCIS and ILC (Intra lobular carcinomas) are found in less than 5% .Ca breast spreads by lymphatics and by hematogenous route. Metastasis to axillary lymph nodes are found in almost 40-50% cases at time of presentation, though internal mammary chain and supraclavicular nodes may be involved in less than 5%.

Common sites of distant spread are liver, lung, bone and brain. Pelvic deposits may be seen in advanced cases due to transcoelomic spread.

Prognostic Factors

Though there is a long list of prognostic factors today, age nodal status and tumor size remain the three main prognostic factors.

Young age, large tumor and involvement of axillary nodes, gravely effect prognosis.

Histological type and grade, lymphatic and vascular invasion, proliferative index, S phase fraction, ploidy are other factors that effect prognosis.

Over expression of c-erb B-2 ECG factor, Cathepsin D and mutated P53 are poor prognostic factors, while over expressed bcl 2, Nm 23 gene and PS2 factors improve prognosis.

Clinical Presentation

Lump breast is the most common form of presentation of carcinoma breast. Axillary lymphadenopathy, nipple retraction, nipple discharge and skin involvement may be the other presentations. Rarely patient may present only with axillary or supraclavicular nodes only or bone pain rarely.

Investigations

FNAC of the lump and the axillary nodes is the best diagnostic tool. This combined with Tru cut biopsy yields a diagnosis in more that 95%. Mammography and ultrasound are helpful in localizing small tumors and cases presenting with nipple retraction and discharge or axillary lymphadenopathy without a breast lump. However, mammography should be done in all cases of carcinoma breast, specially when breast conserving surgery is being planned to rule out multicentric and bilateral disease and to have a baseline for follow-up of opposite breast. Image guided needle biopsy or lumpectomy with frozen section may have to be resorted to in rare cases for diagnosis where FNAC or Tru cut has been inconclusive. Breast MRI and radionucilide imaging are rarely needed in clinical practice in situation of T0N1 disease.

While X-ray chest and ultrasound of abdomen are adequate for the metastatic work up of early Ca breast, bone scan should be done for all patients of locally advanced metastatic carcinoma breast.

All operative specimens should be checked for ERPR and HER 2 neu receptors, the cases of LABC being managed with NACT (Neo adjuvant chemotherapy), should undergo tru cut biopsy for these tests.

TNM Staging

Primary Tumor (T):
- Tx- Primary tumor cannot be assessed.
- T1S- Carcinoma in site.
- T1- Tumor less than 2 cm.
- T2- Tumor 2-5 cm.
- T3- Tumor more than 5 cm.
- T4-
  (a) Extension of chest wall
  (b) Peau d' orange ulceration or satellite nodule in skin.
  (c) 4a + 4b
  (d) Inflammatory carcinoma breast.

Regional lymph node (N):
- Nx- Regional lymphnodes cannot be assessed.
- N1- Metastasis to mobile ipsilateral lymphnodes.
- N2- metastasic ipsilateral lymphnodes are stuck to each other or other axillary structures.
- N3- Metastatic to ipsilateral internal mammary or supraclavicular lymph nodes

Distant Metastasis(M)
- Mx- Distant metastasis cannot be assessed.
- M0- No distant metastasis.
- M1- Distant metastasis.

Staging Grouping:

Stage	T	N	M
Stage 0	Tis	N0	M0
Stage 1	T1	N0	M0
Stage IIA	T0, T1	N1	M0
Stage IIB	T2	N1	M0
	T3	N0	M0
Stage IIIA	T0 T1 T2	N2	M0
	T3	N1, N2	M0
Stage IIIB	T4	Any N	M0
	Any T	N3	M0
Stage IV	Any T	Any M	M1

Clinical Group Staging:
- This is more commonly used.
- Early Ca breast- T1, T2, N1, M0.
- Locally advanced Ca breast- T3, T4 any N, M0, Any T N2, N3 M0.
- Metastatic Ca breast- Any T, Any N, M1.
- Regional Lymph nodes- There are two groups of lymph nodes that drain the breast.
1. **Axillary lymph nodes:** This group includes the interpectoral (Rotors nodes) and nodes along the axillary vein and its tributaries.

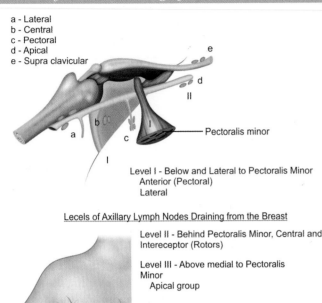

a - Lateral
b - Central
c - Pectoral
d - Apical
e - Supra clavicular

Pectoralis minor

Level I - Below and Lateral to Pectoralis Minor
Anterior (Pectoral)
Lateral

Lecels of Axillary Lymph Nodes Draining from the Breast

Level II - Behind Pectoralis Minor, Central and
Intereceptor (Rotors)

Level III - Above medial to Pectoralis
Minor
Apical group

Circumareolar (Webster Incision)

Submammary (Galliard Thomas)

Different incisions of breast surgery

Levels of axillary lymphnodes are called Berg's levels:

a. *Level I (Low axilla):* Lumph nodes below and lateral to the lateral border of pectorals minor.

b. *Level II (Midaxilla):* Lymph nodes between the medial and lateral border of pectorals minor, (under it) and the interpectoral group.

c. *Level III (Apical axilla):* lymph nodes above and medial to the medial border of oectoralis minor.

2. **Internal Mammary lymph nodes:** in the intercostals spaces, along the edge of sternum.

Management of early Ca breast surgery is the mainstay in management of early Ca breast. There are two options available.

Breast Conservation Therapy (BCT)

BCT is in vogue these days and should be resorted to when ever possible. It includes a lumpectomy with axillary clearance and radiotherapy to breast and boost, preferably with implant, to the tumor bed. One to 2 cm of margins around the lump is adequate and a part of the overlying skin can be excised.

Incision for lumpectomy and axillary clearance should be separate as far as possible.

The only absolute contraindications of BCT are:

• Two primaries in different quadrants.
• Small lump breast ratio

• Nonavailability or contraindication to radiotherapy.
• Pregnancy.
• Extensive DCIS.

All patients undergoing BCT should undergo bilateral mammography to rule out multicentric disease.

BCT can be offered to cases of LABC too, after anterior chemotherapy.

Modified Radical Mastectomy

Entails removal of the lump with the complete breast, skin overlying the lump and nipple areolar system and axillary clearance.

ER PR evaluation should be carried out on operated specimen for all patients.

Management of axilla

Axillary lymph node dissection is an integral part of surgical management of Ca breast for following reasons:

• Gives accurate staging.
• Provides useful prognostic information.
• Assists in planning adjuvant therapy.
• Gives potential therapeutic gain.

The extent of axillary clearance is debatable but as on date removal of Level 1 and II nodes is minimum, desired and considered optimal. Level III is included for optimal clearance because minimum ten nodes are required for proper staging and same may not be available in level I clearance, and secondly the skip lesions in level II nodes, sparing level I is upto 15%.

Removal of level I and II nodes provide adequate clearance in absence of extra capsular spread or numerous nodal metastases and there are survival benefits in subsets of patients who have only microscopic nodal metastasis. These are removed completely as part of Level I and II dissection and it seems that axillary clearance improves 10 year survival rates. Many surgeons include removal of level III nodes in routine axillary clearance, as it does not add to morbidity or increase operative time in expert hands. Apical node clearance is beneficial in node positive axilla and can be omitted in node negative patients.

Sentinel Lymph Node Biopsy (SLN)

Sentinel node biopsy may be the ideal approach to select patients with negative axilla who require conventional lymphadenectomy. The rational of SLN biopsy is that each breast cancer has its unique lymph node draining preference. The SLNs represent the first draining nodes that are most

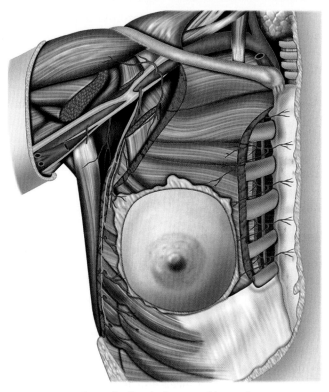

Lymphatic drainage of breast

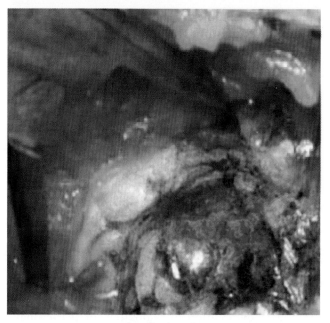

Sentinel node

likely to be involved in tumor matastasis. When SLNs are free of cancer, it is assumed that the remaining lymph nodes are not involved by metastasis. SLN mapping can be achieved by injecting radio labeled tracers or vital dye. Radioisotope activity is then picked up by Gama camera.

Though the detection rate of SLNs in the axilla in most reports is 90% or higher and false negative prediction or skip metasis is approximately 5% or less, SLN mapping has not yet become the standard of care.

Adjuvant Therapy in Early Ca Breast:

Chemotherapy - indications for adjuvant chemotherapy in early Ca breast are:
- All premenopausal and perimenopausal women.
- All node positive cases.
- Tumor size more than 1 cm.
- Young post menopausal ER/ PR negative women even with T1b, No disease.

Infact most patients need adjuvant chemotherapy, except postmenopausal lady with ER/PR positive, T1b,N0 diseases, or elderly ladies with node negative disease favorable history like mucinous tubular or papillary carcinoma.

Chemotherapeutic Regimes

Commonly used chemotherapeutic regimes are - anthracyclin, (Adriamycin, or epirubicin) based four to six cycles of CAF (Cyclophosphamide, Adriamycin and 5-FU), AC, FEC or EC are normally given.

Radiation

External beam radiation to the chest wall recommended for following situations:
- Involvement of skin or muscle.
- Residual disease.
- Positive margins.
- TX or PT3 lesion.
- More than four nodes positive.
- Perinodal spread.
- Vascular or lymphatic spread.
- More than 25% of nodes positive of the lymph nodes cleared.
- Axilla is included in radiotherapy field if:
  – N2 disease.
  – Residual nodal disease.
  – Posterior axillary boost given if more than 10 nodes positive.

Radiotherapy in BCT is part of primary treatment.

Sequence of chemotherapy and radiotherapy:

- If radiotherapy is to be given for residual disease or positive margins, then it should be given after one cycle of chemotherapy, and followed by remaining chemotherapy.
- If radiotherapy is indicated for nodal involvement or T3 T4 lesion, or muscle or skin involvement, then 3-4 cycles or all cycles of chemotherapy should be given before radiotherapy.
- It is however preferable to give radiotherapy within 14-16 weeks after surgery.

Hormonal Therapy:

Tamoxifen is the most common hormonal treatment used. Indicated in all patients who are ER PR positive, irrespective of menopausal status, in doses of 20 mg OD for five years. Tamoxifen preferably to be started after completion of chemotherapy and radiotherapy where indicated. Aromitase inhibitors like letrozole to be given to these patients for 2-5 years after completion of tamoxifen, or if they have recurrence while on or after tamoxifen.

Locally Advanced Breast Carcinoma (LABC):

LABC (T3 or T4 with any N or Any T with N2 or N3 and M0) are managed with all three modalities, surgery, chemotherapy and radiotherapy. The sequence of these to be tailor made to suit the patient.

If the tumor is operable then the patient undergoes surgery (Mastectomy or lumpectomy and axillary clearance) followed by chemotherapy and radiotherapy.

Cases which are nonoperable at time of presentation, are given anterior (neoadjuvant) chemotherapy, three to four cycles to downstage and make the tumor operable. Once this is achieved, surgery is performed, followed by radiotherapy and remaining cycles of chemotherapy.

Chemotherapy regimes and indications for hormonal treatment are same as in early Ca breast.

Patients with supraclavicular nodal metastasis are treated as LABC. Anterior chemotherapy is given and once the supraclavicular nodes regress, the patient is offered surgery and radiotherapy and remaining chemotherapy.

Two to three cycles of neoadjuvant chemotherapy may be given to even operable cases of LABC to prevent systemic spread.

Metastatic Carcinoma Breast

There is no role of surgery in patients presenting with metastatic disease at the time of diagnosis. Common sites for metastasis are liver, lungs, bone and brain. (Remember LLB)

These patient are managed with taxol based chemotherapy and hormonal treatment.

Patients with brain metastasis get cranial radiotherapy with or without tablet timizolemide.

Patient with extensive body metastasis require hemi or whole body radiation with monthly injection pamidronate.

Local surgery or radiotherapy can be offered as a palliative measure, in case of pain, necrosis, ulceration, fungation or anxiety of patient for retaining the diseased breast.

Oophorectomy by surgery or radiotherapy can be considered for premenopausal ladies with metasitatic disease.

Recurrent Disease

Local recurrence after BCT needs mastectomy and recurrence over chest wall following mastectomy is treated with wide local excision and local radiotherapy.

Second line chemotherapy to be considered in all these cases.

Recurrent disease at distant sites is managed with salvage chemotherapeutic regims like MMM (Mitomycin, methotrexate, and mitoxantrone) and second or third line hormonal therapy with megace or femera. Other chemotherapeutic agents available are liposomal doxorubi, weekly epirubicin, gemcitabin and vinorelbine with cisplatinum.

Herceptine to be used in recurrent or advanced metastatic cases, which are HER 2 neu positive.

Carcinoma Breast in Males

About one percent of breast cancers are found in males. The initial stage of presentation in males is higher than in females with a large number being diagnosed in stage III.

Management and prognosis is same as in females. Males may have lobular carcinoma too tamoxifen is used in ER, PR cases for hormonal manipulation.

Inflammatory Carcinoma Breast

This is an aggressive form of cancer breast seen in younger patients with extensive involvement of overlying skin and subcutaneous lymphatics. Managed as LABC with only change being that surgery is usually performed after chemotherapy and radiation.

Carcinoma in Situ

Ductal Carcinoma *in Situ* (DCIS)
DCIS or intraductal carcinoma is a distinct identity and its detection and incidence has markedly increased due to widespread use of screening mammography.

An abnormal mammographic report of clustered micro calcification is the most common presentation DCIS, however, it can also present as a lump, nipple discharge and an incidental finding in a breast biopsy. Involvement of lymph nodes in DCIS is very rare, found in about three percent of cases.

Treatment of DCIS is lumpectomy with radiotherapy. Axilla is normally spread, unless in cases with a large lump where axillary sampling can be done. Postoperative use of taoxifen reduces chances of ipsilateral or contralateral recurrences.

Patients of DCIS with large lumps or nodal deposits to be treated as early carcinoma breast.

Lobular Carcinoma *in Situ* (LCIS)

LCIS is an incidental finding in biopsy of breast tissue removed for some other cause. LCIS has low proliferative rate and most carcinomas that develop in women with LCIS are infiltrative ductal carcinomas and not infiltrative lobular carcinomas, LCIS hence is considered as a risk factor for breast cancer.

Close observation is all that is required for these patients, however, those who do not want to undertake the risk of developing cancer breast (1%) can undergo Bilateral simple mastectomy with immedeiate breast reconstruction.

Management of High Risk Patients

Patients with LCIS, strong history, women who carry mutations in BRCA 1 or 2 and those with atypical hyperplasia on biopsy of breast tissue, are high risk patients.

These patients should be under close observation and annual mammography.

Follow-up

Patients with Ca breast should be observed closely after treatment for metastasis and second primary on opposite breast. Besides routine work up, they should undergo annual mammography of the opposite breast, ultrasound abdomen and pelvis for endometrial carcinoma and bone scan every 2 years.

CASE 20

A Case of Solitary Nodule Thyroid (SNT)

My patient Anil Kumar, a 29 year old male, resident of Ghaziabad, UP, presented with a complaint of swelling infront of neck for last 3 months.

HISTORY OF PRESENT ILLNESS

My patient was apparently asymptomatic before 3 months back. When he noticed a pea nut size nodule infront of his neck which is gradually painlessly progressive and attained its present size approx. 3 x 3 cm.

i.   But there is no history of pressure symptoms in the form of:
     1. Difficulty in swallowing.
     2. Difficulty in breathing.
ii. No features suggestive of hypothyroidism in the form of:
     •   Weight gain.
     •   Fatigue.
     •   Intolerance to cold.
     •   Low memory etc.

Or hyperthyroidism in the form of:
     •   Increased appetite but weight loss
     •   Palpitation
     •   Weakness
     •   Intolerance to heat or
     •   Any difficulty in (eye function) vision.
iii. There is also no history of any other swelling in the neck.
iv. No history of bone pain, chest pain, hemoptysis, cough etc. (to exclude metastasis)

MULTINODULAR GOITER (MNG)

Case history in case of MNG—My patient Maina, a 35 years old female presented with a swelling infront and left side of her neck which is gradually progressive for last 5/6 years and attained its present size of approx 6 x 4 cm.

But there is no history suggestive of hypo/hyper-thyroidism.

On examination- general survey is essentially normal. On local examination, there is a swelling infront and left side of her neck which moves with deglutition. The swelling measures 6 x 4 cm. All the borders including lower border is well palpable, surface is nodular, firm and nontender. Carotid pulsation is well felt. No cervical lymph node palpable.)

CASE HISTORY IN CARCINOMA THYROID

My patient, Mina Kumari, a 40 years old lady, presented with a neck swelling for last 2 years which was initially increasing slowly in size but for last 5/6 months the swelling in rapidly increasing in size. Patient also complaints of feeling of heaviness in her neck along with change of voice for last 2 months.

No features suggestive of hypo or hyperthyroidism.

On examination, general survey is essentially normal. On local examination, there is diffused enlargement of thyroid; left lobe is more enlarged than the right measured 6 x 4 and 3 x 2 cm respectively.

Swelling moves with deglutition.

Surface is nodular, hard in consistency, all borders are well palpable but irregular. Not fixed to the underlying structure or overlying skin.

Pemberton sign—negative.

But there is multiple cervical lymph node palpable which are firm in consistency, mobile. Systemic examination is essentially normal.]

PAST HISTORY

•   Not contributory.
•   No history of HTN, DM.
•   No history of Long term drugs intake or any exposure to radiation.

FAMILY HISTORY

No relevant family history.

O/E-

- Patient is on average built, well nourished.
- P- 78/ min. normal volume, rhythm is regular.
- No pallor, Icterus, oedema or generalized lymphadenopathy noticed.

LOCAL EXAMINATION

I. **On inspection:** there is a spherical swelling approx 3 x 3 cm in the thyroid region just left to the midline.
- The swelling moves with deglutition but not with protrusion of tongue.
- Skin over the swelling looks normal not erythematous.
- No other swelling noticed at the neck.

II. **Palpitation**
- Inspectory findings are confirmed.
- Temperature not raised.
- Non tender.
- The swelling is round shaped 3×3 cm (site shape size).
- Firm in consistency, smooth surface.
- Lower border well palpable by Criles method the swelling is proved as a thyroid swelling Kocher's method shows- no pressure effect.
- It is a mobile swelling moves side to side, up and down. Not fixed to the skin or surroundings structure.
- Carotid pulsation felt at the normal site.
- No other swelling felt at neck.

III. **Percussion:** On percussion - in case of a large thyroid swelling - retrosternal prolongation of thyroid dull on percussion.

IV. **Auscultation:** No bruit is available.

Cervical lymph nodes: no lymph nodes palpable.

SYSTEMIC EXAMINATION

Essentially normal.

Summary

My patient 29 years old male, presented with the complaint of swelling at left side of thyroid region for last 1 month.

Which is painlessly progressive without any history of pressure effects or features suggestive of hypo/ hyperthyroidism or without any other swelling in the neck.

On Examination

Vitals are essentially normal. There is a 3 x 3 cm globular swelling at left side of thyroid region, moves with deglutition, firm in consistency, smooth, mobile lower margin well palpable, not fixed to the surrounding structure and without involvement of any lymph node in neck

Differential Diagnosis of solitary thyroid nodule are-
- Colloid goiter - up to 50%
- Cystic swelling in thyroid in 30% cases.
- Dominant nodule of MNG.
- Adenoma of thyroid.
- Malignant thyroid nodule 10-15% cases.

How will you present in this case?

Sir, first, I will confirm my diagnosis by doing
i. FNAC- for tissue diagnosis.
ii. USG- Neck- when cystic swelling is suspected.
iii. Thyroid profile test (T3, T4, and TSH) to exclude subclinical hypo/ hyperthyroidism.

How will you differentiate between follicular adenoma and follicular carcinoma in FNAC?

In FNAC, the picture may be same in both adenoma and carcinoma. In follicular carcinoma, capsular and vascular invasion is there my malignant follicular cells which cannot be identified from FNAC.

Can you try trucut biopsy in solitary nodule thyroid?

Trucut biopsy is not recommended for thyroid nodule.

The relative indications are:
i. When repeated FNAC is inconclusive and thyroid nodule is larger.
ii. In advanced carcinoma thyroid, trucut may be done for tissue diagnosis before giving chemotherapy.
iii. To diagnose lymphoma when it is suspected if FNAC is inconclusive.
iv. Anaplastic carcinoma thyroid if FNAC is inconclusive.

By FNAC, what are the conditions of thyroid are diagnosed?

Thyroid conditions that may be diagnosed by FNAC include, colloid goiter, thyroiditis, papillary Ca thyroid, medullary carcinoma, anaplastic carcinoma and lymphoma.

What are the indications for surgery of a SNT?

- All malignant nodules.
- Follicular neoplasm.
- Symptomatic thyroid nodules.

- Cystic nodule which does not disappear following three times aspiration.
- Non functioning or hyper functioning nodule.
- For cosmetic purposes.

In a case of thyroid malignancy how will you decide total or hemithyroidectomy?

In low risk group of patients I will do have or sub total thyroidectomy and in high risk group I will do total thyroidectomy.

How will divide low and high risk group?

Remember- AGES.

Low risk group	High Risk group
A- Age [Men < 40 years Female 16-45 yrs	[Men > 40 years Female< 16 years
G- Grade- Low grade tumor	or > 45 years.
E- Extension- Intra thyroid disease With or without minor capsular involvement Or extra thyroid spread.	High grade tumor major capsular involvement
S- [Papillary Ca < 1 cm Follicular Ca < 4 cm	[papillary > 1 cm Ca Follicular > 4 cm Ca

What are the risk factors of developing thyroid malignancy?

The risk factors are

i. Past history of exposure to radiation in the neck (example–radiation therapy for Hodge Kin's lymphoma in adolescent).

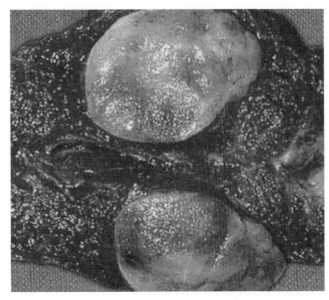

Follicular carcinoma thyroid

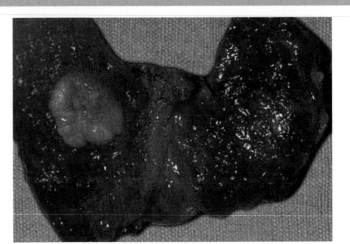

Medullary carcinoma thyroid

ii. Family history of thyroid malignancy. Example- 6-8 % of papillary carcinoma is familial. 15-20% of medullary carcinoma is familial.

Clinically how will you suspect malignant change from a benign SNT?

- Rapidly increasing size.
- Thyroid nodule with development of hoarseness of voice, dysphagia or dyspnea,.

    [Involvement of Recurrent laryngeal nerve, involvement of oesophagus and trachea respectively].

- Hard and fixed nodules.
- SNT along with pretracheal (Delphic), para tracheal lymph nodes (level 7) involvement.

What is thyroid paradox?

In case of papillary carcinoma thyroid cellular neoplasm is soft, cystic in feeling on palpation where as the cystic swelling is firm (tense cystic) in feeling - this is called thyroid paradox.

You know the WHO classification of thyroid swelling?

Yes Sir,

- Grade 0- no visible or palpable thyroid swelling.
- Grade I- there is a palpable thyroid swelling which is not visible.
- Grade II- there is visible and palpable thyroid swelling.
- Grade III- Large thyroid swelling.

How 'Berrys' name is related with thyroid?

Berry is related by the name of

i. **Berry Ligament**- the false capsule is cervical fascia. It is thin along the posterior border of the lobes, but thick on the inner surface of the gland where it forms suspensory ligament of Berry which connects the lobe to the cricoid cartilage.

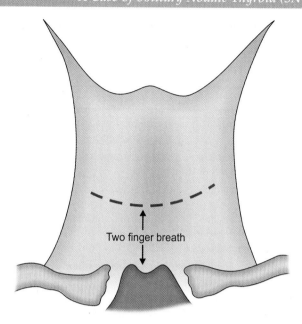

The location of parathyroid glands

Incision for thyroid operation

ii. **Berry sign**- In benign thyroid swelling carotid artery is displaced but pulsation is palpable. [normally carotid pulsation is felt at the level of upper border of thyroid cartilage at the anterior border of sternocleidomastoid muscle].

But in malignant lesion carotid sheath and surrounding tissue may invaded by thyroid malignancy as a result carotid pulsation may not be palpable. This is called Berry's sign.

iii. **Berry picking**- cervical nodes, along with thyroid malignancy are removed by a small incision over the individual lymph node - this is called Berry picking. It was being done before the concept of neck dissection initially

How l-thyroxine helps in malignant SNT?

It has been reported from different study that l thyroxin reduces, significantly the size of malignant thyroid nodule. But many other studies contradict this opinion.

But it is commonly accepted that l thyroxin is effective in patient of Hashimoto's thyroid in regression of goiter.

Can you define solitary Nodule thyroid (SNT)?

Yes sir, Solitary nodule can be defined as a discrete swelling (nodule) in one lobe with no other palpable abnormality in both the lobes of thyroid is termed as SNT.

[Discrete swelling with evidence of abnormality elsewhere in the gland are termed as dominant].

Can you tell be why all types of goiter more common in the female than in the male?

All types of goiter are more common in the female than in the male owing to presence of oestrogen receptors in thyroid tissue?

What are the types of thyroidectomy?

i. **Hemithyroidectomy**: Removal of one lobe and entire isthmus. It is usually done in benign disease of one lobe.

ii. **Subtotal thyroidectomy**: Removal of all thyroid tissue, keeping 8 grams of functional thyroid tissue at lower pole (4 grams may be kept at each lobe and it is measured by the size of pulp of patient's thumb or the amount of tissue in trachea oesophageal group.

iii. **Partial thyroidectomy**- Removal of thyroid tissue infront of trachea after mobilization.

It's commonly done in non toxic multinodular goiter. It is role is controversial.

iv. **Near total thyroidectomy**- Rim of thyroid tissue to be kept at lower pole of one or both the sides to save recurrent laryngeal nerve and parathyroid glands.

v. **Total thyroidectomy**: Entire thyroid gland is removed. Usually done in a case of papillary follicular carcinoma and medullary carcinoma of thyroid.

Other common questions - on thyrotoxicosis

How will you differentiate between primary and secondary hyperthyroidism.

Primary	Secondary
Symptoms appear first, swelling later	Swelling appears first symptoms later after a long time.
Usually thyroid swellings Diffuse, smooth, soft or firm	Swelling is large nodular.
Features are much more slowly	Features are less prominent and
prominent and rapidly progressive compared to secondary thyrotoxicosis.	progressive compared to primary thyrotoxicosis.
Ex ophthalmos and different eye signs are common	Eye signs are not common
CNS (central nervous system) signs like tremor, irritability, insomnia, weakness of muscle.	CVS (Cardiovascular symptoms) are common like palpitation, ectopic beats, dyspnea, chest pain etc.

What are the eye signs in toxic goiter?

i. **Von Graefe's sign:** Lid lag sign[Remember-VLDL] The upper eye lid lags behind the eye ball when the patient is asked to look downwards.

ii. **Jofroy's Sign:** Absence of wrinkling of forehead when the patient looks upwards including the face downwards.

iii. **Stellwag's sign:** Infrequent/absence of blinking of eyes- so there is a starring look as there is a widening of palpable fissure. This is due to contraction of levator palpebrae superiors. Remember this is the first sign to appear.

iv. **Moebius sign:** Lack of convergence of eye balls.

v. **Dalrymple's sign:** here the retraction of upper eyelid causes visibility of upper sclera.

vi. **Gifford sign**- difficult in everting upper eyelid in primary toxic goiter - it can differentiate between exophthalmos with proptosis. In exophthalmos it's very difficult to evert the eyelids but in proptosis you easily everts.

In exophthalmus in primary toxic goiter as the upper eyelids are tracted owing to increase partial sympathetic stimulation of levator palpebrae of upper eyelids. So eyelids are difficult to evert. Here eye ball is not pushed forward but looks like that.

But in proptosis, the eye ball is pushed forwards due to increase oedema, fat deposition or cellular infiltration in the retro orbital space. So there is no problem in upper eyelid. Sympathetic innovation is normal so eye lids can be everted easily.

vii. **Jellinec K's sign:** Increased pigmentation of eyelid margins

viii. **Enroth sign:** Oedema of eyelids and conjunctiva.

ix. **Rosenbach's sign:** Tremor of closed eyelids.

x. **Nafziger's sign:** In sitting with eye ball of the patient can be visualized when it is observed from behind.

What is exophthalmos?

Exophthalmos is mimicking forward protrusion of eye ball where potion of sclera is visible both above and below the cornea.

Causes of exophthalmos- Retraction of eyelids by any cause like increase sympathetic stimulation of upper eyelid, mimics forward protrusion of eye ball but actually eye ball is not protruded. [but commonly the term exophthalmus is used as like as proptosis where forward protrusion of the eye ball occurs due to increased retro orbital fat, infiltration of retrobulbar tissue with fluids and round cells.

So, exophthalmos and proptosis are different clinical conditions which can be differentiated by the sign called 'gifford sign'- described earlier.

What is thyroid acropathy?

In a case of primary thyrotoxicosis when there is clubbing of fingers and toes appear that clinical condition is called thyroid acropathy. This is one of the late signs to appear in thyrotoxicosis.

What are the surgical treatment modalities for the patient of thyrotoxicosis?

If possible subtotal thyroidectomy is the better way to treat the patient as no further thyroxin (eltroxin) treatment to be given life long but in severe disease like Grave's disease with eye signs better to do total or near total thyroidectomy where better control of thyrotoxicosis is achieved and eye signs are regressed relatively earlier. But the patient will need life long thyroxine treatment.

What are the advantages and disadvantages of surgery?

Advantages:
- Surgery gives rapid cure from the disease by removing hyperactive tissue.

Disadvantages:
- Recurrence though rare, after surgery still chance is 9-10%.
- Life long thyroxin therapy to be given after total/ near total thyroidectomy.

How to prepare a patient of hyperthyroidism for surgery?

My aim is to make the patient euthyroid state and to maintain it for long time.

So I will start

1. Tab Carbimazole (Neomarcazole) 10 mg. TDS to QAS for 6-8 weeks to relieve form symptoms and for biochemical improvement.

   Last dose to be given day before surgery evening [Mechanism of action- inhibits coupling of iodotyrosine residues to from T3 and T4.

2. I will give propranolol 20-40 mg twice/ thrice daily to reduce cardiovascular symptoms.

   [Mechanism of action- Reduce peripheral conversion T4 to T3].

3. I will give potassium iodide tab 60 mg TDS for 10 days prior to reduce vascularity of thyroid gland, there by minimizing bleeding during surgery.

   [Initially Lugol's iodine used to be given 15 drops thrice daily for 10 days prior to surgery.]

What is Pandered syndrome?

When goiter is associated with severe sensorineural hearing impairment and abnormality of the bony labyrinth.

This is observed in CT scan of temporal bones.

What is thyrotoxicosis factitia?

High dose of thyroxine (more than 25 mg/day) may induce hyperthyroidism which is called thyrotoxicosis factitia.

What is Jod Basedow thyrotoxicosis?

Large dose of iodide given to a hyperplastic endemic goiter that is iodine avid may produce temporary hyperthyroidism and very occasionally, persistent hyperthyroidism - this is called Jod- Basedow thyrotoxicosis.

Wolf-ChaiKoff effect-Excess iodine transiently inhibits thyroid iodide organification. This phenomenon of iodine dependent transient suppression of thyroid causes hypothyroidism.

In post operative patient after thyroidectomy when do you look for para thyroid insufficiency?

Most cases present dramatically 2-5 days after operation but very rarely, the onset is delayed for 2-3 weeks.

Incidence less than 5 %. [Parathyroid insufficiency is due to removal of parathyroid glands or due to the damage to the parathyroid end artery.

How will you manage the patient of thyrotoxic crisis?

- IV fluid.
- Cooling of the patient.
- O2 (Oxygen) inhalation.

- Diuretics for cardiac failure.
- Digoxin for uncontrolled atrial fibrillation.
- I V hydrocortisone.
- I V propranolol (1-2 mg) - slowly carefully under precise ECG control.

Next- Carnimazole 10-20 mg 6 hrly lugol's iodine 10 drops 8 hrly or potassium iodine tab 60 mg 8 hourly propranolol 40 mg 6 hrly.

What is pemberton's sign?

This is performed to exclude retrosternal prolongation of goiter. Patient is asked to

i. Raise both arms over the head touching the ears for 2/3 minutes.

   (Narrowing of thoracic outlet by contraction of scalenus anticus).

ii. To hold the breath- (which causes increase flow in great vessels.)

   If there is retrosternal prolongation of goiter, there will be congestion of face, enlargement of neck veins and patient may have breathing difficulty.

Why thyroid swelling moves with deglutition?

i. Posterior lamina of pretracheal fascia which forms the false capsule of thyroid is attached with larynx and trachea which move with deglutition so thyroid moves along with.

ii. Ligament of Berry on either side of thyroid is attached with cricoid cartilage which moves with deglutition.

iii. Sometimes up to 50% cases, levator glandulae thyroidae- the fibromuscular band- connects the isthmus and hyoid bone which moves with deglutition.

What all thyroid swellings do not moves with deglutition?

i. Large thyroid like big colloid goiter.

ii. Carcinoma thyroid, infiltrated ligament of Berry.

iii. Anaplastic carcinoma thyroid.

What are the causes of respiratory difficulty in a patient of goiter?

Respiratory difficulty may be due to

i. Long standardizing multinodular goiter causes tracheomalacia and difficulty in breathing.

ii. Carcinoma thyroid may involve recurrent laryngeal nerve, causing respiratory difficulty.

iii. Mechanical compression huge benign thyroid or by carcinoma thyroid may case breathing difficulty.

iv. Retrosternal prolongation of goiter may cause respiratory distress.

v. In thyrotoxicosis, there may be cardiac failure which itself causes respiratory distress.

What are the causes of dysphagia in a case of thyroid swelling?

Pseudo dysphagia is the commonest as the patient may have a feeling of difficulty in deglutition because of the swelling lying above Malignant infiltration to the food pipe.

Riedel's thyroiditis due to its fibrosis may cause narrowing of the food pipe.

MNG

What all investigations you like to do in MNG?

i. FNAC from dominant nodule and different sites of palpable nodules.

ii. USG neck to see
   - Multiple nodules even as small as 2-3 mm nodules.
   - Can detect solid or cystic component or both components (complex cyst) which give suspicion of malignancy.

iii. USG guide FNAC can be done from a small nodule.

iv. To see the cervical lymph nodes involvement.

v. Thyroid profile T3, T4 TSH as usual to exclude subclinical hypo or hyperthyroidism.

Without doing FNAC can you do surgery in a nodular goiter?

Surgery can be done without FNAC when there is a suspicious thyroid malignancy clinically and based on history in the following conditions.

   i. Thyroid swelling which is fixed and irregular.

   ii. Thyroid swelling with hoarseness of voice due to recurrent laryngeal nerve palsy.

   iii. Thyroid swelling with cervical lymph nodes involvement.

   iv. Thyroid mass with past history of radiation.

How multinodular goiter develops?

In increased demand of thyroid hormone, in iodine deficiency area, during puberty or pregnancy

↓

There is diffuse hyperplasia of follicular cells to fullfil the demand.

↓

as a result hyperplastic goiter is formed.

↓

If there is fluctuation of TSH stimulation a mixed pattern develops as follicular cells are more sensitive to response, some don't. Thus multinodular goiter develops.

↓

The nodules are multiple may be colloid or cellular gradually there may be cystic degeneration and gradually there common in these nodules.

How colloid goiter is formed?

In increased demand of thyroid hormone there will be diffuse hyperplasia of follicular cells occurs.

↓

In late stage when TSH stimulation stops many active follicles become inactive and become full of colloid material.

What are the complications of multinodular goiter?

   i. Development of secondary thyrotoxicosis where the CVS symptoms will be the manifestation.

   ii. Tracheal compression may be caused by large swelling or retrosternal prolongation.

   iii. Malignancy, though uncommon, may develop. Example- Follicular carcinoma in endemic area.

MNG- indications for surgery-

   i. Suspected Neoplastic MNG.

   ii. Retrosternal prolongation of thyroid with compression symptoms.

   iii. Large goiter with tracheal or oesophageal compression causing difficulty in breathing and difficulty in swallowing respectively.

   iv. Rapidly growing thyroid swelling.

   v. Over all cosmetic purpose.

What are the opinions of surgery for a patient of MNG?

   i. MNG involving one lobe (through rare)- hemithyroidectomy.

   ii. MNG involving both the lobes subtotal thyroidectomy.

   iii. If one lobe is more affected than other, total lobectomy on the more affected side and subtotal thyroidectomy on other side done. This is called **'Dunhill Procedure'**.

   iv. Total or near total thyroidectomy may be considered when both lobes are equally affected and hardly ever any normal tissue.

In haemithyroidectomy why isthmus is to be removed?

As

   i. The junction of isthmus and lobe is prone to develop MNG including malignancy.

   ii. It is easy to perform tracheostomy, post operatively if required, after isthmusectomy.

   iii. For more effectiveness of radio therapy on malignant bed isthmusectomy is required.

How you will care post operative patients after thyroi-dectomy?

1. Look for persistent voice change -visualize the card.
2. Transient hypocalcemia (25% patient develop) - if symptoms are severe I V calcium gluconate 10 mg state

and 8-12 hourly. Next switch over to oval calcium. Serum calcium to be measured at the first review attendance 4-6 weeks after operation.

3. Most patients develop thyroid failure within 2 years of surgery (20-45% incidence ultimately regain normally).

CARCINOMA THYROID

What is leteral aberrant thyroid?

There is no evidence of aberrant thyroid, occurs in the lateral position, but in a case of occult papillary carcinoma thyroid metastatic cervical lymph node may be palpable laterally-called lateral aberrant thyroid.

What do you mean by occult carcinoma?

The term occult carcinoma is applied to all papillary carcinomas less than 1.5 cm in diameter. Prognosis is very good.

Can you tell me the course of recurrent laryngeal nerve?

In left sided recurrent laryngeal nerve arises from the vagus nerve where it crosses the aortic arch.
↓
Loops around the ligamentum arteriosum
↓
Ascends medially in the neck within the tracheoesophageal groove.
↓
Right recurrent arises from the vagus at its crossing with the right subclavian artery.
↓
The nerve passes posterior to the artery before ascending in the neck. Its course is more oblique than the left RLN.
↓
Along the course in the neck, RLN, may branch pass anterior, posterior or interdigitate with branches of inferior thyroid artery.
The right RLN may be non recurrent .5-1% of individuals and often is associated with vascular anomaly.
Non recurrent left RLN is rare.
↓
To identify the nerves and their branches, often lateral and posterior extent of thyroid gland, tubercle of Zucker Kandi, at the level of the cricoid cartilage are required.
↓

Last segments of the nerves often course below the tubercle and are closely approximated to ligament of Berry.
↓
Branches of the nerve traverses the ligament in 25% of individuals and are particularly vulnerable to injury at this junction.
↓
The RLNs terminate by entering the larynx post to the cricothyroid muscle.

Remember-
[RLNs innervate all the intrinsic muscles of larynx except Cricothyroid muscle which innervated by the internal laryngeal nerves].

What happens in case of injury of unilateral and bilateral recurrent laryngeal nerve?

Injury to one RLN leads to paralysis of the ipsilateral vocal cord, which comes to lie in the paramedian or the abducted position (Wagner-Grossman Hypothesis)
↓
The paramedian position results in a normal but weak voice, where as the abducted position leads to a hoarse voice and an ineffective cough.
[Semon's law- Abductor fibres of RLN is more susceptible and paralysed Bilateral RLN injury may lead to airway obstruction].
↓
It requires emergency tracheostomy.
Bilateral injury may lead to loss of voice also.

Remember- If both cord come to lie in an abducted position, air movement can occur, but the patient has an ineffective cough and that may increase the risk of repeated respiratory tract infections from aspiration.

What are the indications of radio iodine scan in a patient of Carcinoma thyroid?

Routinely it is not done for pre operative evaluation of patient but when the follicular lesion is there - Radio Iodine scan may be done.

It shows 'hot' nodule [Treatment either RAI Ablation/ Thyroidectomy]

Or 'cold' nodule [treatment thyroidectomy].

What do you mean by cold nodules and hot nodules?

The areas that trap less radio activity than the surrounding gland termed cold".

Where as areas those demonstrate increased activity are termed 'hot'.

The risk of malignancy is higher in cold lesion (15-20%) than in hot or warm lesions (5-8%).

What are the primary sites from where carcinoma may spread to thyroid?

The common sites are: Colon, Kidneys and melanomas.

What is TNM staging in carcinoma thyroid?

- Tx- Primary can not be assessed.
- T0- No evidence of primary tumor.
- T1- tumor < = 2 cm greatest dimension and it is within thyroid gland.
- T2- tumor 2-4 cm at greatest dimension and within thyroid gland.
- T3- tumor > 4 cm or minimal extra thyroid involvement.
- T4- Extending beyond capsule any size.
    a. involvement beyonds capsule, i.e. subcutaneous soft tissue.
       Fine plastic carcinoma within RLN.
    b. Involves prevertebral fascia, carotid artery and mediastinal vessels.
       Extra thyroid anaplastic carcinoma.
- N0- No evidence of metastasis.
- N1- Regional node metastasis.
    a. Involvement of level VI.
    b. Unilateral / Bilateral or contra lateral cervical or sup mediastinal LN (level VI).
- M0- No evidence of metastasis.
- M1- Metastasis present.

What is the role of radio iodine in metastatic disease of carcinoma thyroid?

Metastasis from thyroid carcinoma, takes up radioiodine and it may be detected by radioiodine (I 133) scanning (usual dose is 5 micro curie).

For effective scanning the following things to be done prior to scanning are:

i. All normal thyroid tissue must have been ablated either by surgery or preliminary radio iodine. [Dose is average 80 micro curie].
ii. Patient must be in hypothyroid state i.e. if patient is on thyroxine it is to be with drawn minimum 1 month prior to the scanning.

What are the indications of radio iodine scan?

Indications are:

- Suspected unresectable disease.
- To detect local recurrence if suspected.
- To detect metastatic disease.
- To detect ectopic thyroid tissue.
- Retro sternal/ goiter etc.

How will you treat the metastasis in a case of carcinoma thyroid?

If metastasis take up radio iodine- it is likely to be suppressed by thyroxine as effectively as by radio iodine.

It metastases have been treated the scan should be repeated annually and further therapeutic dose of radio iodine given as necessary.

Solitary distant metastases may be treated by external radiotherapy.

What is the role of thyroglobulin in Ca-Thyroid?

The measurement of serum thyroglobulin is of value in
i. follow up
ii. detection of metastatic disease in a patient
    Who has undergone surgery for differentiated thyroid cancer.

Radioactive iodine scan, there after will confirm and locate the disease.

[The presence of circulation anti thyroglobulin antibodies interferes with and invalidates thyroglobulin as serum marker for recurrence. In such cases careful clinical exam of neck will detect local recurrence in the presence of low thyroglobulin (normal level <5 mg/ ml).

Have you heard the word 'thyroid steal'?

In thyrotoxicosis, patient is taken to operation theatre daily for few days before doing surgery - aim is to reduce the anxiety a fovea regarding operation.

What is MIVAT?

MIVT means Minimally Invasive Video Assisted Thyroidectomy.

It is becoming popular for a small nodule and gland without thyroiditis. But it costly.

What are the complications of thyroidectomy?

i.   Hemorrhage-
Primary- during surgery reactionary- due to slipping of ligatures either of superior thyroid artery or other pedicies.
A subcutaneous hematoma and collection of serum undersurface of skin flap should be evacuated as early as possible. Life threatening deep tension hematoma to be tackle at the earliest.

ii. Respiratory obstruction- due to either or due to laryngeal oedema for which emergency endotracheal intubation is to be done along with steroid injection. Often tracheostomy is required as a life saving procedure.

iii. Recurrent laryngeal nerve palsy- transient or permanent.
Transient is around 3% and it is usually recovered in 3 weeks to 3 months. Often steroid therapy and speech therapy are required.
Permanent- rare if it is identified during surgery. Treatment is described above.

iv. Hypothyroidism incidence is around .5%.
Mostly it is temporarily due to vascular spasm of parathyroid glands, occurs in 2nd to 5th post operative day- presented with weakness, carpopedal spasm, convulsions, muscle weakness ais the earliest symptoms. Chvostek's sign +ve.
Serum calcium estimation <9 mg%. (Normal level 9-11 mg %)
Treatment- 10 ml 10% calcium gluconate 8 hrly.
$$\downarrow$$
Shifted to oral calcium 500 mg BD to TDS for 4-6 weeks.
$$\downarrow$$
Serum calcium is estimated.

v.   Thyrotoxic crisis (thyroid storm): as described earlier. Other complications are:

vi. Injury to external laryngeal nerve.

vii. Hypothyroidism- revealed clinically after 6 months.

viii. Wound infection.

ix. Stitch granuloma.

x.   Keloid formation etc.

What is Chvostek-Weiss sign?

In case of parathyroid tetany a gentle tap on the facial nerve, infront of the external auditory meatus, invites a brisk

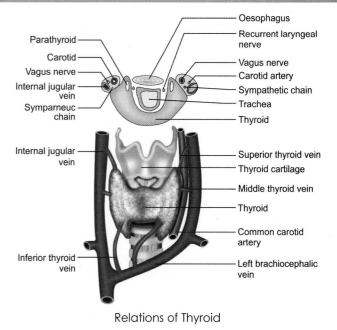

Relations of Thyroid

muscular twitch of the same side of the face- this is called chvostek sign.

Trousseau's sign: When blood pressure is raised around 200 mm Hg in sphygmomanometer within few minutes' typical contraction of hand can be seen - so called 'obstetrician hand'.

IMPORTANT SHORT NOTE ON THYROID:

THYROID

a) Anatomy:

- Development of thyroid
- Parts.
- Blood supply
  1. Superior Thyroid Artery (Branch of External Carotid Artery)
  2. Inferior Thyroid Artery (Branch of Thyrocervical Trunk which arises from Subclavian Artery)
  3. Artery Thyroidema (Arises from Brachiocephalic Trunk or directly from Arch of Aorta)
- Venous drainage
- Lymphatic drainage.

Relations of thyroid gland:

i.   Recurrent laryngeal nerve lies in the tracheoesophageal groove, in relation to ligament of 'Berry'.

ii. Superior laryngeal nerve which gives a branch external laryngeal nerve supplies cricothyroid muscle. It accompanies superior thyroid artery.

iii. Parathyroid glands- four in number from each side embedded in thyroid.

The superior parathyroids are cephalad to inferior thyroid artery and are usually located at the posterior lateral aspect of upper half of thyroid gland i.e. it is dorsal to the plane of the nerve (RLN).

The inferior parathyroid gland is frequently adherent to or within the cord of thymic tissue / sited anterior to the recurrent laryngeal nerve at the lower pole of thyroid. It is ventral to the plane of RLN.

b) Physiology of thyroid gland:

Thyroxin synthesis:
1. **Trapping:** Thyroid has special capacity to trap the iodide from circulating blood The iodide is mainly derived from drinking water.
2. **Oxidation:** The iodide is converted into iodine by a peroxidase enzyme.

$$\text{Iodide} \xrightarrow{\text{Peroxidase}} \text{Iodine}$$

3. **Binding:** Iodine combines with essential amino acid tyrosine to form
   a) Monoiodotyrosine
   b) Di-iodotyrosine
4. **Coupling:**
   a) Monoiodotyrosine + Di-iodotyrosine = Try iodotyrosine (T3)
   b) Di-iodotyrosine + Di-iodotyrosine = Thyroxin (T4)
      T4 (Thyroxin) is formed far in excess to T3
5. **Reversible conjugation**-Thyroxin (T4) and (T3) immediately get attached to thyroglobulin which is a special protein secreted by thyroid cells.

   The conjugated material is called "Colloid substance" and stored in thyroid acini.

As per the requirement of system the conjugation breaks alfa (a) thyroxin (T4) and (little amount T3) is liberated into the circulation.

Half life of T4 is 4-14 days and T3- few hrs to days.

Thyroid Hormone Synthesis
Ant Pituitary

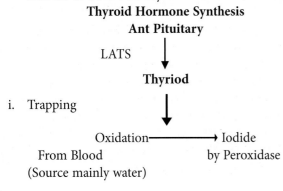

ii. Binding   Iodine + Tyrosine

   • Monoiodotyrosine
   • Di-iodotyrosine
iii. Coupling

   • Monoiodotyrosine + Di-iodotyrosine =

   Try iodotyrosine (T3)
   • Di-iodotyrosine + Di-iodotyrosine =

   Thyroxin (T4)

vi. Next   T3/T4 + Thyrogloghoin

   o Conjugated to form Colloid substance
     Conjugation breaks on demand

T3/T4 Released

iv. In the circulation
   (a) Found to Serum Protein
   (b) Face T3 and T4
   T4 (Thyroxin) T ½   4 - 14 days
   T3 ------------ T ½   Few hrs to days

Classification of Goiter

1. Simple Nontoxic Goiter

Diffuse hyperplastic.
   i. Physiological -
   • Puberty
   • Pregnancy.
   ii. Primary iodine deficiency- endemic goiter.
   iii. Secondary iodine deficiency-
   • Intake of goitrogens of brassica family - like cabbage kale rape, soybean, etc.
   • Excess dietary fluoride.
   • Drugs PAS, lithium, phenyl butazone, thiocyanates, potassium perchlorate. And thyroid drugs radioactive iodine.
   • Dyshormonogenic goiter.
   b. Colloid goiter.
   c. Multinodular goiter.
   d. Solitary nodular goiter (non toxic).
   e. Recurrent nontoxic nodule.
2. Toxic goiter:
   a. Primary diffuse goiter- Grave's disease.
   b. Multinodular (secondary) - Plummer's disease.

c. Toxic nodule- solitary.

d. Recurrent toxicosis.

3. Neoplastic -

a. Benign- Adenoma, Papillary, follicular, Hurthle cell, colloid.

b. Malignant-
- Carcinoma-Papillary, follicular, medullary, anaplastic.
- Lymphomas, secondaries.

4. Thyroiditis, Acute bacterial, Granulomatous, Hashimto's Auto immune, Riedel's.

5. Other causes- Bacterial, Amyloid.

Colloid Goiter

- Age 20-30 years i.e. after physiological hyperplasia has subsided.
- Whole gland becomes enlarged, soft, elastic.
- Pressure effects are the problems i.e. dyspnea, difficulty in swallowing.

MNG

- Age 30-40 years.
- 6 times commoner in females than males.
- Slow growing painless lump in the thyroid.
- Sudden enlargement with pain suggestive of hemorrhage into the inactive nodule or malignant transformation.
- Pressure effects may be the manifestations when it is quite large, otherwise asymptomatic.
- Secondary thyrotoxicosis occurs in approximately in 25-50% cases.
- Multiple nodules of different sizes are formed in both lobes and isthmus which are firm, nodular, nontender, moves with deglutition.
- Complications include-
  1. secondary thyrotoxicosis.
  2. follicular carcinoma of thyroid.
  3. hemorrhage inside the nodule.
  4. tracheal obstruction.
  5. cosmetic problem.
- X-ray neck may show ring or rim calcification.
- Nodular goiter is an irreversible condition. So, surgery is the treatment of choice.

SNT

A discrete nodular swelling in one lobe with no palpable abnormality elsewhere is termed as solitary thyroid nodule.

DIFFERENTIAL DIAGNOSIS

- Colloid goiter—50%.
- Simple cyst thyroid.
- Dominant nodule of MNG.
- Adenoma - Papillary, colloid, adenoma.
- Papillary carcinoma thyroid 10-15%.
- Types are nontoxic and toxic.
- C/F- Palpable solitary nodule in thyroid.
- Common site - at the junction of isthmus and lateral lobe.

Treatment

- SNT (non toxic)- Haemithyroidectomy.
- Papillary ca thyroid- total thyroidectomy with suppressive dose of L- Thyroxine. 3 mg OD.
- Toxic SNT- Radio active iodine I131 - 5 micro curie given orally if age > 45 years.
- Age < 45 years- anti thyroid drugs heme/ subtotal thyroidectomy.

Carcinoma:

Papillary carcinoma-
- Hormone dependent tumor.
- TSH level is high.
- Commonest carcinoma thyroid 60%.
- Common in female and younger age group 15-20 years.
- Exposure to radio therapy or past history of radioactive iodine therapy.
- It contains brownish black fluid.
- Microscopy- shows papillary projection with psammoma body, malignant cells with ' orphan annie eye' nuclei.
- Slow progressive, less aggressive tumor.
- Usually no blood spread, only lymphatic spread.

Treatment -
- <1 cm haemithyroidectomy and regular follow up.
- >1 cm total thyroidectomy.

Follicular Carcinoma

- 17% common.
- Female predominant.
- Occurs de novo or in pre existing MNG.
- Types are- Noninvasive 50% and invasive-Blood spread common 50%.
- Aggressive tumor- spreads mainly through blood into bones, lungs, liver.
- Bone secondaries are typically vascular, warm, pulsatile, localized commonly in the skull, long bone, ribs.
- Lymphatic spread is occasional.

Clinical features:

- Thyroid swelling- firm to hard and nodular.
- Tracheal compression and stidor may be present .
- Recurrent laryngeal nerve involvement may cause hoarseness of voice.
- Infiltration into carotid sheath may cause absence of carotid pulsation - called Berry's sign it signifies advanced malignancy.
- Pulsatile secondaries may be found in skull and long bones.
- Dyspnea, hemoptysis, chest pain suggestive of lung secondaries.

Investigations

- FNAC cannot differentiate between follicular adenoma and follicular carcinoma as capsular and vascular invasion cannot be detected by FNAC.
- Frozen section biopsy may be useful.
- USG abdomen, chest X-ray, X ray bones etc.

Treatment

- In low risk group hemi/sub total thyroidectomy.
- In high risk group total thyroidectomy to be done along with block dissection of neck nodes.
- Tap L thyroxine 100 mg OD for life long.

Follow up

Radio isotope (I 123) scan to be done at regular interval (6 monthly) to exclude secondaries.

Estimation of thyroglobulin is a essential follow up method to decide for radio isotope study (normal value 0-5 micro gram/L

>50 microgram/L is suggestive of malignancy).

- If secondaries are detected therapeutic dose of radio active I 131 is given orally (L-Thyroxin has to be stopped 4-6 weeks prior to this treatment).

Dose of radio active I 131 is 50-150 m curie, average dose 80 m curie. Secondaries in bone are treated by external radio therapy.

[Remember - there is no role of chemotherapy in follicular carcinoma thyroid].

Hurthle cell carcinoma

A variant of follicular carcinoma.
- It contains abundant oxyphil cells.
- It spreads more commonly to regional lymph nodes than follicular carcinoma thyroid.
- It does not take up I 131.
- It secretes thyroglobulin.
- Poorer prognosis than follicular carcinoma.

CASE 21 — Cervical Lymphadenopathy

My patient Ranvir, a 30 year old male, resident of Haryana, presented with multiple swelling both side, of his neck for last 6 months.

He noticed a single swelling in his left side of neck first graduate multiple swelling appeared both side of his neck.

Swelling are gradually progressive, and painless. So he did not care about it initially but gradually he has got his history of weight loss, loss of appetite for last 3 months and Fever for last 2 months. The fever with swelling stay for 5-7 days and followed by a period of apyrexia.

History of Abdominal pain and swelling in the lower limb (IVC obstruction)

Features suggestive of TB like evening rise of temperature

History of Exposure [to exclude sexually Transmitted Disease (STD)]

History of Salivary gland swelling, conjunctivitis, dyspnea, cough, to no preauricular swelling (for Sarcoidosis)]

GENERAL SURVEY: Patient is anaemic; pallor look, like white -coffee poorly/averagely nourished.

On local Examination-There are multiple ovoid Swellings, more in the posterior triangle of neck, no swellings, moves with deglutition. No dental caries, oral hygiene Waldeyer's ring appear normal.

On palpation-The swellings are 2-4 cm in size nontender, discrete, rubbery in consistency, smooth surface mobile, free from overlying skin and underlying structure, Axillary, Inguinal lymph nodes not enlarged

Systemic Examination

- GIT- There is splenomegaly and hepatomegaly. Spleen is 14 cm on its axis
- Liver is 4 cm enlarged on mid clavicular line.
- No abdominal hymphadenopathy noticed.
- Both testis appear normal, (to exclude testicular malignancy)
- Others examination are essentially normal.

So my provision diagnosis is - this is a case of Hodgkin's lymphoma but I like to put differential diagnoses for this case. It may be.

1. Tubercular Lymphadenopathy
2. Secondary syphilis
3. Chronic pyogenic lymphadenitis
4. Secondary metastatic lymph node.

Why is you considering Hodgkin's lymphoma as your first diagnosis?

Sir my patient is a Young male, presents with slowly growing painless lymph nodal mass in the neck-especially in the posterior triangle. He has been having fever for last 2 months which occurs in a periodic fashion and he has got the history weight loss, anorexin, night sweats, etc.

On exam patient is anaemic, the pallor is like white-coffee. The cervical lymph nodes are ovoid, smooth, discreate these are solid, firm and rubbery in consistency nontendor, mobile (rarely may be fixed occasionally the lymph nodes may be matted in late stages called **pseudo matting**)

There is hepatosplenomegaly also. So this is clinically a case of Hodgkin's lymphoma.

[**Differential Diagnoses** (i) **tubercular lympha-denopathy**

- It may occur at any age (but common in children).
- persistent enlargement of lymph node and this most common cause of cervical lymphadenopathy in our country
- Feature of tuberculosis along with -like evening rise of temperature, weight loss, anaemia, cough etc.

On Examination: the enlarged lymph nodes are firm in feel and initially discrete but later it's become matted (due to periadenitis)

Often slightly tender

- Evidence of Tuberculosis may be present in the lung.

ii. Chronic pyogenic lymphadenitis

- History of chronic infection in oral cavity like Dental caries
- Painless, persisting for along.
- Lymph nodes are firm, tender not matted
- Antibiotics reduce the size of the lymph node again it appears.

iii. Secondary Syphilis:

- Young age (20-30 yrs)
- History of exposure present
- Ulcer may present in mouth, genitalia,
  - Fever, arthritis, various skin rashes (pleomorphic)
  - On Exam-Mucocutaneous lesion may be present ulcer in dorsum of tongue angular fissure, condyloma.
- Generalized enlargement of superficial group, firm, desecrates and shotty, non tender most characteristically there is enlargement of epitrochlear and suboccipital groups.

iv. Metastatic lymphadenopathy

- Common in elderly male, few cancers like papillary Carcinoma thyroid occurs in young adults.
- Patients present with painlessly enlarged swellings enlarged in the neck.

Slowly progressive

- General symptoms like anorexia, weight loss, and weakness may be present along with primary lesion.
- Metastatic nodes are common in the nodes of anterior triangle. These are deep to the anterior edge of the sternomastoid (sternocleidomastoid)

On examination-Lymph nodes are stony hard, mobile, may be fixed, non tender, usually at initial stage nodes are smooth and discreate and variable sizes, later on it has got irregular or bosselated surface.

- Primary lesion almost always presents example, head and neck cancer, carcinoma oral cavity ca oesophagus, lung, stomach, pancreas, testes breast etc.
- Presence of enlarged metastatic lymph nodes in left supra clavicular fossa is called Virchow's gland. It is usually associated with abdominal malignancy and called Torisier's sign.

Other causes of lymphadenopathy are:
- Non Hodgkin's lymphoma
- Chronic lymphatic leukemia
- Sarcoidosis etc.

1. Non Hodgkins lymphoma

- Common in younger
- Lymph nodal involvement is from centripetal, i.e. involvement is from periphery to towards centre.
- Rapidly growing swelling
- Constitutional symptoms like weight loss, anorexia, fever, night sweats are present in 25%, cases.

On examination- Lymph nodes are variegated consistency, soft, firm or hard
Extranodal site of origin is common 10-35%

2. CML (chronic lymphatic Leukemia)

- Above 50 years commonly in mates
- Presence of constitutional symptoms like fever, gross weakness, weight loss, recurrent upper respiratory tract infection.
- Lmph node enlargement is slowly growing painlessly progressive cervical lymphadenopathy.

On Exam-Anaemia ++
- Lymph nodes discreate, firm, mobile, nontender.
- Skin thickening or nodules may present (due to leukaemic tissue infiltration)
- Hepatosplenomegaly- firm smooth nontender.

Sarcoidosis:

- Young adult and middle aged person.
- May present with enlarged superficial group of cervical lymph node with variable constitutional symptoms like fever, bone pain paroxysmal dyspnea, pain full eyes, etc.

On examination

Superficial group of cervical lymph nodes are enlarged more characteristically Pre auricular groups. These are firm, discreate, nontender.
- Parotid gland enlargement
- Facial nerve palsy, uveitis, conjunctivitis may be present.

How will you proceed in this case of cervical lymphadenopathy?

Sir, I will confirm my diagnosis first
I will do
1. FNAC/ Excision biopsy of lymph node. Lymph node biopsy confirms the diagnosis.
   [Macroscopically cut section shows fish flesh appearance Microscopically-Red stern berg's giant cells-Pleomorphism of cellular tissue is characteristic feature]

2. Chest X Ray- may show enlarged mediastinal shadow with pleural effusion.
   • Chest and abdomen to stage the disease.
3. CT Scan may show
   • Mediastinal, Retroperitoneal lymphadenopathy, liver spleen enlargement.
   • Sometime exploratory laparotomy may be required for retroperitoneal lymphadenopathy and involvement of liver, spleen, particularly where CT scan not adequate or not available.
4. Blood test-Anaemia, Pancytopenia, Leucocytosis with lymphocytopenia eosinophilia.
5. Bone marrow Examination- to stage the disease.

How will you differentiate between Hodgkin's's and Non Hodgkin's's Lymphoma?

S. no HODGKIN'S			NON-HODGKINS
1	Site of Origin	Nodal	Extranodal 10- 35% (most common site by GI Tract)
2	Nodal distribution	Centrifugal (centre to periphery)	Centripetal (periphery to central)
3	Nodal spread	Contiguous	Non contiguous
4	Lymph cells affected	B-Lymphocytes characterized by the Reed-Sternberg's giant cell's	B-Lymphocytes T Lymphocytes and NK Cells
5	Liver involvement	Uncommon	Common > 50%
6	Bone marrow involvement	Uncommon <10%	Common > 50%
7	Role of chemotherapy	Curable	Not curable

How will you classify Hodgkin's disease?

• An Artor classification since 1971
• The Cotswolds modification in 1988.

Principal stage-

• **Stage I** Involvement of single lymph node region (I) or single extralymphatic site (Ie)
• **Stage II** Involvement of two or more lymph nodal regions on the same side of the diaphragm (II) of one lymph node region and a contiguous extra lymphatic site (II e)
• **Stage III** Involvement of lymph node regions on both sides of the diaphragm which may include spleen (III s) and or limited contiguous extralymphatic organ or site (IIIe or IIIes)

• **Stage IV**- Disseminated involvement of one or more extralymphatic organs.
• Modifications A and B- The absence of constitutional symptoms is denoted by adding an A to the stage, the presence is denoted by adding B to the stage.
• E: is used if the disease is extranodal or has spread from lymph node to adjacent tissue.
• X: is used if the largest deposit is > 10 cm (bulky disease) or whether the mediastinum is wider than 1/3 rd of the chest (on chest X Ray)
• Type of staging-CS-Clinical stage and PS-Pathological stage.

What are the adverse prognostic factors in a case of Hodgkin's lymphoma?

The international studies of prognostic factors are
1. Age> 45 years, Male > female.
2. Stage IV disease
3. Hemoglobin < 10.5 gm%
4. Lymphocyte < 600/cnmm or <8%
5. WBC count > 15,000/cnmm
6. Albumin < 3 mg%

How will you treat the patient?

Sir, the treatment depends on the stage.
i. In early stage (IA and II A) -Radiotherapy is very effective treatment

Chemotherapy may be given
ii. In late stage (III, IV A or IV B)-combined chemotherapy alone
iii. Hodgkin's lymphoma at any stage if there is mass in chest that is usually treated with combined chemotherapy and radiotherapy.

What chemotherapy regime is the gold standard for treatment of Hodgkin's's disease?

Currently ABVD chemotherapy is the gold standard for treatment of Hodgkin's lymphoma.
• A-Inj Adriamycin 25 mg/m2
• B-Inj Bleomycin 10 mg/m2
• V-Inj Vinblastin 6 mg/m2
• A-Inj Dacarbazine 37 5mg/m2
   On D1-D15 4 weekly X 6 cycles. Over 85% Hodgkin's lymphoma cases are curable with this regimen.

Why it is called Hodgkin's lymphoma.

Formerly this lymphoma was known as Hodgkin's lymphoma cases are has been described by Thomas Hodgkin in 1832.

What is the subtypes of classic Hodgkin's lymphoma (CHL)

i.   Nodular Sclerosis- most common subtype world wide.
ii. Lymphocytic predominant-relatively uncommon but has better prognosis

iii. Lymphocyte depleted- Uncommon subtype. Bad prognostic.
iv. Mixed Cellularity-This most common in Indian and it and most common subtype world wise wide.

SHORT NOTES ON CERVICAL LYMPHADENOPATHY

Lymph nodes are arranged in the neck in two groups.

1. Superficial groups-these are few and scattered superficial to investing layer of deep cervical group.
2. Deep group [vertical group/Circular group]

    - Vertical group-Level I to level VI [as described in Neck nodes management]
    - Circular group-anterior to posterior-
        - Submental
        - Submandibular
        - Pre auricular
        - Post-auricular
        - Occipital

CERVICAL LYMPHDENOPATHY

CAUSE: A------ACUTE
            B----CHRONIC

A ---Acute   (i)   acute pyogenic lymphadenitis
             (ii) Acute lymphatic leukemia
             (iii) Acute Infectious mononucleosis

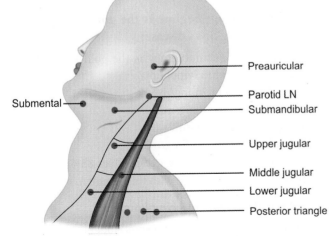

Different levels of neck nodes

Preauricular
Parotid LN
Submental
Submandibular
Upper jugular
Middle jugular
Lower jugular
Posterior triangle

B---Chronic Inflammatory:
- Chronic pyogenic lymphadenitis
- Tubercular lymphadenopathy
- Secondary syphilis
- Sarcoidosis
- Brucellosis
- Blastomycosis

II NEoplastic

Primary

- Hodgkin's lymphoma.
- Non Hodgkin's lymphoma
- Chronic lymphatic leukaemia
- Burkit's lymphoma.

Secondary

- Metastatic lymphadenopathy

III Autoimmune disorders

- SLE (Systemic Lupus Erythematosus)
- Still disease (Juvenile rheumatoid arthritis)

CAUSE OF GENERALIZED LYMPHADENOPATHY

- Tubercular lymphadenopathy
- Hodgkin's and Non Hodgkin's lymphoma.
- Secondary Syphilis
- Chronic lymphatic leukemia (CML)
- Metastatic lymphadenopathy
- Sarcoidosis
- HIV with generalized lymphadenopathy

1. TUBERCULOUS LYMPHADENITIS

Characteristics of lymph node enlargement
- Cervical group is involved initially common in upper deep cervical group (Jagulo-di-limapulu)

- The lymph nodes are firm in consistency and discrete initially but gradually with the passage of time lymph nodes become matted (due to periadenitis)
- May be slightly tender
- Tonsils may be studded with tubercles.
- Stage of tuberculous Lymphadenitis
    - Stage (i) Infection and lymphadenitis
    - Stage (ii) Periadenitis with matting
    - Stage (iii) Caseating necrosis and formation of cold abscess
    - Stage (IV) Formation of collar stud abscess
    - Stage (v) Discharging sinus formation which discharges yellowish caseating material
- look for associated pulmonary TB always.

2. LYMPH NODE'S PATHOLOGY

- Macroscopically looking solid, matted and cut section shows yellowish caseating material.
- Microscopically-caseating material at the centre surrounded by epithelioid cells and then Langhan's type of giant cells.

3. INVESTIGATIONS

- Hematocrit/ ESR
- FNAC from lymph node and smear for AFB (Acid fast Bacilli)
- Chest X Ray PA view to exclude pulmonary Tuberculosis
- PCR (Polymerase chain Reaction) and KP 90 are useful method for detecting tuberculosis.
  If HIV is suspected, do ELISA and Western blot test.

TREATMENT

If the diagnosis is established start Antitubercular drugs.
1. Tab Rifampicin 10-15 mg/kg body weight (450-600 mg/day)

Before breakfast OD
2. Tab INH (Isoniazid) 5-10 mg/kg body Weight OD after breakfast (300 mg to 450 mt./day)
3. Tab ethambutol 5 mg /kg body weight. (800 mg/day)

OD after breakfast
4. Tab Pyrazinamide 20-30 mg/kg body weight OD after breakfast. (1500 mg/day)
5. Tab pyridoxine 10 mg OD along with INH to reduce neuritis.
    - Duration of treatment is usually 6-9 months
    - All 5 tablets are to be taken for first 2 months.

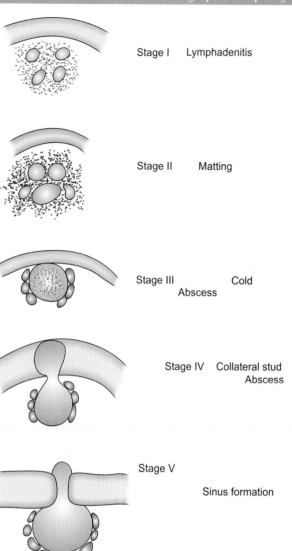

Stage I — Lymphadenitis

Stage II — Matting

Stage III — Cold Abscess

Stage IV — Collateral stud Abscess

Stage V — Sinus formation

Different stages of tubercular lymphadenopathy

- Next only Rifampicin and INH along with Pyridoxine long OD for 6-9 months depends on the extensiveness of the disease.

4. Side effects of antitubercular drugs

- Rifampicin, Hepatitis is a major adverse effect.
- Flu like Syndrome chills fever headache
- Cutaneous syndrome-flushing, pruritus + rash, Respiratory syndrome'-breathlessness shock
- Abdominal syndrome-Abdominal cramps with or without- diarrhoea, nausea, vomiting.
- Urine and secretions may become orange-red but this is not harmful.
- .INH+ Peripheral

- – Neuritis and variety of neurological manifestations-paresthesia, numbness, mental irritation etc.
  - – Hepatitis is a major adverse effect.
- .Ethambutol - Loss of visual acuity /color vision, field defects due to optic neuritis
  - – GI intolerance, fever, rash, few neurological changes
- .Pyrazinamide-Hepatotoxicity is most important dose related side effect.
  - – Arthalgia, flashing, rash, loss of diabetic control etc.
  - – Second line antitubercular drugs are:
  - – Thiacetazone
  - – Para amino salicylic Acid (PAS)
  - – Ethionamide
  - – Cycloserine
  - – Kanamycin
  - – Amikacin
  - – Capreomycin

The newer Antitubercular drugs are

- Ciprofloxacin
- Ofloxacin
- Clarithromycin
- Azythromycin
- Rifabutin.

Management of cold Abscess

Cold Abscess

⬇

Antigravity aspiration

(Needle to put in a nondependant site along a 'z' Track in a zigzag pathway to prevent sinus formation)

If it recurs

⬇

To be drained all the caseating material (Through a non dependant incision)

Wound to be closed without any drain.

Role of Surgery for removal of tubercular Lymph node

There are few indications for removal of tubercular lymph node

1. Lymph nodes to be removed if there is no local response to drugs.
2. In case of persisting sinus
   Procedure-Skin flap to be raised and remove all lymph nodes along with caseating material.

SECONDARIES IN NECK LYMPH NODES

- Common primary sites are:
  - – Oral cavity, tongue, tonsil
  - – Salivary glands
  - – Pharynx-nasopharynx
  - – Larynx, oesophagus
  - – Lungs, GI+, Thyroid
  - – Testes
- Feature of secondaries in neck
  - – Commonly in elderly male
  - – Commonest presentation

Usually slowly progressing, painless swelling in the neck.

May progress rapidly like Non Hodgkin's lymphoma.

On exam- Hard in consistency, nodular surface and often fixed at presentation though it would be initially mobile.

Exception-secondaries from papillary carcinoma thyroid-usually occurs in young adults and secondaries can be soft cystic

- – Evidence of primary growth may be there at above mentioned sites.
- – Different symptoms to be clarified like
- – Dysphagia-carcinoma posts 1/3 rd of tongue, pharynx, and oesophagus.

Hemoptysis, cough, dyspnea

- – carcinoma lung

Hoarseness-Carcinoma larynx, thyroid.

Ear pain, deafness, nasopharyngeal carcinoma.

- Spinal accessory nerve involvement-drooping of shoulder
- Involvement of Hypoglossal nerve-Tongue deviates to the same side with wasting of tongue muscles.
- Sympathetic chain-Involvement
  - – Horner's syndrome consisting of
  - i. Miosis (due to contraction of pupil owing to paralysis of the dilator papillae)
  - ii. Anhidrosis (absence of sweating in face, neck of that side)
  - iii. Ptosis (dropping of upper eyelid due to paralysis of the levator palpebrae superiors)
  - iv. Enophthalmos (regression of eye ball due to paralysis of muller's muscle)
  - v. Loss of celio - spinal reflex.

Types of Secondaries in the neck

1. Secondaries in the neck with known primary
   - The name it self suggests that primary has been identified along with secondaries in any of the above mentioned sites.

- Biopsy from the primary site and FNAC from the secondaries to be done.
- Treatment primarily depends upon the stage, surgery/ chemotherapy, radio therapy or combine therapy as required.
- For Nodes-It mobile, operable
- MRND otherwise palliative chemo/radio therapy.

2. Secondaries in Neck with unknown primary also called CUPS (Carcinoma Unknown Primary Sites)
   - Where primary sites has not been identified clinically
   - FNAC from secondaries to confirm the metastasis.
   - Look for primary sites by various investigations like
   i. Triple endoscopy   Nasopharyngoscopy
                                Laryngoscopy
                                Bronchoscopy
                                Esophagoscopy
   ii. Biopsy from suspected occult primary sites like: Pyriform fossa, Nasopharynx, Base of tongue, Subglotic Other sites are: fossa of Rosenmuller, lateral wall pharynx, thyroid, Para nasal sinus, Bronchus, oesophagus etc.
   iii. .CECT scan face, neck, chest, and abdomen

Treatment- If primary site is detected treatment is surgery, chemotherapy and or radiotherapy as per pre planned treatment protocol. Secondaries are to be treated either by Modified radical Neck Dissection or chemo/radio therapy whichever is suitable for the patient.

3. Secondaries in Neck with an occult primary
   - Occult primary sites which can cause secondary in neck are mentioned above.
   - Here the secondaries are confirmed by FNAC but primary has not been identified by various investigations as mentioned above. So it is called occult primary.
   - This variety is usually less aggressive and relatively has better prognosis.
   - Here initial treatment is MRND. If MRND type 1 (spinal accessory is spared only) done in one side and other side minimum type II MRND to be done because along with spinal accessory one sided Internal jugular vein to be preserved.
   - Regular follow up at 3 months interval is mandatory to reveal the primary site as early as possible.
   - Once primary site is identified biopsy to be performed to confirm the diagnosis there after treatment will depend upon the stage of the disease.
   (Details treatment written in the chapter of carcinoma oral cavity and management of neck nodes).

Hodgkin's disease

- Bimodal incidence curve
- First being young adult 20-35 yrs
- Second being over 60 years.
- All verities are more common in male except nodular sclerosis variant which is more common in female.

Symptoms and signs

i. Painless, progressive lymphadenopathy in a centrifugal manner.
ii. Systemic symptoms (B symptoms) like fever, night sweets, weight loss, pruritus, fatigue, bone pain may be present Bone pain may be induced/ enlarged by drinking alcohol

    Fever with or without rigors occurs in a periodic fashion.

    Period of High grade pyrexia (fever) for 7-10 days alternating with nearly a similar period of apyrexia which may continue for several months called Pel-Ebstein fever
iii. Hepatosplenomegaly

    Diagnosis, types, classification, prognostic factors are described in question and answers part.

Non Hodgkin's lymphoma

NHLs are tumors originating from lymphoid tissues, mainly of lymph nodes. NHL represents a progressive clonal expansion of B cells or T cells and/or natural killer cells. 85% NHLs are B-cells origin.

Male: female= 1.4:1, i.e. incidence is slightly higher in male. Age > 50 years.

1. Clinical feature—slowly progressive

- Painless peripheral adenopathy.
- Centripetal in distribution is the most common presentation.
- B' symptoms (fever) > 38o c, night sweats, weight loss > 10% from base line within 6 months occurs in 30% cases.
- More than 1/3rd of patients present with extra nodal involvement. The commonest site is GI Tract
- Others involvements are skin, bone marrow, sinuses, genitourinary tract, CNS, thyroid etc.
- Hepatosplenomegaly with bone narrow involvement also common >50% cases.

2. Investigations

- Complete blood count, Hb% platelet count may show Anaemia, secondary to bone narrow infiltration, autoimmune hemolysis, bleeding and anaemia due to chronic disease.

- Elevated LDH (Lactate dehydrogenase) - related with increased tumor burden. Abnormal LFT- secondary to hepatic involvement.
- Imaging studies
  - Chest X-ray- PA view
  - USG abdomen and pelvis
  - CT scan neck, chest Abdomen and pelvis to see the extent of the disease.
  - Bone scan is indicated in patients with bone pain and or elevated alkaline phosphatase.
- MRI—If primary CNS lymphoma, lymphomatous meningitis, para spinal lymphoma.

How to perform bone narrow aspirate and biopsy

In a case of Non-Hodgkin's lymphoma.

- Bone narrow aspirate and biopsy should be performed on both the side, i.e. bilaterally as bone narrow involvement is patchy.

- Neoplastic cell infiltrate in a focal, interstitial. Or diffuse pattern.
- Biopsy of extramural sites: approximately 30-35% patients with NHL, the extra nodal sites are the primary presenting sites and the most common site is GI tract.

Treatment

Chemotherapy is the main stay of treatment CHOP is the main regime

- C---Cyclophosphamide
- H---Hydroxydaunorubicin
- O---Oncovin
- P---Prednisolone

Other option is:--

- Stage I and II NHL-treated with involved field (if) radiation.
- Whole body radiation (WBR) is used if field therapy is failed.
- Stage III and IV-chemotherapy is the treatment of choice.

My patient Sandhya, a 40 years old lady presented with history of swelling around her left ear lobule for last 4 years.

Since last 4 years my patient having the swelling below front and back of her left ear lobule which is

- Slowly progressive
- It is painless.
- attains its present size approximate 4 × 3 cm from its initial size of a peanut.

[Keep in mind the following negative history but do not utter except very important relevant points].

There is no history of

- Trismus.
- No history of sudden increase in size.
- No history of facial weakness.
- No history of dysphasia.
- Or recurrent snoring.
- Paresthesia. | Metastases.
- Hoarseness of voice.|

No other swelling found in the face or neck, floor of mouth etc.

No features suggestive of facial nerve involvement.

On Examination

General survey

Essentially normal.

Local examination

- There is a 4 x 3 cm swelling in the left parotid region.
- There is obvious loss of left submandibular furrow.
- Left lobule lifted up.
- Overlaying skin approximate normal.
- No facial deformity / asymmetry noticed.
  - The lump is non tender, local temperature not raised firm in consistency.
  - Mobile, well defined margin, smooth surface.

- Not fixed to the masseter/SCM or overlying skin.
- No paresthesia over the face/ ear lobule.
- Facial nerve's function is intact.
- Parotid duct -NAD.
- Bidigital palpation reveals the involvement of superficial lobe only, not the deep lobe.
- No other lump or lymph nodes are palpable in the neck.

Clinically my diagnosis is

Left parotid tumor most probably benign.

[Remember-

- Mixed parotid tumor, i.e. pleomorphic adenoma or parotid carcinoma is typically around the ear lobule, i.e. in the parotid region.
- Adenolymphoma (Warthin's tumour)- usually arises from the lower pole of the gland and lies at or below the angle of mandible.
- Accessory parotid tumor arises at the region of cheek also.]

Why do you say it is a benign parotid tumour?

- It is a slowly progressive tumour.
- ON examination well defined margins, smooth surface underlying muscle or overlying skin is not involved.
- Facial nerve is not involved.
- Mixed parotid tumor is the most common benign parotid tumour.

How can you say it is a parotid tumour?

Sir,

i. The swelling is in the parotid region.
ii. The ear lobule is pushed upwards.
iii. Retromandibular furrow is obliterated.
iv. The swelling cannot be moved above the zygomatic bone 'curtain sign'.

These are typical findings of parotid swelling.

What do you mean by parotid region?

The parotid region is bounded by
  i. Anteriorly, the posterior border of mandible.
  ii. Posteriorly, the mastoid process and attached sternocleidomastoid muscle.
  iii. Superiorly the zygomatic arch.
  iv. Inferiorly, posterior belly of digastric muscle.

What are the other possibilities of this type of swelling?

Sir, from history and clinical examination I will keep benign parotid tumor as my provisional diagnosis.
But I will keep in mind the following differential diagnosis
- Adenolymphoma of parotid.
- Chronic sialoadenitis.
- Carcinoma parotid.
- Cervical lymphadenopathy - Tubercular, Metastatic, Lymphoma. Pre auricular lymphadenopathy

Features of

i. **Adenolymphoma (Warthin's tumour, papillary cystadenoma lymphomatosum)**
  - Elderly patient mean age of 60 years
  - M:F ratio 4:1.
  - Usually arises from lower pole of parotid and lies at the level or below angle of mandible.
  - It is often bilateral.
  - Slow growing, soft, cystic, and smooth and fluctuant swelling.

Investigations
- Adenolymphoma, produces a 'hot spot' in 99 technetium pertechnetate scan (due to high mitochondrial content)- it is diagnostic.
  FNAC-> it composed of double layer of columnar epithelium.
- Right adenolymphoma does not turn into malignancy.

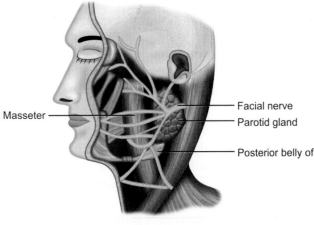

Masseter —
— Facial nerve
— Parotid gland
— Posterior belly of

Anatomical relations of parotid gland

ii. Chronic Sialoadenitis:

Calculi are more common in submandibular gland 80% because
- The gland secretion is viscous.
- Contains more calcium.
- Non dependent drainage.
- Stasis.
  – Pain is more during mastication due to stimulation.
  – Gland size is increased during mastication owing to increase salivary secretion.
  – Firm, tender swelling is palpable bidigitally.
  – In submandibular salivary gland, the stones are multiple with inflammation of gland (sialoadenitis).

Investigations:
- Intra oral X-ray (dental occlusion films) to look for radio opaque stones.
- FNAC of the gland to rule out other pathology.

iii. Carcinoma Parotid:
- Mucoepidermoid tumor is the commonest malignant salivary gland tumour. (In major salivary gland).
- It is slowly progressive, often attains a big size and may spread to neck lymph nodes.
- Facial nerve involvement is only in few advanced cases, usually facial nerve not involved commonly.
- Swelling is usually hard, nodular, irregular margins.
- It often involves skin and lymph nodes.

iv. Cervical and preauricular lymphadenopathy:
Tubercular- Common in upper deep cervical (jaugulo-digastric group of lymph nodes 54%)
  Next common is post triangle lymph node 22%.
- Swelling is firm, matted.
- Features of lymphadenitis- matting - cold abscess-> collar stud abscess-> sinus formation.
- Tonsils may be studded with tubercles.
- Pulmonary TB may be associated with.

Metastatic
" Common in elderly people.
- Presenting with rapidly increasing -painless lump in the neck.
- Nodular, hard in consistency, in advanced stage it may be fixed.
- Features of adjacent structure involvement like skin changes, sympathetic chain involvement causing Horner's syndrome, etc.
- Dysphagia, hemoptysis, dyspnea, hoarseness of voice, ear pain are the features depending on the primary site.

Lymphoma:

- Hodgkin's Lymphoma.
- Common in male.
- Bi modal presentation- seen in young people 20-30 years as well as elderly > 60 years.
- Painless progressive enlargement of lymph nodes.
- Lymph nodes are smooth, firm, nontender, rubbery in consistency.
- Cervical lymph nodes involvement is the commonest site 82% (lower deep cervical group and posterior triangle).
- Hepatosplenomegaly may be associated weight loss may be present which signifies stage 'B' which has got poor prognosis.

  Stage 'A' - absence of these symptoms- signifies better prognosis.]

How will you proceed in this case?

Sir, I will do FNAC from the swelling if it is a benign tumour. I will prepare the patient for surgery by doing all base line investigations and I will do Superficial parotidectomy.

How will you exclude the deep lobe involvement?

I will take the history of difficulty in swallowing and recurrent snoring to exclude deep lobe tumour.

On examination- there will be a swelling in the lateral wall of the pharynx, soft palate and posterior pillar of the fauces if deep part of parotid gland is involved.

(this tumor with the component in the neck and lateral pharyngeal bulge is called dumb bell parotid tumour).

In every case of parotid swelling will you do FNAC?

Sir, it is still a topic of controversy.

Earlier large number of surgeons did not prefer FNAC thinking that there is a fair chance of tumor cells implantation into the tract in a case of malignant parotid tumour.

But present days evidence suggests that using 18 gauge needle for FNAC does not cause viable tumor cells implantation in the needle tract.

Is there any role of incisional biopsy in a case of parotid tumour?

Incisional biopsy is not indicated in parotid tumours as there is a fair chance of tumor cells implantation and parotid fistula formation.

But in a case of inoperable malignant tumor for tissue diagnosis and in a case of minor salivary gland tumor incisional biopsy can be done.

What is superficial parotidectomy?

Removal of Superficial part of parotid gland along with the tumor is called superficial parotidectomy.

The superficial part of parotid gland is the part which lies superficial to facio-venous plane of patey.

[Superficial part lies over the posterior part of the ramus of mandible.

Deep part- lies behind the mandible and medial pterygoid muscle].

What is the incision called for superficial parotidectomy?

The incision for superficial parotidectomy is called Bailey's modification of Blair's incision. This is also called Lazy 'S' incision.

(Incision starts below the zygomatic process just in front of the tragus- it curves around the ear lobule and then descends downward along the anterior border of upper one third of sternocleidomastoid muscle).

Can you offer enucleation for pleomorphic adenoma (mixed salivary tumour)?

No Sir, enucleation is not the surgical procedure for pleomorphic adenoma though it is capsulated as because tumor may come out as Pseudopods and extend beyond the usual limit of the tumor tissue.

So, enucleation is not the ideal way for pleomorphic adenoma.

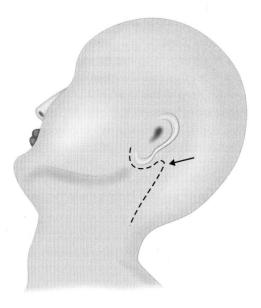

Incision for parotidectomy

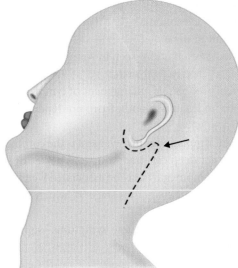

Submandibular
salivary gland

2-4 cm

Incision

Incision for excision of submandibular salivary gland. It should be 2-4 cm below the margin of the mandible to avoid injury to the marginal mandibular nerve

'S' shaped incision for parotidectomy

How will you identify the facial nerve during surgery?

Facial nerve emerges from stylomastoid foramen. The land marks for identification of facial nerves are following:

i. The inferior portion of cartilaginous part of auditory canal, called Conley's pointer 1 cm deep and inferior to its tip facial nerve can be identified.

ii. The nerve lies at the junction of cartilaginous and bony part of external auditory canal.

iii. The medial border of posterior belly of digastric near its insertion into the mastoid process, the facial nerve may be identified.

iv. There is a palpable groove between the bony external auditory meatus and the mastoid process. The facial nerve lies deep to this groove.

v. Identify styloid process, superficial to the stylomastoid foramen, just lateral to the styloid process, facial nerve can be identified.

Why ear lobule is lifted in parotid swelling not in submandibular or parotid lymph node swelling?

As the parotid grows in the parotid region and owing to obstruction by the bony and cartilaginous part of auditory canal, the parotid swelling grows upwards and medially there by ear lobule is lifted up.

But in case of submandibular or parotid lymph nodal swelling the ear lobule can not be lifted up as the swellings

are deep to sternocleidomastoid muscle and deep to cervical fascia.

Is there any indication of CT scan for parotid tumour?

The indications of CT scan are:
• Recurrent parotid tumour.
• Involvement of deep part of parotid.
• Lymph node involvement.

Can you tell me how facial nerve gives it branches inside the parotid?

Yes Sir, Facial nerve emerges from the stylomastoid foramen, lying between external auditory meatus and mastoid process 2 cm inside the parotid the nerve trunk divides into the two:

i. Upper divisions and

ii. Lower division also called zygomaticofacial and cervicofacial respectively.

Zygomaticofacial division gives two branches
• Temporal.
• Facial.

Cervicofacial division gives three branches
• Buccal upper and buccal lower.
• Marginal mandibular.
• Cervical.

Within the parotid the nerve branches and the branches again rejoin to form a plexus. It appears like a Goose foot and known as **'Pes anserinus'**.

Can you tell me why benign pleomorphic adenoma can be recurrent excision?

Yes Sir,

Though the tumor pleomorphic adenoma is well capsulated but the tumor cells may penetrate this tumor capsule with multiple finger like process called 'pseudopods'. So simple excision may leave behind the pseudopods resulting in local recurrence. So enucleation is not indicated in a case of pleomorphic adenoma, i.e. the mixed parotid tumour.

How can you diagnose clinically that the benign tumor is going to transform into malignancy?

- Sudden/ or rapid increase in size of the swelling which was slowly progressive.
- Fixity to the skin or underlying structure.
- Along with facial nerve palsy.
- Tumour becoming hard, painful or causing skin ulceration.
- Cervical lymphadenopathy along with.

Tell me the venous relationship in the parotid gland?

Retromandibular vein, formed by joining, superficial temporal and maxillary vein, enters into the parotid gland and joins the plexus of vein in the substance of the gland. The vein inside the gland divides into anterior and posterior division. Anterior division of retromandibular vein joins with anterior facial vein to form common facial vein and the posterior division joins with posterior auricular vein to form the external jugular vein.

What is arteries relation to the parotid gland?

i. The external carotid artery on it courses, pierces the posteromedial surface of the parotid gland and divides into its terminal branches - superficial temporal and maxillary artery which leaves the gland through its anteromedial surface.
ii. The posterior auricular artery may arise within the gland.

How the nerves are related to the parotid gland?

Three nerves are related to parotid gland.
i. Facial nerve - the relationship already described.
ii. Auriculotemporal nerve, branch of mandibular division of trigeminal nerve, comes in relation to the upper part of parotid gland and it supplies secretomotor fibers to the gland.
iii. Greater auricular nerve- it lies on the superficial fascia, does not enter into the parotid gland. It supplies at the

angle of mandible and there is a chance of injury during parotid surgery.

What are the relationships of Artery, veins, nerve in the parotid gland?

The retromandibular vein and facial nerve lies between the superficial and deep part of parotid gland- this dividing plane is called Facio venous plane of Patey.

The arteries lie in the deepest part.

What is the differential diagnosis of parotid swelling?

Differential diagnoses are:-
  i. Pre auricular Lymph node
   - Features, the lymph node is in front of tragus this usual site.
   - Size is usually small not so large like parotid.
   - Sub mandibular furrows is not obliterated and ear lobule never be lifted up.
   - Clinical Exam may recall same site of primary infection.
  ii. Pre auricular lipoma, fibroma are the other differential diagnosis.

Why pleomorphic adenoma is called mixed parotid tumour?

It is a mixed tumor as because it contains cartilage along with the epithelial cell myoepithelial cells and mucoid material with myxomatous changes.

Classify salivary neoplasm

I. Epithelial Tumours
   a. Adenomas
     i. Pleomorphic
       - Pleomorphic adenoma
     ii. Monomorphic
       - Adenolymphoma (Warthin's tumours)
       - Oxyphil adenomas
   b) Carcinomas
     i. Low grade
       - Low grade mucoepidermoid carcinoma
       - Acinic cell carcinoma
       - Adenoid cystic carcinoma, carcinoma in pleomorphic adenoma
     ii. High Grade
       - High grade mucoepidermoid carcinoma
       - Adenocarcinoma
       - Squamous cell carcinoma

II. Non Epithelial Tumours
- Hemangioma
- Lymphangioma
- Neurofibroma, and neurilemmomas

III. Lymphomas
a. Primary
- Non Hodgkin's lymphoma
b. Secondary
- Lymphoma in SJOGREN syndrome
- HIV patients, etc.

IV. Secondary Tumour
a. Local
- Tumours of head and neck
b. Distant
- From dermatological tumours bronchus.

V. Unclassified tumours

VI. Tumour like lesions
a. Solid lesions
- Adenomatoid hyperplasia
- Benign lymphoepithelial tumour
b. Lystic lesions
- Salivary gland cysts

What is Warthin's Tumour?

It is adenolymphoma of parotid gland
- A benign lesion. It is also called Papillary cyst adenolymphomatosum.
- Often bilateral up to 60% cases because it is said to be due to trapping of jugular lymph sacs in both the parotid during developmental period.
- It is composed of double layer of **columnar** epithelium with papillary projections into cystic spaces with lymphoid tissue in the stroma.

What is the confirmatory diagnostic procedure of adenolymphoma?

99 Technetium pertechnetate scan is diagnostic for adenolymphoma as it produces 'hot plate' due to high mitochondrial of the tumour.

How will you confirm that deep part of parotid gland is involved.

Deep part involvement is mainly diagnosed from patients complain of snoring and difficulty in breathing along with parotid swelling and deviation of Uvula and pharyngeal well towards midline in case of deep lobe tumour.

If any doubt MRI of parotid can be done it reveals deep lobe parotid tumour, usually.

Occupying the parapharyngeal space.

It also shows the facial nerve status and vascular relationship of parotid gland.

What are the complications of parotid surgery?

Complications of parotid gland surgery include: -
- Hematoma formation
- Infection
- Temporary facial nerve weakness (Neuroparexia)
- Transection of the facial nerve and permanent facial weakness
- Sialocele
- Facial numbness
- Permanent numbness of the ear lobule related with greater auricular nerve transaction.
- Permanent facial weakness after radical parotidectomy
- Frey syndrome

What is Frey syndrome?

Frey syndrome is gustatory sweating and it is considered as an universal sequel after parotidectomy.

It results from damage of the innervations of the parotid gland during dissection, in which there is in appropriate regeneration of Para sympathetic autonomic nerve fibres which thus stimulate the sweat gland of overlying skin.

What are the clinical features of Frey syndrome?

The clinical features include swelling and erythema over the region of surgical bed of parotid as a consequence of autonomic stimulation of salivation by the smell or teste of food.

How will you clinically demonstrate the gustatory sweating?

The test is called starch iodine test. This involves painting the affected area with iodine which is allowed to dry first. Then dry starch if applied which turns blue on exposure to iodine in the presence of sweat.

How can you prevent to develop Frey syndrome?

Frey syndrome can be prevented by
i. Applying sternomastoid muscle flap
ii. Applying temporalis fascial flap
iii. Insertion of artificial membranes between skin and parotid bed.

All these methods place a barrier between the skin and the parotid bed to minimize inappropriate regeneration of autonomic nerve fibers.

How will you manage an established Frey syndrome?

The methods include:-

- Antiperspirants, usually astringents such as aluminium chloride.
- Denervation by tympanic neurectomy.
- Injection of botulinum toxin into the affected skin. This method is simple and effective method and can be performed on an out patient basis.

In pleomorphic adenoma why radiotherapy is indicated after surgery?

Pleomorphic adenoma is a benign condition, even though after surgery radiotherapy is indicated as the adenoma has finger like projections (pseudopods) which usually extended beyond its capsule which sometime may not be removed during surgery. So, to prevent the recurrence of the tumor radio therapy is to be given.

My patient Ranjan, 2 years old male child parents presented with complain of
- Swell in the left side of neck for last 1 ½ years

Since last 1 ½ years the child having the swelling at left side of his neck which is gradually progressive, painless and attained its present size approximately 8 × 6 cm.

The swelling becomes more prominent when the child cries and on strain, sometimes it reduces spontaneously. No other swellings noticed anywhere.

General survey is essentially normal on local examination

Inspection - the swelling is 8 × 6 cm arising at the root of left side of posterior triangle neck extending upwards towards the ear and below towards the axilla.

The swelling becomes more prominent when the child cries but strains over it (simple ask the patient to pretend like cry or ask the mother to make the baby cry)

On palpation: Temperature not raised, non tender the swelling is cystic
- Fluctuation positive
- Surface lobulated -overlying skin is free from the swelling
- Margins are diffused all most (as it furrows into tissue space)
- Partially compressible (because of inter communication)
- Trans illumination - brilliantly positive (very distinctive sign)
- Regional lymph nodes not enlarged
- No swelling palpable in axilla, groin etc.
- This is a case of Cystic hygroma in the left side of neck of a 2 years old child.

What could be the other possibilities?

From history, clinical features and clinical examination I feel this is a case of cystic hygroma but I would keep in mind the following possibilities
- Branchial Cyst
- Solitary simple cyst
- Cold abscess in the neck

BRANCHIAL CYST

- Though congenital but usually it appears at the age of 20 - 25 years, even it may appear at the age of 50 years [Fluid accumulation in the cyst is a very slow process]
- Usually the painless slow growing lump appears in upper lateral part of neck (junction of upper 3rd and lower 3rd of anterior border of sternodeidomastoid
- The swelling below the angle of the jaw, below the sternocleidomastoid partly, bulges forward around the anterior border of the muscle into the carotid triangle.
- Tense cystic swelling, ovoid shaped, margins are distinct, not very mobile.
- Fluctuation positive but it is not always easy to elicit
- Trans illumination negative because of its thick contents
- On aspiration material may show fat globule and cholesterol crystals.

SOLITARY SIMPLE CYST

- This is single cyst develops in the same way of cystic hygroma
- Surface smooth, not lobulated
- It usually appears in adult life
- Common site is supra clavicular area
- Others all like cystic hygroma

COLD ABSCESS IN THE NECK

- Children, young, adult and elderly are the victims
- The swelling in the neck is gradually progressive and painless but there may be a history of solid swelling in the neck and features of tuberculosis may be present.
- Site commonly found upper half of anterior triangle of the neck
- Soft cystic swelling
- Surface is rough over lying skin changes may be obvious margins are distinct

- Matted lymph nodes may be palpable
- Fluctuation positive
- Trans illumination negative
- Aspiration may show caseous material

What are the usual sites for cystic hygroma?

- Root of neck in the posterior triangle is the commonest site
- Axilla, groin/inguinal region
- Mediastinum
- Even tongue and buccal mucosa of cheek
  (All these sites are to be examined during examination of cystic hygroma in the neck)

What are the diagnostic criterias of cystic hygroma?

- Infant or young children are the victims
- Commonest site at root of posterior triangle of neck, deep to sternocleidomastoid
- The swelling becomes prominent on cry/strenuous activity
- Soft cystic swelling, surface lobulated margins not well defined on all sides.
- Partially compressible
- Trans illumination brilliantly positive (multiple septae are noticed as the cyst is multilocular)

What are the complications of cystic hygroma?

- During birth it may cause obstructed labor in the size is big
- Recurrent infection as the cyst is surrounded by a shell of lymphoid tissue. Patient may present with
- Respiratory distress - sudden increase in size of the cyst may cause respiratory distress
- Chance of rupture with a neck trauma

What investigations you would like to do in this case?

Sir, it's basically a clinical diagnosis but I would like to do

- Aspiration from the cyst for cytology and Biochemical examination it may show,
  - Clear, watery or straw colored fluid which does not coagulate
  - Cholesterol crystals and lymphocytes are characteristic findings
- USG neck to see - the extent of the swelling - soap, bubbles, mosaic appearance are characteristic features
- Chest X ray to exclude mediastinal cystic hygroma
- All base line investigations.

What is your plan in this patient?

Sir, my patient is 2 years old so, no question of waiting for spontaneous regression

The size is moderate 8 6 cm. So I will try for conservative management initially

What is the conservative management you like to do?

I will do, Aspiration followed by bleomycin injection into the cyst.

Once in a month for 5-6 months

Why bleomycin?

Sir, in present day practice, bleomycin is the agent of choice to diminish the size and destroys its activeness.

If it does not destroy totally by causing fibrosis it definitely reduces the size of the cystic hygroma which will be more localized there by excision of the lesion will be easier.

What are advantages and disadvantages of bleomycin injection

Advantages are

- Destruction of the hygroma causing fibrosis
- It reduces the size, even it may diminish the size
- Localizes the cyst so easier to dissect.

Disadvantages

- A side effect of bleomycin is well known that is pulmonary fibrosis. So proper dose and chest X ray before next dose is recommended.

Any alternate way of treatment?

Sir, aspiration followed by injection of sclerosing agents, like polidocanol, sodium tetradocyl sulphate, even hypertonic saline, hot water, cause fibrosis and the size diminishes.

- Cyst becomes more localized there by dissection will be easier.

  Disadvantage of sclerosant agent may destroy the tissue plane, causing curative surgery difficult. Aspiration alone may give relieve of pressure symptoms.

Suppose sclerosing agents fail to diminish the size what will you do then?

I will do complete excision of the cyst. Care to be taken so that all finger like projections from the cyst wall along with the entire cyst wall to be excised

What are the complications of in complete removal?

- Fluid, electrolyte imbalance leading to dehydration which is difficult to tackle
- Chance of wound infection is high
- Recurrence of the cyst is not uncommon.

Is there any role of radiotherapy in cystic hygroma?

Cystic hygroma is not much radio sensitive. But in case of recurrence and when the part of cyst wall could not be removed completely radiotherapy may be used to take care situation.

Can the cystic hygroma be recovered spontaneously?

It is believed that some kind of cystic hygroma may recover spontaneously and it takes 2 years to be re covered. It is believed that infection of cystic hygroma causing inflammation may lead to fibrosis and spontaneous regression of the cyst.

Why cystic hygroma is also called hydrocele of neck?

Because cystic hygroma has the typical features of hydrocele like
- Fluctuation and
- Brilliant transillumination
  So it is called hydrocele of neck.

Can you tell me what are the cyst is our body which contains cholesterol crystal?

The cysts containing cholesterol crystals are
- Branchial cyst
- Thyroglossal cyst
- Cystic hygroma
- Old hydrocele
- Dental cyst
- Dentigerous cyst

Why cystic hygroma is more prone to develop infection?

Because the wall of the cyst is covered with a shell of lymphoid tissue.

SHORT NOTE ON CYSTIC HYGROMA

A cystic hygroma is a collection of lymphatic sacs containing clear, colorless lymph.

It arises from the congenital lymph sacs which are precursors of adult lymphatic channels it is considered a variety of lymphangioma and broadly this is a hamartoma.

Pathophysiology: 6th week of Intra uterine life 3 pairs of lymph sacs appear in embryo
- One pair in the neck jugular lymph sac
- One pair in retroperitoneum
- One pair near the inguinal region below the bifurcation of common iliac vein

It is believed that cystic hygroma develops from the abnormalities of the primitives sacs. In the neck cystic hygroma develop as a result of sequestration of a portion of the jugular lymph sacs.

The cyst is lined by single layer of columnar epithelium a covered externally with a shell of lymphoid tissue.

SHORT NOTE ON SWELLING IN THE NECK

The most common swelling in the neck are of lymph nodes origin.

Neck swelling

- Lymph nodal swelling 80 - 85%
- Thyroid swelling 8 - 10%
- Other swelling 7 - 10%

Surgical Anatomy of Neck

Triangles of Neck

- Anterior
- Posterior

The anterior triangle is bounded by anteriorly midline from chin to manubrium posteriorly by anterior border of sternocleidomastoid

Above by lower border of mandible

The anterior triangle is subdivided by the digastric muscle and omohyoid muscle into submental, sub mandibular, infrahyoid carotid and muscular triangle.

The posterior triangle is bounded anteriorly by posterior border of the sternocleidomastoid and posteriorly by anterior border of trapezius and below by the middle third of the clavicle.

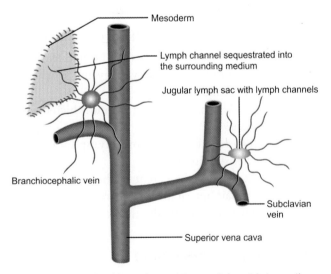

Different levels of lymph sacs in neck in which cystic hygroma develop

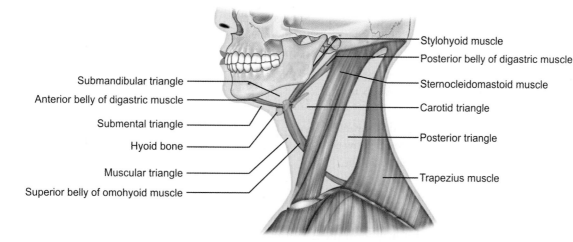

Triangles of the neck

Commonest Midline swelling in neck are

a. Cystic swellings
- Ranula
- Cervical dermoid
- Subhyoid bursal cyst
- Thyroglossal cyst
- Cold abscess aneurysm of innominate artery

b. Solid swelling
- Lymph nodal swelling
- Thyroid swellings (move with deglutition)

Lateral Swellings

a. Cystic
- Plunging ranula
- Branchial cyst

- Cold abscess
- Carotid aneurysm
- Laryngocele
- Cystic hygroma
- Solitary lymphatic cyst
- Cold abscess
- Pharyngeal pouch

b. Solid Swellings
- Lymph nodal swelling
- Submandibular salivary gland tumors
- Carotid body tumour
- Swelling of lateral lobe of thyroid
- Sternocleidomastoid tumor etc.

Ranula is a mucous retention cyst arising from the mucous glands of floor of mouth and under surface of tongue.

It is a soft, bluish swelling mimicking frog's belly [The term Ranula derived from the Latin word Rana which means a little frog]

Plunging type of ranula extends from oral cavity to neck (specifically in sub mandibular area)

Diagnosed by bidigital palpation one finger in oral cavity, other in the neck. If pressure is given by one finger, other finger will be moved, showing the extension of oral ranula in the neck.

Transillumination positive.
- Fluctuation positive

Treatment is complete excision or partial excision with marsupialization

Cervical Dermoid

- Cystic swelling just below the symphysis menti gives rise double chin appearance
- Bi digitally palpable

Triangles of Neck

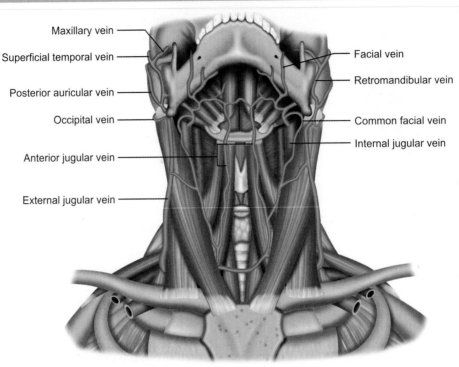

Structure in the midline of neck

- Fluctuation positive but
- Transillumination negative
- Does not move with deglutition (cystic fibrosis thyroid swelling)
- Or does not move with protruding the tongue (cystic fibrosis thyroglossal cyst)
- Fluctuation positive
- Transillumination negative
- Treatment complete excision

Thyroid Cyst

Cystic swelling arises from the remnant of thyroglossal duct. It's a kind of tubule dermoid.

The course of the duct: It starts from foramen caecum of tongue, descends through genioglossi muscles up to the hyoid bone.

At the level of hyoid bone either it descends in front of the bone, through the bone or hooks and behind below the hyoid and descends at upper border of thyroid cartilage.

The fate of the duct

- Usually it undergo complete atrophy except at lower part if forms the is thymus of thyroid and it may form the pyramidal lobe up to 50% cases.

- The tact from foramen caecum to hyoid bone disappears and rest of the duct persists as levator glandulae thyroidal.
- The duct may present at the region of foramen caecum or below it forms lingual thyroid, looks like a flattened strawberry sitting at base of tongue.
- A portion of duct may give rise to cystic swelling called thyroglossal cyst.

Sites of thyroglossal cyst

Subhyoid region is the commonest site otherwise it may occur anywhere along the course of the duct like in the floor of mouth. Suprahyoid region, in front of thyroid or cricoids cartilage.

The cyst content is thick, jelly, like fluid and cholesterol crystal.

How to diagnose
- Common in children - may occur at any age, more common in female
- Mid line cystic painless swelling usually around the hyoid and it's long axis along the long axis of the neck
- Moves with deglutition and protrusion of tongue (because through persistent obliterated thyroglossal duct the swelling is attached to tongue)

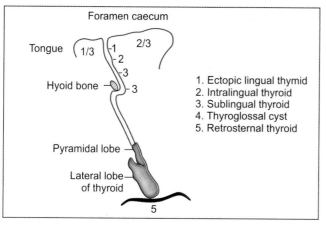

Ectopic sites of thyroid

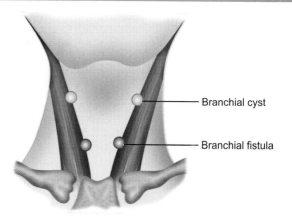

Position of branchial cyst & fistula

- Moves sideways but not up and down
- Cyst may be fluctuant by Paget's test but not always(because it contains thick material inside)
- Transillumination negative

Commonest differential diagnosis of subhyoid thyroglossal cyst is subhyoid bursal cyst but subhyoid bursal cyst moves but not with protrusion of tongue with deglutition other features are painful on set transversely elongated fluctuation positive. Transillumination negative

The swellings moves with deglutition are:
- Thyroid swellings
- Cyst of thyroid isthmus
- Any ectopic thyroid
- Thyroglossal cyst only moves with protrusion of tongue
- Sub hyoid bursal cyst
- Enlarge pre tracheal, pre laryngeal lymph nodes and
- Laryngocele [Thyroglossal fistula is midline fistula of neck which moves with protrusion of tongue]

Complications of thyroglossal cyst are
- Recurrent infection (as the cyst is surrounded by a shell of lymphoid tissue)
- Fistula formation
- Malignant transformation rarely

Treatment of thyroglossal cyst (and fistula) is Sistrunk's operation which consists of
- Complete excision cyst (or the fistulous tract) with removal of every remnant of thyroglossal tract up to base of tongue to avoid recurrence.
- A portion of hyoid bone to be excised for a clear dissection.

Branchial Cyst and Branchial Fistula: A cystic swelling arising from the persistent cervical sinus which is formed due to the fusion of over growing 2nd branchial arch with 6th branchial arch

SITE OF BRANCHIAL CYST

FORMATION OF BRANCHIAL CYST AND FISTULA

How its formed: (please study branchial arches in details) As usually 2nd branchial arch migrates towards the surface and grows over the 3rd, 4th arches (5th arch disappears completely) and fuses with the 6th arch forming a cavity called cervical sinus which usually disappears. If it persists, accumulation of fluid occurs inside the sinus and gives rise to the Branchyal cyst

Sometimes the 2nd arch fails to fuse with the arch and thus form a branchial sinus/fistula

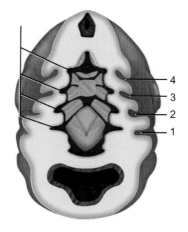

Formation of branchial cyst and fistula

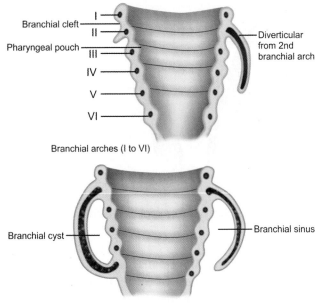

Branchial arches (I to VI)

Development of branchial cyst and sinus

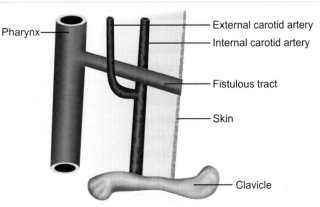

Course of branchial fistula

Branchial cyst usually lies superficial to the structures derived from 2nd , 3rd branchial arches i.e. lesser cornu of hyoid bone, posterior belly of digastric muscle, facial nerve, external carotid artery etc.

How to diagnose

- Infant or young children are the victims
- Commonest site at root of posterior triangle of neck, deep to sternocleidomastioid
- The swelling becomes prominent on cry / strenuous activity
- Soft cystic swelling, surface lobulated margins not well defined on all sides.
- Partially compressible
- Trans illumination brilliantly positive (multiple septae are noticed as the cyst is multilocular)

Branchial fistula

- **Types:** Congenital commonest but usually seen in growing adults
- May be acquired.
- Incomplete type is the commonest
- It does not communicate with the cavity of pharynx called branchial sinus
- Complete it communicates with cavity of pharynx called branchial fistula

- **Site:** external opening is situated at the junction of upper 2/3rd and lower 1/3rd of anterior border of sternocleidomastoid

Course of fistulous tract

The tract pierces the deep fascia at the upper border of the thyroid cartilage, and then it passes between the fork of the common carotid artery, superficial to internal carotid artery and deep to external carotid artery.

Towards the pharynx, the tract lies superficial to stylopharyngeus muscle and glossopharyngeal nerve and deep to hypoglossal nerve and stylomandibular ligament.

Complete excision of the tract is the treatment of choice

Pharyngeal pouch

- It is protrusion of pharyngeal mucosa through Killian's dehiscence, a weak area of posterior pharyngeal wall between thyropharyngeus (oblique) and cricopharyngeus (transverse fibre)
- It is a pressure diverticulum also called pulsion diverticulum
- Mechanism - In appropriate relaxation of cricopharyngeus, particularly during swallowing which leads to protrusion of mucosa through Killian's dehiscence causing pharyngeal pouch.

How to diagnose

- Common in middle or old age men
- Symptoms are according to pathological stages (stage 1 - stage of initial bulging Stage 2 - stage of well formed diverticulum Stage 3 - big diverticulum)
- Gurgling sounds in the neck, especially when patient swallows
- Dysphagia - recurrent respiratory infection
- Visible neck swelling in usually in the left side and behind the sternocleidomastoid below thyroid cartilage

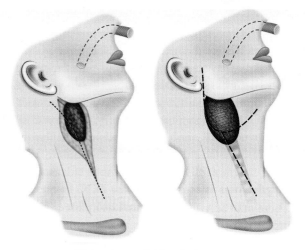

Sites of carotid body tumour

- Fluctuation may be positive
- Transillumination negative
- Barium swallow lateral view shows pharyngeal pouch.

Treatment
- Stage 1 - wait and watch
- Stage 2 and 3 excision of diverticulum

Laryngocele: it is a diverticulum due to protrusion of laryngeal mucosa through thyrohyoid membrane containing air.

How to diagnose:
- Mostly acquired and commonly occurs in professional trumpet players, glass blower and people with chronic cough
- It becomes more prominent when the patient is asked to blow or on Valsalva manoeuvre over thyroid cartilage
- Resonant on percussion
- Excision of the sac is the treatment of choice It moves up with larynx on swallowing
- X ray neck, laryngoscopy, CT scan.

Carotid Body Tumour: Chemodectoma / potato tumour

Tumor arising from chemoreceptor cells of carotid body situated at the bifurcation of common carotid artery.

Sites of other chemoreceptor

- Aortic bodies near origins of left coronary artery innominate artery
- Glomus jugular bulb of jugular vein

- Glomus intravagale ganglion no do sum of vagus nerve
- Para ganglion typanicum along the tympanic ramus of glossopharyngeal nerve.

Site of carotid body tumour

How to diagnose

- Age 40 - 60 years
- Presentation is painless slowly growing lump in the upper anterolateral part of the neck, occasional fainting attack
- Lump is mostly unilateral, potato size surface smooth or bosselated, margin is well defined, solid swelling farm to hard also called potato tumor because of consistence shape and size
- Nontender hot, mobile from side to side but not up and down
- The lump is deep to deep cervical fascia and below the anterior border of sternocleidomastoid
- Carotid angiogram shows the displacement of carotid fork
- Surgery is the treatment of choice
  - Lymph nodal swellings, cold abscess in the neck already discussed in the topic of cervical lymphadenopathy
  - Congenital wry neck (Torticollis)
- A deformity where turning of neck at the affected side with chin pointing towards opposite side
- Factors causing this condition are sternocleidomastoid tumour, trauma infection, ischemia, spasmodic reflex, burns, rheumatic and congenital squint, etc.
- Clinical features : restricted neck movements chin pointing towards opposite side, squint, etc.
- Treatment : cause to be treated

Sternocleidomastoid Tumour: it's actually not a tumour, a misnomer
- It is seen in infant at 3-4 weeks of age.
- The swelling is smooth, hard, nontender
- Chin pointing towards opposite side, head towards the same side (scolis capitis)
- Later age group it causes hemifacial atrophy due to compromised blood supply as a result of compression of external carotid artery by this tumor compensatory cervical scoliosis, squint, etc.
- Early case exercise, developed cases division or excision of sternocleidomastoid.

CASE 24   Inguinal Hernia

My patient, Jitendar a 30 years old, manual labor resident of Bihar, presented with complaints of
- Swelling right groin and upper part of scrotum for last 1 year
- Pain over the swelling off and on for last 4 months
  [Right sided hernia generally precedes that of the left side]
  The swelling was insidious onset and gradually progressing and attained its present position at right side of scrotum.

The swelling automatically /spontaneously reduces on lying down and reappears on standing and walking. The size increases on coughing, sneezing or on strenuous work.

He complains pain off and on for last 3/4 months pain is dull aching. The pain is more on strenuous work and subsides with rest.

Bowel and bladder habit are not normal. He is constipated for a long time, but there is no history of difficulty in micturition. No history of chronic coughs (All precipitating factors to be excluded)

No history suggestive of intestinal obstruction ever (To exclude complications)

No past history of any lower abdominal operation [lower abdominal incision may divide nerves that may lead to weakness of the lower abdominal wall muscle at inguinal region and subsequent direct inguinal hernia may appear].

General survey is essentially normal

On Local Examination: First examine in the standing position and then in the supine position.

On Inspection: There is a swelling in the right inguinoscrotal region extending from right inguinal region to upper part of right side of the scrotum.
- The swelling is pyriform in shape. Skin over the swelling appears normal.
- There may be visible peristalsis (only in thin built patient)
- Expansile cough impulse is visible over the swelling
- The swelling is reducible on lying down.
- The penis is in normal position (A large hernia may push the penis to other side)

- (There may be visible peristalsis seen only in thin built patient when the hernial content is intestine)

The left inguinoscrotal area appears normal on palpation
- Temperature not raised over the swelling and it is non tender
- The swelling is above and medial to pubic tubercle
- Extends from deep inguinal ring to scrotum and
- 'Get above' the swelling in not possible ('Get above' the swelling is possible only in scrotal swelling, not in inguinoscrotal swelling)
- Palpable **expansile cough impulse** over the swelling and over the swelling is reducible [two most important signs of uncomplicated hernia are Impulse on coughing and reducibility)
- The swelling is soft and elastic
- The **content** of the swelling reduces with a gargling sound
- The spermatic cord is not felt separately (As inguinal Hernia remains in front and sides of spermatic cord)
- Deep ring occlusion test (contents of Hernia to be reduced first, keep your thumb on deep ring and ask the patient to stand-up and cough) No swelling appear there by suggestive of **indirect inguinal hernia** (as indirect hernia comes through deep inguinal ring and so on occlusion of deep ring it does not pass through but direct inguinal hernia appears medial to the ring as it passes through Hesselbach's triangle).

Fallacies of deep ring occlusion test are:
 i. Very large deep ring and
 ii. Pantaloon hernia.
   - **On Invagination Test:** Superficial ring is patulous and the cough impulse is felt at the tip of the little finger, suggestive of indirect inguinal hernia (In direct hernia the impulse is felt at the pulp of the finger).

Direction of finger is also important, if the finger goes directly backward it suggests direct hernia. If the finger goes upwards, backwards and outwards suggestive of indirect hernia)

On Percussion — Tympanic sound over the swelling
On Auscultation — Bowel sounds are audible.

Left Inguinoscrotal area is normal.

Systemic examinations are essentially normal

Digital per Rectal Examination is normal (Mandatory to exclude BPH)

So this is a case of

   i. Right sided

  ii. inguinal Hernia which is

 iii. Indirect

 iv. Incomplete

  v. Reducible

 vi. Containing intestine–enterocele.

vii. Without any features of complications

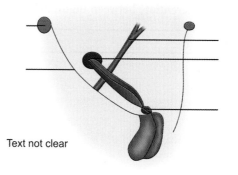

Text not clear

Surgical Anatomy of Indirect Hernia

How will you say this is a case of inguinal hernia?

Sir, 30 years old young man presented with gradually progressive inguinoscrotal swelling which is reducible and expansile cough impulse is visible and palpable. So it is a case of inguinal hernia only.

On examination

– Deep ring test and invagination test suggestive of indirect inguinal hernia.

– Content is soft elastic and bowel sound present in it.

So, this is a case of right sided, indirect inguinal hernia which is incomplete, reducible containing intestine without any complications at present.

What are the differential diagnosis of this case?

Sir, on history and clinical examination it appears a right sided indirect hernia but it should be differentiated from:

   i. Direct Inguinal Hernia

  ii. Femoral Hernia

 iii. Lipoma of the cord

 iv. Epididymal cyst

  v. Congenital Hydrocele

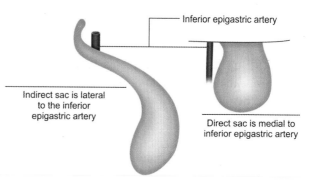

Inferior epigastric artery

Indirect sac is lateral to the inferior epigastric artery

Direct sac is medial to inferior epigastric artery

Difference between Indirect and Direct Sac

How will differentiate between direct and indirect hernia?

What do you mean by an incomplete hernia?

In this case the hernia extends up to upper part of right hemiscrotum and testis is felt separately so it is an incomplete hernia (In complete hernia is extended up to the bottom of the scrotum and testis and epididymis cannot be felt separately).

		Indirect Hernia	Direct Hernia
i.	Age of onset middle	Usually in young individuals	Most commonly seen in aged and elderly person
ii.	Shape	Pyriform in shape may extend upto bottom of the scrotum and called complete	Spherical in shape and shows little tendency to enter into the hernia scrotum so, it never becomes Complete.
	Direction of the Hernia outwards	When little finger enters the superficial Inguinal ring, it goes upwards, backwards	In case of direct hernia the finger goes directly backwards and
i.	Deep Ring Occlusion test	No bulge appear on occlusion of Deep Ring finger	A bulge appears medial to the occluding
ii.	Invagination test	The cough impulse is felt on the tip of the Little finger	The cough impulse is felt at the pulp of the finger

How will you differentiate between inguinal and femoral hernia?

Enterocele		Omentocele
	On inspection	
Peristalsis		
	Peristalsis may be visible	Peristalsis never visible
	On palpation	
Consistency		
	Soft and elastic	Doughy and granular
Reducibility on taxis	Gargling sound may be heard	Not heard
	First part is often difficult to reduce but last part slip easily	First part goes easily but last part is often difficult to be reduced
	On percussion	
Tympani tic note over the swelling		Dull note over the swelling
	Auscultation	
Peristaltic sounds may be heard		Peristaltic sound never heard

Inguinal Hernia	Femoral Hernia
i. Relation with pubic tubercle Inguinal hernia lies above and medial to pubic tubercle	Femoral Hernia lies below and lateral to the pubic tubercle
ii. On Zieman's technique Impulse is felt at index finger	Impulse is felt at ring finger over the
Over the deepring	saphenous opening

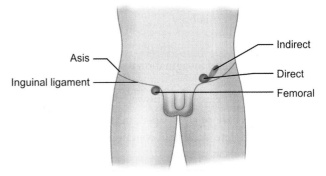

Sites of Direct and Indirect Femoral Hernia

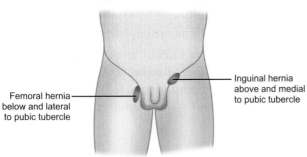

Difference Between Inguinal and Femoral Hernia

What are the parts of a hernia?

Hernia has three parts
Neck
Body
And fundus

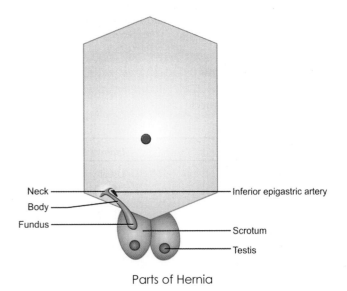

Parts of Hernia

How lipoma of the cord has come as differential diagnosis of inguinal hernia?

As it

i. Appears as inguinal or inguinoscrotal swelling but
ii. The cord is felt soft and lobulated
iii. The swelling is irreducible
iv. No cough impulse is felt and
v. It is relatively a rare condition

What's about congenital hydrocele?

– It appears as inguinoscrotal swelling but
– The swelling is tense cystic /soft
– Fluctuation may be positive and
– It is transilluminant
– It reduces slowly on lying down position due to 'inverted ink 'bottle' effect

What about epididymal cyst?

  It may appear as inguinoscrotal swelling but usually it appears as upper scrotal swelling
– Soft cystic swelling in relation to the head of epididymis
– The swelling has lobulated surface
– It is felt like a bunch of grapes
– Testis can be felt separately from the swelling
– It is transilluminant

What is Malgaigne's bulging?

  Malgaigne's bulging appear as an oval shaped longitudinal Bilateral bulge above and parallel to the medial half of the inguinal ligament, i.e. along the inguinal canal

  It indicates poor tone of oblique muscles of abdomen and demonstrated by observation in profile and by shoulder rising test.

What are the types of hernia?

A. Anatomical type:

1. According to site of exit:

i. *Indirect (oblique) hernia*—when the hernia comes through deep inguinal ring and the neck of hernial sac is lateral to the inferior epigastric artery.
ii. *Direct hernia*—when the hernia comes out through the Hesselbach's triangle which is bounded medially by lateral border of rectus abdominis laterally by the inferior epigastric artery and below by the inguinal ligament. Here the neck of the sack lies medial to the inferior epigastric artery.
iii. *Pantaloon hernia* in which both direct and indirect hernial sacs are present.

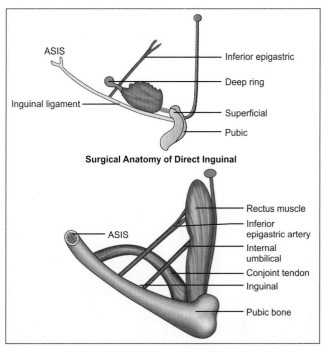

Surgical Anatomy of Direct Inguinal

Anatomy of inguinal region

2. According to extent of Hernia:

i. Bubonocele is an incomplete inguinal hernia in which hernial sac is confined within the inguinal canal, i.e. between deep and superficial inguinal ring.
ii. Funicular—here hernial sac goes beyond the superficial inguinal ring and reaches up to the upper pole of testis. The testis, epididymis can be felt separately from the hernial contents.
iii. complete hernial here the hernia extends up to the bottom of the scrotum.
   The testis, epididymis cannot be felt separately

3. According to the contents:

i. Enterocele—when the sac contains intestine (enteron)
ii. Omentocele—when the sac contains omentum (epiploon). It is also called epiplocele
iii. Cystocele—when sac contains urinary bladder. It is relatively rare.

4. Clinical type

i. Reducible—contents can be returned to abdomen
ii. Irreducible—contents cannot be returned but there is no other complications
iii. Obstructed—bowel lumen is obstructed but blood supply is intact, i.e. there is no interference to the blood supply to the bowel.

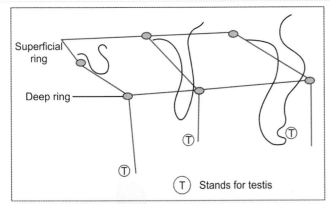

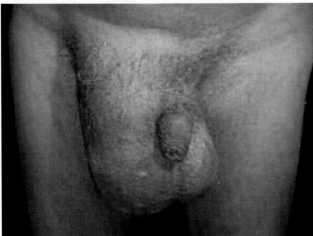

Complete inguinal hernia

iv. Strangulated — where blood supply of the bowel lumen is impaired

v. Inflamed — where the contents of the sac becomes inflamed.

e.g : Littre's hernia where content of the sac is inflamed Meckel's diverticulum.

What is Incarcerated Hernia?

It is one kind of obstructed hernia where the lumen of that portion of the colon occupying hernial sac is blocked with faeces.

What is the basic difference between obstructed and strangulated hernia?

Obstructed Hernia—this is an irreducible hernia containing intestine which is obstructed either from out or from within but there is no interference to the blood supply to the bowel.

The onset is gradual and the symptoms i.e. colicky abdominal pain and tenderness over the hernial site are less severe

Strangulated hernia: When in an irreducible hernia blood supply of its content is seriously impaired and there is a high chance of ischemia.

Symptoms are more severe and gangrene may develop as early as 5-6 hours after the onset of the symptoms.

Urgent intervention is required.

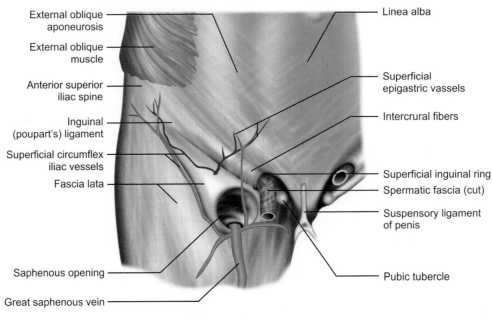

Anatomical relations of lower abdominal structures

Usually there is no clear distinction clinically between obstructed and strangulated hernia so it is always better to assume that strangulation is imminent and treat accordingly.

Know the following tests clearly and practice repeatedly please.

- To get above the swelling
- Deep ring occlusion test
- Invagination test
- Taxis test for reducibility
- Demonstrate expansile impulse on coughing
- Zieman's test

Tell me Gilbert classification of Hernia

Type I: Hernia has a snug internal ring through which a peritoneal sac of any size passes. When the sac has been surgically reduced, it will be contained by the existing internal ring.
            The sac does not re-appear on cough or strain

Type II: Hernia has moderately enlarged internal ring it admits one finger but is smaller than two finger breadths. After reduction of indirect peritoneal sac, it will protrude when the patient coughs or strains.

Type III: Hernia has a large internal ring, two finger breadth or more as is often with large scrotal sliding hernias. The reduced indirect peritoneal sac will prolapse out immediately without effort on the part of the patient.

Type IV: Hernia is typically direct hernia characterized by a large / full bulge out of the posterior wall of the canal. The internal ring is intact.

Type V: A direct hernia protruding through a punched out hole in the transverse fascia. The internal ring is intact.

ROBIN'S modification: along with the above I-V types there are type VI pantaloon hernia and type VII femoral hernia are added.

Can you tell me the Nyhus classification of groin hernia?

Yes sir,

Type I: Indirect inguinal hernia- internal inguinal hernia normal (e.g. paediatric hernia)

Type II: Indirect inguinal hernia—internal ring is dilated and but posterior inguinal wall intact.

Type III: Post wall defect

ABC   A   Direct inguinal hernia

B   In direct inguinal hernia internal inguinal ring dilated, medially encroaching on or destroying the transversalis fascia of Hesselbach's triangle (e.g. massive scrotal, sliding or pantaloon hernia)

C   Femoral Hernia

Type IV: Recurrent Hernia
A   Direct
B   Indirect
C   Femoral
D   Combined

How will you manage this case?

I will do the base line investigations to make the patient fit for anaesthesia and surgery then I will do Lichtenstein tension free mesh repair in this patient.

What are the different types of hernia repair?

i. Herniotomy removal of hernia sac is termed as Herniotomy done in children and teenagers.

ii. Herniorrhaphy it consists of herniotomy + repair of posterior wall of inguinal canal by apposing the conjoint tendon to inguinal ligament.

iii. Hernioplasty consists of reinforced repair of the posterior wall of inguinal canal by filling the gap between conjoint tendon and inguinal ligament by auto or heterogenous material.
    Nowadays most commonly used prosthetic material is **mesh.**
    Autogenous material like fascialata can be used as well.

What is Lichtenstein tension free mesh repair?

Lichtenstein described this very useful technique in 1993 for repairing both direct and indirect hernia.

The placement of mesh in the defect of inguinal canal, without any tension, thereby closure of the defect done without direct suturing.

Fix the mesh at pubic tubercle first. The superior edge is sutured to the conjoint tendon. Lateral edge of the mesh is split around the cord. Two split arch of the mesh are crossed over each other and fixed with 1, 0 polypropylene. Lateral edge is sutured down to the inguinal ligament it creates a new deep ring. External oblique aponeurosis is sutured in front of the spermatic cord.

Still many surgeons prefer anatomical repair of the defect and Little's repair (narrowing of deep ring) before placement of mesh.

What is Rives Prosthetic repair of inguinal hernia?

Placement of mesh in the preperitoneal space is recommended by Rives.

The fascia transversalis is split often and dissected all around widely to create preperitoneal space.

Lower margin is fixed to the Cooper's ligament and fascia iliaca.

The mesh is passed upward behind the cord, transversalis fascia, transversus abdominis aponeurosis and rectus sheath and there by placed into preperitoneal space and fixed all around by interrupted poly propylene suture.

What is Stoppa's procedure for hernia repair?

Giant prosthetic reinforcement of visceral sac (GPRVS) is known as Stoppa's procedure.

This is useful for:
- Elderly people with bilateral
- Hernias—larger defect producing
- Large hernia—recurrent hernias
- Patients with collagen, vascular diseases.

What is the procedure of GPRVS, i.e. Stoppa's procedure?

Here a larger sheet of mesh is placed between peritoneum and anterior, inferior and lateral abdominal wall i.e. in the pre peritoneal space by either midline incision or pfannenstiel's incision.

Unilateral mesh placement may be done by inguinal incision.

After placing the mesh pre peritoneally it is fixed by a single suture to umbilical fascia.

Practically, when the large mesh is placed properly, no anchoring suture is required.

What size of mesh is required for Stoppa's procedure?

Width of the mesh is 2 cm less than the distance between the two anterior superior iliac spines. The length of the mesh should be equal to the distance between the umbilicus and the symphysis pubis.

Ultimately what happens with the mesh in GPRVS (Stoppa's procedure)?

The mesh stretches in the lower abdomen and pelvis from one end to other. The enveloping mesh over the lower half of parietal peritoneum ultimately it gets incorporated by scar tissue and thereby strengthening anterior abdominal wall to prevent herniation.

What is original Bassini's operation?

In 1884, Bassini started Herniorrhaphy. He dissected the hernia sac up to deep inguinal ring and ligated the neck of the sac at that site. He used to divide/split the fascia transversalis from superficial to deep ring. His idea was to reinforce the posterior wall of the inguinal canal by apposing conjoint tendon and inguinal ligament along with both leaves of fascia transversalis (Bassini's famous 'triple' layer using interrupted non absorbable silk suture).

What is modified Bassini's operation?

In modified Bassini's herniorrhaphy two things have been modified:
  i. Fascia transversalis is not divided/splited at all
 ii. Instead of silk suture other non absorbable monofilament sutures like polypropylene is used interruptedly.

Tension is relieved by Tanner's slide

[Procedure—Herniotomy is done first. The lower edge of transversus abdominis aponeurosis and conjoint tendon with fascia transversalis are sutured with inguinal ligament with interrupted polypropylene suture. The tension may be relieved by Tanner's slide]

What is Tanner's slide operation?

To reduce the tension in the repair area, relaxing incision is made over the lower rectus sheath so that conjoint tendon is allowed to slide downward.

What is shouldice repair of hernia?

The shouldice repair utilizes an initial approach that is similar to the Bassin repair.

Here hernial sac is dissected and ligated at the deep inguinal ring and transversalis fascia is divided from deep ring to pubic tubercle.

The lower flap of fascia transversalis is sutured behind the upper flap of the fascia.

Then the upper flap of fascia transversalis is sutured with inguinal ligament from deep inguinal ring to pubic tubercle

The double breasting of fascia transversalis form a stronger posterior wall of inguinal canal. The posterior wall is further strengthened by double layer of suture opposing conjoint tendon to inguinal ligament. First layer from pubic tubercle to deep ring and second layer from deep ring to pubic tubercle.

[Shouldice hernia operation is by the name of Late EE shouldice. In 1945, he opened a private hospital in down town, Toronto, Canada. His practices was limited to the repair of hernia]

Why absorbable sutures are not used for hernia repair?

Following hernia repair, the healing process is continued about a year. 75% of wound tensile strength is achieved in initial 5/6 months. Absorbable sutures lose their tensile strength very early within weeks. So it is not at all ideal suture for hernia repair.

What are the different techniques of mesh repair?

i. Inlay graft: Here the appropriate size of mesh is sutured to the edges of the defect as an inlay graft.

ii. Under lay graft: The mesh is placed deep to peritoneum and it is sutured to a very larger area of inner surface of abdominal wall

iii. Over lay graft : A large sheet is placed below subcutaneous tissue covering the defect

iv. Combine underlay and overlay graft: In this technique one large mesh is placed deep to peritoneum and another over the musculoaponeurotic abdominal wall i.e. just below subcutaneous tissue.

v. Rive's stoppa's technique: In such technique mesh is placed between posterior rectus sheath and the rectus muscles.

What are the common types of mesh used in hernia repair?

i. Polypropylene mesh is most commonly used and considered as an ideal mesh

ii. Dacron mesh

iii. PTFE (Polytetrafluoroethylene) mesh

iv. Polyglycocolic acid mesh (vicryl mesh)

v. Combined polyglycocolic acid (vicryl) mesh and polypropylene mesh (vipro mesh)

{The ideal mesh should relatively cheaper, easily available, flexible, easy shape cutting inert and should have minimal tissue reaction, not easily reject able, less irritant thereby non carcinogenic and reluctant to develop infection}

What are the types of laparoscopic inguinal hernia repair?

There are two methods for laparoscopic inguinal hernia repair

i. Transabdominal preperitoneal repair (TAPP repair)

ii. Totally extraperitoneal repair (TEP repair)

[The non controversial indications for laparoscopic hernia repair are: (i) Bilateral hernia and (ii) Recurrent hernia]

What are the causes of hernia recurrence after mesh repair?

- The cause of early recurrence is technical failure
- Late recurrences is due to tissue failure

Other causes of recurrence of hernia are:

- Hernia repair under tension
- Wound infection
- Wound hematoma
- Use of absorbable suture etc.

(Over all hernia recurrence is 1-5% only)

What is PHS?

PHS stands for proline Hernia system. It is a combined technique of both **underlay** and on lay type of graft. One layer of joint mesh is placed in **preperitoneal space** and another layer is placed below external oblique aponeurosis and few fixation sutures are put in conjoint tendon one site and inguinal ligament other side like Lichen stein repair.

Some surgeons avoid the fixation suture as it is not required logically.

There is a connecting plug between the two.

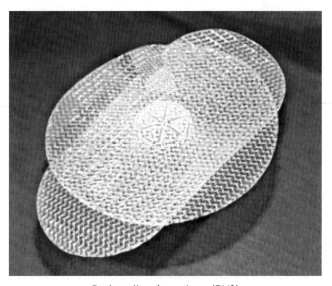

Prolenelternia system (PHS)

What is 3D Max Mesh?

It is a true three dimensional, anatomically formed mesh for use in Laparoscopic inguinal hernia repair.

Three dimensional, anatomically curved shape, sealed edge and medial orientation is marked as 'M'

It easier to put as a rolled mesh, no need to spread it as it spreads automatically and placed properly. No fixation is required. No postoperative neuralgia, very less post operative pain. Recurrence rate of hernia is < 1%.

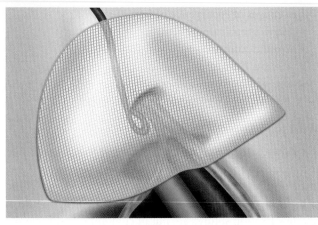

3D Max Mesh

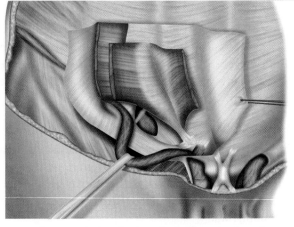

Lower abdominal wall and inguinal region

SHORT NOTES ON INGUINAL HERNIA

Hernia – means in Greek 'to protrude' or 'to bud' in Latin hernia means 'rupture'

Hernia is defined as abnormal protrusion of a part of viscus or whole viscus through an opening, either natural or developed with a sac covering it or through the walls of its containing cavity.

- Inguinal Hernia even in female is the commonest hernia approximately 15%
- Second common hernia in practice is incisional hernia
- Femoral hernia is 15%
- Umbilical hernia is 8.5% and others 1.5%

Aetiology

Chronic straining like constipated patient

- Chronic cough
- Lifting heavy weight
- Difficulty in micturition like cases of BPH, carcinoma prostate, etc.
- Obesity
- Lower abdominal surgery like appendicectomy causing ilioinguinal nerve damage mated to inguinal hernia
- Smoking, collagen vascular disorders are other causes.

INGUINAL CANAL

Surgical anatomy:

Inguinal canal is an oblique passage in the lower part of abdominal wall approximately 4 cm long

Site above the medial half of inguinal ligament

Extending from deep ring to superficial inguinal ring

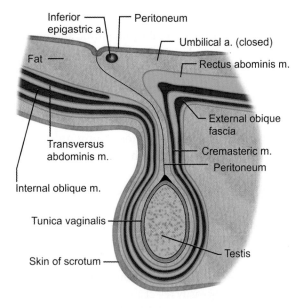

Anatomy of Inguinal Canal

[**Remember:** In infant superficial and deep rings are superimposed without obliquity of inguinal canal]

Superficial inguinal ring is a triangular opening in external oblique aponeurosis and 1.25 cm above the pubic tubercle.

BOUNDARIES OF INGUINAL CANAL

Anterior wall

i.   In its whole extent skin superficial fascia and external oblique aponeurosis

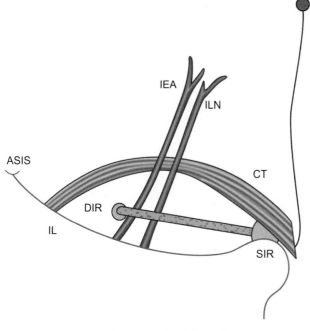

Anatomy Inguinal Canal

ii. In its lateral one third the fleshy fibres of the internal oblique muscle

Posterior wall

i. In its whole extent fascia transversalis, extraperitoneal tissue and parietal peritoneum

ii. In its medial two thirds conjoint tendon at its medial end by the reflected part of inguinal ligament over it is lateral one third by the interfoveolar ligament.

Roof is formed by the arched fibers of the internal oblique and transversus abdominis muscle.

Floor formed by a grooved upper surface or the inguinal ligament and the medial end by the lacunar ligament.

Coverings of Inguinal Hernia

Indirect Inguinal Hernia

Coverings from inside out are:
- Extraperitoneal tissue
- Internal spermatic fascia
- Cremasteric fascia
- External spermatic fascia
- Skin

Lateral direct hernia from inside out
- Extraperitoneal tissue
- Fascia transversalis

- Cremasteric fascia
- External spermatic fascia
- Skin

Remember: covering are like indirect inguinal hernia except instead of internal spermatic fascia there is fascia transversalis.

Medial direct hernia from inside out
- Extraperitoneal tissue
- Fascia transversalis
- Conjoint tendon
- External spermatic fascia
- Skin

Remember: know how the direct hernia is divided into lateral and medial part.

Direct hernia passes through Hesselabach's triangle. The triangle is divided into lateral and medial parts by obliterated umbilical artery.

Direct hernia is called medial or lateral direct hernia when it passes through medial or lateral part of the triangle respectively.

Mechanism of inguinal canal to prevent herniation through it.

i. Obliquity of the inguinal canal the two inguinal rings do not lie opposite to each other. When the intra abdominal pressure rises, the anterior and posterior walls of inguinal canal are apposed thus obliterating the passage. This is known as **Flap Valve Mechanism**.

ii. The deep inguinal ring guarded from the front by fleshy fibers of internal oblique.

iii. Superficial inguinal ring is guarded behind by the conjoint tendon and by the reflected part of inguinal ligament.

iv. **Shutter mechanism of internal oblique:** Internal oblique has a triple relation to the inguinal canal. It forms anterior wall roof and posterior wall of the canal. So when it contacts the roof is approximated to the floor, like a shutter.

v. **Ball valve mechanism:** Contraction of cremaster helps the spermatic cord to plug superficial inguinal ring.

vi. **Slit valve mechanism:** Contraction of the external oblique result in approximation of two crura of the superficial inguinal ring. Thereby preventing herniation through it.

Clinical Features

- Male : Female 20:1 practically more than this
- Commonest presentation is the groin swelling and may have dragging pain better visible on standing and coughing

- May present with feature of intestinal obstruction and that is either by obstruction or by strangulation.

Examination are already described but this is never to forget to examine for:
- Opposite side inguinal hernia
- Digital rectal examination
- Abdominal muscle tone and
- Chest

Different other Type of Hernias

Hernia En Glissade

Sliding hernia also called hernia en glissade. The posterior wall of the sac is not only formed by parietal peritoneum but also by the wall of the viscera.

In the left side by sigmoid colon and caecum on right side and urinary bladder for both the sides. Five out of six sliding hernias are situated on the left side.

Clinical Features

- Sliding hernia occurs exclusively in male over 40 years of age. The incidence rises with the age
- May present with huge, irreducible, complete hernia usually globular in shape.

Treatment: Surgery is the only way of treatment, basic things to remember that posterior wall of the sac should not be separated from the visceral wall, thinking that this is adhesions.

If this is attempted, peritonitis and faecal fistula may result from necrosis.

Here partially excised sac is pushed into the peritoneal cavity with posterior wall and hernioplasty. Or cheilectomy may have to be performed in order to effect a secure repair.

So, **special consent to be taken for orchidectomy.** Remember no role of truss in sliding hernia

Pantaloon Hernia

Pantaloon hernia also called double hernia or saddle hernia.

This hernia clinically presents as direct hernia but it contains both direct and indirect sacs i.e. one medial (direct) and one lateral (indirect) to the inferior epigastric artery.

Both hernia sac straddle the inferior epigastric artery.

Surgery: In such case principles of hernia repairs same except here the hernia sac can usually be simply inverted after the sac has been dissected free and the fascia transversalis is reconstructed in front of it. Then mesh repair to be done as usual.

Maydl's hernia (Hernia-in-w) the loop of bowel in the form of 'w' lies in the hernia sac. The centre portion of the 'W' loop is strangulated and lies within the abdominal cavity

Local tenderness over the hernia is not usually prominent. Hernia gets reduced with the strangulated loop in the centre of 'W'.

Strangulation is often missed also by the expert surgeon and as a result peritonitis and gangrene develops in the loop progressively.

Remember the terms

- **Richter's Hernia** : Part of circumference of bowel wall is obstructed /strangulated
- **Littre's Hernia:** When the content of the sac is Meckle's diverticulum.
- **Phantom Hernia**: Localized muscle bulge following muscular paralysis as a result of nerve damage following an operation
- **Little's Hernia:** Appendix in hernia sac
- **Gibbon's Hernia:** It is hernia with hydrocele
- **Petti's Hernia:** It is a lower lumber triangle hernia

Only **conservative** management for hernia is advisable for elderly people who are not fit for anaesthesia and surgery

Truss usually Rat tailed sprung truss is used and measurement is taken form the tip of greater trochanter to third piece of sacrum circumferentially

The complication of using truss, or discomfort ulceration, inflammation and obstruction, etc.

It is to be avoid absolutely in sliding as well as in femoral hernia.

LAPAROSCOPIC HERNIA REPAIR

Anatomy

The myopectineal orifice of Fruchaud: Fruchaud's contribution to inguinal herniology was to examine the common anatomic etiology of direct, indirect and femoral hernias.

He used the termp Myopectineal orifice as the name suggest what it is

The area bounded
- Superiorly by the arched fibre of internal and transverses abdominis muscles:
    - Medially by lateral border rectus Muscle and sheath
    - Laterally by the iliopsoas muscle and
    - Inferiorly by cooper's ligament (pectin pubis), iliopubic tract.

The funnel shaped orifice is lined entirely by the transversalis fascia

Inguinal ligament spermatic cord and the femoral vessels are contained within the area.

Fuchayd's concept is that the fundamental causes of all groin hernia is failure of the transversalis fascia to retain the peritoneum.

So, in laparascopic groin hernia repair the main aim is to restore the integrity of the transfer salis fascia whether a groin hernia is direct, indirect or femoral hernia becomes irrelevant, because the abdominal wall defect does not need to be addressed.

Space of Retzius: The preperitoneal space behind the pubis in the midline and it is in front of urinary bladder called space of Retzius

Space of Bogros: It is the preperitoneal space lateral to the space of retzius

This space is important because many of the hernia repairs are performed in this area. The important land mark is inferior epigastric artery

Triangle of Doom: Bounded medially by the vas deferens and laterally by the gonadal vessels.

Dissection should be avoided in the 'triangle of doom'. Containing external iliac vessels.

The sac should be divided at deep ring and proximal part should be divided off the cord structure.

In case of complete indirect hernias, no attempt should be made to reduce the sac completely as it increases the risk of testicular nerve injury and hematoma and seroma formation.

- TAPP [Transabdominal preperitoneal repair]

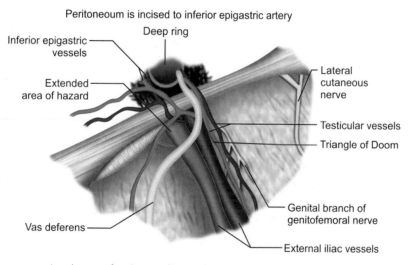

Anatomy of extra peritoneal space for TEP hernia repair

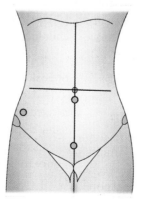

Ports for TAPP Repair

Procedure

Pneumoperitoneum is created

↓ camera port is umbilical port (10 mm)

Working ports

Right / iliac fossa port (10 mm)

↓ [some surgeons like left iliac fossa port (5 mm)]

The peritoneum is incised cephalad to inguinal floor (from medial umbilical ligament to lateral umbilical ligament)

↓ Preperitoneal space delineated.

Hernia defect is dissected and reduced (large sac is usually transacted and the distal sac left in situ)

↓

Placement of polypropylene mesh

A large piece of mesh 15 × 10 cm or larger is introduced into abdominal cavity through umbilical cannula and is positioned over the myopectineal orifice

The land marks for fixing the prosthesis are the pubic symphysis and Cooper's ligament on the same side and Anterior superior iliac spine above iliopubic tract for the medial edge and the posterior rectus sheath and transversalis fascia and at least 2 cm above the defect of the hernia superiorly.

↓

The polypropylene mesh may be secured to cooper's ligament and the under surface of the conjoint tendon.

↓

The mesh is secured by sutures or stapling avoiding any fixation to the 'triangle of doom' and the triangle of nerves'

↓

After fixation of mesh, the peritoneum is sutured back to prevent mesh adherence.

TEP : Total extraperitoneal repair

In this method peritoneal cavity is not entered at all.

The extra peritoneal space is made possible by the fact that peritoneum in supra pubic region can be easily separated from anterior abdominal wall, hereby creating enough space for dissection.

↓

The port of entry

Third port in between two 5 mm

Infraumbilical port (10 mm—1st port)

Second port 2 cm above the pubic symphysis (5 mm)

All ports are in the midline (However some surgeons put one port in right iliac fossa in place of conventional port)

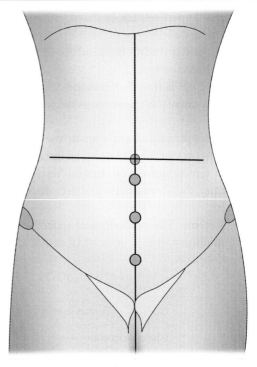

Ports for TEP Repair

↓

By using balloon trocar, the rectus sheath is divided transversely a little lateral to the midline under lying rectus muscle is then retracted laterally and extra peritoneal space is accessed.

↓

Identification and separation of sac from cord structures and dissection for creation of lateral space

(Lateral limit of dissection is anterior superior iliac spine and inferior limit laterally is the psoas muscle. Dissection should be avoided in the **'triangle of doom'**

↓

Sac, after being reduced/transected, is ligated using an endoloop.

↓ (if Bilateral hernia same procedure to be done in the opposite site)

Next mesh fixation: 15 × 12 cm mesh is placed and which is fixed medially over the cooper's ligament and pubic bone using a spiral tacker.

It should not be fixed lateral to cord. Structures to prevent injury to lateral cutaneous nerve of thigh.

↓

The mesh in the position covers the direct, indirect and the femoral defects.

Comparison between TAPP and TEP repair

Criteria	TAPP	TEP
Entry into peritoneal cavity	Yes	No
Anatomy	Relatively familiar	unfamiliar
Diagnosis of bi lateral hernia	Easy	Need efforts
Mesh fixation	required all around	only medial fixation is Required
Port site hernia	common	extremely rare
Learning curve	less steep	very steep

Laparoscopy was first introduced as:

1901	Kelling	Ist Laparoscopy examination of abdominal cavity
1911	Jacobeus	Ist Laparoscopy examination in humans
1929	Kalk	Dual trochar obturator
1938	Veress	Spring loaded obturator
1966	Hopkins	Rod lens optical system
1960-70	Sem	CO2 insufflator, laparoscopic instruments
1973	Wittsomar	Laparoscopy for retroperitoneum
1980	Wittsomar	TV chip camera
1987	Mauret	Ist laparoscopic cholecystectomy
1992	Gaur	Balloon technique for retroperitoneum surgery

Laparoscopy Instruments

1. Endovision camera-silicon Chip (CSC) which is an element which receives light and converts it in to video signal. Each silicon photoreceptor creates a pixel and number of pixels determines the resolution and ½ inch chip consists of 25000 to 38,000 pixels. Single chip camera has composite transmission with red, blue &green compressed into single chip with resultant resolution of 300-400 lines. Three chip camera has RGB transmission with increase pixels with resolution range of 600-1000 lines with increase color and light sensitivity.

2. Video Monitor-Good resolution camera with standard TV with horizontal lines of 100-300 lines.

3. Telescope-Hopkins Rod Lens Telescopes
   a. Eye piece lens
   b. Fibre optic light cable
   c. Jacket Tube

Herniography: just know the term. It is proposed by Gullmo.

Contrast injection is pushed into peritoneal cavity and films are taken in supine position to diagnose small protrusions of peritoneal sac. This is called herniography.

It was earlier used to diagnose undescended testis. It is rarely used nowadays.

SHORT NOTE IN LAPAROSCOPIC SURGERY

Term keyhole surgery is minimal access surgery and is future of general surgery but learning curves are longer and are gaining popularity because of better cosmetics, lesser pain and earlier return to work.

Green A   0 Degree, Red B   30 Degree

4. CO_2 Insufflators - Can delivers 15-30 liters per minute but average rate is 9 liters per minute to achieve a pressure of 12-15 mm Hg. Veress needle delivers 1.5-2 liters CO2 per minute. CO_2 gas used for insufflators has advantage of being inexpensive, easily available and suppresses combustion, but causes hypercarbia.

5. Suction Irrigation system- Ideal for dissection with simultaneous irrigation and suction. 28 mm or 58 mm diameter.

6. Energy sources.

7. Maintenance of laparoscopic instrument either by gas sterilization, chemical and steam sterilization. Gas sterilizations done by ethylene oxide. Hydrogen peroxide starred can be used for metallic and non-metallic instruments. Chemical sterilization by glutaraldehyde 2.4% (cidex) and orthophtaldehyde cidex require 12

minute time for reprocessing. Peracetic acid has bactericidal, tuberculocidal, fungicidal viricidal and sporicidal effect.

8. Laparoscopic cholecystectomy is done with 4 ports. 10 mm camera port is placed just below umbilicus. 10 mm port at xiphisternum and 5 mm port just below the right costal margin on midclavicular line used for dissection and 5 mm post on anterior axillary line at level of umbilicus for retraction of fundus of gall bladder. Calot's triangle is to be dissected first by separating the adhesions. Cystic artery and cystic duct are dissected, clipped and separated. Gallbladder is removed from liver bed by energy source like monopolar cautery and removed through xiphisternal port (remember in laparoscopic cholecystectomy-if the gall bladder is blue you are through, if it is white you have to fight).

My patient, Kamla Devi a 50 years old multipara lady resident of Rajasthan, labor, presented with:
- Right lower groin swelling for last 2 years
- Pain over the swelling for last 7/8 months
  [Right sided femoral hernia two times commoner than the left]

The groin swelling is slowly progressive, initially painless from below upwards and attained its present size approximately 4 × 3 cm from a size of a marble for last 2 years.

She also complains that for last 7/8 months. She have been having pain over the swelling off and on and that is mainly dragging type of pain.

But there is no history of pain abdomen, vomiting or constipation (to exclude intestinal obstruction)

General survey is essentially normal.

Local examination on standing.

- **Inspection:** There is an approximately 4 × 3 cm oval shaped, lower groin swelling in the right.
  - No expansile cough
    Impulse is visible (Neck of femoral hernia is usually so narrow and the contents are adherent to peritoneal sac expensile impulse cannot be transmitted)
  - No visible veins over the swelling (femoral hernia visible veins is a sign called Gours sign)
  - No swelling noticed in the opposite groin.

[Remember in short case only tell the positive history and findings negative history and findings to be avoided except, very relevant one has to be told example in femoral hernia. You have to say there is no expansile impulse on coughing as this is very relevant history to establish yours diagnosis]

On palpation
- Inspectory findings are confirmed
- Local temperature not raised, non tender
- 4 × 3 cm oval swelling, situated below and lateral to pubic tubercle
- Soft well-defined margin

- Non mobile
- No expansile impulse felt over the swelling
- Not reducible
- Ring occlusion test does not suggest direct or indirect hernia
- Zieman's technique cannot be performed as the hernia is not reducible
  On percussion - Dull not heard over it
  On Auscultation - No bowel sound heard inside it

Systemic examination are essentially normal. So, my provisional diagnosis is, this is a case of right sided irreducible uncomplicated Femoral Hernia, most probably containing omentum.

What are the differential diagnosis in this case?

Sir, It may be:
  i. Inguinal Hernia
 ii. Enlarged Inguinal lymph node
iii. Saphena varix
 iv. Lipoma
  v. Psoas bursal cyst
 vi. Femoral aneurysm
      [In male encysted hydrocele of the cord, lipoma in the cord will come as **differential diagnosis**]

- **Inguinal Hernia:** It is in the inguinal region but:
  - Usually reducible automatically or manually
  - Cough impulse positive [except in strangulation which is usually not given in examination]
  - Deep ring occlusion test usually show either direct or indirect
  - Inguinal hernia is above and medial to pubic tubercle
- An enlarged Cloquet's lymph node
  - there may be a cause of this lymph node enlargement
  - antibiotic and rest may reduce the size of the swelling
  - otherwise it is very difficult to distinguish from a femoral hernia

- Saphena varix
  - It is an enlarged terminal part of long saphenous vein associated with varicose vein usually
  - It is very soft
  - Disappears on lying down
  - Impulse on coughing present
  - Fluid thrill, venous lump may be auscultated
- Lipoma
  - As it is universal tumor, painless
  - Slipping sign is very characteristic
  - Soft solid tumor, lobulated surface
  - Freely mobile on both axis
  - It is never reducible and cough impulse can never present
- Femoral aneurysm
  - Below inguinal ligament
  - Compressible cystic swelling
  - Expansile impulse corresponding with the radial pulse
  - Bruit may be heard on auscultation
- Psoas bursal cyst
  - Rare it disappears on hip flexion

In male specially

- Encysted hydrocele of the cord
  - Smooth elongated, tense cystic swelling
  - Not reducible
  - Cough impulse absent
  - On traction of the testis the swelling comes down and becomes fixed - called traction test.
  - Transillumination is positive
- Lipoma of the cord
  - The features are the same as above but the swelling is soft solid
  - Lobulated surface
  - Slipping sign may present
  - Transillumination negative

How will you proceed in this case?

Sir, I will confirm the diagnosis first:
- I will do USG groin to see the origin and the nature of the swelling (solid or cystic)
- If it is still inconclusive, I will explore the swelling to diagnose it and as well as to treat it as the surgery is the only definitive treatment.

Suppose it is a femoral Hernia. How will you tackle it?

Sir, as the Hernia is relatively small and uncomplicated, I will prefer to do low or sub inguinal operation this is called lock woods operation.

What is Lockwood's operation?

Here the sac is approached below the inguinal ligament through groin crease incision.

↓

So, Fundus of the sac is dissected by direct vision

↓

Repair is done from below

Here inguinal ligament is sutured to cooper's ligament [Remember/IC-Inguinal ligament Cooper's ligament] Nowadays mesh repair is preferable.

What are the advantages and disadvantages of this operation?

Advantages of Lockwood operation are:
- A direct approach to the swelling hence the sac
- Simple method and suitable for small and complicated femoral hernia

Disadvantages are:
- Slightly difficult to repair the femoral ring
- Difficult to resect a gangrenous bowel so it is not a suitable procedure if any obstruction /strangulation observed.

Then what is suitable operation for a strangulated femoral hernia?

Sir, in strangulated femoral hernia McEvedy-high operation.

Here an incision is made over the femoral canal extending vertically above the inguinal ligament

↓

Sac is dissected from below but neck from above and the repair is done from above

To Repair here the conjoint tendon is mobilized and sutured to cooper's ligament.

(Mesh repair should not be done as there is high chance of infection)

What are the advantages and disadvantages of McEvedy operation?

Advantages are - easy to deal with gangrenous bowel and to repair the femoral ring
- It does not damage the inguinal canal

Disadvantage—Access to the fundus of the sac is not sufficient

Removal of the sac with its content is difficult.

What is Lotheissen's operation in femoral hernia?

Approaches through inguinal canal like in inguinal hernia
↓
Transversal is fascia is opened and the neck of the sac is identified in the femoral ring
↓
Sac is dissected from above and neck is ligated
↓
Repaired conjoint tendon is sutured toilio pectineal ligament by interrupted non absorbable mono filament sutures

what are advantages and disadvantages of lotheissen's operation?

Advantages
- Easy to deal with gangrenous bowel
- Anatomy of inguinal canal is well known

Disadvantage
- It causes weakness of inguinal canal and its posterior wall, thereby chance of developing inguinal hernia after this operation
- Chance of injury to femoral vein, pubic branch of obturator artery, bladder, etc.

Have you heard the name of AK Henry's approach?

This operation is meant for bilateral femoral hernia through lower abdominal transverse abdominal incision.

What is the role of polypropylene mesh in formal Hernia operation?

Nowadays, the polypropylene mesh is buttressed over the femoral canal to close the defect but it should not be used in a strangulated femoral hernia as there is a very high chance of mesh infection.

What is Hydrocele of femoral hernia?

When femoral hernia contains omentum, which is adherent to the sac, which secrets fluid in the sac forming hydrocele which is so called hydrocele of femoral hernia.

What is sliding femoral hernia?

When a portion of bladder forms the posterior wall of the femoral hernia sac, and its often on medial side called sliding Femoral Hernia.

Is there any role of Truss as a conservative treatment procedure for femoral hernia?

No sir, like sliding hernia, femoral hernia is one of the contraindications for Truss.

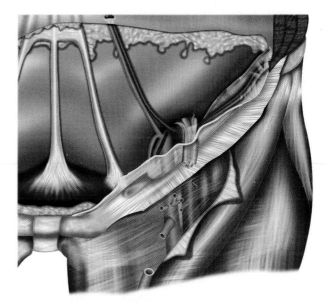

Anatomy of inguino femoral region

SHORT NOTE ON FEMORAL HERNIA

ANATOMY FEMORAL HERNIA

- It is the medial most compartment of the femoral sheath which extends form femoral ring to saphenous opening.
- It is 1.25 cm long and 1.25 cm wide at the base. Below it is closed by cibriform fascia. It contains fat, lymphatic and Cloquet's lymph nodes.
- Femoral ring is bounded:
    - Anteriorly by inguinal ligament
    - Posteriorly by iliopectineal ligament of cooper, pubic bone and fascia covering the pectineus muscle
    - Medially by the lacunar ligament (also called Glimbernat's ligament)
    - Laterally by a thin septum separating from femoral vein.

Aetiology of Femoral Hernia

i. Wide femoral canal in female
ii. Multiple pregnancies
iii. It is always acquired, never congenital

Content of the sac
- Extraperitoneal tissue, peritoneum most commonly
- A part of omentum
- A loop of small bowl

Covering of the sac
- Skin
- Superficial fascia
- Cribriform fascia covering the saphenous opening
- Fascia transversalis- representing the anterior femoral sheath
- Extraperitoneal fat
- Peritoneum - the hernia sac

Course of Femoral Hernia

Through femoral canal the hernia sac descends vertically down up to saphenous opening and then comes out into the loose areolar tissue to expand out like a retort.

The sac cannot pass-down the thigh as superficial fascia of the abdomen (fascia scarpa) to the fascia lata of the thigh at the lower border of the fossa ovalis.

As the neck of sac is narrow and the course is irregular there is more chance of obstruction and or strangulation.

What is femoral hernia?

Femoral hernia can be defined as a protrusion of extraperitoneal tissue, peritoneum and sometimes abdominal contents through the femoral canal.

Clinical Features

- Middle aged, obese elderly
- Male : Female 1:2 ratio
- Common in females, common in multipara
- 20% occurs Bilateral and two times common in the right side
- Presents as swelling in the groin below and lateral to the pubic tubercle
- Rounded or oval shaped below the groin crease
- Dragging pain is usual features
- Cough impulse may present and may be absent also as most cases the contents are adherent to the peritoneal sac
- Reducibility - mostly irreducible as the neck is narrow but it may be reducible if it is small and when the femoral ring is wider.

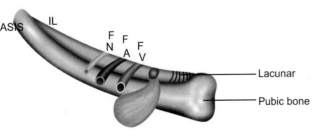

Surgical anatomy of femora hernia

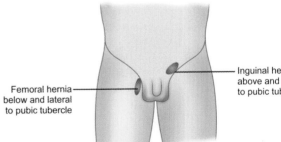

Difference between inguinal and femoral hernia

- Femoral hernia can be often associated with inguinal hernia.

Different forms of femoral hernia

- **Femoral hernia:** Occurs medial to femoral vein
- **Narath's femoral hernia:** In congenital dislocation of hip, femoral hernia occurs behind the femoral vessels
- **Serofinis hernia;** When femoral hernia occurs behind femoral vessels

- **Teale's hernia:** When hernia occurs in front of femoral vessels
- **Laugier's femoral hernia:** Hernia through a gap in the medial part of lacunar ligament almost always strangulated (Remember L for L)
- **Cloquet hernia:** When the femoral hernia is through pectineal fascia i.e. the saclies under the pectineal fascia
- **Hesselsbach's hernia:** When hernia occurs lateral to femoral artery.

CASE 26

Paraumbilical Hernia (Supra- or Infraumbilical Hernia)

My patient, Sushma a 50 years old lady presented with complain of
- Swelling around umbilicus for last 4 years
- Pain over the swelling for last 6 months

The swelling is painlessly and slowly progressive and attained its present size approximately 2.5 1.5 cm from its initial size like a marble. The swelling increases in size during walking or on physical exertion/strenuous work.

She starts having pain which is more or less dull aching in nature over the swelling for last 6 months.

On Examination

General examination is essentially normal on local examination
- The swelling is in the umbilical region
- 2.5 1.5 cm in size, firm, round, knobby and pendulous mass
- The umbilicus is stretched and thinned out/skin with the umbilical cicatrix hangs over the swelling like a festoon
- Cough impulse is present in most cases.
- most hernia is reducible partially (May be irreducible when the contents are adherent to the sac or the neck of the sac is very narrow)
- the defect of linea alba can be felt as firm fibrous edge
- recti may be felt divarticated
- dull on percussion
- no bowel sound heard
  Systemic examination are essentially normal
So my diagnosis is:
- This is a case of para umbilical hernia which is partially reducible, uncomplicated, containing omentum most probably.

How do you say this is para umbilical not an umbilical hernia?

Adult hernia usually does not occur through umbilical cicatrix/scar. The adult hernia usually occurs through the linea alba either above or below the umbilicus.

What may be the content of para umbilical hernia?

Commonest content is greater omentum other contents may be:
- Small intestine
- Transverse colon even
- Urinary bladder, etc.

What is the basic pathophysiology of para umbilical hernia?

The para umbilical hernia occurs through the weak area in the linea alba which is resulting from repeated stretching and thinning out of the linea alba together with wide separation of the recti.

What are the contributory factors for para umbilical hernia?

- Middle aged / elderly women (female : male 5:1)
- Obesity
- Multiparity
- Persistent source of straining, e.g. chronic cough, BPH, constipation, etc. leading to increase tension of abdominal wall
- Flabby abdominal wall

What is the treatment for para umbilical hernia?

Sir, surgery is the only way to treat the hernia.

Any pre operative measures will you take for this hernia patient?

Sir, I will advise for:
- Weight reduction
- Correction of contributory factors like chronic cough, constipation, etc.
- Cleaning the skin pre operatively is important as the skin creases below the swelling is often infected/ulcerated.

What surgery will you prefer to do for this patient?

Sir, Mayo's operation is still preferable.

Through a transverse elliptical incision made encircling the umbilicus

↓

Sac identified, dissected

↓

Neck of the sac to be opened first

↓

Adherent content, omentum /intestine separated carefully and return it back to abdominal cavity

↓

The redundant sac, along with overlying skin is excised and the peritoneum of the neck is closed with absorbable suture

↓

Double breasting of rectus is applied to close the defect by interrupted non absorbable sutures

↓

Put a suction drawn in subcutaneous tissue and skin is closed

What is the role of mesh repair now a days?

If the hernia as well as the defect is larger > 3 cm, umbilectomy along with mesh placement is advisable. Mesh is fixed to the anterior rectus sheath by interrupted unabsorbable sutures but placed at pre peritoneal space.

What should be the post operative management for this patient?

Post operative managements are

- Antibiotics (Cephalosporin and Aminoglycosides)
- Analgesics
- Nasogastric aspiration
- Abdominal binder
- Early ambulation
- Wound care - drain care
- Control of all precipitating factors

Is surgery essential for para umbilical hernia?

Yes sir, as the chance of development of complications are more with para umbilical hernia as the neck is narrow and the chance of obstruction / strangulation is more particularly when the patient is symptomatic i.e. having dragging pain over the swelling, irreducibility of the hernia is there.

My patient, Manmohan SINGH 35 years old manual labor, resident of UP, presented with complaint of:
- Swelling in the upper part of mid abdomen for last 2½ years
- Pain over the lump for last 6/7 months.

For last 2½ years my patient having a swelling in upper part of mid abdomen. The swelling was painless and slowly progressive and attained its present size approximately 3 × 3 cm from a marble size (1 × 1 cm). The swelling used to reduce in size on rest initially but it is not so now a days.

For last 6/7 months he has been having dragging pain over the swelling which is more after eating and aggravated on physical exertion and relieved on rest.

There is no history of previous operation to exclude incision hernia or any history of severe pain abdomen, vomiting, abdominal distension, constipation, etc. (to exclude intestinal obstruction)

On examination: General survey is essentially normal.

On local examination: Inspection there is a swelling at epigastrium approximate 3 × 3 cm, globular. No visible impulse on coughing (cough impulse on palpation may be seen) not spontaneously reduced on lying down.

On palpation: Temperature not raised and the mass is nontender 3 × 3 cm globular and firm in consistency. Smooth surface.
- Slight cough impulse if felt
- The lump is not reducible and no defect at linea alba is felt as such skin is free from the lump.
- Slightly mobile side to side not vertically
- Systemic examination is essentially normal.
- So this is a case of epigastric hernia non reducible but uncomplicated.

Why do you think it is epigastric hernia?

Sir,
- My patient is a 35 years manual labor
- Presented with painless swelling for 2½ years with dragging pain over the swelling for last 6/7 months

- There is an epigastric swelling where expansile cough impulse is present.
- (Reducibility and defect at linea alba are supportive if present.)

What could be the other cause of this swelling?

Sir, commonest differential diagnosis is Lipoma. The points in favor are:
- Firm in consistency
- No visible cough impulse though in palpation the cough impulse is slight, not so obvious
- No defect at linea alba is felt as such
- This is not reducible
- Overlying skin is free

But the negative point is:
- No characteristic slipping sign
- Not freely mobile on both axes
- Surface is not lobulated
- Cutaneous dimples do not appear on the surface when the swelling is pushed away (dimples appears in lipoma as the fibrous strand which traverses the lipoma and it is attached to the overlying skin).

Why the pain is aggravated after meal?

It is observed that the epigastric hernia is often associated with peptic ulcer and pain may be due to peptic ulcer which is usually aggravated after food.

How will you confirm the diagnosis?

Sir, If any doubt in the diagnosis, I will do
(i) USG abdominal wall to see:
- The defect at linea alba
- What is the content of the hernia
- It excludes other diagnosis like lipoma
- To exclude acid peptic disease.

(ii) I will do upper GI endoscopy to exclude an underlying peptic ulcer disease (Done only when USG is normal).

How will you manage the case?

Sir, as the patient seeks medical help definitely I will prefer to offer surgery. If the defect is 3 cm, I will close the defect anatomically after tackling the content.

If it is ≥ 3 cm I will offer mesh repair for the patient.

Can you tell me in short what will do during operation?

Sir, If the defect is less than 3 cm I will make transverse incision. If it is more than 4 cm I would like vertical incision over the swelling

↓

Linea alba is exposed

↓

The protruding extra peritoneal fat is cleared from the hernia orifice by gauge dissection

↓

Pedicle to be separated on all the sides of the defect by blunt dissection and ligated

↓

Then defect to be closed either anatomically or by mesh repair depending on the size of the defect

Where will you place the mesh to repair the hernia?

The mesh to be placed in pre peritoneal space and the facial defect is closed with non absorbable suture usually. But it can be placed inlay, onlay, overlay.

Suppose no mesh is available or patient cannot afford what will you do then?

Sir, if the gap, i.e. defect in linea alba is large it is to be repaired by double breasting to rectus sheath using interrupted non absorbable suture material called Mayo's operation if mesh repair is not possible.

Can you tell me the stage of epigastric hernia?

Sir, there are three stages in epigastric hernia, better to say pathological stages.

First stage. It is just a sacless hernia of the extraperitoneal fat through a defect in the linea alba.

Second stage. A pouch of peritoneum is protruded the defect with the extraperitoneal fat.

In third stage. A small tag of omentum or small part of omentum is protruded through the defect along with extra peritoneal fat and peritoneum. At this stage patient complains of dragging pain and discomfort.

Short Note on Epigastric Hernia

- Epigastric hernia is also called:
  - i. Fatty hernia in linea alba
  - ii. Epigastric lipoma (A misnomer)
  - iii. Pre peritoneal lipoma
- By definition - Epigastric hernia is the protrusion of extraperitoneal fat through a defect in the linea alba any where between xiphoid and the umbilicus
- Contributing factors :
  - Always acquired
  - More common in manual laborers between 30 and 45 years
  - Sudden strain may cause tearing of the interlacing fibre of the linea alba.
- Clinical features:
  - 10% common among all hernias
  - Up to 20 % epigastric hernia is multiple
  - It is a sacless hernia. Often symptomless
  - Swelling may be tender
  - Often symptomless
  - Pain in epigastric region mainly dragging pain
  - Epigastric hernia is often associated with peptic ulcer disease and or gall stone disease
  - Defect is so tight the epigastric hernia does not have cough impulse

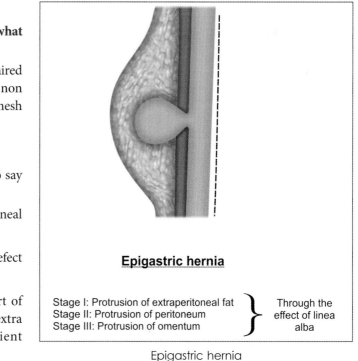

Epigastric hernia

Stage I: Protrusion of extraperitoneal fat
Stage II: Protrusion of peritoneum   } Through the effect of linea alba
Stage III: Protrusion of omentum

Epigastric hernia

- – May or may not be reduced depends on the size of the defect
- – Defect may be palpable and measure.
- True epigastric hernia : with the protrusion of extra peritoneal fat a pouch of peritoneum may follow. When in epigastric hernia content is extraperitoneal fatty tissue having a peritoneal covering then it is called True Epigastric Hernia (and when the protrusion is only extra-peritoneal fatty tissue without having a peritoneal covering called false epigastric hernia)
- Probable causes of pain in epigastric hernia
  - – It may be traction on the parietal peritoneum
  - – Pain may be due to obstruction or strangulation of the content

- – Pain may be due to associated underlying peptic ulcer or gall stone disease
- Basic pathophysiology of development of Epigastric Hernia : Epigastric hernia occurs any where in between xiphoid process and the umbilicus, usually mid way between the structure.

The Hypothesis is that protrusion of extraperitoneal fat occurs at the sites where small blood vessels pierce the linea alba vertically as there are weak spots at the sites of piercing of linea alba.

- Epigastric Hernia
  - – Too small to contain bowel
  - – Only need surgery if painful

CASE 28

Incisional Hernia

My patient, Sushma a 54 years old obese lady presented with

- Swelling at lower abdomen in the line of the scar mark for last 11 months
- pain over the swelling for last 2 months
- My patient underwent abdominal hysterectomy 1 year back. After a month of operation she noticed that there was a swelling at the operative scar
- The swelling is gradually progressive, painless becomes prominent on standing and walking onlying the swelling is reduce automatically
- Now a day for last 2 months, she feels dragging pain over the swelling off and on
- The post operative period after hysterectomy was eventful. The surgical abdominal wound was infected. It took long time to heal after secondary suturing. But there is no history suggestive of intestinal obstruction (pain, vomiting, constipation and abdominal distension) (In case of male history of BPH, etc.)
- General examination is essentially normal
- On local examination: on standing position there is a diffuse swelling in lower abdomen at the scar region. There is well healed transverse scar at supra pubic area.
- The skin over the swelling is thin
- Expansile impulse on coughing is visible
- Swelling is reduced on lying down
- No visible peristalsis seen under the skin.

On Palpation

- The local temperature not raised and non tender
- There is a diffuse swelling at suprapubic area 8 × 6 cm. Margins are diffused
- There is a 4 cm defect in the abdominal wall (The edge of the defect can be delineated)
  [Defect is to assess by leg lifting test (Carnet test) or rising test. Fingers to be placed over the scar horizontally to assess the defect]

- The expansile cough impulse is felt
- The swelling is reducible with gurgling sound
- On percussion dull note heard. An auscultation no bowel sound heard over the swelling
- Divarication of recti is also noticed [In male DRE to be done to exclude BPH] systemic examinations are essentially normal
- So, this is a case of **incisional hernia** through lower abdominal **Pfannenstiel incision**, reducible and uncomplicated, containing most probably intestine.

How will you proceed in this case?

Sir, form history and clinical examination. I am sure that this is an incisional hernia.

But I would like to do:

- (I) USG abdomen to see:
  - the size of the defect
  - whether multiple defect are there or not
  - can confirm where it is really a hernia or muscle bulge only
  - to exclude BPH in male
- (II) Chest X-ray to exclude any COPD and for anaesthesia checkup.
- (III) I will do all base line investigations to prepare the patient it for anaesthesia and surgery

How do you manage this case?

Sir, If the patient is fit for surgery I will do mesh repair in this case as this is the method of choice as the defect is 4 cm.

Why do you not prefer anatomical repair in this case?

In this case the defect is large. The general recommendation is if the defect is 3 cm or less than this anatomical repair can be done.

The defect more than 3 cm mesh repair is preferable.

So, I will prefer mesh repair in this case.

What are the anatomical repairs you know for incisional Hernia?

Sir,
  i. Mayo's technique (double breast technique)
 ii. Muscle pedicle flap repair
iii. Inlay or patch grafting
 iv. Lattice or darning
  v. Keel operation

Remember MILK

Other operation is Nuttall's procedure and most recently laparoscopic incisional Hernia Repair.

What is Mayo's operation?

- The technique is called double breasting technique.
- After reducing the hernia content in usual way the repair is done by double breasting of rectus sheath where one flat of rectus sheath overlaps the other using interrupted non absorbable sutures like polypropylene give a GOOD strength to the scar and defect area.

What is cattle's operation?

- The hernia is repaired in layers which aims to anatomical restoration.
- The method is suitable in small defect where scaring is minimum.
- After tackling the sac and its contents the repair is done in 6 layers.
- Layer I - neck of the sac with an interlocking suture of 2,0 vicryl
- Layer II - The cut edges of the base of the sac with proline
- Layer III - matted tissue and fascia around the sac
- Layer IV- Muscle
- Layer V - Anterior rectus sheath
- Layer VI- Skin

What is keel operation?

Keel operation is done in a large hernia. Sac is not opened rather it is widely inverted within rectus sheath layer by layer with non absorbable interrupted sutures until a firm rectus layer is formed together. It appears ultimately like a 'keel of a SHIP i.e. the bottom of the ship.

What is Nuttall's procedure?

It is done in lower abdominal hernia. Rectus muscles, both sides, are detached from its attachment to the pubic bone and cross over to the opposite side and attached to the opposite pubic bone with non absorbable sutures.

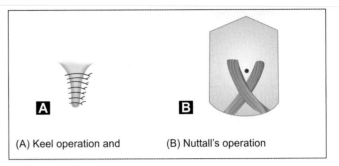

(A) Keel operation and   (B) Nuttall's operation

Different operations for incisional hernia

How will you care the patient postoperatively?

- Antibiotics broad spectrum like CEFTRIAXONE sodium (CEPHALOSPORIUM) + Amikacin (Aminoghcoside)
- Analgesics
- Nasogastric aspiration
- Abdominal binder suitable size for support
- Early ambulation
- wound care Aseptic dressing, etc.
- correction of anaemia, malnutrition, etc.

Next patient to be asked to
- Control obesity
- Stop smoking and
- Control of other precipitation factors.
- Would you offer surgery in all cases of incisional hernia?
No Sir, not every cases.

The indications for surgery are
- Discomfort , pain with the hernia
- Hernia with complications like irreducibility, intestinal obstruction, etc.
- Cosmetic reasons
- Patient's choice and last but not the least

Any preoperative measures will you take for incisional hernia?

Few preoperative measures are essential -
- Control of obesity
- Correction of contributory factors like anaemia, cough, hypoproteinemia, hypertension, diabetes, etc.
- Correct malnutrition
- Causes which increase intra abdominal pressure like BPH, constipation, stricture urethra, etc.

What is the essential principles of Anatomical repairs of incisional hernia operation?

After dissecting and cleaning the neck of the sac, the sac is pushed back into the abdominal cavity by a series of inverting and pleating layers of unabsorbable sutures. Lastly the anterior sheath and skin are repaired.

What is the role of laparoscopy in the repair of incisional hernia?

This modern technique is gradually coming up for incisional hernia like groin hernias.

The mesh repair is called IPOM (Intraperitoneal Onlay Mesh Repair).

The Dual Mesh (Absorbable material on visceral surface and non absorbable material in peritoneal side or composite mesh is used.

SHORT NOTES ON INCISIONAL HERNIA

I.   **Definition:** It is the herniation through a weak abdominal scar resulted from previous abdominal surgery.

II. Predisposing factors:
   a. Poor surgical technique
      - Vertical scar, midline scar, lower abdominal scar may injury the nerves of the abdominal muscles
      - Scar of major surgeries
      - Scare of emergency surgeries
      - Faulty technique of closure
      - In appropriate suture material suture under tension etc.
   b. Pre operative uncontrolled straining factors
      - Chronic cough—BPH, stricture urethra, etc.
   c. General factors
      - Tuberculosis
      - Jaundice
      - Anemia
      - Malnutrition
      - Elderly
      - Obesity
      - Smoking
   d. Malignancy, immune compromised patients
   e. Tissue failure—abnormal collagen formation is related with late development of hernia.

III. Clinical Features
   - Swelling in the scar line
   - Dragging pain
   - Bowel moments (peristalsis) may be visible under the skin
   - Irreducibility of the hernia
   - Features of intestinal obstruction strangulation, etc.

Lattice or darning procedure: After tackling the sac and its content, the defect in the abdominal wall is closed with fascial sutures in an interlacing manner between muscle and aponeurosis of either side. The interlacing sutures is made in the form of lattice work on darn.

Inlay Graft: When the defect is very large cannot be closed anatomically (The mesh is placed, preferred polypropylene mesh). The mesh is placed beneath the recti muscles and sutured all around with polypropylene sutures without tension. The rectimuscles and anterior rectus sheath should cover the mesh completely.

Recurrence after incisional hernia repair: After anatomical repair chance of recurrence is up to 30% after mesh repair recurrence is about 10%.

My patient, Satish Kumar, a 30 years old male, presented with a swelling and heaviness with ache in right side of his scrotum for last 6 months.

The swelling was gradually progressive in size initially but for last 4 months the swelling is rapidly increasing and attained it's present size along with dull aching pain without any reduction in size or any swelling in the groin, abdomen or in neck. There is no history of undescended testis or orchidopexy in the past.

On examination, general survey is essentially normal.

On local examination there is a right scrotal swelling, firm in consistency, globular in shape; get above the swelling is there. The swelling is irreducible. There is loss of testicular sensation.

Both spermatic cords are normal on palpation. Left testis appears normal.

Abdominal examination—NO lump detected.

No abdominal and supra clavicular lymphadenopathy noticed.

What is your diagnosis?

Sir, this is case of right sided testicular tumor without any clinical evidence of distant metastasis.

Do you have any differential diagnosis?

Other than testicular tumour, the differential diagnosis are:
1. Epididymo-orchitis—as patient having pain along the swelling.
2. Lymphadenopathy—no other palpable swelling or lymph node palpable.
3. Old hematocele—because there is possibility of unnoticed trivial trauma to the patient that can lead to the swelling. No clinical evidence of infection or malignant lymphadenopathy.

How will you manage this patient?

Sir, I will confirm my diagnosis first. The investigations required to confirm the diagnosis are:

i. Ultrasound of the scrotum to identify the nature of swelling. USG commonly shows a homogeneous hypoechoic intra testicular mass (larger lesions may be more inhomogeneous). Calcification and cystic area more common with NSGCT (Non Seminomatous Germ Cell Tumour) than seminoma.

ii. Ultrasound-abdomen and groin—to exclude abdominal and inguinal lymphadenopathy.

iii. Serum markers:
  1. Alpha feto protein (AFP)
  2. Lactate dehydrogenase (LDH)
  3. Human chorionic gonadotropin (hCG)

iv. Chest X-ray to exclude metastasis.

v. CECT abdomen—to stage the disease, to see the retroperitoneal lymphadenopathy and to exclude intra abdominal metastasis.

Other than these special investigations, all routine investigations are to be done for preoperative fitness.

What is the significance of tumor markers?

- If AFP and hCG both are elevated, the probability of having NSGCT is 90% (any one of them is elevated in 90% of cases, both will be elevated in 40% of the cases).
- hCG elevated in 5% cases of seminoma.
- Raised AFP indicates the presence of teratomatous element.
- In follow up cases these markers are very useful.
- Increase serum markers indicate active metastasis before the disease gets manifested.

Why have you taken the history of cryptorchidism?

As because, 10% of the testicular tumors are associated with cryptorchidism. Patients having 5-15% chance of developing testicular tumour.

NB: Orchidopexy does not prevent carcinogenesis, only it helps to give early diagnosis.

What are the tumor markers having high diagnostic specificity?

B-HCG for choriocarcinoma. Calcitonin for medullary carcinoma thyroid.

Will you do tissue diagnosis by FNAC in this case?

In testicular tumor most of the surgeons do not do FNAC because there is a chance of seeding of tumor cells in the scrotal skin and thereby inguinal lymph nodes may be involved, more over diagnosis is settled by tumor markers. If serology is inconclusive, FNAC may be considered.

Suppose a patient presents with a recurrent testicular tumor with involvement of scrotal skin. What will you do?

Sir, to reduce the tumor burden, I will excised whole tumor along with scrotal skin and I will give chemotherapy for better survival.

How will you manage the excised raw area after ilioinguinal dissection?

Careful anatomical reconstruction of the lower abdominal wall is mandatory.

The Hasselbach triangle is repaired like direct hernia repair. The free margin of conjoint tendon and fascia transvarsalis are approximated to the iliopectineal line by non absorbable suture (1, 0 proline preferable).

Sartorius muscle is to be transected adjacent to the anterior superior iliac spine and reattached medially to cover femoral vessels.

After completion of deep closure, skin flaps are inspected. If skin flaps are well vascularized, primary suturing to be done without tension and suction drain placed. Heavy dressing to be avoided.

Where the skin cannot be closed primarily, split skin graft may be applied. It the skin disease is large, and then it can be closed by tensor fascia lata, rectus abdominis myocutaneous flap. Scrotal skin flap, random flaps can be used.

Can you tell me the staging of testicular tumour?

TNM staging:
Tumor:
- Tx- tumor cannot be assessed.
- T0- No evidence of tumor.
- Tis- Carcinoma in situ (intratubular)
- T1- tumor invades testis and epididymis without any lymphovascular invasion but tunica albuginea is invaded.
- T2- tumor invades testis, epididymis with lympho-vascular involvement. It may invade tunica vaginalis through tunica albuginea.
- T3—tumor invades spermatic cord with or without lymphovascular invasion.

- T4—tumor invades scrotum, with or without lymphovascular invasion.

Lymph node:
- N0—no evidence of lymph node involvement.
- N1—lymph node < 5 in number and Diameter < 2 cm.
- N2—lymph node more than 5 in number and diameter 2-3 cm.
- N3—lymph node mass more than 5 cm in size, irrespective of number.

Metastasis:
- Mx—met cannot be assessed.
- M0—no evidence of met.
- M1—distant met.

How will you stage testicular malignancy?

Modified walter Reed	TNM	Description
Stage I	N0	N0 regional LN metastasis.
Stage II A	N1, N2	Minimal Retroperitoneal disease, <5 positive nodes, no nodes >2 cm. Elevated serum marker but
normal		pre operative CT scan
Stage II B	N2	Moderate retroperitoneal disease, > 5 +ve nodes, nodes > 2 cm in
size.		
		Mass <5 cm on pre operative CT scan.
Stage II C	N3	Palpable abdominal mass, mass > 5 cm or CT without involvement of viscera or without any spread above diaphragm.
Stage III	M+	Lymphadenopathy above the diaphragm. With pulmonary visceral, CNS or bony disease.

[NB: No stage IV]

What is the group staging of TNM?

The TNM group staging is as follows:
- Stage I- (T1-T4, N0 M0).
- Stage II- Any T, any N, M0 (two types- bulky and non Bulky)
- Stage II   → A- Any T, N1, M0
                  → B- Any T, N2, M0
                  → C- Any T, N3, M0
- Stage III—any T, Any N, M1.

Can you briefly tell me the treatment modality of testicular tumour?

Treatment modality is slightly different for seminoma from non seminomatous germ cell tumour.

A. **Treatment of s eminoma:**
- Stage I (T1-T4, N0M0)—External beam radiotherapy.
- Stage II (any T, Any N, M0)—Radiotherapy on tumor and RPLND (Retroperitoneal lymph nodes dissection)
- Non bulky Disease- over 3 weeks 25 gy in a hockey stick field.
- Stage II–Bulky disease—Radial high inguinal orchidectomy followed by 4 cycles of BEP chemotherapy.
- Stage III

B. **For NSGCT**
- Stage I (T1-T4, N0, M0)   } High inguinal orchidectomy with retroperitoneal lymph nodes dissection.
- Stage II → A (Any T, N0, M0)
           ↘ B (any T, N2, M0)
- Stage II C (Any T, N3, and M0)   } 3-4 cycles BEP chemotherapy
- Stage III (Any T, Any N, M1)
  [BEP: B-bleomycin, E-etoposide, P-cisplatin]

If patient does not respond to two different regime of chemotherapy what will you do?

In such a case autologous bone marrow transplantation with high dose chemotherapy to be given.

What is the pattern of retroperitoneal lymph nodes involvement in a case of testicular tumour?

Lymph node metastasis is common to all forms of germ cell tumor (except choriocarcinoma) which has got a predilection of metastasis by vascular invasion.

The primary drainage of right testis is in the following retrograde pattern:
[Remember Indian Railway—I-Inter aorta caval, R-Stands for right].

Interaortocaval
Level L2 vertebra
↓
Pre caval
↓ Pre Aortic [not Para Aortic]
↓ Para caval

Right common iliac
↓ Right external iliac-LNs.

The primary drainage of left testis is in the following retrograde pattern.

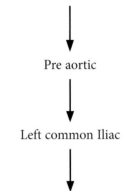

Para Aortic at the level of hilum
↓
Pre aortic
↓
Left common Iliac
↓
Left external iliac lymph nodes

[NB: Cross metastasis occurs more commonly (up to 50%) with right sided tumor because of lymphatic drainage from right to left]

How do you do the high inguinal orchidectomy?

Orchidectomy is to be done through inguinal approach. An inguinal incision like hernia cases, is made and skin, subcutaneous tissue are incised
↓
External oblique aponeurosis is incised
↓
The spermatic cord is exposed
↓
A vascular clamp applied to the spermatic cord as close to internal ring.
↓
Testicular tumor is mobilized form the scrotum and delivered into the wound.
↓
The spermatic cord is divided in between clamp as high as possible in the inguinal canal. (Keep the suture slightly long for future identification in case if any lymph adenopathy arises)
↓
The testis and spermatic cord delivered through the wound.
↓
The wound closure is done in layers.

IMPORTANT NOTES ON TESTICULAR TUMOUR

Carcinoma testis is the most common malignancy in males between 20-40 years of age but it is one of the most curable neoplasms and serves as a paradigm for the multimodality treatment, cure rate in stage I is nearly 100%. Even patients with advanced disease may achieve complete remission rates over 90%.

ETIOLOGY

Congenital

Cryptorchidism—10% patients with testicular tumor have a history of cryptorchidism. An estimated 5-10% of patients with past history of cryptorchidism develop a malignancy in the normal contra lateral testis.

Acquired

Hormonal: Alteration of sex hormone levels are contributory to develop testicular tumour- utero exposure of males to diethyl stilbestrol (DFS), it may cause maldescent and dysgenesis of testis which may lead to testicular tumour.

Atrophy: Non specific or mumps related atrophy of the testis has been suggested as a causative factor in development of testicular cancer.

TESTICULAR Tumor Classification

1. Germ cell tumour:
A. Seminomatous (40%) → Classical (Typical)
                        Atypical
                        Spermatocystic
B. Nonseminomatous
     E—Embryonic Carcinoma
     T—Teratoma -32%
     C—Choriocarcinoma
        Yolksac tumor.
2. Sex cord stromal tumor (Interstitial stromal tumor)
   - Sertoli cell carcinoma—responsible for feminization
   - Leydig cell carcinoma—responsible for masculinization.
   - Granular cell carcinoma
   - Mixed tumor.
3. Mixed germ cell stromal tumor Gonadoblastoma.
4. Adnexal and para testicular tumor
   - Mesothelioma
   - Adenocarcinoma rete testis.

5. Miscellaneous
   - M—Metastasis.
   - L—Lymphoma- 7%
   - C—Carcinoid.

CLINICAL PRESENTATION

Symptoms

Most common gradual painless enlargement of testis. Most of the patients complain of dull ache or heavy sensation in the lower abdomen, perianal area or scrotum.

Acute testicular pain due to intra testicular hemorrhage or infarction is seen in about 10% cases.

In about another 10% cases, the presentation of metastasis disease such as

    i. Cough and dyspnea chest pain, etc. (Pulmonary metastasis)
   ii. Anorexia, nausea, vomiting, malaise (liver met)
  iii. Neck mass (supraclavicular lymph node met)
   iv. Lower limbs swelling (Iliac/ IVC Obstruction)
    v. Low backache - (Bulky retroperitoneal met)
   vi. Gynecomastia in about 5% cases.
  vii. Bone pain (Skeletal met).
viii. Features of gastric outlet obstruction (Retroperitoneal met)

Around 10% cases patients are asymptomatic at presentation where the tumor may be detected incidentally following trauma or detected by patient's sexual partner.

Signs

Locally

   i. Diffuse enlargement of affected testis which is firm and nodular.
      10-15% cases epididymis may be involved with probably of nodularity.
  ii. Secondary hydrocele may be present which shows brilliant Trans illumination.

Per Abdomen

   i. Bulky retroperitoneal lymph nodes may be palpable.
  ii. Inguinal/supra clavicular lymphadenopathy in advanced cases.

Chest Examination

- Gynecomastia.
- To exclude pulmonary involvement.

Lab Findings

- Anaemia present in advanced cases.
- Renal function test is deranged in bulky retroperitoneal disease causing ureteral obstruction.
- Liver function test may be deranged in presence of hepatic metastasis.

How does testicular tumor spread?

Testicular tumor spread by three ways

  i. Direct spread.

  ii. Lymphatic spread.

  iii. Blood spread.

  i. Direct spread is late because the tumor is confined by tough tunica albuginea. It may spread to the epididymis and the spermatic cord. Scrotal skin involvement signifies advanced stage.

  ii. Lymphatic—common involvement of Retroperitoneal lymph nodes is different in right and left testicular tumor (described earlier). Mediastinal lymph nodes may be involved.

Supra clavicular lymph nodes involvement is not uncommon.

[Seminomas more commonly spread by lymphatic]

  iii. Blood Spread—Teratomas particularly embryonal carcinoma and choriocarcinomas spread more commonly by blood stream.

Metastasis may occur to the lungs, liver, brain, bones.

Investigations: Described earlier.

TREATMENT

Seminoma

The different modalities have been implemented in the initial treatment of seminomatous tumour. Seminoma is most sensitive to radiotherapy.

Currently following radical orchidectomy

a. Patients with low stage seminomas (stage I and IIA) treated with therapeutic /adjuvant radiotherapy to abdomen and pelvis.

Radiation is delivered to the para aortic and inguino-pelvic lymphatics.

Dose- 25 gy over 3 weeks.

b. Patients with high stage seminoma (IIB, IIC, and III) commonly treated with 4 cycles of BEP (Bleomycin, Etoposide and Cisplatin) chemotherapy.

↓

About 90% patients remaining disease free up to 4 years after this treatment.

If there is no response to chemotherapy

Salvage RPLND (Retroperitoneal Lymph node Dissection) or Radiation may be offered.

c. For Residual masses
- Mass <3 cm- should be observed.
- Mass> 3 cm- surgical excision / Radiation.

Nonseminoma

- Nonseminomatous germ cell tumor is not radio sensitive.
- Patients with low stage (I, IIA) disease treatment is RPLND.
- Various reports suggest up to 70% of patients with stage I disease are cured by radical orchidectomy alone.
- So, RPLND is controversial. Some suggest that surveillance should be the rule rather than exception. Because RPLND may over treat the patient.

Thereby current recommended therapy for clinical stage I and IIA of NSGCT is limited RPLND and the cure rate is approximately 90%.

↓

Patients with relapse have a high cure rate with cisplatin based salvage chemotherapy.

In clinical stage IIB, IIC, and III NSGCT:

Generally treated with 4 cycles of BEP therapy. Most patients respond to this treatment without any additional therapy.

↓

Partially responded patient to this protocol require post chemotherapy RPLND

↓

Followed by second line chemotherapy (vinblastine, Ifosfamide and Cisplatin)

↓

Autologous bone marrow transplantation with high dose chemotherapy.

- RPLND- (Retroperitoneal Lymph node Dissection)

Types:

  i. Standard RPLND

  ii. Limited RPLND

  iii. Nerve Sparing RPLND.

i. Standard RPLND:
- Standard RPLND includes a full bilateral dissection.
  Boundary—Above—Renal veins
                Below—Aortic bifurcation.
- For full Bilateral dissection:
  a. Left sided dissection:
     - Superior boundary- the left adrenal vein, both renal veins and below the SMA (Superior mesenteric artery).
     - Inferior boundary- Aortic bifurcation and the IMA (inferior mesenteric artery) which is sacrificed routinely.
     - The medial boundary is the medial aspect of right ureter.
     - The lateral boundary is the soft renal hilum, left ureter and the iliac bifurcation.
  b. Right sided dissection:
     - **Superior boundary** includes the right adrenal vein, both renal veins and below the SMA.
     - **Inferior boundary**- Aortic bifurcation. The IMA is sacrificed routinely.
     - **Medial boundary** medial aspect of left ureter.
     - **Lateral boundary** - right renal hilum, ureter and the iliac bifurcation.

The drawback of standard RPLND, ejaculation failure rate is 100% because sympathetic ganglia are sacrificed routinely. Now a day this procedure is not wisely practiced.

ii. Limited RPLND:
  a. In limited left sided dissection the boundaries are:
     - Superior—left adrenal vein, left renal vein, below SMA.
     - Inferior—above IMA (IMA is spared.)
     - Medial—mid vena cava.
     - Lateral—left renal hilum, ureter, and iliac bifurcation.
  b. Limited right sided dissection:
     - Superior—right Adrenal vein, renal veins, below SMA.
     - Inferior- above IMA (IMA spread)
     - Medial—lateral to aorta.
     - Lateral—left renal hilum, ureter, and iliac bifurcation.

In this limited setting, the area overlying the aorta below the IMA is spared. Because post ganglionic sympathetic fibers are preserved; so ejaculation is preserved in 80-90% of patients.

iii. Nerve Sparing RPLND:
- This is the latest modification of RPLND. In this setting, the branches of sympathetic chain that course over aorta are preserved. So the ejaculation preservation is almost 100%.
- This technique is routinely performed in combination with limited RPLND for better results.
- **Contraindications:** This technique is contraindicated in patients with grossly positive nodes.
- In nerve sparing RPLND—the dissection varies depending on which disease stage is being tackled.

Nerve sparing RPLND I
- This dissection is performed in patients with no clinical signs of spread to retroperitoneum and there is no surgically visible disease, i.e. clinical stage I disease.
- The surgical technique employed is either the template or nerve sparing technique.
- In the modified template technique, the dissection is complete above the level of the IMA but is limited to the ipsilateral side below the level of IMA.
- In this nerve sparing RPLND, the lumber sympathetic nerves are prospectively identified and preserved and the node bearing tissue around these nerves are then removed. Both techniques preserve ejaculation in most of the cases.

Nerve sparing RPLND II
- This is performed in a patient with low volume, clinically demonstrable disease or with visible disease at surgery i.e., clinical stage IIA, IIB disease.
- The surgical boundaries are generally wider than RPLND and usually Bilateral above the IMA and in most cases Bilateral below the IMA as well.
- The lumber sympathetic nerves and hypogastric plexus are carefully preserved, resulting in the preservation of ejaculation is over 90%.

Nerve Sparing RPLND III
This is a cytoreductive procedure performed after chemotherapy. Only in highly selected cases, nerve sparing boundaries utilized—Up to 50% of patients may have preservation of ejaculation following the procedure.

3. Lymphoma
Treatment: Radical and adjuvant chemotherapy is the treatment of choice.

SIDE EFFECTS OF PLATINUM-BASED CHEMOTHERAPY AND OTHERS

- Fertility: approximate 40-70% patients are hypo fertile.
- Secondary leukemia's- secondary acute leukemia, non lymphocytic leukemia may be developed.

- Renal function creatinine clearance may be decreased.
- Hearing deficits - Bilateral hearing deficits occur with cisplatin based chemotherapy.
- Bleomycin has 90% toxic effect on lung may cause lung fibrosis.
- Radiation therapy- may be associated with secondary cancers of different organs a decade or later.

Recurrent Testicular Cancer

Treatment depends on
- Specific cancer.
- Prior treatment.
- Site of recurrence.
- Individual patient considerations.

(i) Salvage Regimens

Ifosfamide, cisplatin can induce long term completer responses in about ¼ of the patients.

↓

In refractory disease- autologous bone marrow transplantation with high dose chemotherapy are effective in refractory cases.

↓

In some highly selected patients with chemorefractory disease confined to a single site surgical resection may yield long term disease free survival.

↓

Surgical resection is also practiced in a recurrent bulky disease to reduce the tumor burden.

FOLLOW UP

Very important aspect of management of testicular tumour. Patients underwent RPLND or Radiotherapy are followed at 3 monthly interval for 2 years and then 6 monthly interval till 5 years and then yearly.

Follow up protocol includes-
- Examination of testis, abdomen and lymph nodes.
- Tumour markers AFP, HCG, and LDH.
- Chest X-ray.
- CECT abdomen if required.

PROGNOSIS

Five years disease free survival rates are as follows:
- Seminoma:
  – Stage I - 98%.
  – IIA- 92-94%.
  – IIB and III- 35-75%.
- NSGCT-
  – Stage I- 96-100%.
  – Stage IIA and IIB- 90%.
  – Stage III- 55-80%

CONCLUSION

Testicular tumor is fairly common tumor in young males (20-40%). It is tackled with a combination of surgery, radiotherapy and chemotherapy and it carries a good prognosis present days. Clinical suspicion is very important so that it can be detected in early stages where it is 100% curable.

My patient Suresh, a 45 Years old man, presented with complaint of swelling in his right side of scrotum for last 2 Years.

The swelling of scrotum is gradually progressing and painless. Now a days, the patient feeling discomfort with the size of the swelling. The size is not changeable with straining or lying down position.

[Take the history of following but no need to tell the negative history to the examiner except very relevant one. Take history of trauma, infection (epididymo orchitis) neoplasm to exclude secondary hydrocele, history of previous operation in the scrotum, etc.]

On examination: General survey is essentially normal.

On local examination:

- The scrotal swelling confined to right side of the scrotum.
- Rugosity of skin over the swelling is reduced compare to the scrotal skin in the side.
- Penis is slightly deviated to the left.

Palpation:
- Get above the swelling present
- No rise of temperature, Non tender on palpation.
- The swelling is tense cystic in feeling.
- It is not reducible
- Fluctuation is positive.
- Transillumination is brilliantly Positive.
- Right sided testis cannot be felt separately (as it is surrounded by a bag of fluid).
- Spermatic cord is felt above the swelling. Other sided testis and left side of scrotum are felt normal.

So this is a case of Right sided Primary Hydrocele without any complication.

How do you say it is a primary Hydrocele?

Middle aged/elderly patient with a scrotal swelling which is tense cystic, larger in size and both fluctuation and transillumination are positive. It is the commonest variety of hydrocele.

What is the differential diagnosis in a case of scrotal swelling?

Sir,

Apart from Hydrocele, the swelling may be.
- Epididymal cyst
- Spermatocele
- Chylocele
- Encysted hydrocele of cord
- Hematocele, etc.

(i) Epididymal cyst

Features

- Usually found in middle life.
- Very slowly progressive scrotal swelling is the presenting complain
- This swelling is situated at the head of the epididymis and hence above and behind the testis.
- It is a multi locular swelling- felling or palpation is like a branch of tiny grapes (as it consists of multiple small cysts)
- Fluctuation is positive
- Transillumination positive.
- Presence of multiple septae giving rises to Chinese lantern or marble floor appearance
- On aspiration crystal clear fluid without having sperm is characteristic.

[Treatment: Elderly people—excision

Younger people—better to avoid excision as it may lead to infertility by the blockage in sperm conducting pathway.]

Spermatocele
- Soft cystic swelling
- Situated in the head of epididymis and thereby, it is above and behind the testis.
- Fluctuation is positive
- Transillumination is poorly positive (as fluid contain is opalescent)

- Aspiration shows: whitish, barley water like fluid with dead spermatozoa.

(Treatment small—can be left alone. It is symptomatic or larger-excision is the answer through scrotal route)

How will you differentiate between spermatocele, epididymal cyst and hydrocele?

Both spermatocele and epididymal cyst are situated above and behind the testis—but

- Spermatocele is unilocular
- Epididymal cyst is multilocular
- In both cases testis can be felt separately but in case of hydrocele testis cannot be felt separately.
- Both cysts are softer in feel but hydrocele is tense cystic in feeling.
- Transillumination, positive and presence of Chinese Lantern appearance or marble floor appearance in epididymal cyst.
- Spermatocele it is poorly positive.
- Hydrocele it is uniformly positive i.e. brilliantly positive

On Aspiration

- Epididymal cyst—crystal clear fluid.
- Spermatocele—white opalescent (Barley water like) fluid.
- Hydrocele—amber color (urine-like).

What is encysted hydrocele of the cord?

Elongated cystic swelling in relation to the spermatic cord.

- Site of the swelling may be inguinal, Inguino scrotal or in the scrotal (Depending on which part, the funicular process present.)
- Swelling is limited both above and bellow and the testis can be felt separately from it.
- Fluctuation positive
- Transillumination positive
- Traction test: Positive–when a gentle traction is given, the swelling comes down and becomes less mobile.
- Nonreducible
- Cough impulse present.
  (Treatment- Excision)

What is chylocele

- – Presence of chylous fluid in the tunica vaginalis.
- – Previous history of fever or diagnosed filarial epididymitis
- – Chylocele is usually large and sac is thickened.
- – Clinically it is very difficult to differentiate from primary hydrocele.
- – Transillumination is negative.

Fluid—Aspiration contains fat, rich in cholesterol and microfilariae may present.

(Treatment—Subtotal excision of sac-as-sac is usually larger and thickened).

4. Hematocele

- Usually, it is slowly progressive and painless (due to spontaneous hemorrhage into the tunica vaginalis without any proper history of trauma) but trauma can precipitate the Hemorrhage.
- Firm in consistency
- Non tender
- Non fluctuant
- Transillumination negative
- Testicular sensation may be absent (Because of constant pressure on the testis and testis may become functionless) (Remember—It mimics testicular malignancy in many aspects).
  (Treatment—Acute hematocele-clot evacuation and wound is closed with a drain.
  Chronic—Orchidectomy as the testis is atrophied and functionless.)

How will you proceed in this case?

Sir, I will do all the base line investigations to make the patient fit for Anaesthesia and Surgery. Then I will do Jaboulay's operation.

What is Jaboulay's operation?

Jaboulay's operation is nothing but eversion of sac- this is commonest practised operation for medium size Hydrocele.

Here vaginalis is incised anteriorly and the fluid is drained out. The sac is everted behind the testis and epididymis and closed by continuous suture.

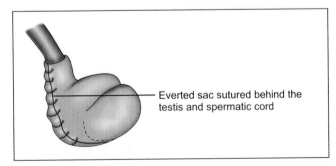

Everted sac sutured behind the testis and spermatic cord

Jaboulay's operation: Evertion of sac

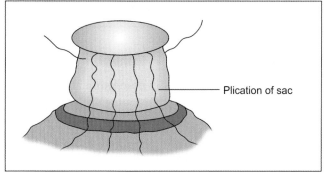

Lord's operation

What are the other operations for Hydrocele?

Excision of sac: When the is sac is thick, in a case of very large sac, chylocele, hematocele, etc. subtotal excision of the sac is done.

Subtotal excision to be done, not complete excision, because tunica vaginalis is reflected on the cord structures and epididymis posteriorly. Total excision of Sac includes division of cord with orchidectomy.

Lord's Operation: Usually, performed in a small hydrocele where sac is small, thin and contains clear fluid.

Here the edges of the sac are plicated around the periphery with interrupted sutures, when the sutures are tied the whole tunica is bunched into a ruff at the periphery of the testis, there by potential space for hydrocele is obliterated.

What is the role of tapping in hydrocele?

This is a temporary measure and chance of infection, hematoma formation, testicular injury and recurrence rate are higher, so, it should be avoided as far as possible.

Relative indications are:
  i. In case of large hydrocele tapping may be performed to relieve acute discomfort.
  ii. As an alternative to Surgery.

Do you know about Sharma and Jhawer technique?

After evacuation of fluid, the sac along with the testis is placed in a newly created pocket between the fascial layers of the scrotum. This is not a highly accepted technique. So rarely done.

What are the surgical complications of hydrocele?

The complications of Surgery are:
- Reactionary hemorrhage
- Infection
- Pyocele
- Sinus formation
- Recurrent hydrocele.

SHORT NOTE ON HYDROCELE

DEFINITION

Hydrocele is a clinical condition which is formed due to collection of fluid in the sac of tunica vaginalis.

How Hydrocele Develops

Here the fluid is collected in tunica vaginalis due to
  i. Excessive secretion of fluid as in secondary hydrocele.
  ii. Defective absorption of fluid by tunica vaginalis which may be due to damage to the endothelial wall by any means like infection, trauma etc.
  iii. Defective lymphatic drainage by lymphatic vessels of spermatic cord.
  iv. Communication with peritoneal cavity through the patent processus vaginalis.

Primary Hydrocele

When there is no obvious cause is known for the hydrocele is called primary hydrocele or idiopathic hydrocele.

It is thought that there is an imbalance between secretion and absorption in the layers of tunica vaginalis.

Types

The primary hydrocele is five types.
  i. Vaginal hydrocele - commonest
  ii. Congenital hydrocele
  iii. Funicular hydrocele
  iv. Infantile hydrocele
  v. Encysted hydrocele of the cord.

Vaginal Hydrocele

Here the fluid collection between the visceral and parietal layers of the tunica vaginalis of the testis.

[Diagnostic criteria, differential diagnoses and treatment have been discussed above.]

Complications:

- Rupture
- Hematocele
- Infection
- A trophy of testis
- Hernia of the hydrocele sac through dartos muscle.
- Calcification of the sac
- Inconvenient for the patient personally, cosmetically and socially.

Congenital Hydrocele

Here the processus vaginalis communicates with the peritoneal cavity. As this communicating orifice is too small that bowel loop cannot come through and thereby hernia is usually not developed.

"Inverted ink bottle" effect in congenital hydrocele where fluid cannot be emptied by digital pressure as it cases inverted ink bottle effect.

Features:

- Appears since childhood
- Presents as an inguinoscrotal/scrotal swelling
- becomes prominent on walking or standing.
- Fluctuation positive.
- Cough impulse present as communicating with peritoneal cavity.
- Transillumination positive
- Partly reducible due to inverted ink effect.
- Testis may or may not be palpable separately.

Funicular Hydrocele

Here the processus vaginalis is shut off from tunica vaginalis just above the testis.

- **Features** - all features are similar to congenital hydrocele except that here the testis can be palpable separately.

Infantile Hydrocele

Here tunica vaginalis and processus vaginalis are continued up to the internal ring not beyond that thereby no communication with peritoneal cavity.

Infantile hydrocele is a misnomer as it is not a hydrocele of an infant.

Encysted Hydrocele of the Cord.

When the portion of funicular process fails to shrink into a fibrous cord and persists isolated i.e. it is cut off above from peritoneum and below from tunica vaginalis (Details in differential diagnosis of Hydrocele above)

Processus Vaginalis: It is a peritoneal diverticulum which is dragged down by the testis during it descent from retroperitoneal space to scrotum.

Soon after birth, processus vaginalis is obliterated at two points one at deep inguinal ring and other just above the testis.

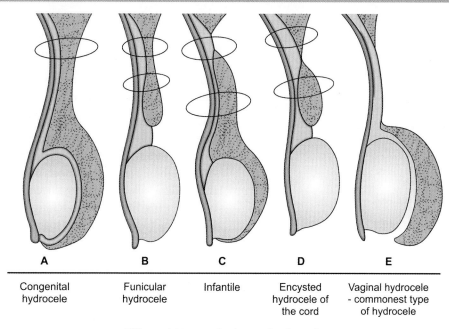

A	B	C	D	E
Congenital hydrocele	Funicular hydrocele	Infantile	Encysted hydrocele of the cord	Vaginal hydrocele - commonest type of hydrocele

Different types of primary hydrocele

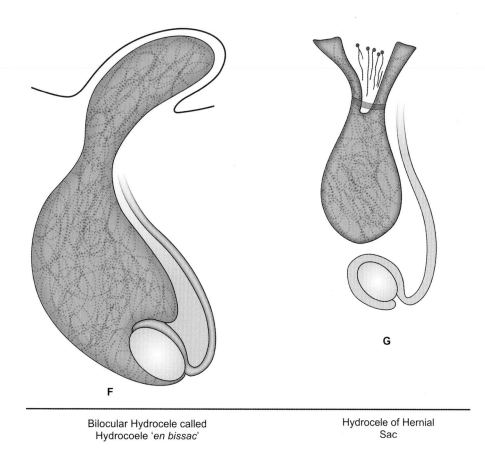

Bilocular Hydrocele called Hydrocoele 'en bissac'

Hydrocele of Hernial Sac

Different types of hydrocele

The portion of processus vaginalis in between two occlusion points is known as funicular process which usually forms a fibrous cord being obliterated.

The processus vaginalis around the testis is called tunica vaginalis.

In some cases the processus vaginalis does not obliterate and this persistent processus vaginalis is the principal causative factor in the development of different varieties of hydrocele as mentioned the types above.

Secondary Hydrocele: Here the hydrocele is secondary to some pathological processes like.

- Trauma
- Epididymo orchitis
- Tubercular
- Syphilitic
- Filarial
- Testicular
- Lymphatic obstruction.

Few Important terms:

"Hernia of the hydrocele" - Here the hydrocele sac is protrude through the dartos muscle.

Hydrocele-en-bisac (Bilocular hydrocele). Here the hydrocele has got two inter communicating sacs, one above and one below the neck of the scrotum. Here cross fluctuation is positive.

- Hydrocele of the canal of Nuck.
  - Hydrocele forms around the round ligament in a female and it is always lying within the inguinal canal.

Practice: All the tests for Hydrocele like fluctuation, transillumination perfectly.

Fluctuation Test: hold the upper part of scrotal swelling between thumb and index finger in one hand to make the hydrocele tense and steady. These two fingers are called watching fingers. Another thumb and index fingers to be placed at lower part of the swelling called displacing fingers. When pressure is given by displacing finger the watching finger will be lifted up. Fluctuating to be repeated at the right angle to the previous axis.

[You know why Fluctuation test to be performed in both the direction?

Think.

See a relaxed muscle or soft tissue can show the fluctuation in one direction without containing any fluid. So, bidirectional fluctuation test is mandatory to demonstrate the fluctuation of a cystic swelling]

Transillumination: a roll of x-ray film is to be placed on one side of the swelling and a pencil torch is to be placed from the other side of the swelling, i.e. at the horizontal plane and see the red glow through the roll if red glow is there this is called transillumination positive.

My patient, Dindayal a 28 years old unmarried male, Army soldier presented with complain of:

- Swelling in the left side of scrotum for last 3 year
- Pain in the swelling for last 6/7 months

The left sided scrotal swelling started 3 years back and gradually increasing in size from bottom of the scrotum to root of the scrotum.

The swelling is reduced or less prominent on lying down and becomes prominent on standing or walking.

Initially, the swelling was painless but for last 6/7 months he complains dragging pain in the affected side. The pain is slightly more in the evening.

But there is no history of constipation (10 added pelvic colon may cause varicocele) no history of urinary problem like hematuria, etc. (to exclude renal cell carcinoma which causes varicocele).

On examination: General survey is essentially normal local examination - left testis lying at lower level than the right, multiple dilated veins are seen in the left side of the scrotum. When the patient lies down or the scrotum is elevated the swelling reduces in size. On standing the swelling reappears and fills up from the bottom of the scrotum.

- No expansile cough impulse is seen
- The swelling becomes more prominent on Valsalva maneuver.

On palpation: The mass of scrotum is felt like a bag of worms from bottom of scrotum to the level of superficial inguinal ring.

- No expansile cough impulse is felt but the swelling gives a fluid thrill like impulse
- Testicular volume is less
- Fluctuation and trans illumination negative.

Bow sign positive: The mass is held between the fingers and the thumb and patient is asked to bow down the tension within the dilated veins will be less and the size of the swelling will be reduced.

Abdominal examination reveals no lump in the abdomen. No loaded pelvic colon found.

So this is a case of left sided varicocele.

What could be the other possibilities?

Sir, from history and clinical examination I feel it is nothing but a varicocele but I will keep the differential diagnosis like:

- Inguinal hernia
- Lymph varix
- Congenital hydrocele
- Epididymal cyst, etc.

Differential Diagnoses

Inguinal Hernia

- Expansile cough impulse both visible and palpable
- Reducible unless complicated and when the swelling appears on standing it fill up from above downwards
- Reduction occurs abruptly not at all so slowly like varicoses during reduction there may be gurgling sounds (enterocele or the sac feels doughy (omentocele).

Lymph varix

- History filariasis
- Feels soft and doughy
- On lying it reduces very slowly than varicocele.

Congenital Hydrocele

- Swelling usually present since birth
- Testis cannot be felt separately from the swelling
- Cystic swelling fluctuation positive
- Cough impulse present
- Reducible partly on lying down and partly on gently pressure
- Transillumination—positive

Epididymal Cyst

- Usually found during middle life
- Very slow growing swelling usually above and behind the testis. The testis can be distinctly felt apart from the swelling
- Swelling feels like branch of tine grapes
- Fluctuation the transillumination
- Positive but is finely tessellated giving Chinese lantern or marble floor appearance.

How will you differentiate between primary and secondary varicocele?

In primary, i.e. idiopathic varicocele, on elevation of scrotum (while patient is lying down) varicocele disappears as the veins will be emptied by the gravity.

But in secondary varicocele, the varicocele will remain same as some secondary cause is there like renal lump causing obstruction of testicular venous drainage.

What is Bow sign?

The mass of varicocele is held between the fingers and the thumb and the patient is asked to bow down.

The tension within the venous plexus will be less and size of varicocele will be reduced in size because bowing will cut off the continuity of the blood inside the varicocele mass with the testicular vein.

OK, how will you proceed in this case?

Sir, basically it is a clinical diagnosis. But if there is any doubt. USG scrotum and abdomen color Doppler study is helpful for diagnosis of varicocele.

USG—Testicular volume to be measured
- To exclude any renal lump, etc.
- Semen analysis to be carried out.

Why testicular volume is measured in varicocele?

Testicular volume is measured because one of the important effect of varicocele is loss of testicular volume which may lead to male infertility, particularly in Bilateral varicocele. Oligospermia is very common with this case.

Next what will you do?

Sir, I will grade the varicocele for further management.

What are the different grades of varicocele?

- Grades of varicocele are based on physical findings
- Grade I—small varicocele which becomes prominent and palpable only on Valsalva maneuver
- Grade II—size is moderate and easily palpable
- Grade III—large varicocele, visible prominently
- Grade IV—severely tortuous

What is the plan of management of your patient?

Sir, my patient has grade III varicocele loss of testicular volume and patients is symptomatic, having dragging pain.

So I will choose surgery for this patient.

What surgery will you like to do?

I will do high ligation of testicular vein through inguinal approach.

What will you do through inguinal approach?

I will,
- Open the inguinal canal through inguinal incision like a case of hernia
- Spermatic cord is delivered, coverings are incised
- The vas deferens with its supplying vessels are separated.
- Testicular artery is identified and separated—two pairs of clamps applied proximally and distally at a gap of 5 cm and the intervening segment of veins are excised.
- This removes the main mass and also shorten the spermatic cord.

Why high ligation of testicular vein is required?

Sir, the aim of this operation is to reduce to a minimum the number of veins in the pampean form plexus.

At the level of deep inguinal ring the testicular veins only two in number so this is the right place to ligate the veins.

What are the advantages and disadvantages of the inguinal approach?

Advantages: Easy approach to occlude most of the dilated veins. Shortening of the cord brings back the testis to a higher level
Disadvantages: Chance of damage to the testicular artery, cremasteric artery, etc.

What happens if testicular artery is ligated by mistake during the procedure?

If the testicular artery is ligated by mistake testis can still survive as artery to vas and artery to cremaster will supply the testis.

But the chance of testicular atrophy is as high as 50%. Commonly testicular atrophy occurs 20-30%.

What is Palmo operation in varicocele?

Palmo operation is for high ligation of testicular vein.
- A small oblique incision is made 3 cm above the level of deep ring

- Splitting of parietal muscles is done in gridiron manner
- Extra peritoneal fat and peritoneum are swept medially upwards
- The testicular vessels are seen on the posterior abdominal wall lateral to - external iliac artery
- The testicular vein is identified, separated, ligated and divided.

What are the advantages and disadvantages of Palmo's method?

Advantages

- Less chance of testicular artery injury
- Venous drainage of testis is maintained as cremasteric vein anastomoses with testicular vein.
- Relative by simple and can be done under local anaesthesia

Disadvantage

It may aggravates varicocele in about 10% cases.

Is there any other approach for varicocele?

Sir, Scrotal approach is there where through the scrotal incision the varicose veins are exposed right down to the level of testis

Most of the tortuous and varicose veins are divided and ligated individually keeping behind few veins for venous drainage of testis.

What are the advantages and disadvantages of this procedure?

Advantages

Easy approach, Local anesthesia is adequate

Disadvantages

- Separation of individual veins at the level of testis are very difficult where a free anastomosis exists.
- Chance of bleeding and damage to testicular artery is high.

What is the role of laparoscopy in the case of varicocele?

In present days, laparoscopic approach became popular for this operation also.

Ligation of testicular vein in the retroperitoneum by laparoscopy through transperitoneal approach. In laparoscopic approach what is the landmark for varicocele.

'Triangle of Doom' is the landmark in laparoscopic approach for varicocele as well as hernia.

The triangle is bounded:
- Medially by the vas deferens
- Laterally testicular vessels
- Above the joining of these two structures
  The external Iliac vessels are the content of this triangle.

What are the complications of varicocele surgery?

Complications are:
- Testicular artery injury which may lead to testicular atrophy
- Secondary hydrocele formation, which is mainly due to lymphatic obstruction
- Chance of recurrence of varicocele.

How surgery is beneficial for this patient of varicocele?

i. Patient will be symptomless. Cosmetically, it appears better
ii. Testicular volume may be returned to normal and normal function of testis is regained.

In all cases varicocele should be operated?

Not in all like if the patient is asymptomatic and small varicocele (grade I) is there surgery is not required in such a case but the indications for surgery are
i. Grade II, III and or symptomatic varicocele
ii. Testicular volume is less in compare to normal site history of sub fertility or infertility
iii. For recruitment problem
iv. Cosmetic purpose and ofcourse patient's choice

SHORT NOTES ON VARICOCELE

- **Definition**: Varicocele is a condition of dilation, elongation and tortuosity of the veins of pampiniform venous plexus.

  Varicocele may present only cremasteric veins which anastomose freely with the testicular veins.
- Surgical anatomy of pampiniform plexus:

  Pampiniform plexus is nothing but a bunch of veins which forms the main bulk of the spermatic cord. Pampiniform plexus consists of thee groups of veins

  i.   Veins from the testis and epididymis
  ii. Veins of vas deferens
  iii. Veins of cremaster muscle

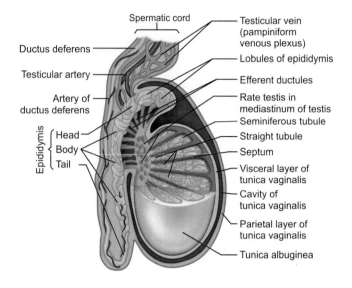

Struture of tests

Anastomosing of these groups of veins forms the plexus of veins at the upper pole of testis which are about 15-25 in numbers.

↓

As the plexus ascends the number is reduced to 12-15

↓

At the level of superficial ring the number comes down to 1 as they join together

↓

At the level of deep ring the veins further joint to form 2 veins only

↓

These veins enter the abdomen and unite at various level to form testicular vein

↓

The left testicular vein drains in the left renal vein at right angle and the right testicular vein drains in the inferior vena cava at an acute angle

Surgical physiology

The pampiniform plexus around the testicular artery. Serves as a heat exchanger mechanism, constituting a counter current system to reduce scrotal temperature 2.5° C lower than core temp to keep the testicle cool and it plays an important role in spermatogenesis

Types of Varicocele

i. Primary or idiopathic (90%) where no definite cause has been found.

   Usually it occurs in young unmarried men and it is due to chronic venous congestion as a result of unrelieved sexual stimulation.

ii. Secondary: The formation of varicocele is due to some specific reasons like Renal cell carcinoma, loaded pelvic colon, etc. which obstruct testicular vein.

Etiology: 90% cases no specific aetiology is found called idiopathic

1. Age : Varicocele is mostly seen in teen aged and early twenty. Tall thin men 10 to 25 years are frequently

2. There may be absence or incompetent terminal testicular vulvae causing varicocele.

3. Left side is most commonly affected (95%) for the following

   i.   The left testicular vein is longer than the right as left testis lies at lower level

   ii. Left testicular vein joins the left renal vein at right angle but right testicular vein drains the inferior vena cava at acute angle. So left testicular vein has 8-10 cm greater pressure than the right

   iii. Left testicular vein is more likely to be compressed by loaded pelvic colon as it ascends behind the left sided colon

   iv. There is a sandwich effect of left renal vein in between abdominal aorta and trunk of superior mesenteric artery therefore it hinders the venous return of the left renal vein leading to varicocele

   v.   Left testicular artery may arch over the left renal vein and may compress it, leading to varicocele (16-20% cases)

vi. The close association between entry of left supra renal vein and the left testicular vein in the left renal vein. So the circulating adrenaline is responsible to constrict the testicular vein - increase pressure leads to varicocele

vii. Tumour infiltration from renal carcinoma along the left renal vein thus may cause obstruction to left testicular vein.

Effects of Varicocele on the Testis

Effects of varicocele are variable on testis depending on the severity (grades) of the varicocele. The net result is male infertility or subfertility due to its adverse effects on spermatogenesis.

The testicular abnormalities are may be due to:

- Hyperthermia—presence of varicocele hampers the counter current heat exchange mechanism which keeps the test is cool, causing increased scrotal temperature which inhibits spermatogenesis.

- Reduction of testicular volume as a result of varicocele testicular volume is reduced thereby sperm production will be less or grossly reduced leading to subfertility.
- Intratesticular hyperperfusion injury abnormally elevated micro vascular blood flow causing increased intratesticular temperature, increases metabolic activity, depletion of glycogen storage and parenchymal injury.
- Leydig cells dysfunction reduces intratesticular testosterone formation
- Due to unknown reasons unilateral varicocele may cause decreased spermatogenesis, maturation arrest. Leading to subfertility or infertility (Correctable infertility).

Role of Conservative Treatment in Varicocele

- Re assurance
- Scrotal support/front underwear may relieve discomfort
- This is applicable when the discomfort is not constant. Grade I or II varicocele, etc.

My patient, Ram Lal, a 60 years old Hindu male, presented with ulcerative growth at his glans penis for last 1 year.

The lesion started as a small ulcer 12 months back and it is gradually and painlessly progressive and attained its present size and occupying almost whole of his glans penis. He is unable to retract his foreskin beyond corona and having burning/itching sensation under surface of his fore skin.

[Keep the following history in mind but do not tell the negative history to the examiner (Except very important relevant negative history) while you are presenting the short case.

Take history of discharge/bleeding from the ulcer, history of trauma, exposure, urinary retention, difficulty in passing urine (involvement of urethra) history of swelling in the groin (lymph nodes involvement), history of cough, hemoptysis, bone pain, etc. to exclude metastasis].

On Examination

- General Survey is essentially normal except patient having pallor.
- Local examination reveals there is an ulceroproliferative growth involving almost whole of the glans penis but not the prepuce.

    The ulcerative mass has irregular margin, everted and rolled out edge, floor is full of necrotic tissue, base is indurated, bleeds on touch.

    The mass is tender on palpation. Firm in consistency shaft of penis is normal. No bilateral inguinal lymphodenopathy noticed.
- Systemic examination is essentially normal.

So what is your diagnosis?

Sir,

This is a case of carcinoma penis

Most probably squamous cell carcinoma without inguinal lymph nodes metastasis.

Why do you think, this is Carcinoma?

An elderly Hindu patient. Presenting with ulceroproliferative growth which bleeds on touch.

Why are you mentioning Hindu male repeatedly?

Sir,

In Muslim and Jews carcinoma penis is rare as they undergo, circumcision as per the religious norms which prevent to develop carcinoma penis as no smegma can accumulate there.

But in Hindu there is no such norms thereby they are more prone to develop carcinoma.

Anyhow, do you think any other diagnosis?

Sir, I think it is a case of Carcinoma penis but I will keep in mind

i. Giant Condyloma Acuminata (Cauliflower like lesion, arising from prepuce or glans. The cause is human Papilloma virus—The lesion may be difficult to distinguish from well differentiated squamous cell carcinoma.)

ii. Buschke Lowenstein tumor:
   - Uncommon tumor
   - Biological pattern of a verrucous carcinoma.
   - Locally destructive and invasive
   - Usually inguinal lymph nodes not involved]

i. Balanitis Xerotica Obliterance:
   - Whitish patch originating on the prepuce or glans.
   - Usually involving meatus.
   - Middle aged, diabetic patients are more prone to be affected.

How will you proceed in this case?

Sir, I will confirm my diagnosis first.

I will do incisional biopsy taking both from growth and the adjacent normal looking area of the penis to prove the diagnosis.

Suppose the HPE (His to pathological examination) report comes as carcinoma—then how will you proceed?

Sir, I will do other investigations to stage the disease.

I will do USG/CECT abdomen, pelvis and inguinal region to detect lymph nodes if any.

I will do all base line investigations to make the patient fit for anaesthesia.

In this case what will you plan for the treatment?

Here I will do partial amputation of penis where I will keep the proximal line of resection 2 cm away from the proximal margin of the growth.

Suppose the HPE report reveals it is an anaplastic variety of carcinoma what will you do?

Sir, as anaplastic variety has poor prognosis and rapidly progressive I will prefer to offer total amputation with Bilateral orchidectomy.

Why Bilateral orchidectomy?

Sir, the patient will have sexual desire if both testes are kept and that may lead to psychosexual disorder.

No 2. total penectomy patient will have perineal urethrostomy.

So patient will have problem during micturition as both be testes will over hang on the passage So Bilateral orchidectomy is required.

Suppose this patient presented with inguinal lymph node —how will you manage?

Inguinal lymph nodes along with carcinoma penis may be infected (50% cases) or it may be metastatic.

So I will give a course of antibiotics (Doxycyclin 100 mg twice daily for 2-3 weeks)

If the nodes are persistent: I will do FNAC.

If FNAC +ve: I will do inguinopelvic lymph node dissection on the involved site and superficial inguinal lymph node dissection on the other site.

Why will you dissect pelvic lymph nodes?

Sir,
- The penile metastasis spreads on a sequential manner
  - Superficial inguinal lymph nodes
  - Deep inguinal lymph nodes, next
  - Pelvic lymph nodes.

So,

When there are multiple inguinal lymph nodes are involved. Pelvic lymph nodes are likely to be involved, and pelvic lymph nodes involvement is an important prognostic factor. Adjuvant chemotherapy to be given for better survival.

Can you tell me the boundary of inguinal pelvic dissection?

Yes sir,
- In pelvic dissection above up to the bifurcation of common Iliac artery
- Below inguinal ligament
- Laterally genetofemoral nerve and
- Medially obturator nerve.
- In inguinal dissection at femoral triangle.

Base inguinal ligament:
- Apex—the triangle is continuous with the inter muscular space, adductor canal.
- Lateral border—by the medial edge of sartorius muscle
- Medial border - by the medial edge of adductor longus muscle
- Lymph nodes also to be removed from the femoral vessels adventitia.
- The anterior wall is formed by the fascia lata and the superficial fascia of the thigh containing the superficial inguinal lymph nodes.

How will you reconstruct the rare area?

If the inguinal lymph nodes are fixed how will you manage?
- Fixed inguinal lymph nodes suggestive of advanced disease, there by inoperable.
- Chemo and or radiotherapy may make the fixed lymph nodes mobile.
- Inguinal pelvic dissection may be considered for better survival.
- If it is still fixed palliative Radio/chemo therapy is the option.

What's all are the indications for radiotherapy in primary lesion in a case of carcinoma penis?
- Smell lesion usually < 1 cm
- Young patient with small lesion.
- Superficial lesion confined to glans.
- Palliative RT in advanced inoperable disease.
- Patients choice as alternative to surgery.

Can you tell me the premalignant conditions of penis?
- Leukoplakia of glans penis.
- Long standing genital warts (condyloma acuminata)

- Balanitis Xerotica obliterans
- Paget's disease of penis (Erythroplasia of Queyrat)
- Bowen disease (squamous cell carcinoma *in situ*)

How malignancy develops in penis?

Two important contributing factors to increase the incidence of carcinoma penis are

i. **Phimosis:** Either primary or secondary - or due to poor penile hygiene accumulated smegma (desquamated epithelium produced by Mycobacterium smegmatis) has been implicated as carcinogenic agent and one of the important etiological factors to develop carcinoma penis.

ii. **Chronic balanoposthitis:** It is also associated with higher incidence of carcinoma penis.

Do you know other than Ca penis what are the diseases where sentinel lymph node biopsy are usually offered?

Sir, Cabana described sentinel LN biopsy initially for Carcinoma penis.

But it is being followed to treat sentinel node in, carcinoma breast and malignant melanoma too.

What is to do for sentinel lymph node biopsy?

Sentinel lymph node (the first draining LN from the tumor) mapping and biopsy being done in number of ways

i. Isosulfan blue, the dye is injected into the lesion in the penis 2 to 3 hours before surgery and on inguinal explorations sentinel lymph node is identified by this bluish coloration.

ii. **Radioactive:** Sulphur colloid is injected into the lesion and detected by Gamma probe.

Suppose the sentinel lymph node is detected what will you do next?

If sentinel lymph node is positive, an inguinal pelvic lymph node dissection is to carry out along with the primary surgery.

Is there any role of chemotherapy in carcinoma penis?

To tell the truth, systemic chemotherapy has got limited role in carcinoma penis. In advanced disease chemotherapy is used as a combination therapy for palliative procedure. The agents used are, bleomycin, methotrexate, cisplatin and 5 FU, etc.

What are the treatment options in carcinoma penis?

i. Carcinoma *in situ*—Application of 5 fluorouracil cream
Or
Neodymium : YAG laser treatment is effective.

ii. For lesion, involving the prepuce: Simple circumcision is effective.

iii. For lesions involving the glans or distal shaft, partial penectomy with 2 cm margin to decrease the local recurrence.

iv. For lesions involving the proximal shaft or when partial penectomy results in a penile stump of insufficient length for sexual function or directing the urinary stream. Total penectomy with perineal urethrostomy has been recommended.

v. Less aggressive surgical resections, such as Moh's micrographic surgery and local excision directed at penile preservation are the current practice.

What are the other penile tumor?

- Squamous cell CA 98%
- Other 2% includes:
  - Melanoma
  - Basal cell carcinoma
  - Paget's disease, etc.

What important things to study in this case?

- Anatomy of penis
  - Cut section of penis
  - Artery supply and venous drainage.
  - Lymphatic drainage, etc.

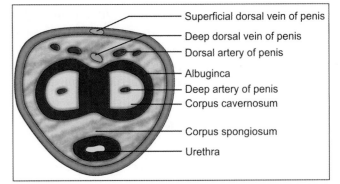

Anatomy of penis on cross section

SHORT NOTE ON CARCINOMA PENIS

INTRODUCTION

Penile malignancies are uncommon, but, when they are diagnosed, they are psychologically devastating to the patient because of its physical and psychological consequences. Benign, premalignant, and malignant conditions must be distinguished from each other. Malignancies are usually squamous cell carcinomas and behave similarly to those occurring elsewhere on the skin.

Epidemiology

Penile carcinoma is rare is men in the USA and Europe, and accounts for 0.4-0.6% of all malignant diseases in men in these regions but can constitute up to 10% of malignant diseases in men in African, South American and South Asian countries.

In India the incidence varies from .7 to 3 per lakh population forming 6% of all malignant diseases in men. It is a disease of older men but the tumor is not unusual in younger men. The disease has also been reported in children.

Causes and Risk Factors

1. **Poor penile hygiene:** Smegma has been implicated as the carcinogenic agent, and although definite evidence has not been established, its association with development of penile cancer has been widely observed.
2. **Phimosis:** Present in 25-75% of patients with penile carcinoma. Circumcision protects against penile carcinoma as evidenced in Jews where carcinoma of the penis is almost nonexistent. Adult and pubertal circumcision though confers no protective effect.
3. **Viral infection:** Associated with sexually transmitted human papilloma virus (HPV), which is present in 15-80% of patients with penile carcinoma, and in 70-100% of biopsy samples of penile intraepithelial neoplasm.
4. **Ultra violet radiation:** Patients with psoriasis who have been given oral 8-methoxypsoralen and ultraviolet. A photochemotherapy (PUVA) have a 286 times higher risk of developing penile and scrotal carcinoma compared with those who do not have this disorder.
5. **Balanitis xerotica obliterans (BXO):** The male genital variant of lichen sclerosus et atrophicus was associated with penile carcinoma in 2.3% of 522 patients.
6. **Premalignant lesions:** Cutaneous horn, pseudoepitheliomatous keratotic and micaceous balanitis, BXO, giant condyloma, and bowenoid papulosis have potential to evolve into cancers. Penile intraepithelial neoplasia is thought to be a precursor of squamous cell carcinoma, but only a small proportion (5-15%) develops into invasive squamous cell carcinoma. Carcinoma in situ of the penis is referred to as erythroplasia of Queyrat when occurring on the glans and Bowen's disease when it involves the follicle-bearing skin of the penile shaft.

Clinical presentation

Penile carcinoma can present as a subtle induration, a small excrescence, a small papule, pustule, or warty growth to an obvious extensive carcinoma with sloughing. The earliest symptoms of penile cancer include itching or burning under the foreskin and ulceration of the glans or prepuce progressing along the penile shaft and involving corpora cavernous. It can also present with bleeding, urinary fistula, or urinary retention. Occasionally, the primary lesion remains concealed in the phimotic sac and inguinal lymph-node metastasis is the initial complaint. Constitutional symptoms like weakness, weight loss, fatigue, and systemic malaise occur secondary to chronic suppuration.

Tumors can originate anywhere on the penis but are most commonly found on the glans (48%) and prepuce (21%) glans and prepuce (9%), coronal sulcus in (6%), and the shaft (<2%)(8). Inguinal lymphadenopathy can be palpated at diagnosis in 20-96% of patients. Of these, 45% will have cancer within the nodes. Distant metastases (1-10%) are unusual in the absence of regional nodal metastasis.

The growth rates of the papillary and ulcerative lesions are similar, but the flat ulcerative lesions have a tendency to metastasize to the lymph nodes earlier and therefore, are associated with a lower 5 year survival rate. Cancers larger than 5 cm and those involving more than 75% of the shaft are associated with a high prevalence of nodal metastases and a lower survival rate.

Starting treatment is delayed for longer than 1 year in 15-50% patients as a result of fear, embarrassment, ignorance, and personal neglect. Without treatment, patients with penile carcinoma usually die within 2 years.

Diagnosis

Incisional biopsy samples should be obtained from the periphery of the lesion, so that healthy tissue is included. Most penile cancers are squamous cell carcinomas that demonstrate squamous cell carcinomas that demonstrate keratinization, epithelial pearl formation, and various degrees of mitotic activity. The normal rete pegs are disrupted, and invasive lesions penetrate the basement membrane and surrounding structures Fine-needle aspiration cytology is useful only to assess suspicious nodes and does not have much use in diagnosis of the primary penile carcinoma. However, clinical suspicion of metastasis should override a negative result on FNAC.

Imaging: Sonography measures penile involvement more accurately than clinical examination, which usually overestimates the extent of tumor enabling better salvage of penile length during surgery, and results that are cosmetically and functionally better than those obtained with other techniques. It is useful in detecting whether the femoral vessels are involved and nodal disease is resectable in patients with large bulky lymph nodes and also be used to assess iliac, pelvic, and para- aortic lymphadenopathy. CT scanning can be used in patients with advanced nodal disease to investigate vascular involvement and identify enlarged retroperitoneal lymph nodes.

General evaluation: Which includes a CBC count; a chemistry panel with liver function tests; and an assessment of cardiac, pulmonary, and renal status, is helpful as a base line and to detect any unsuspected problems. Patients with advanced disease may be anemic, with leukocytosis and hypoalbuminemia. Hypercalcemia has been found in some patients in the absence of metastases.

Differential diagnosis

Penile lesions can be categorized as benign, premalignant, and malignant neoplasm.

Benign lesions include pearly penile papules, papillomas, and coronal papillae.

Premalignant conditions can be BXO, leukoplakia, and viral lesions like condyloma acuminata.

Kaposi sarcoma manifests as a cutaneous neovascular lesion that is raised, usually painful, and often ulcerated with a bluish discoloration Giant condyloma acuminate or a Buschke-Lowenstein tumor differs from the standard condyloma in that it displaces, invades, and destroys adjacent structures by compression.

Malignant carcinoma includes variants of squamous cell carcinoma such as CIS, erythroplasia of Queyrat, or Bowen disease. Erythroplasia involves the glans, prepuce, or penile shaft, while similar lesions on the remainder of the genitalia and perineum are termed Bowen disease.

Staging: The Jackson and TNM systems are used, although the TNM system is preferable. In the Jackson system, characteristics of the primary lesion, such as size and confinement to the epidermis (superficial or invasive), are not used and also the presence and extent of nodal metastases is not addressed.

The Jackson Classification

Stage 1 (A)	:	The tumor is confined to the glans, prepuce, or both.
Stage II (B)	:	The tumor extends onto the shaft of the penis.
Stage III (C)	:	The tumor has inguinal metastasis that is operable.
Stage IV (D)	:	The tumor involves adjacent structures and is associated with inoperable inguinal metastasis or distant metastasis.

UICC-TNM Classification 2002 (11)

Primary Tumor

TX	:	Primary tumor cannot be assessed.
T0	:	Primary tumor is not evident.
Tis	:	Carcinoma in situ.
Ta	:	Noninvasive verrucous carcinoma.
T1	:	Tumor invades subepithelial connective tissue.
T2	:	Tumour invades corpora spongiosum or cavernosum.
T3	:	Tumour invades the urethra or prostate.
T4	:	Tumour invades other adjacent structures.

Regional Lymph Nodes

Nx	:	Regional lymph nodes cannot be assessed.
N0	:	No regional lymph node metastases.
N1	:	Metastasis to a single superficial inguinal lymph node.
N2	:	Metastasis to two or more superficial inguinal lymph nodes on the same side or on both sides of the body.
N3	:	Metastasis to lymph nodes deep within the groin or pelvis on either one or both sides of the body.

Metastasis

Mx	:	Presence of distant metastases cannot be assessed.
Mo	:	no distant metastasis.
M1	:	Distant metastasis has occurred.

Treatment

The aim of treatment being to completely remove the primary tumor , aggressive local therapy can provide good quality of life, long term palliation, and survival even in patients with advanced disease. Partial or total penectomy is the gold standard of therapy. Recently efforts have been made towards organ sparing techniques such as partial organ sparing techniques such as partial excision. Moh's microsurgery and non-surgical techniques with radiotherapy, lasers, or cryotherapy.

Surgery: Partial penectomy with a 2 cm tumor free margin is done for tumors involving the prepuce, glans, and distal shaft, leaving a stump which permits erect voiding and sexual function. A margin of 1 cm for grade 1 and 2 tumors and 1.5 cm for grade 3 tumors has also been found to be adequate. Local recurrence ranges from 0% to 7% which are managed by total penectomy. In most prepucial lesions, circumcision, along is not effective in tumor control and recurrence after circumcision is common (32-50%). In the absence of inguinal nodes 5 years survival is 80%. In cases where a 2 cm margin cannot be achieved, total penectomy is done with a perineal urethrostomy. A total penectomy and scrotectomy with Bilateral orchidectomy is done when the scrotum is involved. Treatment of advanced disease involving public bone of this nature is pubic by primary chemotherapy followed by radical locoregional treatment in responsive cases.

Moh's Micrographic Surgery (MMS) is a penile tissue sparing technique which employs removal of diseased tissue in thin layers, accurate reconstruction and mapping of excised tissue and confirmation of negative margins by frozen section. This procedure allows preservation of maximum normal penile tissue and is best suited for small lesions involving the distal portion of the glans.

Penile Conservative therapy (PCT): Various conservative treatment modalities including conventional and micrographic surgery, laser and radiotherapy have been tried to preserve maximum functioning phallus in selected patients with early cancers. Penile control rate is in the range of 80 to 90% even in appropriately selected cases. These patients require regular follow up and failures can be salvaged with a penectomy.

Laser surgery: Laser therapy has been used to treat premalignant and small invasive lesions. It should be used judiciously to achieve local control rates comparable with more radical procedures.

Radiation therapy: External beam radiotherapy (EBRT) using megavoltage telecobalt gamma rays or 6 MV photons from linear accelerators or interstitial implantation has been used depending on the tumor location, thickness and proximity to the urethra. Doses ranging from 45-60 Gy are delivered in 30 fractions over 3-8 weeks. Local control rates of about 80% can be achieved by external beam radiation for small, microinvasive lesions (stage T1, T2).

Management of Inguinal Lymphadenopathy

Lymphadenectomy is node positive disease results in 20-50%. 5 year disease free survival. However not all enlarged nodes are metastatic nodes.

In T1-T2 lesions if the nodes are enlarged at presentation, a course of antibiotics should be given with the intention that inflammatory charges will resolve. They are reassessed after four to six weeks. All patients with persistent inguinal lymph nodes, with proven metastasis, or who develop lymphadenopathy should undergo lymphadenectomy. Lymphadenectomy with two or fewer positive lymph nodes has a 5-year survival of 82-88%, compared with 7-50% survival when more than two lymph nodes are positive.

In patients with clinically negative nodes the following is recommended:

In T1 and T2 disease, although the incidence of false negative nodes is 15 to 20 %, metachronous node metastasis after adequate treatment of the primary lesion occurs is only 5 to 11% of patients. These patients are offered close surveillance every 2-3 months for the first years and appearance of nodes should be treated with lymphadenectomy after histological confirmation. Poorly differentiated tumors may be considered for early prophylactic lymphadenectomy.

In patients with T3 and T4 tumors, the incidence of occult nodal metastases in clinically negative nodes increases to as high as 65% of cases. In these, a prophylactic lymphadenectomy is advocated not withstanding the morbidity of the surgery.

Extent of lymphadenectomy

Whether the palpable nodes are unilateral or Bilateral, it is advocated that a Bilateral lymphadenectomy be done due to the fact that 50% of the lymphatics have cross over drainage.

In patients who develop unilateral nodes while on surveillance it may be adequate to perform unilateral lymphadenectomy especially if the metastasis free interval is more than 1 year. Lymphadenectomy is associated with substantial morbidity (24-87%), postoperative wound infection (3-70%), skin necrosis (8-60%), subcutaneous seroma (9-87%) and lower limb lymphoedema (27-100%). It carried a mortality of up to 3%.

Cabanas described sentinel lymph node biopsy on the basis of lymphangiography and labelled the lymph node close to the superficial epigastric vein as the sentinel lymph node. He recommended biopsy of this node and inguinal node dissection that was restricted to the involved side. However, others have reported a high false negative rate and later development of advanced nodal disease.

Positive pelvic lymph nodes are present in 20-30% of patients with involved inguinal lymph nodes and have a poor prognosis. The presence of large nodes (more than > 2 cm) and fixation or ulceration of inguinal nodes increases the risk of pelvic node involvement. Iliac lymph node dissection should be offered to patients with clinically or radiologically positive iliac nodes; those with multiple, positive, large, fixed or ulcerated inguinal lymph nodes; and to young patients and low surgical risk patients.

Patients with fungating nodes can be treated by lymphadenectomy followed by reconstruction with tensor fascia lata myocutaneous or anterolateral thigh flap. Routine use of myocutaneous flaps results in nearly 100% wound healing and shortened hospital stay.

There seems to be no role of primary radiation therapy in patients with confirmed lymph node metastasis. The 5 year survival with primary irradiation is half (25%); that of surgery (50%).

Chemotherapy

Neoadjuvant chemotherapy in advanced disease may make the tumor resectable in 50% of patients. However, no randomized clinical trials have been done to assess the benefit of chemotherapy in either the adjuvant or neoadjuvant situation.

Prevention

Despite the fact that many cases of penile squamous cell cancer can be either prevented or at lease diagnosed early enough to avoid invasion, most patients present with advanced stages of disease. Ignorance regarding penile hygiene, and cultural, educational, and professional factors cause long delays in diagnosis and treatment. A vigilant diagnostic approach including histopathological assessment in patients who have an uncertain diagnosis is important to detect premalignant lesions.

My patient, Ram Vilas, a 45 years old, fisherman (expose to sun rays) resident of Bihar presented with complain of an ulcerative lesion at right nasolabial fold for last 1 year.

Initially approximate 14 months back a firm papule appeared (flat or slightly raised plaque or dark cystic swelling also may appear initially) at the site, gradually the growth became an ulcer for last 1 year. It is slowly progressive and extended right infra orbital region.

On Examination: General survey is essentially normal.

The ulcer is at right side of nasolabial fold extended towards infra orbital region and 1 cm short to lower eyelid - shape is irregular.
- The margins are irregular.
- The ulcer edge is raised and beaded.
- The floor-central part is covered with scab - peripheral part of the scab is dry - Nontender
- Base of the uncer is indurated slightly but not fixed to the underlying structure
- No lymphadenopathy noticed in neck.

So this a case of skin cancer most probably basal cell carcinoma at right side of face.

Why do say it is a basal cell Carcinoma?

- My patient is an elderly (male exposure to sunray)
- Fisherman in occupation regularly)
- Typical site of involvement i.e. above the line going angel of mouth and ear lobule typical progression of ulcer from a firm papule
- The edge of uncer is raised and beaded
- The floor is covered with a scab
- No regional lymph nodes in the neck are not palpable. and it is the commonest malignant skin tumour.

Where from the basal cell carcinoma arises?

- Basal cell carcinoma arises from basal cells of the epidermis of skin.

- It may also arise from adnexal basal layer of hair follicles, sweat glands, sebaceous glands, etc.

Why basal cell carcinoma is called rodent ulcer?

Basal Cell Carcinoma erodes deeply into the local tissues and causing extensive local destruction, i.e., it burrows deep like a rat so it is called Rodent Ulcer.

Why basal cell carcinoma is also called 'Field Fire' cancer?

Sometimes in basal cell carcinoma ulcer tends to heal at one area white breaking out in the adjacent area like 'field fire'. Here ulcer spreads centrifugally.

(it is also called 'Tear Cancer' because it seen commonly in the area where tears roll down.)

What are the predisposing factors causing basal cell carcinoma?

- Late middle life above the age of 40 years
- Male > Female
- It is more common in white skin people and where exposure to UV light is more like people in Australia.
- Occupation factors like it is more prone to develop in agriculture workers, fishermen, dedicated sunbathers etc.
- Chronic exposure to arsenic may develop multiple Basal Cell Carcinomas.

What are the common sites of basal cell carcinoma?

i. Most common site is face above the imaginary line joining angle of mouth and the carlobute. Approximately 9.3% basal cell carcinoma occurs in the region like
   - Inner and outer canthus of the orbit
   - Nose, nasolabial fold, check, forehead.
ii. Other sites are neck, scalp, trunk, extremities even in perianal region etc.

What are the types of basal cell carcinoma?

The common types are:
- Nodular,
- Ulcerative,

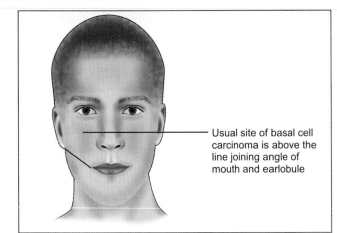

Usual site of basal cell carcinoma is above the line joining angle of mouth and earlobule

Site of Basal cell carcinoma

- Noduloulcerative,
- Cystic
- Pigmented basal cell carcinoma
- Basosquamous type - behaves more like SCC and spreads to lymph nodes.
  Noduloulcerative is the commonest type around 70%.

How will you manage this case?

Sir, I will confirm my diagnosis first.

I will do:

Edge biopsy to see the closely packed islands of uniform basophilic epithelial cells containing a large basophilic nucleus and absent of prickles cells and epithelial pearls are the characteristics of basal cell carcinoma.

  i. X-Ray of face to exclude involvement of surrounding bone.

Suppose this is basal cell carcinoma and bone is not involved, what will do?

Sir, I will do all base line investigations to make the patient fit for surgery and anesthesia and

I will do wide local excision keeping 1 cm can healthy margin all around. In this case as the upper margin is nearer to lower eyelid I will take 0.5 cm, upper margin to save the eye and I will reconstruct the raw area with advancement flap from right sided cheek.

Basal cell carcinoma is radiosensitive why will you not offer radiotherapy to this patient?

The lesion is very close to eye, so radiotherapy cannot be given in this case to save the eye.

What are the other contraindications for radiotherapy?

- lesion adhered to bone or cartilage i.e., over nose, ear to avoid subsequent necrosis
- lesion very close to eye
- lesion on the back of the hand, and
- patient who are living in extreme cold area as the patient are more prone to have frost bite.

What are the indications for surgery?

- Where the radiotherapy is contraindicated as above
- Recurrence after radiotherapy
- Appearance of a new lesion closely adjacent to previously treated area.

What are the modern methods of surgery for Basal Cell Carcinoma?

- Laser surgery—Cryosurgery
- MOHS (Microscope Oriented Histographic Surgery) is useful in places where more tissue to be preserved by giving clearance of tumor free margin. Example in this patient where basal cell carcinoma is close to the eye.

What are the differential diagnosis of basal cell carcinoma?

Differential diagnoses are:
  i. Squamous cell carcinoma (described in SCC topic)
  ii. Melanoma (described in Melanoma topic)
  iii. Keratoacanthoma (described in SCC topic)

How does basal cell carcinoma spreads?

It is a locally invasive carcinoma. It spreads by direct infiltration. It directly spreads to superficial and deep structures (Cartilage, bone, etc.).

Lymph node metastasis usually very uncommon and blood spread is also very rare.

What are the more common sites for recurrence of treating basal cell carcinoma?

Basal cell carcinoma—at centre or more towards the center
- At postauricular region,
- Pinna, forehead are common sites for recurrence.

Know few words about
i. Basis squamous carcinoma
  - the name itself suggests histological features of squamous carcinomatous changes, are seen often at the edge of a basal cell carcinoma.

- Commonly occurs in area of current lesion or the skin destroyed by previous radiation.
- The lesion is friable, more necrotic, and edge of the lesion is mostly wet rather dry.
- Lymphatic metastasis is not very uncommon.
- Edge biopsy confirms the diagnosis.
- Treatment to be done as per the guidelines of SCC

ii. Turban tumor
- called cylindroma of scalp

- locally malignant and an uncommon tumor of the skin - arises from cutaneous nerves of the scalp. It may be multiple.
- grow for a long time (over the span of years) coalescing and involve the entire scalp gradually.
- looks like a wig or turban, hence the name
- scalp skin shows reddish, lobulated lesions with deep crevices.
- Management: Biopsy to confirm the diagnosis and wide local excision and SSG is the treatment.

SHORT NOTE ON BENIGN SKIN AND SUBCUTANEOUS TISSUE TUMOUR

- **TUMOR**: By definition tumor (Neoplasm) is a growth of New cells which proliferate independent of the Body need.
  - Benign tumors proliferate slowly with without evidence of mitosis whereas malignant tumors proliferate fast with evidence of mitosis and invasiveness.
- **LUMP:** Lump is a vague mass of the body which is a three dimensional structure i.e. a well defined growth of the tissue.
- **SWELLING:** Swelling is a vague term which denotes any enlargement or protuberance in the body tissue. It includes lump and tumour.

Tumour may be: (i) Inconsequential, (ii) traumatic, (iii) inflammatory, (iv) neoplastic and (v) miscellaneous like hamartoma

Sign of inflammations are: (i) color-temperature, (ii) dolor-pain, (iii) tumor swelling, (iv) rubor-redness, and (v) functio laesa-loss of function.

I will discuss, following most common and important benign swellings in this chapter:
  i. Dermoid cyst
  ii. Sebaceous cyst
  iii. Lipoma
  iv. Fibroma
  v. Hemangioma
  vi. Neurofibroma

Dermoid Cyst also called Epidermal Cyst.

Varieties
  i. Sequestration dermoid most common and a true variety of congenital dermoid cyst arising from primitive ectodermal cell,

ii. Implantation dermoid - and acquired cyst following a minor prick or trauma epidermis gets buried into subcutaneous tissue,

iii. Tubulodermoid and,

iv. Teratodermoid.

Sequestration dermoid - most common variety:

How to form: during embryonic fusion for ectodermal cells are sequestrated into the deeper layer (Mesoderm). These cells proliferate and liquefy to form dermoid cyst.

MODE OF SEQUESTRATION DERMOID FORMATION

Common Sites: are at the line if embryonic fusion like
  i.   at the midline of the body like root of nose, neck
  ii.   on the scalp (Pteryon and Asteryon) like postauricular dermoid, dermoid at forehead
  iii. at the inner or outer angle of the eye like external angular dermoid internal angular dermoid is near root of nose
  iv.   Sublingual Dermoid.

Pathology: This is a true cyst, lined by squamous epithelium with hair, hair follettetes, sweat and sebaceous glands.

Content is toothpaste like material with or without hair. The paste is a mixture of sebum, sweat and desquamated epithelial debris.

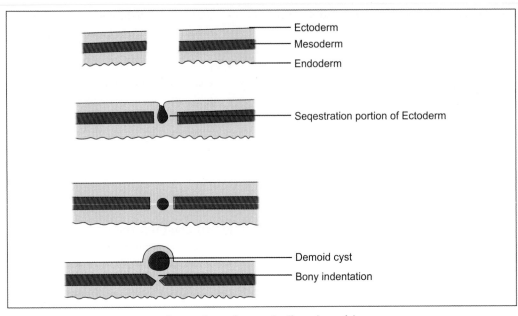

Formation of seqestration demoid

How to diagnosis:

a. From clinical features
   - common in 2nd and 3rd decade onwards
   - painless swelling at the line of embryonic fusion as mentioned above.

b. From Clinical Examination:
   - The swelling is usually 2-3 cm smooth, soft Cystic swelling, ovoid and spherical shaped
   - Fluctuation positive but trans illumination negative, not compressible
   - Skin is free from the tumor (Remember dermoid, derm free)
   - There may be resorption and bone indentation when dermoid is located in relation with bone. Which can be palpable at the base of the cyst.
   - The scalp dermoid only show impulse of coughing when it is partly intracranial and partly extra cranial or it may lie extra-cranially but it is attached to underlying dura by a pedicle or stalk.

c. **From investigations:**
   - X-ray of the part to exclude bone involvement
   - CT scan when intra cranial extension of the dermoid is suspected.

Treatment: Excision is the way - in scalp. If it is external excision is enough but if intracranial extension is there, formal neurosurgical approach is required by raising cranial osteocyte news flap. Rarely craniotomy to be done to excise the intra cranial Cyst.

Implantation Dermoid

- Also called post traumatic dermoid as it is observed common in fingers, toes and feet.
- Common in tailors, woman with habit of swing, gardeners
- Usually painless but may be painful.

Clinical Features

- It is smooth, soft, slightly mobile, tense cystic, 0.5-1 cm.

Size, may be
- Adhered to skin, most often
- Fluctuation may positive on Paget's test
- Trans illumination negative

Treatment

- Excision

Tubulodermoid

- Arises from embryonic tubular structures
- Example are
  - Thyroglossal cyst.
  - Ependymal cyst
  - Post anal dermoid etc.

Teratodermoid

- Arises from ecto-, meso- and endo- dermoid, i.e. from all germinal layers.
- Example:
  - In ovary as ovarian cyst
  - In Testis -as Teratoma,
  - In Retroperitoneal and mediastinal usually as solid swelling
  - It contains hair, tooth, cartilage and muscle
  - It can be benign or malignant

Different Diagnosis

  i. Lipoma
  ii. Sebaceous cyst

SEBACEOUS CYST (WEN, EPIDERMOID CYST)

What it is

- This a retention cyst due to accumulation of sebum due to blockage of the duct of sebaceous gland.
- Common sites are scalp, face and scrotum but it occurs at any site of the body where sebaceous glands exist except palm and sole.
- Cyst is lined by squamous epithelium and containing yellowish white cheesy material (paleface like material) with unpleasant smell. Such material is mixture of sebum, fat and desquamated epithelial debris.
- Rarely in the wall of sebaceous gland, one organism found, on histological section, named Demodex folliculorum.

How to Diagnose

a. From history and clinical features:
  - Scalp, face and scrotum are common sites
  - Usually spherical or globular shaped and .5 cm to 5 cm.
b. Clinical examination:
  - Swelling is smooth, soft, nontenders, freely mobile, adherent to skin especially over the summit.
  - There is a bluish spot at the site of the blockage of the ductal opening called Punctum. It is found in 70% cases. Remaining 30% cases the duct opens into the hair follicle so punctum is not present.
  - Punctum is adherent to the cyst. On squeezing cheesy material comes out through the punctum with unpleasant smell.

- Skin cannot be lifted up i.e., adherent to skin.
- Flactuation by Paget's test may be positive
- Transillumination negative.
- (In scalp sebaceous cyst, usually punctum is not visible and the cystic swelling itself can be indented by a finger trip pressure-this is diagnostic).

Complications

- Infection, suppuration, ulceration, calcification and its look cosmetically ugly.
- Cock's peculiar tumor: It is due to chronic irritation on the surface of the cyst due to escape of sebaceous material from the bursting cyst:

  As a result of chronic irritation there is a granuloma or granulating ulcer looks like a tumor like epithelioma (SCC) called Cock's peculiar tumor. Pathogenesis

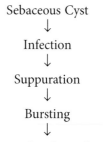

Sebaceous Cyst
↓
Infection
↓
Suppuration
↓
Bursting
↓

escape of cheesy material and purulent material causing
↓
chronic irritation on the surface
↓
↓
Granulating ulcer/granuloma
↓
Cock's Peculiar Tumour

- Sebaceous horn: It is nothing but a horny projection from the hardening of slowly discharged sebum through the punctum.
- Pathogenesis: Inspissated sebaceous materials in the cyst
↓
leaks through punctum. Accumulate on the surface skin in successive layers
↓
It gets dried up and give rise to a horny projection called sebaceous horn.

Treatment

- Excision of cyst: Entire capsule to be removed otherwise cyst will recur.

- If cyst is infected drain the infected material, pus, to control infection, then excise the entire cyst.

(Fordyce's disease is a heterotrophic sebaceous glands in mucosa of the lip and oral cavity)

LIPOMA

What it is: It is called as universal tumor as anywhere it can be occurred where there is a fat, i.e. yellow fat (except in brain)

(Tumor arising from brown fat is called Hypernoma)

- It is the most common benign tumour
- Common sites are, subcutaneous tissue over the trunk, nape of the neck and the limbs
- It can be diffused or capsulated, i.e. localized which is commonest type.

Diffuse variety is called pseudolipoma as it is without a capsule.

- Multiple lipomas are often associate with many syndromes like MEN syndrome

Classification

- Anatomical depends on the sites
  - Subcutaneous
  - Sub fascial or Sub aponeurotic
  - Intramuscular
  - Subperiosteal
  - Subserosal (Retroperitoneal)
  - Submucosal (GI tract)
  - Subsynovial
  - Intra-articular
  - Extradural or sub- Dural
  - Intraglandular, etc.
- Histological

In addition to adipose tissue other tissue presents
  i. Fibrolipoma—adipose tissue and fibrous tissue
     – Firm to hard in consistency
  ii. **NAEVO lipoma**—Adipose tissue and hemangiomatous lesion
     – Lipoma along with bluish discoloration of the overlying skin,
     – It is Blunched on pressure
     – Compressible
  iii. Neurolipoma
     – Adipose tissue and Nerve tissue
     – usually often painful
     – Multiple painful, Tender neurolipoma is called **neurolipomatosis**

- When neurolipoma or neurolipomatosis is associated with painful deposition of gat it is called Dercum's disease also called Adiposis dolorous

It is commonly seen on the trunk, buttocks and thigh and found commonly in female.

How to Diagnose

Features

a. Clinical:

Painless, solid, nontender, lobulated soft morbid, swelling at the common sites as mentioned above

b. Clinical Examination:

Surface is lobulated, lobules can be seen and felt at the surface as well as at the edge.

- Overlying skin is free
- Edge is well defined and may have multiple irregular curves due to lobularity of lipoma
- Slipping Sign - the edge of the
- Swelling slips under the examining finger
- Mobile on both the axis and may show Pseudo/semiflactuation (as in body temperature it remains in semiliquid form)
- When the swelling is pushed away, dimples appear on the surface (due to attachment of fibrous strands between lipoma and the skin

Differential Diagnoses > Dermoid, sebaceous cyst, neurofibroma etc.

Common sites where lipomas are more prone to transfer into malignancy (liposarcoma) are:
  i. Retroperitoneal Lipoma - de novo origin
  ii. Lipoma in the thigh especially intermuscular variety
  iii. Shoulder region and back - Subcutaneously lipoma

LIPOSARCOMA

Features: sudden/rapid growth from a previous lipoma.
- Warm and vascular
- Dilated over the surface
- Infiltration into the surrounding structures and deeper plane
- Mobility is restricted.
- Skin fixation.
- Features of lung metastasis may be there.

Treatment of Lipoma: Excision of lipoma is the treatment of choice if
  i. Lipoma is large, unsightly, and troublesome

ii. Lipoma at the regions of retroperitoneum, thigh and shoulder

Treatment of liposarcoma is wide local excision.

Fibroma

It is a capsulated benign tumor arising from fibrous tissue:

- True fibroma is rare. It is most commonly associated with mesodermal tissue like fibrolipoma, Fibromyoma, neurofibroma, etc.
- Uncapsulated proliferation of fibrous tissue which may be aggressive in nature called aggressive fibromatosis. Commonly seen in abdominal wall and chest wall. It is considered as a locally malignant tumour.
- Fibroma may be also soft or hard
  Soft fibroma contains immature fibrous tissue and hard fibroma contains well formed matured fibrous tissue.
  Desmoid tumor is an example of aggressive fibromatosis.

Desmoid tumor (desmos means tendon and eidos mean appearance)

Arising from musculoaponeurotic layer of abdomen, below umbilicus.

- Common in middle aged person, more common in female (80%) after delivery particularly.
- Present, with an abdominal lump slow growing, commonly in relation to rectus sheath from old hematoma or old incisional scar.
- The mass is parietal on 'CARNETS test', smooth, firm to hard,
- It is often associated with gardener's syndrome (Familial polyposis col:, osteoma, odontomas and epidermal cyst) - clinically it appears like fibrosarcoma
- Diagnosis is confirmed by excision biopsy.

Treatment

- Wide local excision with 2.5 cm clear margin along with mesh repair of abdominal defect.
- Radiotherapy can be given as it is moderately radiosensitive
- Drugs like sulindac, indomethacin, tamoxifen can be given to promote tumor shrinkage.

Hemangioma

The commonest Hamartomata (Hamartomata—a tumor like malformation of various tissue or tissues proper to the part)
Types:
  i. Capillary

ii. Cavernous (venous)
iii. Arterial or plexiform.

[The Word Hamartomata means "missing the mark in spear throughing "]

Capillary hemangiomas are:

- Salmon pink patch—disappears by year since birth
- Port-wine stain strawberry angioma and
- Spider naevus—central dilated Arteriole (red spot) and multiple linear, radiating capillaries like legs of a spider.

Sturge weber syndrome: Port-wine stain at face is associated with - a hemangioma of ipsi.

Lateral cerebral hemisphere:

- Jacksonian epilepsy
- Eye complication like glaucoma buphthalmos, loss of vision, etc.

Cavernous (Venous) Hemangioma

- Common sites are: Any where in the skin—commonly in face, ear and the lip
- Subcutaneous tissue
- Mucous membrane of tongue, mouth, lips
- Internal organ like liver, kidney, etc.
- Present since birth.

How to diagnose:

- Patient presents with appreciable swelling or just an elevated area from the surface
- Presence since birth, smooth, well localized, bluish, soft, compressible, spongy masses
- Gradually increases in size and may be trouble some like looks ugly, hemorrhage, thrombosis etc.
- Emplying sign may present
- It is nonpulsatile. If it is pulsatile, it indicates communication with arterial system.

Treatment

- Therapeutic embolization
- ligation of feeding artery
- Small area of involvement can be excised
- Sclerosant therapy, laser ablation are the recent treatment way.
- Injury to be avoided.

Arterial or Plexiform Hemangioma

- It is a type of congenital arteriovenous fistula
- Diffuse swelling over the part
- Feels like a bag of warms
- Swelling is pulsatile and compressible

- Systolic thrill or part may show bone thinning or destruction.
  Treatment as cavernous hemangioma as above.

Neurofibroma

- It is also regarded as hamartoma arising from connective tissue of the nerve (endoneurium)
- It may appear at any age but common in adult life

Types

i. Solitary or localized
ii. Generalized neurofibromatosis or von Recklinghausen's disease
iii. Plexiform neurofibromatosis
iv. Elephantiasis neurofibromatosis.

i. Solitary neurofibroma
How to diagnose

- Subcutaneous nodule, localized smooth, firm, well defined margin in relation with nerve.
- May be tender, moves horizontally or perpendicular to the direction of nerve, not along the nerve fibre.
- There may be history of pain, and hyperaesthesia in the distribution of the nerve.
- Supplied muscles weakness may be there sometime, so, power of the muscle to check always [Muscle power - Grade 0- No muscle contraction visible]

Grade-1   Muscle contraction visible but no movement
Grade-2   Movement when the effect of gravity eliminated
Grade-3   Movement is sufficient to over come gravity
Grade-4   Movement to over come gravity plus added resistance
Grade-5   Normal power

- Differential diagnosis
  - Fibroma, lipoma, neck node (when at neck)

ii. Generalized neurofibromatosis (Von Recklinghausen's disease)

- It is inherited as autosomal dominant disease and there will be multiple neurofibromas in the body, especially in face, neck, trunk, and the limbs.
- It is usually associated with coffee colored pigmented spots in the skin called 'café au lit' spots and commonly seen in back, abdomen and thigh. More than 6 in number.
- May be associated with different symptoms like MEN type vi B, skeletal deformities of limbs, osteoporosis of the bone etc.

- The nodules consistency vary from soft, firm to hard and may be sessile or pedunculated. In a typical case body surface has a 'Cobbled stone appearance.

iii. Plexiform Neurofibromatosis (Patchy dermatocele)

- Excessive over growth of endoneurium in the subcutaneous tissue, most commonly occurs along the distribution of 5th cranial nerve in the face skin of face.
- It may occur along the distribution of peripheral nerve
- There may be myxomatous degeneration of endoneurium of the nerve and the enormously thickening nerve hangs downwards.
- Over lying skin may be thickened, pigmented and folded skin looks like thrombosed hemangioma which hangs like a festoon.
- On palpation it resembles tortuous thrombosed veins due to plexiform mass (if hemangioma)
- In patchy dermatocele—this type of fibromatoses usually involves neck.

iv. Elephantiasis neurofibromatosis is a congenital lesion where skin of the limb largely thickened and rough like elephant limbs hence the name.

Treatment of Neurofibromatosis

- Solitary—complete excision of neurofibroma keeping the nerve intact and surgery is indicated when
  - Cosmetically looks ugly
  - Symptomatic, i.e. associated with pain, paraesthesia etc.
  - Showing sarcomatous changes.
- Generalized neurofibromatosis—practically it is impossible to remove numerous neurofibroma and it is unwarranted. But surgery may be planned when patient is symptomatic, i.e. pain is constant
  - Pressure symptoms present
  - Showing sarcomatous changes
  - Cosmetically looks very ugly in a particular area like face, neck, etc.

Treatment of keloid—Controversial still

A. Conservative

i. Intra keloid injection of steroid (Triamcinolone) once in a week for 6-8 weeks.
ii. Methotrexate and vit a therapy into the keloid.
iii. Irradiation

Table 32.1: Know the difference between Keloid and Hypertrophic Scar

		Keloid	*Hypertrophic Scar*
I	Definition	– It is a tumor like lesion arising from the connective tissue elements of a scar with proliferation of blood vessels and grows beyond the scar	– It is the hypertrophy or proliferation of mature fibro blast or fibrous tissue with any proliferation of blood vessels and it is confined to the scar
II	Sites	– Chest wall, over sternum upper arm, lower neck, ear.	– Any where in the body common in flexor surfaces.
III	Growth	– There are claw like processes and continue to grant with out time limit	– No claw like process and growth limits for 6 months
IV	Vascularity and collagen synthesis	– There is signs of increased vascularity and collagen synthesis is 20 times more than normal skin	– No sign of increased vascularity and collagen synthesis 6 times more.
V	Genetic Predisposition	– It is genetically predisposed and commonly in blacks.	– No genetic predisposition and no racial relation.
VI	Age and sex	– Adolescents and middle aged female are more prone	– Children are prone but both sexes are equally affected
VII	Treatment and recurrence	– Poor response to treatment and recurrence is very high	– Good response to steroid and recurrence is uncommon.

B. Surgical:

Excision and skin grafting excision with keeping a keloid margin all around.

C. Combine treatment:

   i. Excision and irradiation
  ii. Steroid injection

↓
Excision
↓
steroid injection

Hypertrophic Scar: Often self limiting and it responds steroid injection very well.

Squamous Cell Carcinoma (Epithelioma, Epidermoid Carcinoma)

My patient, Nitish Kumar (male > female) a 50 years old farmer (exposure to Sun rays) resident of UP, presented with complain of ulcerative swelling in his left foot for last one year.

The swelling was insidious in onset, gradually progressive, painless and attended its present size. For last 2 months he notified an ulcer developed over he swelling which is gradually increasing in size with watery discharge without any other swelling in left lowest limb and groin (LN swelling) [But there is no history of trauma, exposure to chemical, burns, etc.]

General survey is essentially normal except the patient having mild pallor.

Local Examination

- There is an ulceroproliferative swelling at dorsum of foot, 4 × 3 cm irregular shape.
- Margins are irregular
- Edge—everted and raised
- Floor is covered with grayish white slough.
- No active discharge seen.

On palpation: Bleeding on touch (characteristic of malignant ulcer)

Base inserted and not fixed to the underlying structures (May be fixed to the deeper structures).

So this is a case of skin carcinoma at left foot, most probably Squamous Cell carcinoma, without any evidence of lymph nodal metastasis.

Why are you telling it is squamous cell carcinoma?

- Elderly people
- Farmer in occupation, so exposure to sun is an important factor there.
- Rapidly developing swelling and ulcer
- Ulcer margin is irregular and edge is everted and raised
- Bleeding on touch

These are all in favor of squamous cell carcinoma.

What are the other possibilities?

Sir, on history and clinical examination I feel this is squamous cell carcinoma but it may be
- Basal cell carcinoma
- Melanoma
- Keratocanthoma, or
- Skin adnexal tumor

[Basal cell carcinoma and melanoma described in respective chapters]

Features of Keratocanthoma (Molluscum Sebaceum)

- Its an overgrowth of hair follicle and subsequent regression
- Commonly seen in adults
- It is rapidly growing, single swelling in the skin, painless with central brownish area, and mobile, non-tender, firm even hard swelling
- It grows for usually 4 weeks and there after it shows spontaneous regression slowly up to 4 months or more
- During regression, central area is separated from the lesion leaving a deeply seated scar
- It never turns into malignancy but looks like Squamous Cell Carcinoma

[Wide local excision is the treatment]

What are the features of skin adnexal tumor?

- Tumors arising from accessory skin structures like hair follicles, sebaceous glands, sweats glands, etc. and may be benign and malignant.
- It appears as protruding well localized swelling in the skin; often with involvement of regional lymph nodes which are hard and modular.
- It mimics squamous cell carcinoma of skin.
- [NB: Wedge biopsy of the swelling and FNAC of lymph node are diagnostic

For benign tumor excision and for malignant tumor wide local excision and block dissection of lymph nodes is the treatment]

OK, how will you proceed in this case?

Sir,

I will confirm my diagnosis first.

I will do-wedge (incisional) biopsy from the margin of the lesion and see the biopsy report.

X-ray of the part to exclude bone involvement and USG groin to exclude any node involvement.

Suppose biopsy report is squamous cell carcinoma what will you do next?

Sir,

I will do wide local excision of the lesion, keeping 1 cm margin all around and in depth up to deep fascia.

And resulting defect will be covered by a split thickness skin graft.

How will you manage the inguinal nodes?

Sir,

In this patient I won't do any inguinal lymph node dissection as there is no evidence of inguinal lymphadenopathy and elective dissection does not provide any survival benefit.

On follow-up if lymph node appears and FNAC proves it is metastatic; I will do inguinopelvic block dissection of lymph nodes.

How will you manage the patient post operatively?

Further management depends on histopathology report. If the margins of the tumor are free and it is well differentiated I will ask the patient for follow up regularly.

- If margins are positive and it is poorly differentiated tumor—I will plan for postoperative radiotherapy or
- Re-surgery with a wider excision 1-2 cm clear margin can be done.

What is the follow up scheduled for this patient?

I will ask the patient for follow up at 3 months interval for first 2 years and next every 6 months for next 3 years, then yearly.

What will you do in follow up?

I will examine the local site to exclude local recurrence and also examine the regional lymph nodes to exclude any enlargement.

What are the courses of lymph nodes enlargement in the patient of SCC?

Lymph nodes may be enlarged either due to (i) infection, or (ii) due to metastasis.

Infective enlargements of lymph nodes respond to antibiotics and metastatic does not, thereby metastatic lymph nodes need block dissection.

How does squamous cell carcinoma spreads?

- Local spread by continuity and contiguity
- Lymphatic spread by both permeation and the process of embolization.
- Blood spread is very rare.

What are the indications for amputation for this patient?

Amputation is indicated when

  i. Wide local excision is not possible as disease is so extensive like in forefoot.

  ii. The deeper structures including bone involvement.

What are the other treatment modalities for SCC?

1. Radiotherapy, as SCC is very sensitive to radiotherapy. The indications for radiotherapy are:
   - Small lesion, lesion in head and neck (T1 and T2 lesions)
   - Muscle, cartilage and bone are not involved.
   - Lesion not close to eye or not in the scalp.
   - Anaplastic carcinoma etc.
     Palliative external radiotherapy is given:
     – In advanced case with fixed lymph nodes
     – To palliate pain, fungation and bleeding.
2. Chemotherapy can be given in:
   - Locally advanced case as neoadjuvant therapy to down grade the tumor before surgery.
   - Along with radiotherapy, when resected, specimen shows margins positive
     Or in case of recurrence of malignancy.
3. Field therapy , for a small size, SCC field therapy with cryo probe, electrodissection or using topical fluorouracil may be effective and more cosmetic.

Where radiotherapy is contraindicated in general?

Radiotherapy is contraindicated:

  i. Near the eye to save the eye from the adverse effects of radiotherapy.

  ii. Over Pinna where radiation necrosis is frequent and painful sequel.

  iii. Over scalp where radiation causes wise depilation and cosmetically very poor sequel.

What are the prognostic factors in SCC?

- Tumor size > 3 cm
- Aggressive and ill-defined margin of the tumour
- Poorly differentiated variety of SCC
  And if, SCC is associated with immunosuppression.

What are the variants of SCC?

- Verrucous carcinoma
  - Slow growing SCC commonly occurs in mucous membrane and mucocutaneous junction.
  - The growth is usually warty type exophytic, dry and indurated.
  - No lymph node metastasis or blood spread usually seen.
  - Wide excision is enough. RT, CT not indicated.

  Few examples of verrucous carcinoma are:
  - Penis: giant condyloma acuminate, Buschke-Lowenstein tumor
  - Oral cavity: Florid verrucous carcinoma
  - Foot: verrucous carcinoma foot called carcinoma cuniculatum.
- Marjolin's ulcer.
  - Low grade squamous cell carcinoma
  - Occurs in chronic scar or ulcer
  - Lymph nodal spread is rare.
    (Details written in post-burns contracture and marjolin ulcer case)

Where from Squamous Cell Carcinoma arises?

- In skin SCC arises from malpighian or spindle cell layer of the epidermis
- In Mucous membrane - arises from stratified squamous epithelium.
- SCC may arise from metaplastic columnar epithelium.

What are the sites for SCC?

- Any part of skin.
- Mucous membrane lined with stratified squamous epithelium like in buccal cavity, pharynx, oesophagus, larynx, tongue, rectum, and canal, vagina, etc.
- Where squamous metaplasia of columnar epithelium occurs like gall bladder, bronchus, etc.
- Where squamous metaplasia of transitional epithelium occurs like renal pelvis, urinary bladder, etc.

What are the premalignant lesions of the skin?

- Radiodermatitis
- Solar Keratosis
- Leukoplakia
- Bowen's disease (see in CA penis)

- Xeroderma pigmentosa
- Chronic ulcer like venous ulcer, non-healing ulcer, etc.
- Old Scar, post burn scar sinuses, etc.
- Chronic irritation in skin due to chemical (Industrial workers), local heat application like Kangri cancer in Kashmiri people.

Sun ray's exposure like in farmers who work in the field in the day etc.
  - Chimney sweep cancer—occurs in scrotum who handles tar regularly.
  - Kang cancer—occurs in bullocks and heel of Tibetans due to sleeping over oven bed to control cold.
- Lupus vulgaris, and
- Due to unknown reason, it is common in immuno-suppressed individuals.

What are the types of SCC?

- Exophytic: This type grows very slowly. It is locally invasive only.
- Ulcerative - or ulceroproliferative
  - This lesion starts as a nodular lesion grows rapidly ulcerates only or along with proliferation it form ulceroproliferative lesion.
- Invades local tissue early, distal metastasis and
- Lymph nodes involvement are common.

What is the histological characteristic features of SCC?

Malignant whorls of squamous cells i.e. 'cell-nests' and keratin pearls are characteristic features.
    Know TNM staging of skin cancer other than melanoma.

T- Tumor
  - T0 - No evidence of tumour
  - T1 - Tumour < 2 cm
  - T2 - Tumour 2 - 5 cm
  - T3 - Tumour > 5 cm
  - T4 - Tumour involving cartilage muscle, bone etc.

N - Nodal status
  - N0 - No evidence of lymph node metastasis
  - N1 - Regional lymph nodes involvement +

M - Metastasis
  - M0 - No evidence of distant metastasis
  - M1 - Distant metastasis +

SHORT NOTE ON SCC

A. Know the layers of skin:
  i. Epidermis: An avascular layer of skin.
  Layers
  - Stratum corneum (Horny cell layer)
  - Stratum granulosum
  - Stratum spinosum (Princkle cell layer)
  - Stratum basal
  - Stratum lucidum—seen in palms and soles.
    [Melanocytes—one melanocyte is seen for every 10 basal cells]
  ii. Dermis contains collagen fibres, elastic fibres, capillaries, venules, arteriotes, lymphatics nerves, sweat glands, sebaceous glands, etc.
  Layers are only two:
    i. Papillary
    ii. Reticular

B. Different types of biopsy—Most important investigation to rule out malignancy. Various methods of biopsy are
  i. Fine niddle aspiration cytology (FNAC) using 23-24 G needle.

  ii. Tru cut biopsy—when FNAC is inconclusive - true cut biopsy is done. Specially designed thicker biopsy needle and more tissue are available for histopathology examination.
  iii. Punch Biopsy—more often used for viscera, hollow or solid viscera. With specially designed punch biopsy forcep tissue are taken from the margin of the tumor along with normal tissue around it and from the base of the ulcer, like ulcer of stomach.
  iv. Edge/wedge biopsy—biopsy taken from the margin
  v. Open biopsy— Excisional biopsy
                  Incisional biopsy
  Excision biopsy is done in a small lesion (usually < 3 cm) where whole of the lesion is excised.
  Whereas, in incisional biopsy a slice of tissue is taken from a larger mass for histopathological examination.
  vi. Drill biopsy—rarely done now a days but it claimed accuracy of more than 90%. Here biopsy is taken using a high speed compressor air drill.

My patient Sonia, a 40 years old lady, agriculture worker (more common in female and exposure to sun light is the most important risk factor) resident of Punjab, presented with complain of a Blackish Ulceroproliferative growth in the sole just below the right 4th and 5th toes for last 6 months.

Six months, back he noticed a black nodule that appeared just below the right 4th toe which was slowly progressive initially and for last 3 months it is rapidly increasing in size painlessly and became large, approximate 3 × 2 cm florid mass which protrudes from and overlaps the surrounding skin.

Gradually, it is ulcerated, along with off and on bleeding and color changes and becomes more dark in appearance.

For last two months, there are multiple small nodules on the dorsum of the foot (satellite nodules characteristics).

On Examination

General survey is normal except pallor is present.

On Local Examination

There is a 4 × 3 cm blackish ulceroproliferative mass at the front of the right sole. Just below 4th and 5th toes. It appears soft, wet and boggy and a hard brown pigment was noticed around the growth. The ulcer is covered with crust of blood, nodular, solid and hard in consistency, non-tender, irregular margins, and elevated edges. It slightly moves with the skin.

Multiple subcutaneous satellite nodules are present on the dorsum of the foot where are hard in consistency and non-tender.

No other lesions present all over the body.

No regional i.e. popliteal and inguinal lymphadenopathy palpabal (should be always examined).

Systemic examinations are essentially normal (exam abdomen for liver, respiratory system for lung and brain for neurological abnormality).

So, this is a case of malignant melanoma at the sole of right foot without any lymph node metastasis.

What are the other possibilities of such a pigmented lesion?

Other possibilities are:
  i. Pyogenic granuloma
 ii. Pigmented squamous cell carcinoma
iii. Pigmented Basal cells carcinoma
 iv. Kaposi's sarcoma
  v. Pigmented senile/seborrhoeic keratosis
 vi. Cutaneous angioma/angiosarcoma

  i. Pyogenic granuloma
   • Its an exuberant over growth of granulation tissue usually 0.5-1 cm only
   • Red or reddish in color
   • Soft to firm, polypoid lesion
   • History of trauma or foreign body insertion which may not be remarkable to the patient
   • Slow growing. Sometimes ulcer develops it is difficult to differential diagnosis is very difficult from malignancy like malignant melanoma (Excisio is the treatment).
 ii. Pigmented squamous cell or
iii. Pigmented basal cells carcinoma—features of SCC and BCC (already described) are along with pigmentations and appear like malignant melanoma.
 iv. Kaposi's sarcoma
   • A low grade soft tissue malignancy. Arises from lymphovascular endothelial cells in the skin (79%), may involve lymph nodes along with or separately (70%), often seen in patients with Acquired Immunodeficiency Syndrome (AIDS) and other immunosuppressed states like organ transplantation.
   • An elevated solid lesion 0.2 to 0.5 cm in diameter, papule is blue or dark-blue or violaceous.
     (Treatment symptomatic. Skin lesion can be treated with radio therapy, intra lesions injection of chemotherapy cryotherapy and excision).

v. Seborrhoeic keratoris (Basal cell papilloma, seborrhoeic wart)
- A benign overgrowth of basal layer of epidemis
- Commonly seen in elderly of both sexes
- Common sites are back, face, neck, and trunk
- It is a slow growing, widening lesion looks like an void, brown plaque stuck on the epidermis and varies few mm to few centimeter.
- Surface is rough, waxy feeling and hyperkeratotic and can be picked off from the skin.

It may become infected or ulcerated with deeply pigmented, it appears like malignant melanoma but change to malignancy is rare (Treatment is excision or cryosurgery, etc.).

What are the risks factors for developing melanoma?

Risk factors are:
- Exposure to sunlight (UV rays exposure)
- Xeroderma pigmentosa
- Albinism
- Junctional naevus
- High socioeconomic group, ethnic factors, climate, fair skin people and exposure to sunlight (more in people of Australia).
- Familial dysplastic meavus syndrome
- Sporadic dysplatic naevi
- Larger congenital naevi (>15 cm)
- Family history of melanoma
- History of earlier skin cancers, etc.

Can you tell which malignancies spread from mother to foetus?

They are:
- Melanoma, and
- Lymphosarcoma

What are the clinical types of melanoma?

i. Superficial spreading—most common type approximately 64%. Can occur in any part of the body with variegated appearance and growth is more radial.
ii. Nodular melanoma (15-25%)
   More malignant common in younger age, can occur in any part of the body. Growth is vertical.
iii. Lentigo maligna melanoma—5-10%
   Least malignant, common elderly people and in face (to his son's freekle)
iv. Acral lentigo melanoma 5%.
   Prognosis is poor. Commonly seen in palms and soles and subungual region.

v. Amelanotic melanoma—the worst type'
   It's a rapidly progressive tumor and mimics like soft tissue sarcoma.

What are the important characteristics of melanoma?

Remember: ABCDE

A-symetrical, B-Border irregular, C-color variation, D-diameter > 6 mm, and E-elevated lesion.

What are the most important clinical features of malignant melanoma?

- Common after puberty, usually 20 - 40 years
  Female > male. In female lower limbs more commonly affected. In male upper limbs and chest involvement is more.
- Starts from pre-existing naevus (commonly junctional naevus) 50-60% or as de novo in normal skin 40-50%.
- The growth is rapid with irregular margin, elevated edges and rough surface with pigmentation, gradually becomes darker.
- It is a nontender, firm and solid swelling fixed to the skin and moves with skin, surrounding skin may show halo of brown pigment around the growth.
- Satellite nodules are secondary nodules within 2 cm of primary and the nodules beyond 2 cm of primary are called Transit's nodule.
- Ulceration of the growth, occasional bleeding, itching, and changes in colour are the important features of melanoma.
- And involvement of regional lymph nodes may be there.

How does malignant melanoma spread?

i. Lymphatic spread to regional lymph nodes by permeation or by embollsation.
   Retrograde spread of dermal lymphatic, produces satellite nodules and transit's nodules.
ii. Blood spread - to lung, liver (becomes very large), and brain, skin, bones and common in black people.

What are the features of lung metastases?

A patient of melanoma may present with history of cough, chest pain, hemoptysis, etc.
- Clinically, the patient may have
  - Pleural effusion
  - Reduce air entry in lungs.
- Chest X-ray may show cannon ball. Secondaries.

How will you investigate a case of melanoma?

- Excision biopsy if the lesion is small
- FNAC from involved lymph node

- USG abdomen to see hepatomegaly (in melanoma huge hepatomegaly is there)
- Chest X-ray to see the lung metastasis (cannon ball appearance in melanoma)
- CECT abdomen, head, chest when metastasis is suspected tumor mark as: MELAN-4, S100, hydroxymethyl bromide 45 (AMB 45).

What will you do in your patient of Melanoma?

In my case the melanoma is a larger one. Here no question of excision biopsy.

There is no clinical involvement of lymph node, so I will do:

- USG abdomen
- Chest X-ray

and all base line investigations to make the patient fit for anaesthesia and surgery. In this case the location of melanoma is such that wide local excision keeping 2 cm minimal margin is not worthy. Here primary area is wide, so amputation one joint above is to be done to clear the satellite nodules also or at least disarticulation of 4th, 5th toes to get at least 2 cm clear margin.

If only disarticulation is done. Satellite nodules are to be treated by superficial electron beam radiotherapy or isolated limb perfusion to be done.

Why incisional biopsy or needle biopsy or needle biopsy are not indicated in melanoma for tissue diagnosis?

In either incisional biopsy or needle biopsy should be avoided in melanoma because there is a high chance of transferring melanoma cells to the subcutaneous fat and thus, superficial melanoma is converted to deep melanoma.

What are the treatment modalities for lymph node involvement from melanoma?

- If clinically palpable mobile lymph nodes
  FNAC positive
  Regional block dissection of lymph nodes like ilioinguinal, axillary, neck dissection to be done as per site of involvement.
- If lymph nodes are fixed. Palliative chemotherapy is the treatment of choice only.

What is sentinel lymph node biopsy?

Sentinel lymph node is the first affected lymph node from the tumor bearing area. If this lymph node is not involved chance of involvement of other lymph nodes are rare; thereby elective lymph node dissection (ELND) is not logical.

In a case of much thicker melanoma (thickness is 1-4 mm), there are high chances of micrometastasis. So some surgeons prefer to do ELND.

- Prophylactic regional block dissection in case of melanoma is still a highly controversial topic.

How will you do lymphatic mapping and sentinel node biopsy?

Radioactive colloid (99m Tc labeled colloid albumin) is injected around the primary site day before or in the morning of the operation.

The sentinel lymph node is detected by hand held gamma probe.

iii. Isosulfan blue or even methylene blue dye is injected into peritumoral area and lymph node can be localized by staining of the lymph node.

[History of sentinel lymph node biopsy in short. Cabana is the person who described sentinel lymph node biopsy on the basis of lymphangiography. He started this method for carcinoma penis to see the sentinel inguinal lymph node involvement.

Gradually the SLN biopsy is practiced in both
- Melanoma, and
- Carcinoma breast widely

The aim of sentinel LN biopsy is to avoid unnecessary lymph node dissection when sentinel lymph node is not involved].

What is the indication of regional/isolated limb perfusion?

Isolated limb perfusion is indicated: (i) when the lesion is confined to one limb along with satellite and Transit's nodule, (ii) for locoregional recurrent melanoma.

Can you tell me how the limb perfusion is done?

Sir,

The vessels (artery and vein) supplying the limb are to be cannulated and connected to an extracorporeal circulation device. The venous blood is oxygenated by passing through the membrane oxygenator and mixed with chemotherapy (commonly used CT is melphalan).

The oxygenated blood mixed with chemotherapy is returned back into the limb through the artery. So high dose chemotherapeutic agents are used.

How will you tackle locoregional recurrent melanoma?

i. In locoregional recurrent melanoma, isolated limb perfusion using oxytotoxic agents like Melphalan (Remember: M for M, i.e. Melphalan for Melanoma)

(The complications are DVT, bleeding, sepsis, etc.)
It is not only used for locoregional recurrent but also used for transit's nodules

ii. Laser ablation can be done for multiple small cutaneous lesions.

What are the indications of chemotherapy in a case of malignant melanoma?

The indications of chemotherapy are:

i. Secondaries in lungs, liver, bones

ii. In case of locally advanced malignant melanoma. It is given as adjuvant therapy after surgery.

Common chemotherapeutic drugs used are:

- Melphalan (phenyl alanine musters)
- DTIC–Diethyl Triamine Aminocaproic Acid (carbox-amide)

What is the role of immunotherapy in a case of malignant melanoma?

Immunotherapy is being tried in treatment of malignant melanoma.

- Intralesional BCG vaccination, specific tumor antibodies to melanoma antigens, tumor vaccines, purified tuberculin, Corynebacterium parvum are proved beneficial.
- Other agents like interleukins, alfainterferons, levamisole are also used as newer challenges.

What about the role of radiotherapy in malignant melanoma?

Malignant melanoma is radio resistant so, this has not much role for radio therapy. Radiotherapy is beneficial only in secondaries involving brain, bones.

What are the prognostic factors for the case of malignant melanoma?

The prognostic factors are:

- Tumour thickness and level of local invasion
- Ulceration of the tumour
- Nodal status, i.e. presence of metastasis
- Transit's nodules.
- Number of mitotic figure and lymphocytic infiltration etc.

Tell me something about 'melanin' now?

Melanin is a pigment produced by melanoblasts which arises either in:

- Surface epithelial cells
- Neuroectoderm of nervous system
- Melanin producing cells lying in the skin, choroid of the eye and rarely meninges, medulla tela choroidea, mucocutaneous junction of vagina, mouth
- Anorectal junction, in nail bed, iris, ciliary body etc.
  Melanin is synthesized from Tyrosine

Tyrosine --------- DOPA---- ---- Melanin
          Tyrosinase Oxidase

How will you follow up the postoperative case of malignant melanoma?

- Follow-up first 2 years 3 months interval
- 3rd to 5th year, 6 months interval
- Next yearly.
- On follow up along with meticulous physical examination, chest X-ray, tumor markers like melan-A, S-100
- USG abdomen, pelvis
- CECT in selected cases like suspected lung metastasis, brain metastasis, etc.

SHORT NOTE ON MELANOMA

MELANOMA

- Melanomas are melanin containing tumors arising from melanocytes and melanoblasts.
- Melanin is sulphur containing iron free black pigment. It is synthesized from the amino acid tyrosine.

$$\underset{\text{Tyrosinase}}{\text{Tyrosine}} \xrightarrow{} \underset{\substack{\text{(Dihydroxy-}\\\text{phynylalamine)}}}{\text{DOPA}} \xrightarrow{\text{Oxidase}} \text{Melanin}$$

- Function of melanin is protective against sunlight.
- Benign Melanoma or Pigmented Naevus or Mole
- Naevus is a general term referring to localized cutaneous malformation of melanocytes due to repeated stimulation.
- Naevus means birth mark, so it may present since birth or appears later in life.

Types of Naevus

i. Hairy mole—mole with hairs on its surface
ii. Non-hairy mole—mole without any hair
iii. Blue naevus—it is a special type of intradermal naevus and common in children, on face, dorsum of hand and foot and buttock (Mongolian spot) are the common sites.
   It is flat or slightly elevated. Surface is smooth and shiny and it disappears by the age of 5 years.
iv. Junctional naevus—it lies in the junction at layers (basal layer) of epidermis as clusters.
   - It's a macular lesion, smooth, flat or slightly raised 1 mm to 1 cm in size. Light brown to dark brown or brown black in colour.
   - It can occur anywhere and anytime in life, but most commonly in soles, palms, digits and genitalia are of junctional type.
   - 90% malignant melanoma begins in junctional naevi but all junctional naevi do not change into malignancy. Change in size, colour, bleeding, ulceration, crusting, satellite nodules etc.
v. Compound naevus—combination of both junctional and intradermal components. Intra dermal part is inactive and junctional part is potentially malignant.
   Light brown to dark brown in colour. Common in older children and adult. It is round, or elliptical or elevated lesions.

vi. Juvenile melanoma—a type of compound naevus
   - Occurs commonly in young children on face
   - Like compound naevus it has a tendency to become completely intradermal
vii. Freekle (Hutchinson's Freckle Lentigo maligna)
   Commonly seen in elderly on face and neck. It starts as a macule and gradually a large area of pigmentation appears.
   - It has three distinct characteristics
   Late development, steady centrifugal enlargement and, high in cedens of malignant changes.
viii. Halo naevus, dermal naevus are others rare varieties.

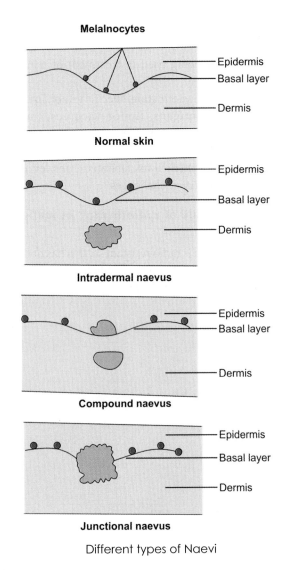

Different types of Naevi

Treatment is total excision when indicated like

- Cosmetically looks ugly
- Transferring into malignancy
- Junctional naevus, freekle, compound naevi which are more prone to develop malignancy - Naevi on sole, palm digits, genetalia where repeated trauma is more likely.
- Laser excision, cryosurgery are the modern ways of treatment.

Giant Naevus: Naevus occupying more than 1% of body surface area and or more than 20 cm is called giant naevus.

MALIGNANT MELANOMA

Classifications

A. Breslow's classification based on thickness of invasion measured by optical micrometer
- Stage I—thickness < 0.75 mm
- Stage II—thickness 0.76 mm to 1.50 mm
- Stage III—thickness 1.51 mm to 4 mm
- Stage IV—thickness > 4 mm

B. Clark's level
Melanoma
- Level 1: involved in epidermis only
- Level 2: extended into papillary dermis
- Level 3: Filling of papillary dermis completely
- Level 4: Extended into reticular dermis
- Level 5: Extended into subcutaneous tissue.

C. TNM Staging—TNM staging updates at 2009 by AJCC
T0 - No evidence of tumour
Tis - Carcinoma in situ

T - Thickness
T1 < 1 m Tia without ulceration mitosis < 1 m^2
T1b with ulceration with mitosis > 1/m^2

Thickness

T2	1-2 mm	a.	without ulceration
		b.	with ulceration
T3	2-4 mm	a.	without ulceration
		b.	with ulceration
T4	> 4 mm	a.	without ulceration
		b.	with ulceration

N

N0	No evidence of lymph node metastasis		
N1	1 Node metastasis	a.	micrometastasis
		b.	micrometastasis
N2	2-3 nodes metastasis	a.	micrometastasis
		b.	micrometastasis
		c.	Satellite or transit nodules without metastatic nodes

N3   4 or more metastatic node or matted nodes or transit/satellite nodules with metastatic nodes.

M

M0   No evidence of distant metastasis

M1
a. skin, subcutaneous or nodal metastasis
b. Lung metastasis
c. All other visceral metastasis or any distant metastasis with elevated LDH.

Updated later in January, 2010.

REMEMBER

- A history of loss of an eye from a disease longback and an enlarged liver (huge) is diagnosed recently - suggestive of an ocular melanoma.

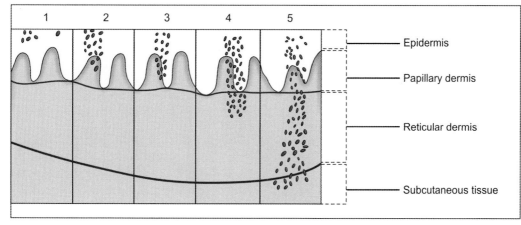

Clark's level of melanoma

- Extensive visceral involvement may cause melanuria
- Occult malignant melanomas are commonly found in anas, scalp, external auditory cannel and genetalia, nail bed, eye, adrenal medulla.
- Prognosis of malignant-melanoma depends on pathological type, site, tumor thickness, clinical staging, and level of invasion.
  - 5 years survival low risk patient 95-100% intermediate risk 85-95% and high risk group 15-50%.
  - Lymph node metastasis, ulceration of melanoma lowers the survival rates. Melanoma face has better prognosis. Overall have a 10% survival advantage.

- Treatment of malignant melanoma in other sites like
- Anorectal melanoma - abdominoperineal resection
- Melanoma vulva - treated by vulvectomy with reconstruction.
- Melanoma of the eye - choroids melanoma
- Enucleation of the eye, conjunctival melanoma can be treated with radioactive strontium plate.

Peutz-Jeghers syndrome: Multiple circum oral melanoses is associated with multiple intestinal polyposes. It's a familial condition.

Upper Limb Ischemia

My patient a 40 years old lady (ULI common in female) smoker, resident of Bihar, farmer in 2occupation presented with complain of

- Pain in left upper limb for last 6 months.
- Blackish left little finger for last 1 month.

Since last 6 months my patient is having pain in her left upper limb off and on. The pain appears when she works at field for a while and she initially used to manage to continue the work but for last 2 months she has to take rest frequently to continue the work. Nowadays, at the evening she has to take pain killer for her pain and for last 1 month she has been developing blackish discoloration at her left little finger which is gradually progressive and attained its present condition. It started with sudden onset of pain at night 1 month back.

[Keep in mind—the following negative history, no history of trauma, syncope (to exclude TIA).

- No history suggestive of Raynaud's syndrome.
- No history suggestive of any collagen disorder like myalgia, rashes, arthralgia etc.
- No neurological or joints problem.
- No history of exposure to vibratory tools or chemicals (vinyl chloride may produce vasospastic disorder)].

On Examination

General survey is essentially normal except mild pallor.

On Local Examination

- Patient looks slightly tense.
- No gross wasting in the left upper limb.
- Look for signs of ischemia like thinning, diminished hair, loss of subcutaneous fat, brittle nail with transverse ridges, etc.
- There is obvious gangrene at left little finger and line of demarcation is well visualized.

Palpation

i. **Peripheral pulses**

	Right upper limb	Left upper limb
Subclavian	++	++
Axillary	++	+
Brachial	++	+
Radial	++	-
Ulnar	++	-

ii. **Capillary filling-less than 3 seconds is normal.**

iii. **Venous filling (Harvey's sign) - less than 10 seconds is normal.**

iv. **Test:** Buerger's postural test < 30° indicates severe ischemia

[Adson's test (scalene maneuver) positive in case of cervical rib and scalenus anticus syndrome due to compression of subclavian artery.

This case radial pulse not palpable in the left so, this test is not relevant here.

If radial pulse palpable then do the test to exclude cervical rib or scalenus anticus syndrome.

How to perform the test: stand in front of the sitting patient. Ask her to take deep breath and to turn the face to the affected side. Check her radial pulse. This may be obliterated due to compression of subclavian artery]

- Elevated arm stress test (Modified Roos test) to exclude thoracic outlet syndrome.
  [How to perform the test: ask the patient to keep the arm in 90° abduction and external rotation position and she is asked to make a fist and release repeatedly for few minutes. Normal people can continue this thing for a long time but the patient of upper limb ischemia will have pain and stop the maneuver]
- Costoclavicular compression manoeuver (Falconer test) to check radial pulse.

How to perform: Ask the patient to draw her shoulders backwards and downwards like 'sabdhan' position in military. In this position subclavian artery is compressed in between first rib and clavicle, so radial pulse will be absent or feeble.

- Hyperabduction maneuver (Halsted test) to check the radial pulse.

  How to perform: Ask the patient to hyperabduct the arm and check the radial pulse. Radial may be absent or feeble as the artery gets compressed by the pectoralis minor.

- **Allen's test:** To see the patency of radial and ulnar arteries.

  How to perform: Aim to find out the patency of both radial and ulnar arteries. The patient is asked to clench his fist tightly. You press both the arteries at the wrist. After a minute she is asked to open the fist. The palm appears white. Now the pressure on the radial artery is removed keeping pressure on ulnar artery. If the radial artery is blocked the white color will remain, but if it is patent the palm assumes normal reddish color.

  Again the test is repeated, now the pressure on ulnar artery is removed keeping pressure on radial artery. If the ulnar artery is blocked the hand remains white if it is patent the hand assumes normal color.

In this case as radial and ulnar pulse absent - so no value of this test. These test to be done when radial and ulnar pulses are palpable even feeble.

So this is a case of left upper limb ischemia most probably due to thromboembolic episode just above the bifurcation of left brachial artery.

Why are you telling most probably the upper limb ischemia is due to thromboembolic episode?

- She is a chronic smoker.
- History of sudden onset of severe pain and gradually progressive gangrene in her left little finger.
- Both the radial and ulnar pulses are not palpable. It suggest the clot is lodged somewhere just above the bifurcation of brachial artery.
- Thromboembolism is the second most common cause of upper limb ischemia.

What are the causes of subacute and chronic upper limb ischemia?

A. Obliterative causes:
  - Atherosclerosis.
  - Thromboembolism

- Trauma
- Dissection
- Thoracic outlet obstruction
- Vasculitis- giant cell arteritis.
- Buerger's disease.
- Takayashu's disease.
- Thrombosed aneurysm.
- Extrinsic compression by tumour.
- Drugs related causes, etc.

B. Vasospastic causes:
  - Raynaud's disease.
  - Vibration finger- acrocyanosis.

How will you proceed in this case?

So, I will like to do few investigations to establish the diagnosis.

First I will do

i. Color Doppler ultrasonography to establish
  - Presence of ischemia.
  - Site of obstruction
  - Nature of obstruction- fixed/ spastic
  - Extent of obstruction
  - Status of proximal and distal vessels.
  - Identifies collateral pathways.

ii. Computed tomographic angiography (CTA)

  Best of evaluating of-
  - Atherosclerotic sterno-occlusive disease.
  - Embolic phenomenon.
  - Traumatic or iatrogenic injury
  - Vasculitis.
  - Aneurysm etc.

  Other valuable investigations are MRA—Magnetic Resonance Angiography for better delineation of artery, vein, and nerve separately and clearly.

  Apart from this I would like to do.

iii. Complete blood count—ESR.
  - Blood sugar- lipid profile.
  - RA factor
  - ECG
  - X-ray of the upper limb
  - Chest X-ray to exclude cervical rib etc.

What is the role of digital subtraction angiography (DSA) in upper limb ischemia?

Digital substraction angiography still remains the gold standard for arterial imaging.

DSA uses image substraction so that the bone does not obscure vascular detail and has the advantages of the ability to manipulate the images. But it is invasive. So present day's non invasive imaging techniques like CTA/ MRA are preferable.

What do you do in this patient?

In this patient the left brachial pulse is palpable but both artery and ulnar artery pulses, not palpable. So probable, site of occlusion is just above the bifurcation of brachial artery. I will confirm it by color Doppler and I will see the site of occlusion.

It's been already a month and only gangrene is found at the distal phalanx of finger.

Sir, if I find any thrombus/embolus at brachial artery I will remove it by Fogarty's catheter to get instant relieve from obstruction and I will definitely do 'Ray's amputation for the gangrene of left little finger.

Here it is been already 1 month but left upper limb is still viable only distal pulses are absent. In such a case could you advise for any other method instead of Fogarty's catheterization?

Sir, I can also do intra arterial thrombolysis as the ischemia is not acute and so severe.

I will use tissue plasminogen activator (TPA) which is the agent of choice today because of its relative rapid action and freedom from allergic side effects.

(Streptokinase, Urokinase has now become obsolescent in this purpose).

Tell me, in your case, distal pulses are not palpable but whole limb is viable except the gangrene in little finger. How it could be happened?

Sir, the symptoms are usually mild in case of upper limb ischemia. The viability of the limb sustained only because of liberal collateral circulation. Rest pain and ulceration are exceedingly rare and indicate multilevel occlusion.

How will you manage a case of upper limb ischemia due to atherosclerotic occlusion?

Medical management of atherosclerosis is very essential. Abstinence from tobacco, aspiration, statins, etc.

Many patients with left subclavial occlusion do not require surgery as symptoms are mild.
Surgical options include:
- Carotid subclavian by pass using PTFE graft transposition.
- Subclavian common carotid.

- Extra anatomic bypass like axilloaxillary bypass.
- Alternatively angioplasty and stenting of the lesion can be performed. The results are comparable to surgery and with very low comparable to surgery.

What is Raynaud's syndrome?

It's an episodic digital ischemia occurring in response to cold or emotional stress. The patient present with typical triphasic color changes. The syndrome has been divided into two subgroups: (i) Raynaud's disease, and (ii) Raynaud's phenomenon.

What is the difference between Raynaud's disease and Raynaud's phenomenon?

Raynaud's disease refers to the patient with intermittent digital ischemia in the absence of an associated disease. It is an unknown vasospastic condition occurring in young female. Where a Raynaud's phenomenon refers to the patients who manifest digital ischemia due to an underlying disease; usually associated with a connective tissue disorder.

What are the typical triphasic color changes in Raynaud's syndrome?

- First phase—white or pale, stage of blunching.
- Second phase—blue or cyanosed, stage of dusky anoxia.
- Third phase—Crimson or red, stage of red engorgement.

What is the pathophysiology behind the triphasic color changes?

Stage I: Local syncope/ pallor- due to spasm of digital arteries.

Stage II: Local asphyxia—cyanosis due to slowing of circulation with accumulation of reduced haemoglobin.

Stage III: Stage of red engorgement: Due to release of spasm of the digital arteries.

If such attacks are repeated—gangrene appears at fingertips called stage IV- local gangrene.

Practice the following tests repeatedly please:
1. Venous filling
2. Capillary filling
3. Buerger's postural test
4. EAST [Elevated Arm Stress Test].
5. Falconer (Costoclavicular compression manoeuver).
6. Halsted Test (Hyperabduction maneuver).
7. Adson's Test
8. Allen's Test.

SHORT NOTE ON UPPER LIMB ISCHEMIA

Anatomy: Arteries of upper limb.

Left subclavian artery directly arises from the arch of aorta but right subclavian artery arises from branchiocephalic trunk (innominate artery)

From underneath sterno clavicular joint subclavian artery arches over the pleura and apex of the lung about 2.5 cm above the clavicle and after reaching the lateral border of the first rib it continues as axillary artery.

Subclavian artery is divided into three parts by pectoralis minor muscle.

V i)   Vertebral artery.

I ii) Internal thoracic artery.

T iii) Thyrocervical Trunk   [inferior thyroid artery
                                Suprascapular artery
                                Transverse cervical artery]

C iv) Costocervical trunk [superior intercostals
                                Deep cervical arteries]

D v) Dorsal scapular artery—occasionally.

  Axillary artery is divided into three parts by pectoralis minor muscle.

First part gives one branch-   i. Superior   thoracic artery.

Second part gives two branches- i. Thoracoacromial
                                 ii. Lateral thoracic

Third part gives three branches- i. Subscapular
                                 ii. Anterior
                                 iii. Posterior.
                                ↓
                Circumflex humeral artery.
                                ↓
at the lower border of teres major muscle it enters the arm
        and continues a branchial artery.
                                ↓
about 2.5 cm below elbow crease the brachial artery
bifurcates into radial and ulnar arteries which run in the
                forearm.
                                ↓
Ulnar artery forms the superficial palmar arch which is
completed by superficial palmar branch of radial artery.
                                ↓
radial artery form the deep palmar arch and completed by
        deep palmar branch of ulnar artery.

Cervical Rib: Different types: The cervical rib arises from the transverse process of the 7th cervical vertebra. It may be

No. 1. A complete rib articulating with manubrium sterni or the first rib

No. 2. The rib is incomplete and the free end expands into a bony mass.

No. 3. The rib is incomplete and the free end is connected to the first rib by a fibrous band

No. 4. There is no bony rib but a fibrous band passing from the transverse process of 7th cervical vertebra to first rib. Neurovascular bundle may be compressed by this band.

SUBCLAVIAN STEAL

As a result of atherosclerotic stenosis of the subclavian artery, proximal to the site of the origin of vertebral artery, there is reduction of pressure in the subclavian artery beyond the stenosis results in retrograde flow from the brain stem down the vertebral artery to the axillary and brachial artery. This phenomenon is called subclavian steal syndrome as the blood is stolen from the brain.

Symptoms: Patients may have syncopal attacks due to ischemia to the brain stem particularly when the patients use the affected arm more like weight lifting, exercise etc. there may be visual disturbances as well.

On examination: Pulse volume will be decreased in the affected site, BP will be also decreased.
There may be localized bruit in the supraclavicular space.

Embolism and Thrombosis

Embolism is the commonest cause of acute limb ischemia in developing countries.

Causes

i. Cardiac emboli 80-90% of cases of all embolism. Myocardial infarction, cardiac valve prosthesis are the other causes of embolism.

ii. Non-cardiac embolism
    Atherosclerotic disease (plaques) in proximal arteries is the commonest cause.
    Other causes are aneurysms in proximal arteries, non cardiac tumors. Primary or metastatic lung cancers invading pulmonary vasculature.

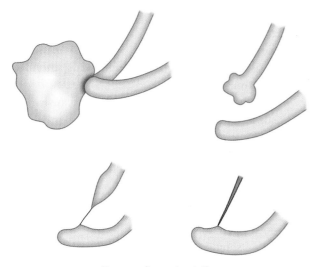

Types of cervical ribs

Table 35.1: Difference between embolism and thrombosis

		Embolism	Thrombosis
i.	Source	Identification source frequently detected	Identifiable Source is not detected.
ii.	Claudication	rare	Frequent
iii.	Physical findings	proximal and contralateral pulses normal	Epsilateral or contralateral examination of PVD
		Temperature changes more marked	Temperature changesless marked.
iv.	Angiography	minimal disease sharp cut off few collaterals	diffused disease tapered and irregular cut off collaterals well developed.

Paradoxical Embolism

It occurs when patient has got a history of heart disease, like patent foramen ovale, develops pulmonary embolism following deep vein thrombosis. Recurrent pulmonary embolism creates pulmonary hypertension. This phenomenon is called paradoxical embolism.

Peripheral arterial thrombosis

It usually occurs at the sites of underlying arterial stenosis due to various disorders like atherosclerosis, aortoarteritis, Buerger's disease etc.

Due to slow process of development of a stenotic lesion, collaterals would have developed around the stenosis and there fore in acute thrombosis patient may not present with a severe degree of ischemia.

Thrombosis of a normal artery can occur in certain hypercoaguable states like malignancy, anti phospholipids antibody (APLA) syndrome, protein C, proteins, antithrombin III deficiency, etc.

70-80% cases common sites of occlusion are branching point of arteries like femoral, brachial artery bifurcations and at the site of stenosis.
Histological changes can develop within 4 hours of warm ischemia and irreversible ischemia after 6 hours.

Cardinal Features

Remember 5 'P'.

Pulse lessness, pain ,pallor, paresthesia and paralysis and sixth P namely poikilothermia.

Treatment

A. Surgical
B. Endovascular
C. IVC filters.

A. Surgical

i. Surgical: Exploration and removal of clot by Fogarty catheter still a preferable method for arterial embolism today.
ii. Open thrombectomy with or without bypass procedure.

B. Endovascular therapy is of three types

i. Thrombolytic therapy: Usually intralesional using Urokinase, Tissue plasminogen activator inhibitor etc.
ii. Percutaneous mechanical thrombectomy like suction of clot via catheters, thrombus dissolution by pulverization and aspiration by high speed rational motors or retrograde directed fluid jets.
iii. Ultra sound accelerated thrombolysis—principal of acoustic cavitation to ablate thrombus.

But all types of thrombolysis are contraindicated in recent major bleeding, recent stroke, recent major surgery and trauma, irreversible ischemia to the end organs, intra cranial tumors and recent eye surgery, etc.

In a word, surgery is the treatment of choice for embolism, severely ischemic limb and a high risk patient.

While endovascular therapy is suitable for thrombosis in the distal vasculature with the limb not being severely ischemic.

C. IVC Filters:

It is a modern alternative to open surgical placation of the IVC in patients with contraindications to open surgery

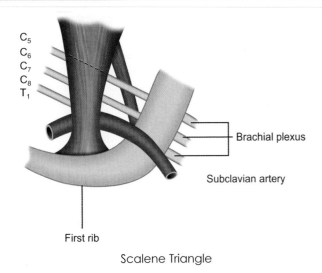

Scalene Triangle

recurrent emboli or fare chance of recurrent emboli despite anticoagulation.

Filters devices are delivered percutaneously from a femoral, jugular or antecubital vein approach.

The filters are: Temporary, removable or retrievable devices.

Infrarenal position is preferable as supra renal placement may cause vena caval occlusion of up to 20%.

THORACIC OUTLET SYNDROME (TOS)

Anatomy

- Thoracic outlet is bounded by
- Anteriorly—upper border of manubrium sterni.
- Posteriorly—superior surface of the body of 1st thoracic vertebra/spine posteriorly—on each side 1st rib with its cartilage.

Two main spaces in the thoracic outlet are:

a. Scalene triangle- most common site for nerve compression boundary—anteriorly-anterior scalene muscle, posteriorly the middle scalene muscle and inferiorly the 1st rib.
b. Costoclavicular space—bounded by:
   - Anteriorly: Clavicle and subclavius muscle.
   - Medially: Anterolateral border of the first rib.
   - Posteriorly: Scapula.
   - This is traversed by all three structures artery, vein, and nerve.

Etiology

A. Congenital
B. Acquired.

A. Congenital

i. Cervical rib 0.45 to 1.5%.
ii. Abnormal first rib.
iii. Soft tissue anomalies (myofascial bands, anomalous scalene muscle insertion).
iv. Brachial plexus anomalies (post-fixed plexus).
v. Postural-sagging shoulder heavy breast.

B. Acquired

- Fracture first rib, clavicle.
- Bony exostosis/tumor or soft tissue tumor.
- Scalene muscle injury/hypertrophy.
- Previous operations/scars.
- Dropping shoulders, etc.

SYMPTOMATOLOGY

Thoracic outlet syndrome by definition as upper extremity symptoms due to compression of neurovascular bundle in the thoracic outlet.

- Each structure may be compressed separately giving rise distinct symptoms complexes i.e. Neurogenic, venous or arterial TOS.
  Neurogenic TOS is the most common form.
I. Neurogenic TOS is the most common form of TOS.
  Age group 20-45 years.
  70% are women.

Symptoms

- Pain is the predominant symptom, pain localized to lateral aspect of arm and shoulder area, ipsilateral headache and facial pain along with it upper brachial plexus roots are involved.

  Pain in inner aspect of the arm and forearm of the ulnar nerve distribution when the lower roots are involved.

  The pain may be aggrevated by elevation of arm or along with daily activities like washing cloths, cooking etc.
- Paresthesia: compression of all nerves of brachial plexus most common.
- Headache: Occipital headaches probably due to reflected referred pain from tight scalene muscle.
- Weakness of the arms and hand is common in patients with TOS.

Investigations

- X-ray cervical spine.
- MRI and Nerve conduction studies.

Treatment

The treatment of neurogenic TOS is mainly conservative like short course of analgesic, followed by an exercise program for 6 weeks. Avoid lifting weights, hyperabducting shoulder.

Therapeutic blockade of scalene muscles using steroid, botulinum toxin has also been tried.

Surgery is reserved for the patient who fails to respond to conservative treatments and continues to be symptomatic like-
- Scalenectomy of scalenus anticus.
- Soft tissue anomalies to be corrected.

CONSERVATIVE MANAGEMENT

1. Structural exercise program:
   - Neck stretching
   - Abdominal breathing
   - Posture exercise

2. Medications:
   - Analgesics
   - Muscle relaxants
   - Anti depressants.

3. Ergonomic evaluation:
   - Avoid heavy lifting
   - Repetitive movements
   - Avoid hyperabduction

4. Physiotherapy:
   - Heat/cold application
   - Ultrasound to supraclavicular region
   - Local massage

5. Brachial plexus block.

SURGICAL MANAGEMENT

Transaxillary Excision of First Rib

The first rib is reached by blunt dissection in the axillary tunnel
↓
The subclavius muscle tendon is divided close to its attachment
↓
The scalenus medius and intercostalis muscle are pushed off the first rib
↓
T1 Nerve root is visualized and protected
↓
First rib is divided and removed

Advantages

- Super cosmetic value.
- Takes care of bony and soft tissue causes of compression.
- Adequate decompression of costoclavicular space.

Disadvantages

- Limited exposure—difficult to operate in deep surgical field.
- Radical scalenectomy is not possible.
- Removal of posterior part of the first rib may be incomplete and there is high chance of long thoracic nerve damage.
- Chance of Brachial plexus damage.

Supraclavicular Scalenectomy

Scalene pad of fat is mobilized laterally and omohyoid scalene anterior muscles are excised.
↓
Neurolysis of C8, T1 is done.
↓
Excision of scalenus minimus is done.
↓
Scalenus medius muscle is resected
↓
The first rib is cleared and excised.

Advantages

It permits good clearance of all soft anomalies as well as the osseous causes.

Combined Approach

Combined supraclavicular and transaxillary approach provides the best exposure to the upper and lower nerve roots of brachial plexus.

The Trans axillary approach is better for 1st rib excision and the supraclavicular exposure facilitates excision of soft tissue anomalies and scar.

In the combined technique the supraclavicualr scalenectomy and neurolysis done first and then trans-axillary resection of first rib is performed.

ARTERIAL TOS

- Older patient.
- Less female predominance.
- Acute/ sub acute presentation.
- Acute upper limb ischemia (pain, pallor, paresthesia, paralysis and absence of pulse) with a pulsatile supra clavicular mass/ or bruit is the classical presentation of arterial TOS.
- Sub acute presentation is painful limb, claudication, color changes, coldness in the hand.

Investigations

- Color Doppler.
- Angiography
- X-ray chest, cervical spine to detect 1st rib.

Treatment

- Severe limb ischemia- emergency.
- Surgery like thrombo embolectomy or bypass.
- Semi emergency situation patient to be given heparin first.
- Scalenectomy and cervical rib resection.
- Excision of aneurismal/ ecstatic portion of subclavian artery and restoration of continuity by suitable graft.
- Cervicodorsal sympathectomy.
- Distal thromboembolectomy or bypass surgery, etc.

III VENOUS TOS

- Young healthy males.
- Sudden onset of arm pain swelling and cyanosis.
- Usually follows by some kind of repeatitive activity like pitching a baseball, house painting, swimming, rowing a boat etc.

This is termed as "effort thrombosis syndrome"- Pain may be periodic and transient arm swelling particularly with abducted arm and hyperextended shoulders.

Investigations

- Color Doppler
- Venography
- X-ray chest, cervical spine to exclude cervical rib.

Treatment

Conservative

Rest, analgesic, heparinization/ anti coagulant etc.

Surgery

Thrombolysis by Fogarty's catheter followed by removal of offending structure.

Raynaud's Syndrome

An episode digital ischemia occurring in response to cold or emotional stress.

The syndrome is divided into two subgroups:
a. Raynaud's disease.
b. Raynaud's phenomenon.

Raynaud's Disease
The patient is with intermittent digital ischemia in the absence of an associated disease.

This is a vasospastic condition. It is seen in young females.

Raynaud's Phenomenon
Patients who manifest digital ischemia due to an underlying disease, usually a connective tissue disorder.

Etiology

- i. Primary Raynaud's disease.
- ii. Connective tissue disorders:
  - Scleroderma
  - SLE
  - Rheumatoid arthritis
  - Sjogren's syndrome
  - Mixed connective tissue disease.
- iii. Drugs:
  - Ergotamine
  - OCP
  - Cytotoxic drugs
  - Beta blocker etc
- iv. Vascular disorders:
  - Atherosclerosis, TAO (Buerger's disease)
  - Thoracic outlet syndrome (TOS).
  - Arthritis, Fibromuscular disease, etc.
- v. Occupation

- Vibration arterial injury
- Cold exposure.
vi. Others—malignancy, neurological, endocrine disorders, etc.

Clinical Features

Typical features are triphasic color changes in the fingers which usually start on cold exposure or under emotional stress.

The color changes occur in the following way-
- Stage I—stage of local syncope or stage of pallor.
- Stage II—stage of local cyanosis.
- Stage III—stage of red congestion.
- Stage IV—stage of ischemic gangrene.

Pathophysiology of COLOR Changes

Stage I (stage of local syncope/pallor):

Exposure to cold
↓
spasm of digital blood vessels.
↓
reduced blood supply to digits
↓
Pallor.

Stage II (stage of local cyanosis):

As a result of reduced blood supply to the digits.
↓
anoxia of these digits leading to accumulation of metabolites.
↓
Capillary dilatation.
↓
filled with de oxygenated blood.
↓
produces local cyanosis.

Stage III (stage of red engorgement):

Pre capillary sphincter relaxation.
↓
but post capillary sphincter still in spasm.
↓
oxygenated blood enters into dilated capillary bed.
↓

Red engorgement.
↓
As a result of repeated attack
↓
Resorption of the terminal pulp space.
↓
Tips of digits appear conical.
↓
persistent spasm of digital vessel leads to ischemic gangrene.

Diagnostic Test

Ice water immersion test and finger temperature recovery time.

Treatment

Conservative
- Main treatment is conservative for majority of patient.
- Avoid cold
- Emotional stress.
- Abstinence from tobacco.
- Wearing gloves, etc. are adequate for the majority of cases. Thermally heated gloves are better.
- Drugs - used are Nifedipine, losartan, fluoxetine, etc.

Surgery
Cervicodorsal sympathectomy - is very effective in relieving vasospasm.

Other techniques include
- Periarterial digital vasospasm.

Epidural spinal cord stimulation.
- Vibration white finger:
  Occurs in steel industry, welders, miners, and road and construction workers.
  After a variable period of exposure these tools patients develop a painful white finger on exposure to cold.
Change of profession, avoid cold, etc. are the only way of treatment.

Acrocyanosis
- Occurs due to cutaneous arterial vasospasm.
- Seen exclusively in females.
- Patients present with oedema, coldness, cyanosis of hands, feet and legs.

Diabetic Foot

My patient, Ravisankar, a 50 years old man, known diabetic, presented with complaint of ulcer in his right foot for last 4 months (Planter aspect is commonest as it is a trophic/ischemic ulcer).

He has got a history of minor trauma 4 months back and few days after that injury the ulcer developed and attained its present size.

The ulcer is spreading gradually, painlessly but there is no history of intermittent claudication and loss of sensation (Relevant negative history only).

General survey is essentially normal, no lymph adenopathy noticed in inguinopopliteal region (right).

On local examination: There is a 5 x 3 cm oval shaped ulcer at planter aspect of his right foot around the heel.
- Edge is punctate (seen both arterial and diabetic ulcer)
- Floor partly granulated, partly full of slough (or exudates and slough)
- No active discharge
- Peripheral area looks blackish, unhealthy.

On Palpation

- Ulcer: Peripheral temperature not raised, mild tenderness
- Inspectory findings are confirmed base of the ulcer indurated, Bony tenderness+, not fixed to under lying structure.
- No bleeding on touch.
- No popliteal and inguinal lymphadenopathy noticed.
- To exclude vasculopathy: Popliteal artery (right) well palpable, anterior tibial pulsation++, post-tibial + artery dorsalispedis+
- To exclude neuropathy: No sensory or motor deficit noticed.
- To exclude arthropathy: No bony deformity is there as such.
- Systemic examination is essentially normal.

So my diagnosis is:
This is a case of diabetic foot right without any obvious complications.

What do you mean by diabetic foot?

Diabetic foot is a syndrome complex involving pain, deformity, inflammation, infection, ulceration and tissue loss of the foot in diabetic patients.

How you will proceed in this case?

I will do:
- Complete hemogram to exclude infection
- Blood for sugar [fasting and post prandial]
- Urine for sugar and ketone body
- Wound discharge for culture/sensitivity
- X-ray foot to exclude features of chronic osteomyelitis (Feature of chronic osteomyelitis are dead bone, (sequestrum), Bony rarefaction surrounded by dense sclerosis and involucrum)
- X-ray chest-[Especially in tubercular and malignant ulcer]
- Color Doppler flow imaging (CDFI)—to exclude vasculopathy. It is not done routinely. It is indicated when clinically vasculopathy is suspected.

What is the role of CT/MRI scan in diabetic foot?

CT scan may be indicated in the assessment of suspected bone and joint pathology not evident of plain radiographs. It offers high anatomic detail and resolution of bone with osseous fragmentation and joint subluxation may be well visualized.

MRI is used in evaluating soft tissue and bone pathology. The scan may be indicated to aid in the diagnosis of osteomyelitis, deep abscess, septic joint, tendon rupture etc. It is highly sensitive for bone infection and it is helpful for surgical planning, despite of its cost,

MRI has gained wide acceptance in the management of diabetic foot infection.

Can you tell me briefly what the pathology behind diabetic ulcer is?

There are three factors play role to produce diabetic ulcer
1. Diabetic neuropathy
2. Diabetic atherosclerosis causing ischemia and
3. Vulnerable glucose laden tissue which is more prone to develop infection and ulcer is due to neuropathy- a trophic ulcer results

When the ulcer is due to ischemia, an ischemic (arterial) ulcer results. But it is relatively less painful than typical arterial ulcer.

Wedge biopsy is required in diabetic ulcer?

Not every case. Wedge biopsy is required but when malignant ulcer is suspected, like irregular, rolled out everted edges, bleeding on touch, etc. then wedge biopsy is to be done to exclude malignant ulcer.

When do you say the patient having sensory neuropathy?

Sensory neuropathy is said to exist when 4 out of 10 sites show absence of sensation when the pin/ware is pressed against the skin. The points of testing are planter aspect of 1st, 3rd and 5th digits, the planter aspect of 1st, 3rd and 5th metatarsal heads, planter aspect of mid-foot medially, dorsally and the planter aspect of heel. Total 10 sites.

What are all will you advice to prevent diabetic foot ulcer?

To prevent ulcer formation and lower extremity amputation in patient with diabetic following protocol to be followed.
*   First and foremost thing to control sugar levels to reduce development of neuropathy and to maintain immunologic function in patient with diabetics.
*   Avoid any risk of foot injury.
*   Any foot lesion should be assessed for infection, debride devitalized tissues and x ray foot to look for foreign body, soft tissue gas and bony abnormalities.
*   Poorly designed and ill fitting shoes to be avoided.

Tissue load management- Create some environment, that enhances soft tissue viability and promotes healing of the pressure ulcer, including proper positioning of the patient, move the patient at least once in an hour.

What all you examine in a case of diabetic foot?

Diagnosis of Diabetic foot must identify and assess all elements of the pathophysiology namely-Vasculopathy, neuropathy, osteopathy and infections etc.

Assessment of diabetic foot:

1. Examination of the foot; staging of foot (Wagner classification) by examining infection-ulcer-skin changes-callus-gangrene-foot deformities etc.

2. Neurologic Examination:
    *   Tendon reflexes
    *   Vibration test
    *   Sensation test [Pain, Touch, Temperature.]
    *   Biothesiometry

3. Vascular examination:
    *   Distal pulses
    *   Ankle Brachial Index
    *   Duplex arterial study of leg
    *   Trans cutaneous oxygen saturation

4. look for infection:
    *   Superficial
*   Deep
    *   Osteomyelitis

How will you treat diabetic foot?

First and foremost- good control of diabetes mellitus
*   **Eliminate infection:** Augmentin is a good broad spectrum antibiotic and then Switch over the antibiotics as per culture sensitivity. Other measures include, removal of infected bone, drainage of abscess etc.

Debridement:

Autolytic: Autolysis uses the body's own enzymes and moisture to re-hydrate and provide absorption, desloughing and debriding to necrotic and fibrotic tissues.

Enzymatic: Tunnelling ulcer is particularly suitable for the products like collagen, protein, fibrin, elastin, etc. as they remove debris.

Mechanical: It allows the ulcer to proceed moist to dry and removal of dressing cause non selective debridement.

Surgical: Sharp surgical and laser debridement under anaesthesia is the fastest method of debridement.

Other adjunct techniques are:-
* H_2O_2, povidone iodine, should not be used as they delay wound healing. Growth factors like human fibroblast, bioengineered skin grafts are used to augment wound healing.
*   Hyperbaric O_2 (HBO): Hyperbaric Oxygen therapy provides a significant increase in tissue oxygenation which influences collagen deposition, angiogenesis and bacterial clearance from the wound; thereby wound healing will be faster.

- **Ultrasound:** It causes degranulation of mast cells resulting in release of histamine- promote healing accelerate wound contraction, increase tensile strength of healing tissue.
- **Whirlpool treatment:** Water temperature range from 33.3° to 33.5° C which is to administer thrice daily vasodilatation causing softening and loosening of necrotic tissue, wound cleaning, exudates removal and reduced infection.

- Disadvantages are skin maceration and wound break down. Hence, it is condemned.

What is the role of Surgery in a diabetic foot?

Other than debridement, drainage of abscess, excision of infected bone and amputation if required.

Revascularization and free flap for extensive tissue loss are important aspects.

SHORT NOTE ON DIABETIC FOOT

Diabetic foot by definition: It is a syndrome complex involving pain, deformity, inflammation, ulceration and tissue loss of the foot in diabetic patients.

Epidemiology

Diabetic foot ulcer and infections are very common in lay man and incidence is 15-20 % ie 15-20% of diabetic develop foot ulcers and infection.

You know presently India have more than 30 million of diabetics.

Unfortunately, diabetic foot infection is more common in India due to bare foot walking, lack of health care facilities, poverty etc.

Atherosclerosis is few folds greater in diabetes. So, the number of diabetics presenting to vascular clinic with ischemia and infection.

Patho Physiology

The important pathogenic factions for diabetic foot ulcer are:-

- Neuropathy
- Vasculopathy
- Hyperglycemia
- Infections
- Injury

33% of diabetic foot ulcerations are neuropathic, 33% are ischemia and 34 % are of mixed in nature.

Neuropathy

Neuropathy is either Sensory,

- Motor or
- Autonomic.

Sensory neuropathy leads to an insensitive foot with tendency to injury as patient does not have pain sensation or lack of pain sensation.

Motor neuropathy: Causes wasting of small muscles of foot. Resultant foot deformity due to unopposed action of long flexors/extensors, deformities like clamming of toes and bunions occur, these deformities produce elevated pressure at metatarsal heads/tips of toes etc. With more severe deformity like charkot's neuro arthropathy, risk of infection increases.

Autonomic neuropathy produces ulcer/crack/fissure.

Vasculopathy

Diabetics have both micro vascular and macro vascular disease and atherosclerosis is accelerated in diabetes.

Micro circulatory changes cause impairment of cellular exchange and macrovascular disease causes reduction in amount and reduction of blood flow reaching extremity. So that foot in diabetic is more susceptible to changes in perfusion. Infra genicular muscle like Posterior Tibial, Anterior Tibial, peroneal are more often severely affected.

Any deficient with diabetic foot ulcer or infection with feeble or non palpable distal pulses to be considered to have significant vascular disease.

Hyperglycemias

Hyperglycemia affects host immunologic defences. Granulocyte adherence, chemo taxis, phagocytosis and bacterial function is impaired with hyperglycemia. Thereby glucose laden tissues are more prone to develop infection.

Infections

The spectrum of foot infections in diabetes ranges from simple superficial cellulitos to chronic osteomyelitis. Infections of diabetic patients are difficult to treat because of impaired micro vascular circulation which limits the access of phagocytic cells to the infected area and results in a poor concentration of antibiotics in the infected tissues.

For this reasons cellulitis is the most treatable and reversible form of foot infection in diabetic patients. Deep skin and soft tissue infections also result in substantial long term morbidity.

Patients can have a combine infection involving bone and soft tissue called fetid foot. The extensive soft tissue and bone infection, if chronic, and usually requires extensive surgical debridement and even amputation.

Identification of organism needs culture of the wound. The organisms for mild to moderate infections are surface staphylococcus aureus and streptococci.

More severe infections are due to polymicrobial including aerobic gram positive cocci (staph and streptococci) Aerobic gram negative rods (like-E-coli, Klebsiella, Pseudomonas and proteus) and anaerobes (like bactericide, Depot streptococci and proteolla etc) .

Injury: Mechanical stress is the precipitator of ulceration in both neuropathic and ischemic foot. The most common sites are the curve of 1st and 5th metatarsal heads. The sole of the foot has a relatively good blood supply and not to ulcerate early. In neuropathic foot ulceration precipitated by direct high pressure injury or gradually through repetitive stress develop under metatarsal heads and heel. Subcutaneous tissue trapped between bone and thick unpliable skin producing high shear forces, leading to sterile deep haematoma.

The deep ulcer then tracks to the skin leading to sinus tract or ulcer.

Charcot foot or neuro arthopathy is a rare outcome seen in diabetics following the action of various factors mainly neuropathy. This is described as a chronic painless degenerative process affecting the weight bearing joints of the foot. Only 1% diabetics are seen with charcots's foot. Other common morphologic changes in foot structure include bony dislocation and collapse of the arch, etc. Anatomic derangement continues the cycle of abnormal weight bearing excessive pressure and ulceration.

DESCRIPTION OF ULCERS

Neuropathic ulcer- Under metatarsal head surrounded by thick hyperkeratosis, pink punched out base, readily bleeds, painless.

Ischemic Ulcer: not surrounded by hyperkeratosis, dull fibrotic base, does not bleed easily and painful to touch.

Infection with ulcer - Surrounding cellulitis, discharge, erythema, and limb threatening infection can be defined by cellulitis extending beyond 2cm from the ulcer margin, as well as deep abscess, osteomyelilits and critical ischemia.

Examination of the Patients

Vascular Examination to Exclude Vasculopathy

Palpation of pulses- dorsalis pedis, posterior tibial, popliteal, femoral.

Absence of pedal pulses in the presence of a palpable popliteal pulse is a classic finding in diabetic arterial disease because of the selective involvement of tibial artery below of the knee
- Venous filling time (normal<10 sec)
- Capillary filling time (normal <3 sec)
- Colour changes, look for signs of ischemia, oedema, etc.

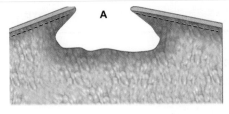

Undermined Edge Seen in Tuberculosis, Amoebic Ulcer, Pressure Necrosis, etc

Punched Out Edge Seen in Syphilis, Trophic, DM, Leprosy, Ischemic Arterial Ulcer.

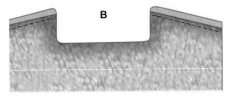

Sloping Edge Seen in Venous and Traumatic Ulcer

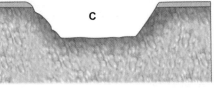

Raised and Pearly-White Bearded Edge Seen in Rodent Ulcer.

Rolled Out (Everted) Edge Typically seen in Squamous Cell Carcinoma.

Diagrams of different types of edges of ulcers

Neurologic Exmination-to Exclude Neuropathy

- Vibration perception
- Light touch
- Two poin discrimination
- Pin prick sensation
- Temperature perception-hot/cold
- Deep tendon reflexes.

Musculo skeletal Examination-to Exclude Osteoarthopathy

Orthopaedic deformity: Hammertoes, bunion, Tailor's funions, flat or arched feet, Charcot deformities, iatrogenic deformities, limited joint mobility, tendo-achilles contracture/eqinus.

- muscle group strength-passive, active.
- planter pressure assessment.

Ulcer Classification

Wagner classification

Grade	Clinical Features
Grade 0	Normal foot but foot at risk. Various degree of neuropathy, joint deformity etc.
Grade 1	Superficial ulcer, cellulitis
Grade 2	Deep ulcer-uncomplicated, may produce osteitis.
Grade 3	Deep ulcer-complicated including deep infection, osteomyelitis and abscess.
Grade 4	Limited necrotising gangrene (digital/planter/heel)
Grade 5	Extensive gangrene.

POINTS TO REMEMBER

- Avoid aminoglycosides in treatment of diabetic patients as it is nephrotoxic
- Avoid fluoroquinolones alone, as they don't have coverge in anaerobes and many gram positive micro organisms
- prolong course of antibiotics are needed in many cases of infection in diabetic foot. (6-8 weeks)
- Osteomyelitis of foot bones can be cured or arrested by minimum debridement followed by prolonged courses of antibiotic therapy (6-8 weeks)
- Infected diabetic foot dressings need to be changed thrice daily.
- Topical application of iodine preparations, astringents, hydrogen peroxide cause damage to the tissue and should be avoided.

- There is no place for foot soaks, whirlpool therapy, pressure cleaning of wounds. These lead to skin maceration and wound breakdown and hence are condemned.
- Topical antibiotics may help to reduce bacterial load and acts as a barrier to exogenous pathogens but remember they also have disadvantages of causing emergence of resistant organisms.
- A variety of dressing materials are available like hydrocolloids, alginates, hydrogels etc suitable dressing with these agents in a moist environment heal the wound faster.
- Antibiotics to be given after suitable specimen have been obtained for culture.

    It mild infection-oral regime of a broad spectrum antibiotics like augmentin (Amoxycillin + clauvilunic acid) or clindamycin alone is sufficient.

For limb threatening infection

Ampicillin + sulbactum or piperacillin + Tazobactam or clindamycin + fluoro qunolons can be initial empiric therapy.

For life threatening infections

Imipenem + cilastin + vancomycin may be suitable.

    Remember that a diabetic may not manifest any indicative symptoms if the patient has neuropathy.

Rocker bottom: High risk diabetic foot patient with foot deformity needs a foot wear extra soft accomodative one that moulds the foot shape while allowing enough space for to movement.

    The sole may need to have recessed heel along with angulation of the sole just behind the metatarsal heads so that a rolling motion is obtained during walking like a rocker bottom.

My patient Surender Singh, 45 years old, farmer, resident of Rajasthan, presented with a non healing ulcer in the left leg for last 4 months.

He had a history of trauma at his lower part of left leg 4 months back while he was working at the field. Within a few days of trauma, the ulcer started along with fever for few days. The ulcer was initially just a papule-pustule type increasing in size for 1 month; thereafter it has remained stationary. It is a considerable and it is accompanied by serosanguineous discharge.

On examination: General survey is essentially normal.

On Local Examination

- An ulcer at the medial side of lower part of leg just above the ankle. The ulcer is 5 × 4 cm in size.
- The edge may be undermined, punched out or slightly raised.
- Copious serosanguineous discharge is there.
- The ulcer appears indolent and refusing to heal.
- Floor of the ulcer is partly full of granulation tissue, partly slough.
- The surrounding skin appears normal. Sensation is normal.
- No bleed on touch and base of the ulcer is not indurated.
- All peripheral pulses are palpable.
- Two left inguinal lymph nodes enlarged, firm and tender. Systemic examinations are essentially normal.
    So this is a case of tropic ulcer at the lower part of left leg in a 45 years old farmer.

What is tropic ulcer?

It is a type of ulcer caused by Vincent's bacterial infection (Bacteroides Fusiformis and Borrelia Vincenti) commonly seen in tropical country.

What are the most characteristic features of trophic ulcer?

- The ulcer starts from a small abrasion as a result of trauma or even after an insect bite.

- The lesion commences as a papule pustule with a zone of surrounding inflammation and induration.
- Considerable pain is accompanied this ulcer.
- The most characteristic feature of this ulcer is after a certain time the ulcer becomes indolent and refuses to heal for months, even years.
- It heals after a long period, leaving a parchment like pigment scar.

What is trophic ulcer then?

It is neurogenic ulcer. This ulcer results from repeated trauma to the insensitive part of the body. So some neurological deficiency in the form of loss of sensation is the cause behind the ulcer formation.

What are the common sites of trophic ulcer?

In ambulatory patient heel and ball of foot and in nonambulatory patient buttock and back of heel are the common sites.

Bed sore and perforating ulcers are the typical examples of trophic ulcer.

What are the causes of Trophic (Neurogenic/Neuropathic) ulcer?

Any form of neuropathy like diabetic neuropathy, leprosy, peripheral, vitamin deficiency, nerve injury neuropathy, ischemic neuropathy are the causes of trophic ulcer.

How will you describe a trophic ulcer?

The trophic ulcer starts with callosity under which suppuration takes place. The pus comes out and the central hole forms the ulcer which gradually burrows through the muscles and tendon and reaches to the bone. So it is called perforating ulcer.

This is a painless callous ulcer and edge is punched out and corny. Floor is covered with offensive slough. Tendons, even bone can be seen and definitely base will be slightly indurated or hardy as bone is underlying.

So surroundings skin has no sensation.

Why the trophic ulcer has punched out edge?

Trophic or neurogenic ulcer is a kind of arterial ulcer. The punch out edges are the result of thrombosis of the end artery at the base causing sloughing and necrosis of the portion supplied by the artery.

What are the types of trophic ulcer?

Trophic ulcers are two types:
- Arterial ulcer.
- Neurogenic ulcer.

What are the characteristics of arterial ulcer?

- Seen in old people.
- Cause is inadequate blood supply to the tissues are skin. So mostly found in atherosclerosis.
- Common sites are anterolateral aspects of leg, toes, dorsum and sole and heel which are subjected to repeated pressure and trauma.
- There may be a history of claudication and the ulcer is painful. Peripheral arterial pulses either diminished or it may be absent.
- The ulcer has punch out edges with slough in the floor.

What are the characteristics of neurogenic ulcer?

- Causes are repeated trauma or pressure in an area which has absent sensation.
- These ulcers present in the patients of diabetic neuritis, peripheral nerve injury, spina bifida, leprosy, tabes dorsalis, syringomyelia. Bed sores and perforating ulcers are the examples of neurogenic ulcer.
- The trophic ulcer starts with callosity under which suppuration takes place. The pus comes out and the central hole forms the ulcer which gradually burrows through the muscles and tendon and reaches to the bone. So it is called perforating ulcer.
- Neurological examination will reveal diminished or absent sensation but peripheral pulses are well palpable.
- Ulcer may have punched out edges with sloughing the floor.

How will you investigate an ulcer?

- Study of discharge for culture sensitivity, cytology, AFB study.
- Edge biopsy. Minimum two biopsies are taken from the edges to exclude any malignant transformation.
- X-ray of the affected part to exclude underlying bone involvement.
- Color Doppler to exclude arterial / venous disease.
- Hemogram. Hb% should be > 10 gm %.
- Blood sugar, lipid profile etc.

What are the aims of management of an ulcer?

Aims of ulcer management are:
- Cause should be found and treated correctly.
- Correction of malnutrition, anaemia, protein deficiency.
- Control of pain.
- Heal the ulcer as soon as possible and the affected part will be made as normal as possible.

How will you take care of an ulcer?

Ulcer to be cared by control of infections:
- Debridement
- Cleaning.
- Dressing.
- Control of infection by giving broad spectrum antibiotics as per culture sensitivity report.

Topical antibiotics application like framycetin, silver sulfadiazine, mupirocin, etc.

Debridement—removal of devitalized tissue all dead, devitalized and necrosed. Tissue is to be removed regularly.

Ulcer cleaning—regular cleaning of ulcer, after separation of slough, to be done by using dilute providone iodine and normal saline. Twice daily dressing is always preferable.

Dressing of ulcer is very important aspect of ulcer management.

Aim of dressing are:
- To keep the ulcer moist.
- To keep surrounding skin dry.
- To reduce pain.
- To protect the wound.
- To soothen the tissue.
- Absorbent for the discharge.
- To make the healing process faster.

What are the different types of dressing available for ulcer dressings?

- Cotton dressing for burns ulcer.
- Paraffin dressing for skin graft harvest site.
- Polyurethane and hydrogel dressing used for heavy exudates in ulcer.
- Type I collagen dressings- causes' hemostasis, proliferation of fibroblasts, improvement of blood supply.
- Foam dressings- highly absorbent, decrease wound maceration.
- Hydrocolloid dressings for separation of slough and autolysis of dead tissues.
- Transparent film dressings are water proof, permit O_2 and water vapor across if and prevents contamination.

Trophic ulcer is a penetrating ulcer. In sole which are the layers it penetrates?

There are four layers in sole:

- First later:
  - Flexor digitorum brevis.
  - Abductor hallucis.
  - Abductor digiti minimi.
- Second layer:
  - Tendon of flexor hallucis longus.
  - Tensor of flexor digitorum longus.
  - Flexor accessories.
  - Lumbrical muscles.
- Third layer:
  - Flexor hallucis brevis.
  - Adductor hallucis.
  - Flexor digiti minimi brevis.
- Fourth layer:
  - interosseous muscles.

– Tendon of peroneus longus.
– Tendon of tibialis posterior.

What are the different types of edges in various ulcers?

1. **Undermined edges:** Seen in tuberculosis, pressure necrosis, carbuncle ulcer, etc.
   Mechanism: The disease spread and destroys the subcutaneous tissue faster than skin. Here, the skin overhangs and forms the undermined edges.
2. **Punch out edge:** Seen in gummatous ulcer of syphilis, trophic ulcer i.e. in both neurogenic and arterial ulcer, (ischemic ulcer), diabetic ulcer, leprotic ulcer, etc.
   Pathology: The disease usually does not spread to surrounding tissue. The edge drops down at right angle to the skin surface and appears like a cut out with a punch.
3. **Slopping edge:** Seen in Traumatic ulcer, venous ulcer and non specific healing ulcer.
   Pathology: When ulcer starts healing, new healthy epithelium gradually fills up the raw area and slopping edge appears as a result.

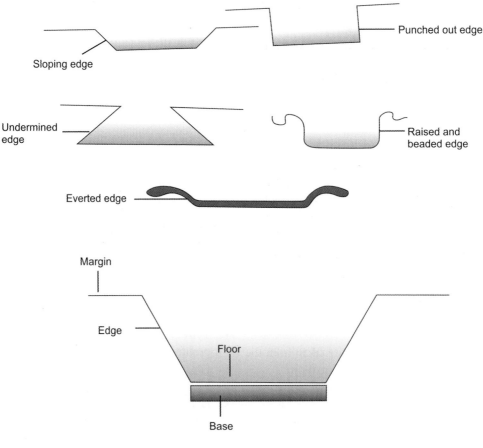

Different edges of ulcers

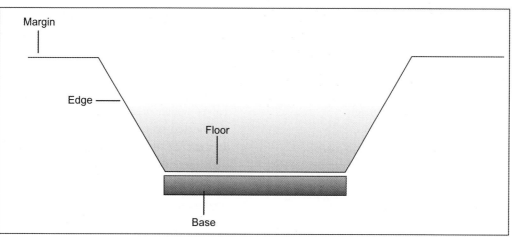

Different parts of an ulcer

4. **Everted (rolled out) Edge:** Characteristically seen in squamous cell carcinoma.

Pathology: In first growing cellular disease, the proliferating malignant tissues heap up and spills over the normal skin, results in an everted edge.

5. **Raised and beaded (Rarely white):** Seen typically in basal cell carcinoma (Rodent ulcer).

5. **Raised, pearly white and Beaded edges** typically seen in basal cell carcinoma.

Pathology: The cellular disease is invasive and becomes necrotic at the centre. Beads are due to proliferating active cells.

What the parts of an ulcer?

1. **Margin:** Is the junction between normal epithelium and the ulcer.

2. **Edge:** Is the area between the margin and the floor of the ulcer.

3. **Floor:** Is the exposed surface of the ulcer. If the floor is covered with red granulation tissue, it seems to be healthy and thereby it's on the process of healing.

4. **Base:** On which the ulcer rests and it is to be felt, on palpation.

[Remember in your house, you can see the floor but can not see the base of the floor like an ulcer]

What are the signs of healing?

Edge becomes more slopping with the bluish epithelium extending gradually from margin to floor of ulcer and covers it up.

There will be three demarcated zones:
  i. Red/pin zone—infinity for healthy granulation tissue.
  ii. Blue zone—for thin-growing epithelium.
  iii. White zone—for fibrosis of the scar in surrounding skin.

Floor contains smooth and even red granulation tissue covered by a single layer of epithelium discharge merely serous.

Base is free.

How will you classify ulcer clinically?

Clinically ulcer is either of three types:

1. **Spreading ulcer:** Edge of the ulcer is inflamed and edematous. Floor may be full of offensive slough. Ulcer is painful and enlarged lymph nodes are tender.

2. **Healing ulcer:** Edge is sloping with healthy pink/ red healthy granulation tissue with serous discharge. Margin is bluish with growing epithelium.

3. **Callous or chronic ulcer:** Edge is indurated with surrounding skin. Floor is covered with pale granulation tissue and ulcer does not show any tendency to heal.

How will you define ulcer?

An ulcer is the break of continuity of the covering epithelium either in mucosa or skin, due to molecular death.

Notes on Martorell's ulcer?

• It is also called hypertensive ulcer as it is seen in hypertensive patient often with atherosclerosis.
• It is commonly seen in calf; often Bilateral and painful.
• There is sudden obliteration of the arterioles of calf skin.

- Necrosis of calf skin with sloughing away results in formation of deep, punch out ulcers into deep fascia.
- It takes months to heal. Peripheral pulses are normal usually.

Treatment

When ulcer granulates, skin grafting is done. Lumber sympathectomy may relieve pain ultimately.

Know about:
- Venous ulcer described in varicose vein case
- Marjolin's ulcer described in post burns contracture case.
- Diabetic ulcer described in diabetic foot case.
- Tuberculous ulcer in cervical lymphadenopathy case.

Diabetic Ulcer

- Commonest site—foot, planter aspect. Others leg, upper limb, back etc.
- It has got the features of trophic ulcer as because the diabetic ulcer is due to neuropathy and/or ischemia.
- It is usually spreading and deep.
- Causes are diabetic neuropathy, diabetic atherosclerosis leading ischemia and glucose laden tissue is quite vulnerable to infection.

Bazin's ulcer (Erythrocyanosis frigida)

- Also called erythema induratum.
- Adolescent girls are affected exclusively.
- The ulcer forms as a result of localized area of fat necrosis.
- Symmetrical purple nodules develop in the ankles and calves which break down forming indolent ulcer with pigmented scars.
- It may be due to tuberculosis and treatment is antitubercular drugs. Sympathectomy is ultimate option.

Meleney's ulcer

- Seen commonly in post operative wounds.
- It is rapidly spreading ulcer with destruction of skin and subcutaneous tissues.
- Common in old age and immunocompromised individuals and surgery for infected cases.
- Common sites are abdomen and thorax.
- End arteritis of the skin leading to ulcer.
- Treatment: Adequate excision, antibiotics, Nutrition, raise haemoglobin etc. ultimately split skin graft.

My patient, Rajnish a 45 years old male presented with—an ulcer over his amputated stump in his left lower limb since last 8 months.

My patient met a Road traffic accident one year back and due to crush injury lower limb underwent below knee amputation, On rehabilitation he started using prostheses and the stump develops ulcer for last 6 month, where the prosthesis was fitted.

But no history of pain in the ulcer. The ulcer is gradually progressing and attended its present size approximate 5 × 4 cm without any history of left inguinal lymph nodal swellings.

General survey is essentially normal except the patient is looking anaemic

On Local Examination

There is a 5 × 4 cm ulcer over the amputed stump thick discharge is there but scanty.
- Margin is indurated. Sourrounding skin is also indurated.
- Edges punch out, mildly inflamed
- Floor is covered with pale, smooth granulation ties (or may be full of slough)
  On palpation base slight induratin is there not fixed to underlying bone non tender and does not bleed on touch surrounding skin is indurated, non tender
  No inguinal lymphadenopathy palpable.
  So, this is a case of Amputated stump with non healing ulcer of left lower limb.

What kind of ulcers this may be?

Sir,
It may be a simple trophic ulcer or may be a marjolin's ulcer.

Why are you saying so?

Trophic ulcer as the ulcer is most probably due to pressure necrosis caused by the ill fitted prosthesis used.

Mechanism: It is due to undue pressure on the stump, there may be compromization of vascularity which it self can cause this ulcer and or it may induce ischemic neuropathy these are leading to this ulcer.

Punch out edge also in favor of trophic ulcer.

Marjolin's Ulcer

As it occurred over the scar of amputated stump and there was a chronic irritation due to the prosthesis, it is slow growing painless as scar does not contain nerves.

It is an indurated, non tender ulcer-edge of the marjolin's ulcer is not always raised and everted.

How will you confirm which type of ulcer this one?

Sir, it will do wedge biopsy from the margin of the ulcer.

Marjolin ulcer is a well differentiated squamous cell carcinoma; usually lower grade.

Why you are telling it as a non healing ulcer?

This ulcers shown the features of chronic or callous ulcer as the:
- Ulcer shows no tendency towards healing for last 6 months.
- Margin and sourrounding skin is indurated, nontender
- Edge is mildly odentous, punchout
- Floor is covered with smooth pale granulation tissue
- Discharge from the floor is slanty.

What are the causes of this type of chronic ulcer?

- Persistent irritation or trauma to the ulcer site
- Malnutrition Anemia peripheral vascular disease due to Atherosclerosis
- Peripheral neuropathy diabetes
- Lack of care to the ulcer, etc.
- Recurrent infection—Malignancy
- Periostitis or osteomyelitis of under lying bone, etc.

How will you manage this case?

Sir, firstly I will rule out marjolin ulcer doing wedge biopsy.

I will do the culture sensitivity test. From the discharge and I will control infection by giving suitable antibiotics.

- Blood sugar. Sugar to be controlled if any. If it is Marjolin's ulcer.
- X-ray of the part to exclude bone involvement.

I will do wide local excision and flap cover to make the contour of the stump.

If it is only a trophic ulcer I will do regular:

- Debridement
- Wound cleaning, and
- Dressings types collagen
- Pulse full, painless and pain head appearance

And when the healthy (red/pink) granulation tissue appears I will flap cover if not possible I will do skin grafting.

[5 P's for granulation tissues. Pink, punctuate hemorrhage, pulseful, painless, pin head granulation]

Why the dressing is with collagen granules?

Sir, dressing with

Type I collagen causes—hemostasis

- Proliferation of fibroblast
- Improvement of blood supply and
- Thereby promotes healing.

How will you manage the patient postoperatively?

- Proper case of the flap
- Regular cleaning to prevent infection
- Proper nutrition and blood transfusion to keep the hemoglobin > 10 gm minimum.
- General care of the patient.
  Coming to amputation.

What are the indications for amputation?

In a ward, dead, deadly and dead loss, limbs are indicated for amputation.

- Dead limb like
  - Developed dry gangrene in limb
- Deadly limb like
  - Wet gangrene, gas gangrene
  - Spreading cellulitis/severe sepsis
  - Arteriovenous fistula
  - Malignancy—Osteosarcoma, melanoma, etc.
- 'Dead loss' limb like
  - Severe rest pain
  - Paralysis

- Severe trauma like crush injury
- Contracture

What is gangrene and what is pregangrene?

Pre-gangrene

- When by any reason, blood supply is inadequate to keep the tissue alive. There with a sequential changes in the tissue and patient presents with:
- Rest pain
- Color changes
- Edema
- Hyperesthesia

With or without ischemic ulcer. But gangrene is microscopy, death of the tissue with or without putrefaction.

What are the types of gangrene?

There are three types of gangrene:

1. Dry gangrene—the gangrene is dry, desiccated, mummified tissue.
   - Caused by gradual slowing of blood stream
   - It is localized and line of demarcation is marked
2. Wet gangrene
   - Spreads proximally from distal part
   - Rapidly progressing
   - No line of demarcation
   - Caused by sudden occlusion of vessel with or without infection and putrefaction.
3. Gas gangrene
   - Caused by clostridium perfringens
   - On phonation crepitus may be present.

How will you manage gangrene?

- Prevention of further development of gangrene by adequate debridement:
  - wound irrigation with hydrogen peroxide, betadine, and normal saline, etc.
  - Prophylactic injection penicillin in adequate dose.
- Curative—Redical debridement if muscle is involved and ultimate option is amputating.

What are the criteria's for ideal stump?

- Healing should be adequate and conical bearing
- Contour of the stump should be gentle, rounded with adequate muscle padding
- Should have adequate length to bear prosthesis
- Should have thin scar which should not interfere with prosthetic function
- Stump should be healthy with adequate blood supply
- Should have adequate joint movement

What should be the ideal length of amputated limb to bear prosthesis?

A. Lower limbs
- For below knee amputation length should be 8 to 15 cm from tibial tuberosity.
- For above knee the length should be 15 to 30 cm from tip of the greater trochanter
B. Upper limbs
  For above and below elbow ideal length of amputated limb is 20 cm.

What are the criterias for conical bearing stumps?

In conical bearing stump:
- There should be no projectile bone, no neuroma
- Stump is myoplastic
- Scar should be thin and non tender
- Proximal joint should have adequate mobility.

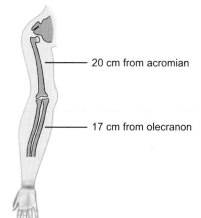

20 cm from acromian

17 cm from olecranon

Ideal levels of amputation upper limb

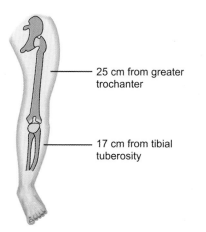

25 cm from greater trochanter

17 cm from tibial tuberosity

Ideal levels of amputation lower limb

What are the types of flaps in knee amputation?

In below knee amputation only posterior flap long posterior flap is marked out and should be of a length 1.5 times the diameter of the leg.

In above knee amputation equal anterior and posterior myocutaneous flaps or with an unequal flaps with a longer anterior flap.

What is 'Skew' flap?

Skew flap is a variation of standard flap technique of below knee amputation; here skin and muscle flaps are fashioned separately. Equal skin flaps are based on the blood supply of the skin.

The flap is related to the venous drainage of long and short saphenous veins and blood supply relies on collateral vessels.

What are the most common indications of above and below knee amputation?

The most common indications of above knee amputation are ischemia and trauma and below knee amputation is peripheral artery occlusive disease (below knee amputations also known as burgess amputation).

What are the types of amputation?

1. –Cone bearing
   –End bearing
2. –Weightbearing
   –Nonweightbearing.

What are the prerequisites to be fulfilled before amputation?

- Evaluate the patient clinically and radiologically, i.e. color Doppler to be done to confirm the need of amputation and level of amputation.
- Prophylactic antibiotics to prevent infection or antibiotics to control suspected infection. Blood transfusion to maintain Hb% above 10 gm%
- Informed written consent must be taken before performing amputation.

Know about few important amputations

- Below knee amputation (Burgess amputation) long posterior flap with scar placement over anterior aspect, prosthetics placement is better with greater range of movements.
- Above knee amputation - Here equal anterior and posterior flaps or with an unequal flap with longer anterior flap

- Syme's amputation
  This is a classical ankle amputation Removal of foot with Calcaneum and cutting of tibia and fibula just above the ankle joint with the dissection of the calcaneum out of the heel flap.
  The incision starts below the tip of the lateral malleolus and is drawn across the sole to a point 2 cm below the medial malleolus. The two ends of the incision are then joined by the shortest route across the front of the ankle joint

Pirogoff's modification - the posterior part of the calcaneum is retained in the heel flap and is opposed to the sawn surface of tibia. So length of the stump is increased here.

- **Gritti stokes amputation:** An amputation through knee. Here the long anterior flap extends down to the patella tendon insertion which is divided and the knee joint entered. A transcondylar amputation where - femur is transacted at an angle to give superior early stability.
- **Ray Amputation:** The most common amputation in the foot. Affected toe with the distal half or head of the associated metatarsal amputation. And in hand, affected finger with distal half or head of metacarpal amputation.
- **Krukenberg amputation:**
  Forearm amputation is done along with a gap between radius and ulna like a claw to have a hold or grip.
- **Guillotine amputation:**
  It is done in emergency condition with sepsis without suturing all tissue and bone is divided at the same level. Suturing done in later period.

What will you advise in post operative period after amputation?

In post amputation period
- Physiotherapy to be started as early as possible post operatively

- Regular aseptic dressing.
- After 3 months suitable prosthesis placed. Before that crutch is used
- Reassurance and Rehabilitation is important
- [prosthesis is the substitution to the part of the body to achieve its optimum function]

What are the complications of amputation?

Early complications are
- Hemorrhage : Primary - Reactionary
- Hematoma, infection etc.

Late complications
- Pain it may be phantom
- Stump ulcer, marjolin's ulcer
- Flap necrosis, painful scar
- Phantom limb- feeling of amputated Portion Toto or part of it with pain over it. Control of pain prior to amputation reduces the chance of developing phantom Limb/ phantom pain analgesics, re-assurance and rehabilitation are the treatment.

Prosthesis
- is used to recover the function of the limb at the most.
- cosmetically it looks near normal

Example of prosthesis

For Below knee amputation - patellar tendon bearing prosthesis (PTB) and solid ankle cushion heel (SACH)

For above knee amputation, suction type prosthesis is used it is placed above the stump, so well tolerated.

Internal prosthesis - the name itself suggests the prosthesis is placed internally by open surgery. Example hip prosthesis in total hip replacement. The prosthesis material should be non reactive and long durable one.

CASE 40

Peripheral Nerve Injury

RADIAL NERVE INJURY

My patient, Mahendra, a 30 years old male presented with complain of inability to elevate his right wrist following removal of plaster for his arm bone fracture for last 1 month.

He also complains of inability to elevate his fingers of the hand.

He sustained an injury in his right arm 2 and ½ months back following a fall from height. After removal of plaster he noticed this abnormality. He underwent open reduction for the fracture.

On Examination

General survey is essentially normal.

On Local Examination

There is right sided wrist drop, i.e. flexion of the wrist joint and metacarpophalangeal joints of right hand.

Wasting of muscles at extensor aspect of the forearm comparing to left side on palpation.

There is a scar in the lateral aspect of right arm

On Palpation

- Patient himself cannot extend the wrist, thumb and metacarpophalangeal joints of the fingers though passive movements are normal.
- The brachioradialis muscle is paralysed. He cannot make the forearm supine.
- Triceps power is normal.
- There is loss of sensation over the anatomical snuff box and dorsal aspect of first web space.
- Elbow joint movements are normal.

Brachioradialis is to be tested by asking the patient to flex the elbow, keeping the forearm in mid prone position against resistance.

In radial nerve injury it can not become a prominent band like structure as normal condition.

Extensor muscles of the wrist joints

Except extensor carpi radialis longus (ECRL) all others extensor muscles of the wrist are supplied by posterior interosseous nerve which is a branch of radial nerve.

Radial nerve directly supplying ECRL which is also an extensor muscle of the wrist joint.

The wrist drop is resulted from the paralysis of the extensor muscle.

Extensor digitorum: It is related to extension of the metacarpophalangeal joints. It also extend inter pharyngeal joints along with interossei and lumbricales. So when the muscle is paralyzed the patient cannot extend the metacarpophalangeal joints but will be able to extend, the interphalangeal joints with the help of intact interossei and lumbricals which are supplied by ulnar nerve. [Please remember this].

So this is a case of right radial nerve injury at the arm due to fracture shaft humerus right.

How do you say this is a case of radial nerve injury?

There is a history of fracture shaft humerus right.

Patient presented with wrist drop and difficulty in extending the joints of fingers.

Brachioradialis muscle is paralyzed and evidence of paralysis of extensor digitorum wasting of muscles at extensor aspect of forearm.

There is a sensory loss over anatomical snuff box and dorsal aspect of first web space.

So this is a case of radial nerve injury right.

Tell me how the radial nerve is supplying?

The radial nerve arises from posterior cord of the brachial plexus. Root value is C5, 6, 7, 8 and T1.

In arm muscular branches to triceps, anconeus brachioradialis, lateral half of brachialis and extensor carpi radialis longus (ECRL).

In the forearm it divides into superficial and deep branch.

Superficial branch supplies the skin over lateral half of dorsum of forearm, over anatomical snuff box and first web space.

Deep branch is posterointerosseus nerve supplies all the extensor muscles in the back of the forearm (Except ECRL which is directly supplied by radial nerve itself).

Practice repeatedly the following tests:

i. Power testing of triceps muscle.

How to perform: Ask the patient to elevate the shoulder against resistance.

ii. Test for wrist extensors.

How to perform: Ask the patient to extend the wrist while you are holding the forearm steadily in prone position. If the patient is able to extend the wrist, apply resistance and ask to extend the wrist and assess the power of wrist extensors.

Remember: The wrist extensors are extensor carpi radialis longus, extensor carpi radialis brevis and extensor carpi ulnaris.

iii. Test for metacarpophalangeal joints.

How to perform: Ask the patient to extend metacarpophalangeal joints, keeping the forearm in prone position. If the patient is able to move the joints, ask him to extend against resistance and assess the power of extensor digitorum

iv. Test for brachioradialis muscle power.

How to perform: Ask the patient to flex the elbow keeping the forearm in mid prone position against resistance and assess the power of brachioradialis.

v. Test for abductor pollicis longus

How to perform: Ask the patient to keep the hand facing palm upwards. Then ask the patient to abduct thumb at right angle to the axis of the palm. If he abducts the thumb, ask to abduct it against resistance and assess the power of abductor pollicis longus.

vi. Test for extensor pollicis longus and brevis.

How to perform: ask the patient to extend the thumb while you try to flex the thumb at the interphalangeal joint and assess the power of extensor pollicis longus.

Why brachioradialis muscle is to be examined in mid prone position?

Brachioradialis muscle helps in flexion of the elbow when the elbow is in mid prone position otherwise, biceps will come into action to flex the elbow.

How will you test the sensation loss in radial nerve injury?

Sensory sensation to be tested by:
- Fine to crude touch.
- Pain, temperature.
- Position and vibration tests.

Fine touch to be tested by touching cotton wool with closed eyes of the patient and deep and crude touch is tested by the blunt end of a pin or any blunt object.

Pain sensation by pin prick.

Temperature sensation by touching of cold and warm water alternatively, keeping in test tubes.

How will test position and vibration sense?

Position test: Move metacarpophalangeal joints or interphalangeal joints up and down (Extension and flexion) with closed eyes and see whether the patient can appreciate the movements or not.

Vibration sense: Vibrating tunic fork is placed over bony prominence of respective part like olecranon process in elbow, medial malleolus in lower limb, etc. or it can be placed over the body surface.

How will you grade the muscle power?

Grade 0 - No contraction of muscle.
Grade 1 - Only flicker of contraction.
Grade 2 - Gravity eliminated movements of the muscle.
Grade 3 - Movements of muscles also against gravity but without resistance.
Grade 4 - Movements of muscles against gravity with some amount of resistance.
Grade 5 - Normal range of movements.

How will you proceed in this case?

I will do

i. Nerve conduction velocity (NCV) of the involved limb to see
- Site of injury of the nerve.
- Degree of damage of the nerve and
- Evidence of regeneration.

ii. Electromyography of involved muscle to see:
- Denervation of the muscle
- Renervation if any.

When do you like to do NCV (Nerve conduction velocity)?

Nerve conduction velocity test to be conducted after 3-4 weeks of nerve injury as Wallerian degenerations—both distal and proximal segments, start after 3 weeks. So NCV is to be done after 3-4 weeks.

How will you repair the nerve?

Sir, the nerve repair to be done without any tension, I will do end to end epineural repair, using 8-0 polypropylene suture, under microscope.

If end to end repair is not possible without tension, I will do nerve grafting.

What are the types of nerve repair?

Three types of nerve repair are there:
1. Individual fascicular repair
2. Group fascicular repair and
3. Epineural repair epineurorrhaphy
4. Epi-peri neurorrhaphy
5. Cable grafting: the nerve graft is cut up so that a number of strands can be used to build up a similar thickness of the nerve trunk being repaired.

What are the nerves used for nerve grafting?

Expandable nerve like sural nerve, medial cutaneous nerve of forearm, lateral cutaneous nerve of forearm are used for nerve grafting.

What are the essentials in immediate postoperative management?

Following nerve repair, limb is to be splinted in plaster cast for 3-4 weeks to prevent contracture of opposing muscles. Passive joint movements are required to prevent joint stiffness.

After removal of splint 3-4 weeks after mobilization of limb with active physiotherapy are essential.

How will you assess the recovery of nerve function following a careful repair?

Tinel's sign is a very useful guide to see recovery.

On percussion over the course of nerve from **distal to proximal** side, patient will have tingling sensation (a sensation of 'pins and needles') or hyperaesthesia, at the site of regeneration.

[Tingling sensation ('pins and needles' sensation) is due to the heightened threshold of the freshly regenerated axons.]

How will you manage nerve injury in a patient with open wound?

The golden rule is early repair of nerve provides the best chance of recovery.

But if the wound is contaminated like in gunshot injury, primary repair may not be logical as chance of infection is more and there by dehiscence of the repair is more likely.

So debride and clean the wound, properly, antibiotics to be given to control infection. Prolene sutures at the ends are tied and the sutures may be fixed to local tissue to prevent retraction of the ends and easy identification of the nerve during re exploration after 3-4 weeks.

What should be the management policy of nerve injury after a blunt trauma?

In blunt trauma induced nerve injury a careful follow up is an important part of management.

Usually, neuroparaxia and axonotmesis type nerve injury recovers with the passage of time. If there is no evidence of recovery after 8-12 weeks, NCV, EMG studies is to be done. If there are no signs of recovery, surgical exploration and nerve repair is indicated.

What are the determining factors for recovery of nerve function after repair?

- Age—children's recovery is faster than adults.
- Type of injury—clean cut nerve injury has better recovery of function where as high traction injury and high velocity bullet injury have worst recovery.
- Type of nerve—recovery is better in pure motor or sensory nerve than a mixed nerve.
- The level of injury—recovery is worse in proximal part of nerve injury than distal.
- Timing of repair—nerve repair at the earliest after injury has better recovery than its repair after 2-3 months.
- Associated injuries—associated vascular, skeletal injury along with nerve injury will have worse recovery than the isolated nerve injury.
- Relation with wound—nerve injury with contaminated wound may have poorer recovery compared to a clean cut injury.

Also know the following about the radial nerve injury.

Sites of radial nerve injury

In axilla
- Crutch palsy, Saturday night palsy due to unusual pressure on the nerve in axilla. It is a neuroparaxia.

- Fracture upper end of humerus.
- Bone or soft tissue growth.

In radial groove at shaft of humerus.

- Pressure on the arm at the edge of operation table.

Saturday night palsy—after excessive consumption of alcohol (usually on Saturday) put his arm over a chair under compression or patient has a blunt trauma over the arm due to fall.

- Fracture shaft of humerus.
- Tourniquet palsy due to prolonged tourniquet application.
- Last but not least—IM injection also may cause radial nerve palsy.
  In the elbow—radial nerve injury due to fracture or dislocation of neck of radius.

II clinical features depending on the sites of involvement:
- Wrist drop, inability to extend metacarpophalangeal joints.
- Inability to extend the forearm.
- Inability to extend the thumb.
- Weakness of brachioradialis muscle.
- Loss of sensation at the back of the arm, forearm, hand, and lateral three and half fingers.
- Dropped fingers caused by the injury of posterior interosseus nerve (deep branch of radial nerve). It is purely motor nerve so no sensory deficit along with.

III muscles of extensor compartment, i.e. back of forearm:
a. Superficial group
  i. Anconeus
  ii. Brachioradialis
  iii. Extensor carpiradialis longus
  iv. Extensor carpi radialis brevis
  v. Extensor digitorum longus.
  vi. Extensor digiti minimi and
  vii. Extensor carpi ulnaris.

The deep muscles are:
  i. Supinator
  ii. Abductor pollicis longus
  iii. Extensor pollicis longus
  iv. Extensor pollicis brevis
  v. extensor indicis

All of the above muscles:
- are supplied by radial nerve
- All muscles cross elbow joint

- Most of them take origin from tip of lateral epicondyl of humerous
- Common extensor origin (front of lateral epicondyle for the attachment of common extensor origin).

IV Structures in 6 compartments under extensor retinaculum:

Compartment I (i) Abductor pollicis longus.
          (ii) Extensor pollicis brevis.

     II (i) Extensor carpi radialis longus.
        (ii) Extensor carpi radialis bravis.
     III (i) Extensor pollicis longus.
     IV (i) Extensor indicis
        (ii) Extensor indicis

Posterior interosseus nerve and anterior interosseous artery:
     V   (i) Extensor digit minimi
     VI (i) Extensor carpi ulnaris.

V carpal bones
- Lateral to medial
- Proximal row—scaphoid, lunate, triquetral, pisiform.
- Distal row—Trapezium, Trapezoid, Capitate, Hamate.
  [You already know the pneumonic to remember this- she looks too preety, try to catch her].

VI triangular spaces:
- Upper
- Triangular space—boundary.
- Medially—Teres minor.
- Laterally—long head of triceps.
- Inferiorly—teres major.
  (Contains – circumflex scapular artery).

  Lower triangular space-boundary.
- Medially long head of triceps.
- Laterally—medial border of humerous.
- Superiorly—teres major.
  (Contains—radial nerve and profunda brachialis artery)
  Quadrangular space—boundary.
- Superiorly- subscapularis in front capsule of shoulder joint and teres minor behind.
- Inferiorly- teres major.
- Medially—long head of triceps.
- Laterally—surgical neck of humerus.
  (Contains—axillary nerve, posterior circumflex humerus vessels).

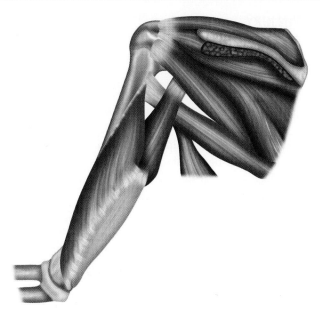

Trangular space

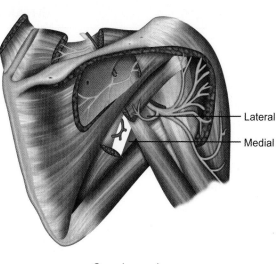

Quadrangular space

VI Treatment of delayed recovery of radial nerve even after repair:

The steps of management are as follows

Step I (i) Neurolysis—excision of fibrous tissue in and around the nerve.

     (ii) Steroid injection and physiotherapy

        ↓ Fail

Step II (i) Intrinsic splint— arrangement, i.e. pronator teres is to be attached with extensor carpi radialis brevis (PT + ECRB acts as internal sphincter)

     (ii) Galvanic stimulation

        ↓ Fail

Step III tendon transfer procedure

(i) Tendon of Palmaris longus to be attached to the tendon of extensor pollicis longus (PL + EPL).

(ii) Flexor carpi ulnaris to be attached to the tendon of extensor digitorum longus (FCU+ EDL).

VII You know, all extensor muscles of wrist are supplied by the posterior interosseous nerve (deep branch of radial nerve) except extensor carpi radialis longus (ECRL) is supplied by radial nerve itself.

How to test the power of ECRL: with the forearm pronated the wrist is extended and abducted against resistance and the muscle is palpated below and behind the lateral side of the elbow.

Action of ECRL

It is extensor and abductor of the wrist and assists in flexion of the elbow. It is indispensable to the action of 'making a fist', acting as a synergist during finger flexion. It assists in flexion of the elbow.

So, if the posterointerosseous nerve is only paralysed patient can abduct the wrist and try to make a fist. This way you can exclude the involvement of extensor carpi radialis longus (ECRL).

VIII Know about extensor digitorum muscle

- Common extensor origin from lateral epicondyle.
- Insertions: The muscles end in a tendon which splits into 4 parts one in each digit except the thumb. Over proximal phalanx the tendon for each digit divides into three slips- one intermediate and two collateral intermediate slip is inserted into the dorsal aspect of the base of the middle phalanx. The collateral slips reunite and insert into dorsal aspect of the base of distal phalanx.
- Supplied by posterointerosseous nerve on the back of the forearm.
- Action—it is an extensor of the wrist, metacarpophalangeal and interphalangeal joints.

Test- with the forearm in pronation and the finger extended, the patient tries to keep the fingers extended at the metacarpophalangeal joints while pressure from the examiner on the proximal phalanges tries to flex there joints.

ULNAR NERVE INJURY

My patient, Deepak, a 25 years old young male, presented with complaints of -inability to move his left little and ring fingers along with the bending of the two fingers.

He has a history of sustaining injury in his left elbow 4 months back following a fall from his bike and elbow was immobilized for 6 weeks. He noticed the problems following removal of plaster.

On Examination
There is claw' hand deformity involving little and ring fingers
- Wasting of hypothenar eminence muscles and interossei

On palpation: There is paralysis of interossei and abductor pollicis muscle - there is loss of sensation in the palmar aspect of little finger and medial half of ring finger.

So, this is a case of left ulnar never injury at elbow region due to medial epicondylar fracture.

What are the clinical features of ulnar Nerve injury?

- Clawhand
- Weakness of all the muscles supplying by ulnar nerve
- Patient cannot hold a card in between two extended fingers as the palmar interossei are weak. [Remember- PAD-palmar interossei are Adductors] this is called '**Card Test**'

How to perform the test: ask the patient to keep a card in between two extended fingers as tight as possible and you try to pull the card and feel the strength the fingers, i.e. the strength of palmar interossei.

- Patient will be unable to spread his fingers it cannot abduct as dorsal interossei are weak [remember-DAB, i.e. dorsal interossei are abductors]
- When patient holds a book between fingers and thumb, patient can hold the book, flexing the thumb instead of keeping straight. This is called **Froment's sign.**

How to perform the test: Ask the patient to grasp a book between the thumb and others fingers and see whether the thumb is extended or flex while holding the book. If ulnar nerve is injured the thumb will be flexed.

Explanation: When we hold book in between fingers and thumb. Thumb will be straight due to the action of Adductor Pollicis and first palmar interosseous muscle if these are paralysed in ulnar nerve injury, grasp is achieved by the action of flexor Pollicis longus and thereby the thumb will be flexed).

- Loss of sensation over medial one and half fingers and hand.

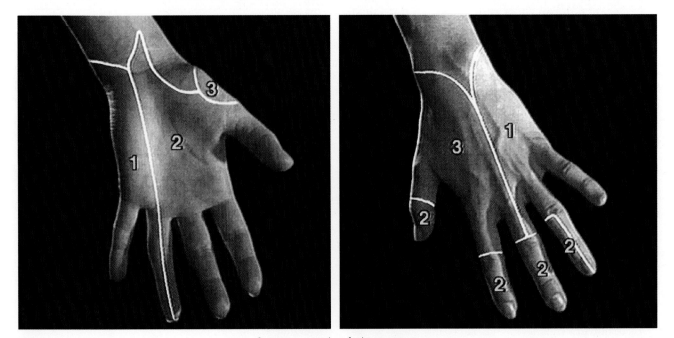

Sensory supply of ulnar nerve

What are the common causes of ulnar nerve injury?

The common causes are:
- Supracondylar fracture
- Injury to medial epicondyle
- Tardy ulnar nerve palsy
- Leprosy and cubitus vulgus are less common causes
  And sites of injury are at the elbow where it passes behind medial epicondyl—at the wrist superficial to flexor retinaculum

What is Ulnar Paradox?

We know usually in peripheral nerve injury, the golden rule is higher the lesion, more the deformity; but in ulnar nerve palsy it is reversed. Higher the lesion lesser the deformity, lower the lesion, more the deformity.

Explanation- in higher lesion FDP (Flexor digitorum Profundus) is paralysed but in lower lesion FDP is intact and causes more flexion due to over action. So 'clawhand' will be more aggravated.

Ulnar nerve supplying which all muscles?

In fore arm—ulnar nerve supplying
- Flexor carpi ulnaris and
- Medial half of flexor digitorum profundus

In hand
  i. Hypothenar muscles
    - Flexor digit minimi
    - Abductor digit minimi
    - Opponens digit minimi
  ii. All palmar and dorsal interossei
  iii. Thenar muscles:
    - Both head of adductor pollicis and deep head of flexor pollicis brevis

What is the sensory supply of ulnar nerve?

Sensory supply of ulnar nerve is in:
- Hypothenar area
- Medial aspect of palm and palmar aspect of little finger and medial half of the right finger.

Following tests to be practiced repeatedly
- Test for palmar and dorsal interossei
  How to perform: do card test to see the power of palmar interossei as described above.
  Ask the patient to fan out (abduct) the fingers and you put the resistance against abduction and feel the strength, i.e. the power of dorsal interossei.
- Test for adductor pollicis and Ist palmar interosseous, i.e. **Froment's sign** as described above.

What is intrinsic minus and intrinsic plus deformity in ulnar nerve palsy?

Intrinsic minus deformity—this is due to intrinsic muscles power loss. 'Clawhand' is the example of intrinsic minus deformity.

Intrinsic plus deformity is due to muscles contracture and fibrosis.

What is 'Claw hand'?

It is an intrinsic minus deformity where there is hyperextension of the metacarpophalangeal joint with flexion of the interphalangeal joints of the hand.

How a clawhand develops?

Flexion of metacarpophalangeal joints and extension of inter phalangeal joins are by extensor hood of interossei and lumbricals. In ulnar and median nerve injury- theses actions are paralysed, claw hand as a result.

Classical claw hand deformity is seen in both ulnar and median nerve injury. Hyperextension of MCP joins due to unopposed action of extensor digitorum which extends proximal phalanx. The IP joints are flexed as a result of paralysis of lumbricals and intersossei. Supracondylar fracture, penetrating injury, blunt trauma elbow may cause both ulnar and median nerve injury).

What may be the causes of claw hand deformity?

Causes are:
- Leprosy
- Trauma
- Entrapment neuropathies
- Tardy ulnar nerve palsy
- Lower brachial plexus injury (Klumpke's paralysis)

Median nerve supplying which muscles?

In forearm

Pronator teres, flexor carporadialis, palmaris longus, flexor digitorum superficialis, flexor pollicis longus, lateral half of flexor digitorum profundus and pronator quadratus.

In hand

Abductor pollicis bravis, flexor pollicis brevis, opponens pollicis, first and second lumbricals.

What is the sensory supply of median nerve?

It supplies lateral half of palm and palmar and dorsal aspect of lateral three and half fingers.

What are the flexor compartments muscles of fore arm?

- Superficial group – Pronator teres, flexor carpiradialis, Palmaris longus and flexor carpi ulnaris.
- Intermediate group—pronator teres, flexor carpi radialis, Palmaris longus and flexor carpiulnaris.

- Deep muscles group—flexor digitorum profundus flexor pollicis longus, and pronator quadratus
  These muslces are supplied by median nerve except flexor Carpi Ulnaris which is supplied by ulnar nerve.

MEDIAN NERVE INJURY

HIGH MEDIAN NERVE INJURY

- Wasting of thenar eminence muscles
- Loss of sensation in lateral three and half fingers, i.e. thumb, index, middle and lateral half of ring finger.
- If patients is asked to clasp the hands, the index finger of the affected hand fails to flex and remains straight called' **Pointing index** [(Known as Oschsner's clasping test). This is due to paralysis of flexor digitorum superficialis and lateral half of flexor digitorum profundus]
- If a pen is held in front of the affected hand, thumb cannot touch the pen (as abduction is not possible due to paralysis of the abduct to pollicis brevis) Ape or simian thumb deformity (due to overaction of adductor pollicis – supplied by ulnar nerve. As all other thenar muscles are paralyzed, thumb comes in the same plane of the Metacarpals.

Lower Median Nerve Injury

Here flexor digitorum profundus not affected so 'pointing index' cannot be seen.

2. Practice the following tests repeatedly please
- Test for Flexor pollicis longus
  How to perform the test: Ask the patient to bend the terminal phalanx of thumb against resistance keeping the proximal phalanx steady. If median nerve is injured flexor pollicis longus is paralysed thereby patient will be unable to flex the terminal phalanx.
- Flexor digitorum superfacilis and lateral half of profundus, i.e 'Pointing index' test, called Ochsner's clasping test.
  How to perform: Ask the patient to clasp the hands. If median nerve is injured the index finger of the affected side fails to flex and remains straight as 'pointing index'
- Abductor pollicis brevis the pen test-
  How to perform: Patient is asked to keep the hand, palm facing up.now the patient is asked to keep the thumb at

right angle to the plane of the palm and asked him to touch a pen held infront. Patient will be unable to do so if Paralysis of adductor pollicis brevis is there due to median nerve injury.
- Opponen's pollicis
  How to perform: Ask the patient to touch the tip of other fingers by the thumb against little resistace. Patient will be unable to do so if opponens pollicis is paralyses. (Remember—slight movement may be possible due to intact adductor pollicis supplied by median nerve.)

3. What are the thenar and hypothenar muscles?
Thenar muscles are:
- Abductor pollicis brevis
- Flexor pollicis brevis
- Opponens pollicis
- Adductor pollicis
  All the thenar muscles are supplied by median nerve except adductor pollicis which is supplied by ulnar nerve.
Hypothenar Muscles
- Palmaris brevis
- Abductor digitiminimi
- Flexor digiti minimi
- Opponens digitiminimi
  All hypothenar muscles are supplied by ulnar nerve.

BRACHIAL PLEXUS INJURY

Anatomy

- Upper brachial plexus consisting of C5, C6 nerve roots.
- Middle brachial plexus—C7 nerve root
- Lower brachial plexus—C8, T1 nerve roots.

Nerves Arise from Different Cords

From medial cord:
- Medial cutaneous nerve of arm and forearm
- Ulnar nerve
- Medial root of median nerve.

From lateral cord
- Musculocutaneous nerve
- Lateral pectoral nerve
- Lateral root of median nerve.

From Posterior Cord (Remember—STAR)
- Sub scapular nerve—upper and lower
- Thoracodorsal nerve
- Axillary nerve
- Radial nerve

III. Important causes of brachial plexus injury

- Road traffic accidents most common cause
- Traction injury due to violent displacement of shoulder girdle, cervical spine like fall from height on shoulder.
- Obstetrics injury during labor
- Operative injury during neck dissection
- Malignant infiltration to brachial plexus like metastasis from 'Pancost' tumour lung.

Types of brachial plexus injury

i. Complete—where all roots of the plexus are damaged. It is rare and occurs only in very severe accidents. There will be complete paralysis of whole upper limb. It will be flaccid and hangs by the side. Loss of all movements, wasting of all muscle groups – sensory loss in the whole upper limb.

ii. Incomplete—where any of the roots involved; most commonly due to road traffic accident, operative injury, stab injury, etc.

Incomplete brachial plexus injury is either
i. Upper brachial plexus lesion called Erb-Duchene Paralysis
ii. Lower brachial plexus lesion called Klumpke's paralysis
i. Upper brachial plexus injury (Erb-Duchene paralysis): Causes—fall from height on shoulder Road Traffic Accident (RTA) – difficult labor
   - Nerve root involved- C5, C6
   - The muscles affected are
     1. Deltoid, biceps, brachialis brachioradialis, supinator
     2. The deformity is called policeman 'taking tip' where the affected limb is internally rotated, extended at elbow and pronated
     3. Sensory loss will be over the outer aspect of arm and upper part of lateral aspect of fore arm.

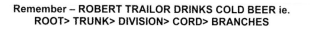

Remember – ROBERT TRAILOR DRINKS COLD BEER ie.
ROOT> TRUNK> DIVISION> CORD> BRANCHES

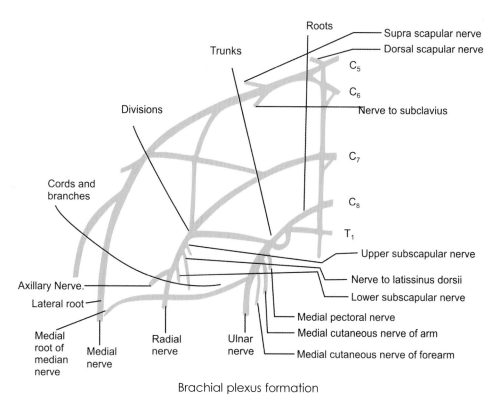

Brachial plexus formation

ii. Lower brachial plexus injury (Klumpke's Paralysis):
- Causes—forceful abduction of the shoulder like in accident
- Difficult breech delivery
- Nerve root involved C8 T1
- Muscles involved
  - Intrinsic muscle of the hand with claw hand (Features of both median and ulnar nerve injury)
  - Sensory loss inner aspect of forearm, hand (ulnar border)
  - Horner's syndrome is usually associated as (cervical sympathetic supply may be affected.

It includes
- Ptosis—dropping of upper eyelid due to paralysis of the levator palpebrae superioris.
- Myosis—contraction of pupil due to paralysis of the dilator papillae
- Enopthalmos—regression of eye ball due to paralysis of Muller's muscles
- Anhydrosis—absence of sweating of face and neck of the affected side.
- Loss of ciliospinal reflex
4. On scratching of the neck, skin pupil dilates usually. This reflex may be lost.

Treatment in Short
- Early surgery and nerve repair is ideal provided the wound is not gross by contaminated.
- Nerve grafting is required when end to end anastomosis is not possible.

Common Peroneal Nerve Injury

- Causes
  - Fracture neck of the fibula
  - Leprosy
  - Lead poisoning
  - Iatrogenic
- Clinical Features
  - Foot drop with high stepping gait
  - Talipes equinovarus deformity
  - Loss of sensation of lateral aspect of leg and dorsum of foot.
- Muscles supplied by common peroneal nerve's branches extensor and peroneal group of muscles and dorsum of the foot.
  Deep peroneal nerve supplies the muscles of extensor compartment of leg, extensor digitorum longus, libialis arterior, extensor hallucis longus, and peroneus tertius

on the dorsum of foot it supplies extensor digitorum brevis.

Superficial peroneal nerve supplies
- Peroneus longus and brevis
- Skin over the peronei and extensor muscles in the lower third of the leg.
- Foot drop—inability to dorsiflex and evert the foot due to paralysis of the peroneal and extensor group of muscles as a result of common peroneal nerve injury.
  - High stepping gait and loss of sensation over lateral and dorsum of the foot.

Treatment: Tendon transfer is the ultimate procedure.

Tibialis posterior muscle is inserted in navicular bone which is detached and inserted to attached tendons in cuboid and cuneiform bones with the help of plantaris tendon graft.

Few important things about nerve and nerve injury

I. Structures of a nerve

Perineurium: Peri means around. It is a sheath of dense connective tissue that envelopes a bundle of nerve fibers.

Epineurium is the covering connective tissue sheath or the outer most layer of connective tissue surrounding a peripheral nerve.

Note: Blood vessels are within the perineurium and epineurium

Axon: Individuals nerve fiber is called axon.

Endoneurium means within or inner. It is the inner most layer of connective tissue in a peripheral nerve, forming an interstitial layer around each individual fiber outside the neurilemma. It is delicate connective tissue around individual nerve fibers inside a nerve. Individual axons within a nerve myelinated or unmyelinated are wrapped in endoneurium.

Fascicle: A group of axons with their endoneurium are arranged in bundles called Fascicle.

II. Nerve Injury

(a) Seddon's classification (Remember—NAN)
  i. **Neuroparaxia:** It is a physiological paralysis of nerve conduction. Example handling of facial nerve during parotidectomy may cause neuroparaxia. Here recovery is complete. There is no reaction of degeneration. Recovery takes few hours to weeks.
  ii. **Axonotmesis:** There is division or rupture of nerve fibers or axons through the nerve sheath remains intact.

Wallerian degeneration occurs only distal portion of broken axon. Quality of regeneration is good and regeneration rate is 2 mm /day first couple of weeks to months, next 1 mm/ per day after that with near complete recovery.

Patient presents with paralysis of muscles, sensory loss and causalgia.

iii. **Neurotmesis:** Here complete division of nerve fibers with nerve sheath occurs.

Wallerian degeneration occurs both proximal and distal segments. In proximal segment retrograde degeneration occurs up to the first node of Ranvier as well as distal to the injury. Recovery is incomplete even after repair.

Patient presents with complete loss of motor and sensory functions with loss of reflexes cut ends of a nerve forms

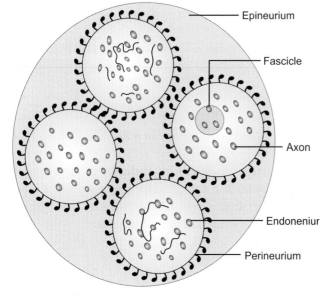

Cross section of a nerve

- Neuroma proximally and glioma distally.

(b) Sunderlands' classification

Grade-I	Conduction block – temporary neural block
Grade-II	Axonotmesis but endoneurium is intact
Grade-III	Axonotmesis with disruption of endoneurium but peri neurium is intact-
Grade-IV	Neurotmesis with disruption of endo and perineurium but epineurium is intact
Grade-V	Neurotmesis with disruption of endo, peri and epineurium.

Addition

- Mc Keown's grade—VI Nerve injury
- Single nerve injury—Neurotmesis at multiple sites.

III. MRC classification of Sensory nerve dysfunction:

SO – No sensation

S1 – Only deep pain sensation present

S II – Pain, touch, temperature sensation present

S III – SII + Accurate localization but no stereognosis

S IV – S III + object and texture recognition but not like a normal person

S V – Normal sensation.

IV. CAUSALGIA

It is a burning sensation of pain with hyperesthesia in the course of peripheral nerve due to in complete injury to the nerve.

- Common site is upper limb and commonly seen in median nerve injury
- Skin over the course of nerve becomes red, shiny and glossy which sweats profusely called 'Weir Mitchell's skin' eventually skin becomes atrophic.

Treatment

- Reassurance
- Analgesics, - Phsysiotherapy
- Tab gabapentine 300 mg BD to TDS
- Inj Guanethisime regionally

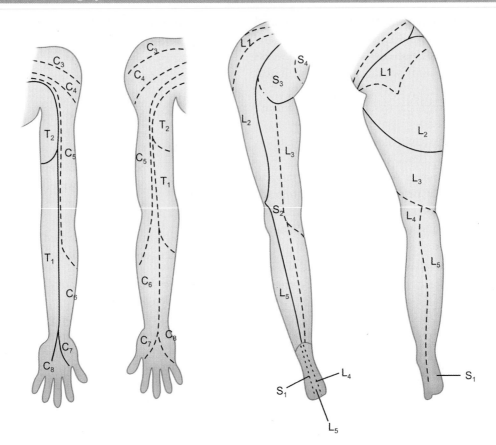

Dermatomes of both upper and lower limbs

- Ultimately sympathectomy - Cervical for upper limb and lumbar for lower limb is the option for pain relief.

V. Autonomous zone of nerve supply

Tip of index finger is only supplied by median nerve. Tip of little finger is only supplied by ulnar nerve. This is called autonomous zone of nerve supply.

Only thumb movements can reflect the actions of three nerves.

Abduction of thumb by Abductor pollicis longus – supplied by median nerve, Adduction by Adductor pollicis supplied by ulnar nerve and Extension by Extensor carpi radialis brevis – supplied by Radial nerve.

CASE 41

Post Burns Contracture and Marjolin Ulcer

My patient Sibani, a 35 years old female cook, presented with complains of:

- Difficulty in movement of neck, difficulty in drinking after burns injury for last 1 year
- Ulcer over chest wall scar for last 6 months.

She sustained flame burns 1 year 3 months back involving face, neck and chest.

The wounds took more than 2 months to heal. Gradually she started feeling difficulty in neck movement, difficulty in drinking and drooling of saliva as scar tissue getting thickened day by day.

She noticed an ulcer over the chest scar for last 6 months which is not healing on conservative management.

On examination: The patient is mildly anaemic, poorly nourished. No lymphadenopathy.

There are grossly thickened scar tissue in the neck, chest and face. The lower lip is everted. There is gross contracture of scar tissue. Drooling of saliva is constant.

Neck movement is grossly restricted.

There is a non healing ulcer over the sternum. Nonhealing margin edge is everted, rolled out, floor is full of necrotic tissue.

Surrounding area is indurated.

Base of the ulcer is also indurated, mild bleeding on touch.

So, this is a case of post burns contracture face, neck, chest with a non healing ulcer over the chest wall scar, most probably Marjolin's Ulcer.

How post burs contracture develops?

Ans. In deep burns involving full thickness of skin and healing occurs by fibrosis, not by epithelialization. Without a proper re surfacing timely the burns ulcer heals by scaring.

↓

All scars mature and contract leading to post burns contracture if superficial burns is infected. It causes sloughing of deeper tissue and healing occurs by fibrosis leading to contracture in spite of superficial burns.

What are the complications of post burns contracture?

Complications depend on sites of involvement.

Face: Disfigurement of face, ectropion of eyelid causing keratitis and corneal ulcer.

Everted lip causing constant drooling of saliva, difficulty in chewing food, drinking properly

Narrowing of mouth- microstomia

Neck: Contracture in the neck causing restricted neck movements, range of vision will be also restricted.

Upper limb: Patient will be unable to put food into mouth, cannot dress, and even cannot comb hairs.

Contracture in shoulder and axilla lead to restricted movement of upper limb, hampering day to day activities. Finger contracture causing inability to write, put bottoms etc.

Joints: Disability and nonfunctioning of joints as a result of contracture.

Other problems are development of hypertrophic scar, keloid, Marjolin's ulcer and cosmetically it looks ugly.

How can you prevent the development of contracture?

i. Appropriate management of primary burns injury
   - Involved joints to be properly splinted
   - When wounds start granulating it is to be covered with split skin graft (SSG) after controlling infection.
   - Infections to be prevented all the ways.
   - Prophylactic antibiotics, antibiotics on culture sensitivity report
   - Regular physiotherapy to prevent secondary graft contracture.
   - Topical silicon sheeting

ii. Secondary management
   - Joint exercise in full range during recovery and post recovery periods.
   - Pressure garments to prevent contracture, hypertrophic scar formation
   - Saline expanders for scars, etc.

What is Marjolin's ulcer?

Marjolin ulcer is a low grade squamous cell carcinoma which develops on a long standing non healing ulcer or in a scar tissue due to repeated breakdown.

What are the characteristics of Marjolin's ulcer?

- It is locally malignant
- Slow growing as scar tissue is relatively avascular
- It is painless as scar tissue is nerveless.
- No lymphatic spread as there is no lymphatics in the scar
- It has raised and everted edge with induration
- Biopsy shows low grade squamous cell carcinoma.

How will you manage this patient?

Sir,

I will do few relevant investigations like wedge biopsy from the edge of the ulcer to exclude Marjolin's ulcer.

I will do all base line investigations to make the patient fit for anaesthesia and surgery. Next I will:

i. Release the contractures by 'Z' plasty at neck
ii. Incise the fibrotic scar tissue till the healthy tissue and raw surface is to be covered with split skin grafting.
iii. For excessive depth flap reconstruction is recommended.

If the ulcer is Marjolin's one, I will do wide local excision, keeping at least 1 cm healthy margin all around and the raw area is to be covered with split skin graft.

Is there any role of Radiotherapy in Marjolin's Ulcer?

As scar tissue is usually an avascular structure so Marjolin's ulcer arising from scar tissue is not sensitive to radiotherapy.

OK, tell me what is the ideal time for release of post burns contracture?

Sir,

The contracture is to be released after maturation of scar tissue only. It takes usually about 6 months to 10/12 months.

How will you identify a matured scar tissue?

Mature scar tissue has a whitish hue and will be relatively soft and supple in texture.

Why consultation of senior Anaesthetist is very important before surgery for this patient?

- Endo tracheal intubation may be very difficult due to contracture in neck
- Fibre optic bronchoscopy may be required to assist endo tracheal intubation.
- Blind Nasotracheal intubation sometimes required.

SHORT NOTES ON BURNS

I. WALLACE'S RULE OF '9'

	Adult	Children	Infant
Head and neck	9%	18%	20%
Front of chest and abdomen	9 × 2 = 18%	9 × 2 = 18%	10 × 2 = 20%
Back of chest and abdomen	9 × 2 = 18%	9 × 2 = 18%	10 × 2 = 20%
Lower limb-front and back	18 × 2 = 3	13.5 × 2 = 27%	10 × 2 = 20%
Upper limb-front and back	9 × 2 = 18%	9 × 2 = 18%	10 × 2 = 20%
Pubic region/ perineum	01% 100%	01% 100%	100%

II. DEGREES OF BURNS

i. As per involvement of skin thickness

a. Superficial Partial thickness burns. This burns goes up to papillary dermis, not deeper than that the clinical features are blistering and or loss of the epidermis. The underlying dermis is pink and moist. The capillary return is clearly visible when balanced. Pin prick sensation is there.

Superficial partial thickness burns heal without residual scaring in 2 weeks without any surgical intervention.

b. Deep partial thickness burns: The burns injury involves reticular dermis and it deeper part.
Clinically: Epidermis is lost. The exposed dermis is not moist. The color does not blanch on pressure sensation is reduced. Difficult/ unable to distinguish sharp and blunt prick on needle examination.

Deep partial thickness burns takes more than 3 weeks to heal without any surgical intervention.

c. Full thickness burns: The whole dermis is involved in this burns injury. Clinically, hard and leathery feel there is no capillary return. Under skin thrombosed vessels can be seen. No pain sensation on deep needle pricking.

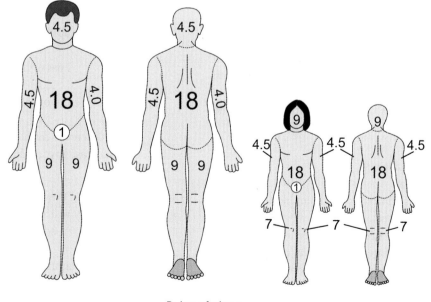

Rules of nines

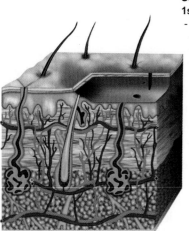

Superficial Burn:
1st Degree Burn
 - Signs and Symptoms
  - Reddened skin
  - Pain at burn site
  - Involves only epidermis

Depth of burns

ii. As per depth of burns (Grading in degree)

First degree burns
- Involves only the epidermis and painful epidermis appears red, no blister, only erythema
- Heals relatively faster in 5-7 days by epithelialization without scaring.

Second degree burns
- Superficial dermal, deep dermal burns.
- Superficial dermal: Involves superficial layers of dermis—forms blister on removal of blisters, the wound is pink, moist, pain sensitive and blanches on pressure
- Heals in 3 weeks by epithelialization.

Deep dermal
- Involves reticular layer of dermis blister formation is there on removal of blister the wound is white, dry capillary feeling may or may not be there pain on pinching pressure is there. Heals in 4-8 weeks with scaring.
  [Remember—blister formation occurs only in second degree burns]

Third degree burns:
- Involves all layer of dermis
- No blisters formation
- The affected area is charred, parchment like
- Painless, insensitive area
- Do not blanch on pressure, leathery feeling
- Eschar (charred, denatured, insensitive, contracted full thickness burns called eschar) formation.
  Grafting is required otherwise heals by scaring and takes more than 8 weeks.

Fourth degree burns: Involves all the layers of skin, subcutaneous fat and variable amount of deeper structures like muscle, bones, etc. The wound is covered with thick eschar. Burns may also be classified simply as:
  i. Superficial burns—includes first degree and superficial dermal burns.
  ii. Deep burns—includes second degree, deep dermal, third degree and fourth degree.

How to assess the depth of burns
  i. Clinically, superficial burns is pain sensitive where as deep burns is pain insensitive
     1st degree—very painful, erythema
     2nd degree—blisters formation
     3rd degree—charred, parchment like leathery feeling eschar formation, painless.
     4th degree—subcutaneous tissue, muscle, bone involvement, thick eschar, etc.
  ii. Radiologically—assessment of blood flow by color Doppler, fluorometry, thermography, etc.

Pathophysiology

Tolerable temperature of human skin is maximum 40°C for a short period.
↓
More than that or even 40°C for a long period causes
↓
Coagulation necrosis of skin and subcutaneous tissue
↓
Release of vasoactive peptides
↓
Altered capillary permeability
↓
Loss of fluid
↓
Severe hypovolemic shock
↓
Decrease cardiac output
Decrease myocardial function
↓

Decrease renal blood flow oliguria lead to renal failure
Altered pulmonary resistance leading to pulmonary edema.
↓
SIRS [Systemic Inflammatory Response Syndrome]
↓
Sepsis

$\downarrow$

Severe Sepsis

$\downarrow$

Septic shock

$\downarrow$

Multi organ Dysfunction syndrome(MODS)

$\downarrow$

MOSF of multi system organ failure

$\downarrow$

Remember MCH [M = metabolic acidosis,
C= coagulopathy and H= Hypothermia]

$\downarrow$

Death

Know the important terms like:

- SIRS
- Systemic Inflammatory Response Syndrome Comprises of
- Hyperthermia (temperature > 38°C)
- Hypothermia (temperature < 36°C)
- Tachycardia - pulse > 90 /minute
- Respiratory rate > 20 / minute
- PCO_2 32 mmHg
- White cells count > 12,000/ lumm or < 4000/lumm of blood
- Neutrophil band > 10%
- SEPSIS = SIRS + Documented infection
- Septic sock—sepsis and compromised cardiac function
- Severe sepsis/sepsis syndrome.
- Sepsis + evidence of one or more organ failure like, cardiovascular, renal, respiratory, etc.

Multi Organ Dysfunction Syndrome (MODS): The effect of infection in whole body, two or more organs are affected
It comprises

- Cellular dysoxia (mitochondrial dysfunction)
- Microvascular occlusion or shunting
- Tissue hypoxia (stagnant/cytotoxic)
- Cellular dysfunction, hibernation and death.

MSOF: Multi system organs failure as a result of uncontrolled MODS.

$\downarrow$

Death (Remember—MCH)
M = metabolic acidosis
C = coagulopathy
H = Hypothermia

- Pathophysiology of shock:
  Any cause of shock:
  - Hypovolemia
  - Cardiogenic
  - Septic shock, etc.

Leads to $\downarrow$

Low cardiac output

$\downarrow$

Vasoconstriction

$\downarrow$

Occurs as a compensatory action to perfuse vital organs (brains, heart, kidney, liver, muscle, etc.)

$\downarrow$

Dynamic circulation increase
- Tachycardia
- Tachyomea as results

$\downarrow$

Activation of sympathetic nervous system
- Release of catecholamine
- ACTH, ADH Cortisol, etc.

Peripheral venous constriction (capacitance vessels)
Leading to
Diverting blood from splanchnic system towards essential vital organs

$\downarrow$

Renal blood flow decreases
$\downarrow$ GFR
$\downarrow$ Urine output
Rennin angiotensin mechanism activated

$\downarrow$

Further vasoconstriction
- Aldosterone release

$\downarrow$

Salt water retention

$\downarrow$

ADH released

$\downarrow$

Further concentration of urine increase

$\downarrow$

Shock persists

$\downarrow$

Cardiac output further decreases

$\downarrow$

Hypotension
- Tachycardia
- Poor perfusion of coronaries

$\downarrow$

Hypoxia
- Metabolic acidosis
- Release of cardiac depressants

$\downarrow$

Cardiac pump failure
- Further hypoxia to tissue

- Anaerobic metabolism
- Lactic acidosis

↓

Cell wall damage

$Na^+ + Ca^+$ ions enter into the cells but K^+ leaks (Na^+ stays K^+ flees)

↓

Hyperkalemia

Hyponatremia

Hypocalcemia

↓

Intracellular lysosomes breakdown

- Release powerful enzymes
- Destruction of own cells

↓

Sick Cell syndrome

- Platelets activated
- Formation of small clots

↓

Disseminated Intra Vascular Coagulation (DIC)

↓

Further bleeding

↓

SIRS

↓

Sepsis → severe sepsis → septic shock → MODS MSOF Death.

- Causes of death in Burns:
  i. Hypervolemia and shock
  ii. Renal failure
  iii. Pulmonary Oedema , ARDS
  iv. Septicemia
  v. Multiorgan failure

Management of Burns

First Aid

- Stop the burning process
- Keep the patient away from burning area
- Cool the area with tap water by continuous irrigation for 20 minutes (Cold water should not be given as it causes hypothermia)
- Cleaning of dirty wounds properly.

Primary Survey and Resuscitation

- Patient to be admitted to the burns unit
- Maintain ABCDEF (Airway, Breathing, Circulation, Disability assessment (CNS). Exposure to a controlled environment, fluid resuscitation)

- Assessment of percentage of burns, depth of burns
- Adequate sedation, analgesics, tetanus toxoid, antibiotics, Ranitidine, Rylestube, catheterization
- Fluid resuscitation indication: Adults with burns over 15%
- Parkland Regime more commonly used the simple formula is fluid requirement in 24 hours = 4 ml X % of burns × body weight ½ of the volume is given in first 8 hours and rest ½ of the volume is to be given by next 16 hours.

Example: 50% burns of a 50 kg women fluid requirement on 24 hours is

4 ml × 50 × 50 = 10,000 ml = 10 L

5 L to be given in first 8 hours and rest 5 L to be given by next 16 hours.

(Maximum % considered is 50%—Remember)

Muir and Burclay regime

$$\frac{\% \text{ of burns} \times \text{body weight (Kg)}}{2} = 1 \text{ Rations}$$

3 rations to be given by first 12 hours

2 rations in second 12 hours and

1 rations is next 12 hours.

Evan's formula

In first 24 hours

- Normal saline/Ringer 1 ml/kg % of burns
- Colloids 1 ml/kg/% of burns
- 5% dextrose, 200 ml in adult

Next 24 hours

- Half of the volume of the total volume given in first 24 hours
- Alternative simple regime is to infuse ringer lactate 1 liter/hour
- Urine out put 40-50 ml / hour (0.5-1 ml/kg body weight/hour) indicates adequate hydration.

Resuscitation in Children

- In children with burns over 10% total body surface area
- In oral fluid can be used salt must be added
- The key is to monitor urine out put.

Fluid Maintenance Therapy: Amount of fluid required in 24 hours is 1500 ml/sqm of body surface + evaporated fluid loss

Evaporated fluid loss = 25 × % of burns × sqm of body surface

In children maintenance fluid is dextrose saline as 100 ml/ kg for 24 hours for first 10 kg, 50 ml / kg for next 10 kg 20 ml / kg for 24 hours for each kg over 20 kg body weight.

[The fluids used are normal saline, ringer lactate Hartman's solution plasma etc. But ringer lactate is the fluid of choice].

Secondary Survey

- Monitor urine output. It should be minimum 40 ml / hour
- Monitor BP, pulse, temperature, PO2, PCO2 Serum electrolytes, Blood Urea, Creatinine O2 nasally or intubation if required
- Ryles tube aspiration and later on feeding purpose
- CVP line care. Total parenteral nutrition (TPN) through it
- Regular wound swab culture and sensitivity
- Antibiotics as per culture sensitivity report (Penicillin, cephalosporin, metronidazole, amino glycosides)
- Inj pentoside 40 mg 12 hourly or Ranitidin 50 mg 12 hourly
- Adequate analgesics (Pethidine + Phenargan (Promethazone) or Fortin (Pentazocin) + compose (Biazepam)
- Maintain Nutrition, Calory requirement 40 k cal/ kg + 25 k Cal/kg extra protein 1 gm/ kg + 2 gm/ kg extra

Local Management

Dressing at regular intervals under sedation/GA using paraffin gauge, hydrocolloid plastic films, amniotic membrane etc.

For head, neck and face and in case of superficial burns - open method with application of silver sulfadiazine without any dressing (other ointments. 5 % silver nitrate, mafenide acetate cream. Silver nitrate, etc.)

Close method is with dressing Idea behind that to smoothen and protect the wound and to reduce pain.

Tangential excision of burn wound with skin grafting can be done at the earliest in patient with less than 30% burns.

In case more than 30% burns, let the wound granulates in 3 weeks then SSG to be done on the raw area.

Slough to be excised regularly. In certain area full thickness graft or flap is required like over joints, eyelids, ear, etc.

Management of Eschar

Eschar is nothing but charred, denatured, full thickness deep burns with contracted dermis.

Circumferential eschar in upper limbs, lower limbs, thorax, neck can cause more oedema leads to venous compression ischemia, gangrene, etc.

So, as per requirement deep tangential full thickness incisions are made at different area to prevent oedema formation and further complications.

This is called echarotomy.

Physiotherapy and psychological supports are very important aspect of burns case management.

Medicolegal and Ethical aspect in burns

- Near by police station is to be informed
- Medical legal documents to be filled up properly mentioning percentage of burns. Superficial, deep, etc.
- High risk consent to be taken in case of major burns > 30%
- Relative along with next of Kin to be informed everything in details like life risk, cost of therapy, prolong treatment, long stay at hospital cosmetic problems etc.
- Special care to be taken in Burns Unit to save the life of the patient.

My patient, Lallu Prasad, a 50 years old, known case of bilateral osteoarthritis knee, presented with a swelling in the back of the right knee for last 10 months. During walking the swelling becomes prominent along with knee pain. Nowadays he is feeling discomfort with the swelling along with mental disturbance.

On examination: General survey is essentially normal.

On local examination

The site of the swelling is situated near the midline of the popliteal loss below the level of the joint line:

- 6 x 4 cm spherical swelling, cystic in feel, fluctuation positive.
    - The swelling is reducible as the fluid can be pushed into the joint and on flexion of the joint.
    - Margins are not well palpable as the swelling lies deep to gastrocnemius muscle.
    - Knee joint examination shows, evidence of arthritis and effusion of knee joint may be obvious (demonstrated by patellar tap)
      All movements of the joint may be restricted and painful with or without crepitus.

So, this is a case of most probably Morrant Baker's cyst.

What is Morrant Baker's cyst?

The cyst develops as a result of herniation of the synovial membrane of the knee joint through the posterior capsule. It is always secondary to the disease of knee joint.

How Baker's cyst develops?

As a result of chronic osteoarthritis or rheumatoid arthritis knee. There is persistent accumulation of synovial fluid which leading to the formation of the cyst.
The cyst comes out through the posterior capsule of knee joint and lies in popliteal fossa deep to gastroenemeious muscle.

What are other swellings in popliteal fossa?

Apart from Baker's cyst, the popliteal fossa may have the followings:
- Semimembranous bursal cyst
- Aneurysm of popliteal artery
- Cystic hygroma
- Popliteal Abscess.

Others swellings are
- Popliteal lymph nodal swelling
- Nerve tumors, etc.

What are the characteristics of semimembranous s bursal cyst?

- Common in children and adolescents.
- Usual site of the swelling is of the posteromedial aspect of knee joint, in between the medial head gastrocnemius and semimembranous.
- The swelling lies above the joint line, slightly to the medial side of popliteal fossa.
- On knee flexion the swelling does not reduce completely, becomes less prominent. But on extension of knee joint the swelling becomes prominent.
- Cystic swelling—fluctuation positive transillumination may be positive.
- Knee joint movements are normal usually.

Treatment: In children, the operation plan may be delayed as the cyst may disappear but if the swelling becomes large, uncomfortable at any time and painful excision of the complete cyst through the transverse incision in the popliteal fossa.
Characteristics of popliteal aneurysm:
- Common in elderly people
- Pulsatile swelling in the popliteal fossa. The pulsation is expansile.
- Compressible but not reducible.
- Transmitted pulse to be excluded by grasping the swelling from both the sides and to be lifted up. If it is pulsatile swelling the pulsation ceases.

Characteristics of cystic hygroma in popliteal region.

- Rare site at popliteal region
- Infants and young children are common victims
- The swelling becomes more prominent on strain i.e. on walking.
- Surface lobulated, margins are not well defined as it burrows into the tissue space.
- Transillumination brilliantly positive, a distinct physical sign.

  During transillumination multiple septae are noticed multilocular cyst.

  [Treatment details written in the topic cystic hygroma under neck swelling]

Characteristics of popliteal abscess.

- It is an acute condition there by painful. Commonest cause is popliteal lymph nodal infection.
- Patient usually tries to flex the knee extension will cause tremendous pain.
- Tender swelling
- Fluctuation positive but trans illumination negative
- Popliteal artery aneurysm to be excluded before making an incision for popliteal abscess.

  Tell me what are the bursae around the knee joint.

  Sir, there are about 12 bursae around the knee joint of which 4 are anterior, 2 posterior and 3 each on medial and lateral sides.

A. Anterior bursae 4 in number
  1. Suprapatellar communicates with the knee joint
  2. Prepatellar
  3. Superficial infra patellar and 4 deep infra patellar.

B. Posterior bursae 2 in number

One between each head of origin of gastrocnemius and the capsule of knee joint. These may often communicate with the knee joint.

C. Medial bursae 3 in number

One lies superficial to medial ligament of the knee, one deep to the medial ligament and one lies between the semi membranous and the medial condyle of the libia called semimembranous burse.

D. Lateral bursae 3 in number

One superficial to the lateral ligament of the knee, one between the lateral ligament and popliteus tendon and lateral condyle of femur, communicates with the joint.

What are the structures of popliteal fossa serially?

- The roof of the fossa is formed by deep fascia or popliteal fossa. The superficial fascia over the roof contains short saphenous vein, those cutaneous nerves, namely posterior femoral cutaneous nerve.
- The floor is provided from above downwards by the popliteal surface of the femur, the capsule of knee joint, reinforced by the oblique popliteal ligament and the popliteus muscle covers by its fascia. The popliteal artery vein and the labial and common peroneal nerves pass through the fossa. A small group of popliteal lymph nodes, i.e. along side the popliteal vein.

What are the boundaries of popliteal fossa?

- The popliteal fossa is a diamond shaped space behind the knee. Above it is limited by semi membranous and semitendinosus on the medial side and biceps femorls on the lateral side, diverging from the apex.
- Boundaries of popliteal fossa are more details as:
  - Superolaterally—the biceps femoris.
  - Superomedially—the semi tendinous and the
  - Semimembranosus, supplemented by graeilis, the sartorius and the adductor magnus.

Inferolaterally, lateral head of gastrocnemius supplemented by the plantaris. Inferomedially medial head of gastrocnemius.

OK, tell me now, how will you manage your case, i.e. the Baker's cyst:

Sir, as the cyst is large enough and causing discomfort to the patient then I will do excision of the cyst with or without synovectomy.

What is about the conservative management of Baker's cyst?

When the cyst is relatively smaller and asymptomatic.
  i. Aspiration and injection of hydro cortisone followed by application of crepe bandage for 6-7 days.
  ii. Treatment of associated joint pathology like rheumatoid arthritis, osteoarthritis, etc.

What is the importance of suprapatellar bursa?

- Suprapatellar bursa is connected with the knee joint and thereby when there is effusion in the joint, fluid goes to the area of bursae and manifested as a swelling above patella. On lying down the fluid goes around the bursa. So during examination of effusion evacuate the fluid, pressing on the supra patellar region and then test for patellar tap.

[Infrapatellar bursitis is called Housemaid knee]

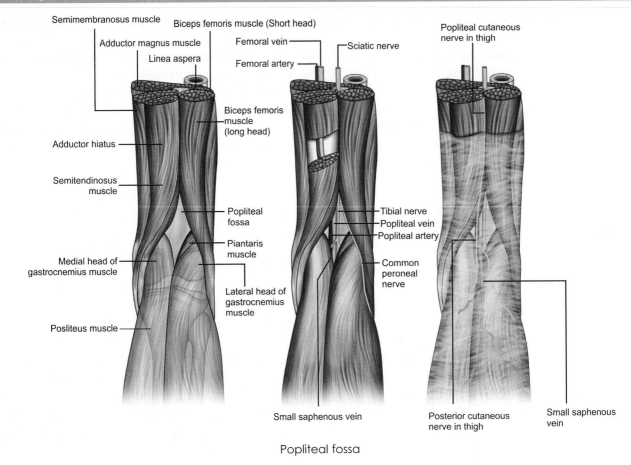

Popliteal fossa

Popliteal fossa

Baker's cyst

What are the common causes of effusion in the joint?

The common causes of effusion are trauma, infection, and tuberculosis and sympathetic effusion.

Why the effusion is seen in tuberculosis?

Tuberculosis of the knee joint is primarily a synovial disease. Synovial membrane is thickened and may be even palpable. Since it is a synovial disease, effusion is the earliest reaction of the synovial membrane.

What is white swelling of the knee?

Tuberculosis of the knee asperse swollen and the swelling is more in presence of muscular atrophy. In this condition skin looks white and puffy. So this is called while swelling of the knee.

How will you investigate the case of tubercular knee joint?

- Apart from ESR, Mantoux
  I will do X-ray knee AP lateral
- Aspiration of fluid for cytology and AFB culture
- Synovial biopsy to confirm the diagnosis.

X-ray will show increased joint space de calcification of arthritic surfaces. In late stage—rarefaction of bone -ground glass appearance. Due to loss of trabeculae. Further late stage—bone erosion and triple deformity (when the knee joint goes into position of flexion, external rotation and backward sublaxation).

What does locking of knee mean?

When patient can only flex the knee cannot extend the knee called locking of the knee.

Why medial meniscus injury is more common?

- It is larger meniscus
- It is a C-shaped meniscus and attached in three places (anterior, posterior and lateral).

What are the loose bodies in the knee?

- Fibrous bodies from effusion
- Melon seed bodies in tuberculosis of knee
- Villous processes of synovial membrane in chronic osteoarthritis.
- Osteophytes—osteochondritis dissecans, etc. arthoscopic removal is the treatment of choice.

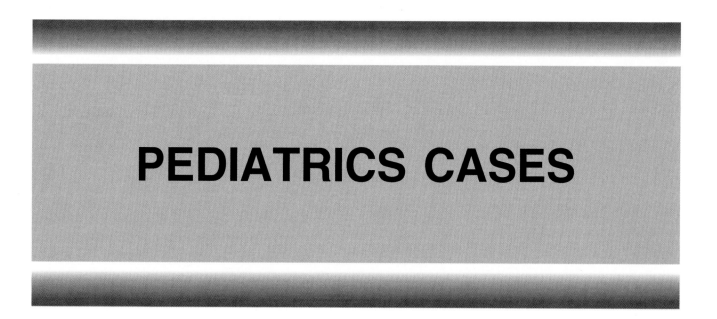

PEDIATRICS CASES

CASE 43 — Cleft Lip and Cleft Palate

My patient, Pabitra, a 6 months old full-term male baby-mother came with complains of slit in the left upper lip, left upper tooth bearing area and roof of the mouth since birth. Milk/ drinks coming through the nose.

But mother denies any history of breathlessness, bluish changes in the face while crying (to exclude congenital cardiac anomalies). No history of other congenital anomalies like hypospadius, undescended testis, vertebral abnormality, etc. in a older baby take history of speech, dental and facial problem). No ear discharge noticed.

Maternal History: Mother, Kushum Kali, a 30 years old married 2½ years back (late marriage), not a known case of diabetes, no history of long term drug intake (like steroid, phenytoin, diazepam may lead to the defect).

No history of malnutrition and infection during pregnancy. No other babies having the same problem in their family.

On Examination

Baby is alert, active and lying comfortably in mother lap general survey is essentially normal weight is 5 kg.

On Local Examination

There is a cleft in the left upper lip.

Lip

- Cupid bow tilted upwards. Pick of cleft side is at higher level to normal side.
- Vermillion is thin, while roll is less prominent towards the cleft.
- Alignment of teeth- underlying teeth are protruding.

Nose

- Allae Nase is flattened, base of the alae attached more posteriorly.
- Nasal opening oval larger.

- Tip of nose is deviated to opposite side of the defect.
- Columella—length of columella is slightly shortened, raised.
- Floor or nose widened.

Alveolus (Tooth bearing area): Wide gap at upper left alveolus. Arch appears collapsed.

Palate

- Cleft in both the hard and soft palate.
- Pre maxilla intact.
- Vomer seen or not (usually not seen as it joined at normal side of the roof of palate).
- Lateral wall—inferior turbinate hypertrophied at cleft side.

Systemic examination

Heart sound S1 S11 (normal), no murmur. Others are essentially normal.

So, my diagnosis is a case of left sided complete cleft lip, alveolus with complete cleft palate in a 6 months old male baby.

Then what will you do in this case?

I will prepare the child for surgery by doing base line investigation and I will repair the cleft lip primarily by rotation advancement method of Millard.

What is Millard's procedure?

Millard's procedure is for repair of the unilateral cleft lip. The repair to be completed in three layers-skin, muscle and mucosa.

Why the Millard's procedure is called rotation advancement flap operation?

The procedure involves the advancement of lateral flap (full thickness of the lip) into the upper portion of the lip combined with downward rotation of the medial segment.

Why the Millard's position is preferable?

- The curved suture line mimics the pillar of the philtrum.
- The Horizontal suture lines in the crease just below the alae.
- Small triangular placed at the junction of the skin.
- Vermilion prevents peaking of the cupid bow.
- Z plasty at the mucosal side of the repaired lip resulted in a deep labial sulcus and an attractive pout to the lip.
- Over all this procedure is relatively easier, more cosmetic and revision can be done who require.

How will you correct the palate cleft in this case?

In present days, anterior palatoplasty, done at the age of 4-6 months (through palatoplasty usually done at 15-18 months) for better development of speech without disturbing mucoperiosteal portion.

My patient, here is 6 months old, so I would like to do anterior (pre maxillary) palatoplasty along with the correction of cleft lip.

What are the principles of cleft palate operation?

- Mobilization and reconstruction of the aberrant soft palate musculature.
- Closure of hard palate to be done by minimal dissection so that scar formation will be minimal.

What are the operative procedures for cleft palate correction?

Most commonly performed procedure is

- Wardill-Kilner-Veau four flap technique—YV advancement of mucoperiosteum of the hard palate and achievement of anteroposterolengthening.
- Von Langen Back- Pedicle mucoperiosteal flaps from hard and soft palate and closed in midline.
- Push back palatoplasty- correction with W shaped mucoperiosteal flap.
- Furlow palatoplasty
- In traveler veloplasty—re-orients the musculus levator veli-palatini which has inserted abnormally on the hard palate.

What are the other procedures for cleft lip?

Apart from Millard operation there are
- Straight line repair - usually it is for a very small cleft.
- Tennison's triangular flap- this is a form of 'z' plasty.
- Delaire's technique—repair of cleft by a lateral quadrilateral flap.
- Mirault Blair procedure- correction is done by using a lateral triangular flap form the side of the cleft.

How will you correct nasal deformity?

Practically every case of cleft palate, except minor incomplete one, requires primary nasal correction.

The simplest way to correct the deformity by separating the alar cartilage from the overlying skin of the affected side and hitching it to the dome of the normal alar cartilage.

Unilateral short columella is lengthened with a 'c' flap.

Can you tell me what are the time scheduled for cleft lip and cleft palate repair?

Defects	Timing
(i) Cleft lip alone unilateral/Bilateral	Unilateral 5-6 months Bilateral 4-5 months.
(ii) Cleft palate	Soft palate at 6 months. Hard palate 15-18 months.
(iii) Cleft lip and palate	**Unilateral:** Cleft lip and soft palate at 5-6 months Hard palate with gum pad with or without revision of lip at 15-18 months. **Bilateral:** Cleft lip and soft palate at 4-5 months Hard palate with gum pad with or without lip revision at 15-18 months.
(iv) Alveolus repair with cortical bone at 15-18 months.	

What is present day concept of anterior hard palate repair?

Now a days, anterior hard palate correction done at the age of 5-6 months by single layer repair. It is done at 5-6 months for better development of speech.

What are the problems develop in cleft lip cleft palate?

Problems with cleft lip are
- Cosmetically it is not desirable.
- Defective suction.
- Defective speech particularly with labial letter BP, FM, VM.
- Defective dentition.

Problems with cleft palate:
- Defective suction.
- Defective speech—particularly with the palatal consonants.
- Defective smell—due to constant irritation of the nasal mucosa by regurgitated food materials.
- Defective hearing.
- Recurrent respiratory tract infection.
- Aspiration bronchopneumonia.
- Defective dentition because of irregular development of alveolus.
- Cosmetically not desirable at all.

How will you manage post operative period?

- Hands of the child to be splinted to prevent pulling of sutures.
- Liquid diet for first few days.
- Aseptic cleaning of the suture line.
- Stitches to be removed 5th to 7th postoperative day.
- Normal diet after 7 days.

Why post operative follow up is very important in a case of cleft lip and cleft palate?

After initial corrective surgery the child to be followed up for

- Further correction of cupid bow.
- Revision surgery for nasal deformity
- For speech therapy.
- Orthodontia to be started around the age of six.
- Ortholaryngologist's advice for hearing loss.
- Correction of maxillay hypoplasia.

What are the complications of early surgery of the patient of cleft palate?

Repair of the cleft palate in early child hood leads to some degree of maxillary hypoplasia as periosteum is taken as flap, as results facial and dental deformities are there.

Late surgery also causes speech deformity for that why, anterior (pre maxilla) palatoplasty done at 5-6 months of age.

What is sub mucous cleft palate?

There is no development of soft palate levator muscles so periosteum is lying next to mucosa leading to Velopharyngeal Incompetence (VPI).

The features of VPI are:
- Prominent notch at the posterior end of the hard palate.
- Zona pellucida.
- Bifid Uvula.

Why there are ear problems in patients with cleft palate?

The levator palatine and Tensor Veli palatine muscles are inserted into Eustachian tube and are responsible for maintaining competence of the tube in preventing the unusual reflux of nasopharyngeal content into the middle ear.

In patient with cleft palate there breakage of this mechanism and middle ear is exposed to nasopharyngeal content leading to otitis media, acute secretory otitis media, chronic secretory otitis media—hearing loss, etc.

What is orthodontic management in this case?

- Regular dental examination.
- Repair of associated cleft lip at 4-6 months.
- Repair of cleft palate by 12-15 months time.
- Obturator placement.
- Postoperative orthodontia to be started around 6 years of age.

What is the optimum timing for isolated cleft lip operation?

Cleft palate should be corrected before primary dentition, i.e. within 6 months form the birth.

A 'Rule of 10' (Millard) to be fulfilled by the baby
- Age 10 weeks minimum.
- Weight—10 Lbs, i.e. 5 kg.
- Hb%—10 gm%.

What are the reasons behind this time scheduled?

- As the lip elements are relatively larger, the repair is technically more precise and easier.
- Post operative dropper feeding facilitating the healing of the lip avoiding sucking with post operative free wound.
- Of course baby would be healthy enough to accept anesthesia as well as operation.

How defective speech is corrected?

By:
a. Speech and language therapy.
b. Secondary palate surgery:
   i. Intravelar veloplasty (muscular reconstruction of soft palate)
   ii. Pharyngoplasty.
   iii. Speech-training devices.

Can you diagnosis cleft lip and palate antenatally?

After 18 weeks of gestation unilateral or bilateral cleft lip can be diagnosed by ultrasonography - isolated cleft palate cannot be diagnosed by USG.

SHORT NOTE ON CLEFT LIP AND PALATE

Cleft lip is the gap in the lip due to failure of fusion of two median nasal processes.

Cleft palate is the gap in the palate due to failure of fusion of two palatine processes.

DEVELOPMENT OF FACE, LIP AND PALATE

To understand the development of cleft lip cleft palate one has to understand and the development of face, lip and palate clearly.

About 6 weeks of intrauterine life, around the primitive mouth (stomodeum) 5 processes appear:
• Frontal process—1
• Maxillary process—2, one on each side.
• Mandibular process—2, one on each side.

Frontonasal Process

Two nasal pits, surrounded by a lateral and medial nasal process, develop in the forntonasal process. The two medial nasal processes merge to form the intermaxillary segment. The median nasal process becomes bluntly bifurcated, forming two globular processes and two globular processes ultimately unite to form the central depressed part of the upper lip called philtrum.

The triangular primary palate (premaxilla) and the nasal septum which develops as a down growth from the fused medial nasal process.

The lateral nasal process forms the side of the nose only.

The Maxillary Process

The maxillary process fuse with the lateral nasal process at the nasolacrimal groove and with the medial nasal processes to form the lateral part of the upper lip.

Two lateral palatine processes, which fuse in the midline to form the secondary palate, develop form inner aspect of maxillary processes. The palate is formed by the fusion of secondary palate to the primary palate.

The mandibular Process

The mandibular process gives rise to the lower lip and jaw. These processes unite around the stomodeum to form the face.

So, cleft lip is as a result of failure to fusion of two medial nasal process and cleft palate as a result of failure to fuse two

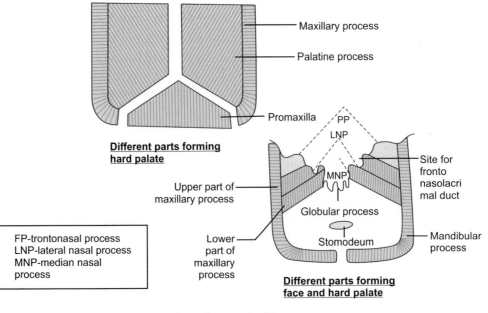

Development of face

lateral palatine process. The mesoderm of the primary palate and the nasal septum.

Incidence

- Cleft lip and palate is 1 in 600 live births.
- Cleft palate alone is 1 in 1000 live births.
- In unilateral cleft lip, left side is more commonly affected (60%).
- Cleft lip and palate together more common in male.
- Cleft palate alone is more common in female.

Etiology

- Both genetic and environmental.
- Family history - among first degree relatives, chance is 1 in 25 live births.
- Maternal late marriage, history of steroid, diazepam, phenytoin intake.
- Pierre Robin Syndrome—comprises
  - Isolated cleft palate
  - Retrognathia
  - Posteriorly displaced tongue (glossoptosis).

- Down, Apert and Treacher Collins syndrome are most commonly associated.

  Nutritional deficiency, endocrine disorder, viral infection, exposure to radiation, stress is the important contributory factor.

Classification

Cleft lip

1. **Central cleft**: It is at center. It is due to a failure of fusion of two globular processes derived from median nasal process.
2. **Lateral cleft**: Common type. It is due to failure to fusion between the median nasal process and the maxillary process.

   It is sub divided into:
   - Unilateral/bilateral
   - Complete/ incomplete.
   - Complete when the cleft extends into the nostril.
   - Simple/compound
     Compound—when the cleft lip is associated with cleft alveolus.

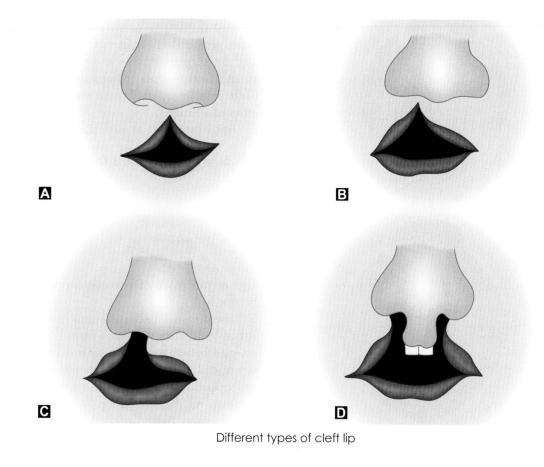

Different types of cleft lip

- Complicated/ uncomplicated. Complicated when it is associated with cleft palate.

CLEFT PALATE

Classification

I. Incomplete

- Bifid uvula—cleft of the uvula only.
- Cleft of soft palate—entire length.
- Cleft of entire length of soft palate and the posterior part of hard palate.

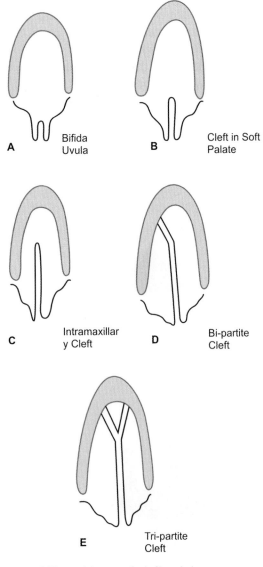

A Bifida Uvula

B Cleft in Soft Palate

C Intramaxillary Cleft

D Bi-partite Cleft

E Tri-partite Cleft

Different types of cleft palate

II. Complete

Cleft of soft palate and entire length of hard palate. So the nose and mouth is one cavity here. Due to failure of fusion between palatine process and pre maxilla.

Bipartite cleft palate

The cleft may extend on one side of the pre maxilla forming bipartite cleft palate.

Tripartite cleft palate

When the cleft extends both the sided of the pre maxilla. Different types of cleft palate.

Indications of operations are simple:
  i. As it looks cosmetically very ugly.
  ii. To prevent important complications like- defective speech, feeding difficulty, hypoplasia of maxilla, mid face deformity, dentition defect, defective hearing, etc.

Principles of Surgery

- To restore normal shape and symmetry of lips, palate and nose.
- Vermillion border should be constructed well.
- Cupid bow should be intact.
- Integrity of orbicularis oris to be maintained.

The basic principles of surgery are:
- Cleft lip surgery attaches and reconnects the muscles around nasal aperture and oral sphincter.
- Cleft palate surgery brings together muscles with minimal scaring.
- Two stage procedure to minimize dissection.

Secondary management for:

  i. Hearing
  ii. Speech
  iii. Dental development
  iv. Facial growth

Hearing:

- Higher incidence of sensorineural and conductive hearing loss.
- ET tube dysfunction causing otitis media.
- All children born with cleft lip and palate should be assessed for both sensory neural and conductive deafness before attaining the age of 12 months.
- Prophylactic myringotomy and grommet temporarily eliminate middle ear effusion.
- Postoperative period of cleft lip/palate also require regular check up for hearing problem.

Speech

Common speech problems are:

- Velopharyngeal incompetence—nasal or hypernasal quality to speech.
- Articulation problems.

Dental

- Too many or too few or problem with eruption of teeth are common.
- Good dentition is essential for successful orthodontic treatment.

Orthodontic management—two phases.

Phase I: mixed dentition (8-10 years) to expand the maxillary arches as a preclude to alveolar bone graft.

Phase II: Permanent dentition (14-18 years) to align the dentition and provide a normal dentition and provide a normal functioning occlusion. It includes surgical correction of a mal positioned/retrusive maxilla by maxillary osteotomy.

Secondary Surgery for Cleft Lip and Cleft Palate

Good result in cleft lip, cleft palate is directly attributable to the quality of primary surgery. Secondary cleft procedures include:

- Cleft lip revision—after 2 years after primary surgery.
- Alveolar bone graft.
- Both cleft lip revision and alveolar bone graft.
- Veloplasty, pharyngoplasty, and closure of palatal fistula, etc.
- Dentoalveolar procedures including transplantation of teeth, insertion of osseo-inegrated dental implants.
- Orthognathic surgery.
- Rhinoplasty, etc.

Truly speaking, cleft lip/ palate appears to be a little problem but it proves ultimately huge one both for the child, parents and doctors too.

My patient, a 3 years old full term baby. Mother presented with complains of baby passing urine from the under surface of penis since birth.

The baby having an abnormal urethral orifice and when he passes urine it starts with spraying then it dribbles, stream is narrow and he soils his under clothes.

But there is no history of difficulty in passing urine. No history of fever with chill rigors (to exclude UTI) and also there is no history of pain and lump abdomen (to exclude hydronephrosis—antinatal period of mother was uneventful and family history is not contributory.

On Examination

Baby active, alert, weight 11 kg.

On local examination

*   The penis appears hypoplastic.
*   External urethral orifice situated at the ventral aspect of corona with a pin whole meatus noticed.
*   There is hood in dorsal prepucial skin.
*   Fore skin is deficient at ventral aspect.
*   Urethral plate grooved and well marked.
*   No chordee is palpable.
*   External urethral orifice is at the ventral aspect of corona with a pin hole meatus.
*   Scrotum well developed.
*   Both testes well developed.   } To exclude other Associated congenital abnormalities
*   No congenital hydrocele or hernia is palpable.

Abdomen—no cystic swelling palpable at lumbar region (to exclude) hydronephrosis which may by developed due to urinary obstructions owing to pin hole meatus in this case) So this is a case of coronal hypospadias with pin hole meatus in a 3 years old boy.

What is Hypospadias?

By definition: Hypospadias is an abnormal ventral opening of the urethral meatus which may be located any where from the ventral aspect of glans penis to the perineum.

What are the important features of Hypospadias?

Apart from the abnormal ventral urethral opening there may be the following important associated features.

Chordae—distal to the ectopic orifice, the urethra and corpus spongiosum are replaced by fibrous cord. During erection of penis contracture of this cord leads to down ward curvature of the penis called chordae.

The more proximal is the ectopic meatus more pronounced the chordae.

– The incomplete ventral prepuce
– The prepuce is deficient on the ventral aspect and excess at the dorsal aspect over the glans giving rise to hooding of the prepuce.

What are the different types of Hypospadias?

Barcat classification of hypospadias is there for the different types of hypospadias.

No I.   Anterior or distal- commonest 70-75%.
*   glandular
*   coronal
*   subcoronal

No II. Middle hypospadias- 10-15%
*   Distal penile.
*   Mid shaft.
*   Proximal penile.

No III. Posterior or proximal hypospadias 20-25%.
*   Penoscrotal
*   Scrotal
*   Perineal

Which are the factors responsible for development of hypospadias?

Two important factors are related with the development of hypospadias:

i.   Endocrine factors and
ii. Enzyme deficiency.

i. **Endocrine factors:** During intra uterine life if there is deficiency of testosterone or dihydrotestosterone or androgen insensitivity syndrome may cause the mal development of urethra leading to hypospadias.

Maternal progesterone therapy during early pregnancy may also cause hypospadium.

ii. **Enzyme deficiency:** There is beta 3 hydroxy steroid dehydrogenase enzyme (B3 hydroxy steroid dehydrogenase) may lead to incomplete masculine development and hypospadias - due to idiopathic local tissue defect and development arrest may also cause hypospadium.

What are the problems with hypospadias which bring the patient to the surgeon?

The problems are:

i. Unusual location of external urethral opening itself along with narrow stream of urine and dribbling of urine may wet the undergarment.

ii. Chordae the fibrous band which bends the penis ventrally which become painful during erection.

iii. Looks ugly as because there is deficiency the prepuce at ventral surface and there is a hood of prepuce at dorsal aspect.

iv. Perineal type hypospadias is mostly associated with undescended testis and ambiguous genitalia. For adult patient

v. Infertility is important problem particularly with posterior (proximal) hypospadias.

vi. Due to chordee, erection of penis will be painful there by sexual intercourse will be a difficult job.

In every case of hypospadias, is corrective surgery mandatory?

Sir, as present days tend every case of hypospadias should undergo corrective surgery except in glandular variety where the abnormal. Wxternal urethral meatus is very close to the normal meatus.

So, no such problem develops with this minor hypospadias. Other than this, all hypospadias in glandular type where the external urethral orifice is situated more proximally, corrective surgery is mandatory.

What investigation you would like to do in this patient?

Sir, I would do USG abdomen to rule out any hydronephrosis or hydroureter.

Base line investigations to make the patient fit for anaesthesia and surgery.

When will you consider for micturating cystourethrography (MCU) in hypospadias?

Sir, if there is a pin whole meatus with hypospadias with suspected chronic retention of urine with vasicoureteric reflux, I will do MCU otherwise it is not required routinely.

How will you accecss the degree penile bending due to chordee?

Artificial erection of penis by injecting PGE or even normal saline into corpora cavernosa will help to assess the degree of penile curvature, thereby the length of chordae. It is useful intra operatively.

Histopathologically what a chordee consists of?

Chordee consists of:

• Smooth muscle cells.

• Highly vascular tissue and

• Fibroblast.

It may be due to shorter penile skin ventrally or a disparity in length of tunica albuginea.

It also may be due to fibrous replacement of corporus spongiosum distal to ectopic external urethral meatus.

What is the ideal time for operation?

Ideally the operation for hypospadius should be completed before the age of 5 years i.e. before class one standard.

Nowadays, with improvement of paediatric anaesthesia, it can be repaired between 6 months to 18 months of age.

What are the basic principles of hypospadius repair?

Hypospadius repairs involves:

i. Arthroplasty—chordee correction.

ii. Urethroplasty—construction of urethra.

iii. Meatoplasty and glanduloplasty reconstruction of meatal stenosis and glans penis.

So, whats all would be the objectives of the surgery for Hypospadius?

• To produce a cosmetically good looking, straight penis.

• To provide a normal or near normal external urethral orifice.

• To achieve a normal urine flowing urethra and meatus.

• To make proper insemination into the vagina.

What is plan for this patient for coronal hypospadius?

Sir, in this case it will do MAGPI procedure which includes simple glanuloplasty with meatal advancement.

I will dissect the glans penis from the coronal site with the development of anterior base, midline flap of glans epithelium. The tubularised neourethra is brought out by the glans incision and neomeatus is constructed at the tip of the glans penis.

What does MAGPI mean?

MAGPI means Meatal Advancement and glanuloplasty Integrated.

This is an ideal procedure for the patient of glandular hypospadius.

It is contemplated in patients with coronal hypospadius with or without a small chordae.

What are the different operative techniques for different types of hypospadius?

Apart from MAGPI there are:
- Snodgrass procedure, i.e. tubularised incised urethral plate.
- A SPOA procedure dorsal free graft inlay.
- Only transverse preputial skin patch.
- Transverse preputial skip tube.
- Two stage repair.

What is Snodgrass procedure?

This is nothing but tubularization of incised urethral plate. This is very suitable for distal penile hypospadius with wide groove, wide distal penile hypospadius with wide groove, wide meatus.
- Healthy, thick urethral plate.
- Healthy skin/ mucosa ventrally.
- Proximal to meatus and
- Without/or minimal chordae.
- Minimal chordae can be corrected by dorsal plication.

What is Asopa's technique of urethroplasty?

- It is the modification of Snodgrass technique, i.e. a dorsal free graft is applied on an incised urethral plate.
- Asopa is described as a similar operation like Snodgrass.
- Tubularisation of incised urethral plate/inner prepuce for neourethra construction and the modification is used to the outer prepuce to make a skin cover.
- The indications are more or less similar to Snodgrass techniques.

What is Onlay transverse prepucial skin tube repair?

It is performed in patients who are having:
- Considerable chordae.
- Conical glans or with a flat shallow glans.
- good adequate prepuce.

Here neourethra is formed by tubularisation of the edges of the inner preputial flap.

What are two stages repair in hypospadius?

Two stage repairs is suitable for the patients with:
- Marked chordee.
- Meatus situated far proximally.
- There is no or inadequate prepuce.

First stage—Orthroplasty is performed, i.e., correction of chordee and the prepuce is repositioned ventrally.

Second stage—after 6 months- neourethra is constructed either by local flap or a tubularized flap.

How will you manage the post operative period?

- Sponge dressing applying medium pressure to prevent Hematoma.
- Penis is kept vertically to make the urethra straight.
- Catheter to be kept *in situ* for 8-10 days.
- Local application of antibiotic ointment and systemic antibiotic for 5-6 days.

What are the complications of hypospadius repair?

Usual complications are:

Early
- Bleeding and hematoma.
- Wound infection.
- Breakdown of repair.

Late
- Urethrocutaneous fistula
- Urethral stricture.
- Urethral diverticulum.
- Meatal stenosis.

What are grafts used for neourethra formation?

The grafts used are:
- Prepuce
- Dartos
- Perineal skin
- Free graft—like skin, buccal mucosa, bladder mucosa, etc.

A Muslim boy having hypospadius came to you for circumcision as per the religious custom, at the age of 4 years. What will you do for this boy?

Sir, I would not do circumcision as in hypospadius, circumcision is contraindicated as prepucial skin is required for urethroplasty.

I will advise for hypospadius repair before completing 5 years of age.

SHORT NOTE ON HYPOSPADIUS

It is common congenital anomaly of urethra.
Incidenceù1 in 350 births.

DEVELOPMENT OF URETHRA

Development of urethra begins at 4th week of intra uterine life.

i.   **Urethral plate:** An outgrowth appears as a thickening form the wall of cloaca and urogenital sinus.
    The thickening is on the anterior wall of the endodermal cloaca called urethral plate.

ii. **Urethral groove:** on either side of urethral plate urethral groove is formed by the developments of urethral folds, on the ventral aspect of the phallic portion of urogenital sinus.

iii. **Definition urethral groove:** The roof of the primary urethral groove disintegrates and forms definitive urethral groove.

iv. In male fetus- at 6-7 weeks the testis develops and the leydig cells start functioning, the urethral folds begin to fuse ventrally in the midline to form the urethra.

The glandular urethra is formed by lamellar ingrowth of surface epithelium which is ectodermal origin which grows towards the extent of the urethral plate and by joining with it, the whole urethra is completed.

Know about Epispadias

*   The external urethral opening is located on the dorsal aspect of the penis.
*   Rare variety, occurs 1, 30000 births.
*   Types—three types—glandular, penile, totalis (where the urethra is deficient throughout it is whole dorsal extent.
*   Commonest site is the abdominopenile junction.
*   It is associated with dorsal chordee, ectopia vesicae, urinary incontinence, and separated pubic bones.

Treatment

Urethroplasty similar in principle of Denis Browne's technique, usually done at the age of three years.

DENIS BROWNE'S TECHNIQUE:

It is a two stage operation.

Stage I: Chordee correction to cause straightening of the penis. Usually, it is done between 1-2 years.

Stage II: Construction of urethra. It is performed between 4-6 years.

My patient Asim, 3 years old male child parents presented with complain of
- Absence of right testis since birth
- Swelling at right groin for last 6 months

Parents noticed the absence of right testis since birth and for last 6 months. There is a swelling in the right groin which becomes prominent when the child crying or standing and it disappears on lying down no other congenital defect is noticed by the parents.

On Examination: The child is sitting comfortably. General examinations are essentially normal.

On Local Examination: Right sided testes is not there in the scrotum and:
- Right side of scrotum is undeveloped looks asymmetrical
- Right sided testes is not palpable in the way of it's descent or it is ectopic position
  [Do leg rising test to make the ectopic testis prominent]
- Left testis and left side of scrotum are normal
- There is an expansible cough impulse in the right groin swelling which is reduced on lying down even on digital pressure.
  (90% cases of undescended testis accompanies congenital hernia)
- The spermatic cord is felt thickened
- No other congenital associated abnormality found like hypospadius.
- Systemic examination is essentially normal.

So, this is a case of right sided impalpable undescended testis with right sided indirect, reducible, uncomplicated inguinal hernia.

How can you say this is a case of undescended testis not retractile?

- In retractile testis: The scrotal sac is normal and well developed

- In retractile testis usually the testis lies either in inguinal canal or in the superficial inguinal pouch
- A retractile testis can be brought down, better say coaxed down in the scrotum, i.e. in its normal position.

But in my case there are typical features of undescended testis like undeveloped scrotum, associated with congenital hernia etc. suggestive of this is a case of undescended testis.

How will you manage this case?

Sir, I will do USG groin, pelvis and retroperitoneal area to localize the testis.

Suppose you are not able to localize the testis by USG abdomen what will you do?

Sir, this is the disadvantage of USG. In majority of cases USG cannot diagnosis the intra abdominal location of testis.

CT/MRI also not very reliable modality so, the choice in such a case is diagnostic laparoscopy.

What all will you see in diagnostic laparoscopy?

Deep ring and associated hernia whether cord structures are remerging from deep inguinal ring or not
- If it emerging it means the testis has descended through deep ring to inguinal canal
- It does not emerge it means the testis still in intra-abdominal location.
- If blind ending vas is found it suggestive of testicular agenesis or vanishing testis, thereby no surgical exploration is necessary.

Suppose on scape you see the testis is inside the abdomen what will you do?

Two things can be done:
  i. Perform an extra-abdominal exploration and attempt to place the testis in scrotum
  ii. Clip/site the testicular vessels and do orchiopexy later date.

When will you consider orchiectomy?

Sir, I will do orchiectomy when I will:

i. Suspect malignancy of the testis
ii. Atrophy of the testis and
iii. The position of the testis is so high in the abdomen that it cannot be brought down

What is the ideal age for orchiopexy and why?

Histological changes may occur as early as 6 months of post natal life, so, in a case of undescended testis. It should be operated at the earliest to prevent the histological changes. The best time for orchiopexy is about 1 year of age.

As the changes are reversible up to 2 years of age. Orchiopexy to be done latest by 2 years.

Your patient 3 years old child. What will you do in this case?

Sir, I will localize the tumour either by USG or by laparoscopy and still prefer to do orchiopexy .

How orchiopexy helps in this patient?

- Chance of normal spermatogenesis
- Risk of tumour development will be less if develops it's earlier to diagnose
- Chance of torsion will be reduced
- Associated inguinal hernia will be repaired
- Mental satisfaction of having both the testes in the scrotum.

What are the basic principles of orchiopexy?

- Mobilization of spermatic cord will be adequate
- Fixation of testis in the scrotum without tension
- Repairing of associated inguinal hernia

Where will you fix the testis in the scrotum during orchiopexy?

Fixation at three points of the tunica albuginea to the tunica vaginalis with fine proline sutures has been recommended.

An alternative method of fixation is to place the testis in a dartos pouch [In case of torsion testis opposite testis should also be fixed as the anatomical variants which predispose to torsion are commonly Bilateral].

What is conventional orchiopexy?

Here approach is through inguinal incision
↓
Hernial sac is dissected from the cord structures and a high ligation of the sac is done
↓

Extra dartos pouch is created in the scrotum and testis is placed in the pouch and fixes it
↓
Adequate dissection is required to avoid tension of the pedicle while placing the testis in the scrotum [Retroperitoneal dissection and careful snipping off lateral peritoneal bands will give adequate length of the cord]

What is Prentiss maneuver?

During orchiopexy if the testis does not reach the scrotum easily then the inferior epigastric artery and vein can be ligated and the testis is brought directly through the floor of fascia transversalis this is called Prentiss maneuver.

What is Fowler Stephen's technique?

In this technique main testicular vessels are ligated and divided.

Artery to vas and cremaster and their collaterals will take care testicular growth and survival. But chance of atrophy is higher. So two stages Fowler Stephen's technique developed.

First stage: ligation of spermatic vessels to gain length and allow developing collateral blood supply. Testis is not mobilized in this stage.

Second stage: After 6 months from the 1st procedure testis is brought to the scrotum through inguinal route.

The blood supply of testis will be through the developed call laterals and artery to vas.

What is Silber procedure?

Orchidopexy by microvascular anastomosis testis is mobilized, testicular vessels are divided and after placement of testis in the scrotal pouch the testicular artery and vein are anastomosed with Inferior epigastric artery and vein respectively.

What is Refluo technique?

In the technique venous drainage is emphasized more. For venous drainage of testis testicular vein is anastomosed with inferior epigastric vein but for blood supply it relies upon the collateral from vas.

What about Ombredanne's procedure?

The undescended testis is placed into the scrotal sac through the scrotal septum.

Do you know the Kettey Torek procedure?

Sir,
This procedure is obsolete now a day. In this procedure the testis is fixed in the thigh with a thread and repeated pulling of thread.

What is the role of Hormonal therapy in undescended testis?

- Human chorionic gonadotrophins (hCG) by injection and gonadotrophin releasing hormones (GnRH) as a form of nasal spray
- It is claimed effective in patients having the testis high scrotal and testis lying in the inguinal canal
- Hormones mainly HCG have been used for the selection of anorchia in a case of impalpable testis (Dose 1,000 IU on alternate days 3 such)
- hCG also used to achieve partial or complete descent of undescended testis and the secondary benefit for re do case as the testicular volume the vessels and the scrotum
- Since the therapy is effective only 20-30% case, it is not widely used
- Not effective in ectopic testis and the will be increased rugosity and pigmentation in the scrotum.

What is the role of laparoscopy in this case?

Paediatric laparoscopy has 95%. Sensitivity for locating a testis or proving it absent particularly when the USG plays no role to detect the testis.

Moreover, it seems to have a reliable diagnostic and therapeutic options for this patient of undescended testis.

It also obviates the need for groin exploration in many cases.

What are the complications of Orchiopexy?

- Failed orchiopexy it self.
- Recurrence of non descent due to in appropriate technique
- Testicular re-ascent quite possible particularly when it is tethered to the operative scar and retracts out of the scrotum with the passage of time and with subsequent increasing growth.
- Testicular atrophy
- Injury to vas
- Injury to testicular vessels, vessels of vas and cremaster.

Suppose during orchiopexy testicular artery is cut through what will happen to the testis then?

Sir, if the testicular artery is injured still the testis may survive as artery to vas and artery to cremaster then take over the supply to testis. But chance of atrophy is as high as 40%.

What are the complications of undescended testis?

The usual complications are: (Remember- SATHI)

S - Subfertility/infertility common with bilateral undescended testis

A - Atrophy

T - Trauma, torsion and tumor development 20 times.

H - Hernia may present up to 90% cases

I - Inflammation and pain

What is the risk of malignancy in undescended testis?

Chance of malignant transformation is as high as 40% and commonest tumour is seminoma but it is more (1, 20) in abdominal testis but less (1, 80) in inguinal testis.

Is there any role of orchiopexy to reduce malignancy?

It is controversial. But orchiopexy before the age of 2 years has definite role. Even study suggests pre pubescent orchiopexy may reduce the risk of developing malignancy.

One definite benefit of orchiopexy is that early detection of cancer if develops.

What changes occur in an undescended testis?

Growth retardation and by the age of six testis becomes hypo plastic. By the time of puberty it would be soft and flabby due to atrophy

Histological changes epithelial elements are grossly immature. By the age of sixteen destructive changes of seminiferous tubules occur which are irreversible.

The number of leydig, Sertoli cells, and germs cells are decreased and defective spermatogenesis.

SHORT NOTES ON UNDESCENDED TESTIS

Undescended Testis: The testis which fails to reach the scrotum but it's descent is arrested somewhere along it's pathway.

Undescended testis is more common in the right side because right testis usually descends later than the left.

Incidence—right-sided UDT 50%, left-sided UDT 30% and bilateral 20% [UDT-Undescended Testis]

Approximately 4% of all full-term newborns have an undescended testis or testes and about 80% are unilateral. Common in premature Infant 30 % and full-term 4% only.

Testicular Descent: Testis develop in the retroperitoneum at the level of L1 Vertebra around 8 weeks of intra uterine life.

↓

Thereafter it traverses the retroperitoneum from 9 weeks to 11 weeks and reaches right iliac fossa by the end of 12 weeks (3 months)

↓

It reaches deep inguinal ring by 6 months of intrauterine life

↓

It traverses inguinal canal between 7 to 9 months

↓

It reaches bottom of the scrotum by the end of 9 months

TYPE of Undescended Testis: [Remember—ARIES]
A—Abdominal testis: In the posterior abdominal wall retroperitoneally

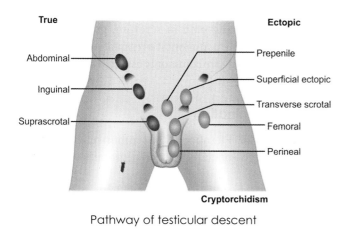

Pathway of testicular descent

R—Retractile testis: Due to contraction of cremaster muscle, the testis is pulled upward either in the inguinal canal or in the superficial inguinal pouch.
I—Iliac, inguinal or interstitial: Iliac deep to deep inguinal ring inguinal or interstitial testis lies in the inguinal canal.
E—Emergent testis: Movement of the testis ranges from the inguinal canal to the superficial ring.

Emergent testis is transiently palpable out side the superficial ring but it slips back to inguinal canal.
S—Simple undescended or high retractile testis: Testis lies at superficial inguinal ring or at upper scrotum.

Ectopic testis: An ectopic testis is one which fails to descend into the scrotum as because it is deviated from its usual path of descent.

Ectopic testis may be found in one of the following positions:
i. Superficial inguinal pouch [the pouch lies above and lateral to the superficial inguinal ring and superficial to the external oblique aponeurosis] is the most common site
ii. Suprapubic region at the route of the penis
iii. Perineum
iv. Femoral triangle (thigh)
v. Opposite scrotal compartment—rarest.

LOCKWOOD THEORY REGARDING ECTOPIC TESTIS

According to 'Lockwood' the gubernacular band (a fold of peritoneum which is responsible for testicular descent called gubernaculam) has four accessory tails called tails of Lockwood.
i. Superficial inguinal tail
ii. Pubic tail
iii. Perineal tail
iv. Femoral tail

Usual way all of the accessory tails disappear except the scrotal tail. In ectopic testis the scrotal tail weakness and ruptures, so the testis is pulled by any of the accessory tails in the above order of frequency.

Cryptorchidism: The term is applied in case of Bilateral undescended testes and clinically impalpable.

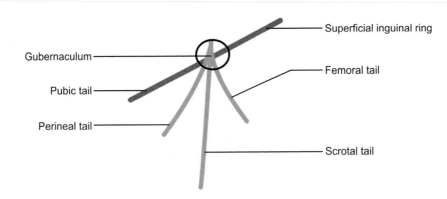

Gubernacular tails of Lockwood

Table 44.1: Difference between undescended testis and ectopic testis

Undescended Testis	Ectopic Testis
1. Descend of testis is arrested any where of its normal path	1. The testis is deviated from it normal path of descent
2. Factors responsible are retroperitoneal adhesion, at deep ring, short testicular vessels, Vas difference, inefficient pull by guberna culum, etc.	2. Weakness or rupture of scrotal tail of lockwood due to unknown oetiology
3. Undescendned testis is poorly	3. Ectopic testis is well developed
4. Scrotum is also poorly developed	4. Scrotum is well developed
5. Inguinal canal it may lie deep in the canal	5. Ectopic testis lies super ficial to inguinal canal at superficial inguinal pouch
6. Spermatic cord is short	6. Cord length is normal
7. Complication are more likely like infertility, tumour torsion, trauma, atrophy, etc.	7. Here only the testis may liable to trauma otherwise normally functioning testis

Clinical differentiation between undescended in inguinal canal and ectopic testis in superficial inguinal pouch:
  i. Ask the patient for shoulder rising, test ectopic testis will be more prominent as it a parietal testis. Undescended testis will be less prominent or impalpable
  ii. Push the testis laterally upwards ectopic testis will be more prominent as it goes to a higher level. Undescended testis will be disappeared as it goes through deep inguinal ring.

Difference between retractile testis and ectopic testis in the superficial inguinal pouch Do 'traction test' retractile testis can be brought down into the scrotum but ectopic testis cannot be.

Tortion of testis: Tortion testis the name itself suggests that the testis is under torsion, i.e. testis twists in its axis compromising its blood supply.

Right testis usually rotates clockwise direction and left testis rotates anticlockwise.

Etiology

- Inversion of testis
- High investment of tunica vaginalis and testis rotates like a clapper in bell
- A wide gap between the body and epididymis so testis twists over epididymis
- Heavy strain, trauma are other etiological factors.

Clinical Features

- Most commonly occurs between 10-15 years
- Sudden agonizing pain in scrotum, groin and lower abdomen are the commonest presentation
- Nausea, vomiting are commonly associated features (90% cases).

Clinical Examination

  i. **Prehn's sign :** Elevation of the scrotum relieves the pain in epididymo or chitis but pain aggravates in torsion of testis
  ii. **Deming's sign:** Tortion testis will be in high position because of twisting of cord and spasm of cremaster muscle.

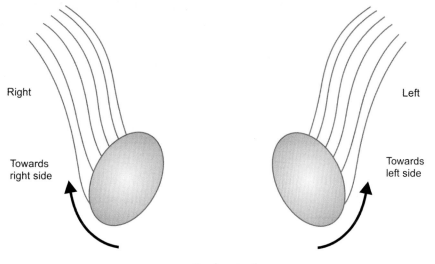

Torsion testis

Angell's sign: Opposite testis will lie horizontally because of the presence of mesorchium.

Differential Diagnosis

1. Epididymo-orchitis
2. Strangulated inguinal hernia

Investigations
- Total WBC count
- Color Doppler to see testicular artery supply (But do not waste much more time for color Doppler)
- USG abdomen another alternative.

Management: Take consent for orchidectomy early exploration (golden time is within 6 hours)

↓

Viability of testis checked put warm saline soaked gauge for 5-10 minutes see the color change

↓

If changed and testis appears viable > 3 points fixation with 3, 0 proline (both the testis)

↓

If no color change testis appears nonviable—orchidectomy is the answer opposite side testis to be fixed

↓

When there is any doubt in viability 50-50 chance—postpone it

↓

Repeat color Doppler and take the final decision

CASE 46

Hydrocephalus

DEFINITION

Hydrocephalus is defined as disproportionate increase in the amount of CST within the cranium, usually in association with a rise in intra cranial pressure.

Or

It can be defined as dilatation of ventricles due to overproduction or failure of resorption or obstruction to CSF flow called Hydrocephalus.

CEREBROSPINAL FLUID

- Volume is around 140 ml.
- It is replaced three times per day.
- Production and re absorption is regulated by ICP.
- Choroid plexus produces 80% of CST.
- CST is a oduction, failure of re sorption or obstruction to its flow leads to hydrocephalus.

PATHWAY OF CST

- Most of CST is produced in lateral ventricles through foramina of Monro.
- CST down through IIIrd ventricle through the duct of sylvius
- Into the 4th ventricle
- Passing laterally through foramina of luschka and inferiorly through foramina of magentie
- Passing over the surface of the cortex for re absorption at the Arachnoids villi.

TYPES OF HYDROCEPHALUS

- **Communicating**: Ventricles are communicated freely into the subarachnoid space.
  Here the defective absorption of CST following an Inflammation, traumas or subarachnoid hemorrhage.

- **Noncommunicating:** Here the obstruction lies in the ventricle or its exit pathway due to any tumor or chronic inflammatory process.

i. It may be :
Congenital: Associated with spina bifida, meningocele or
Meningomyelocele due:
  - Failure of formation of CSF pathway.
  - Arnold Chiari malformation.
  - Congenital stenos are of aque duct of sylvius.

Presentations widening of sutures, tense fontanel's, decreased cortical thickness enlargement of skill occurs either prenatal or postnatal period.

ii. **Acquired causes** are:
  - Chronic meningitis.
  - Trauma—Subarachnoids hemorrhage.
  - Choroid cyst.
  - Brain tumors (cerebellar, pineal body tumor etc.)
  - Archnoid cyst.
  - Colloid cyst of 3rd ventricle

iii. **Clinical features**
  Neonates: Increasing head circumference, tense fortunately, failure to thrives engorged scalps veinsey separatin of suture lines ' Sun setting ' sign- decreased upward gaze.
  Children and adults: Signs of increased intra cranial pressure (ICP), i.e. headache, nausea, vomiting papilloedema, decreasing level of consciousness. lethargy, ataxia elderly-dementia alongwith.

iv. **Clinical Examination**
  - Disproportion of the head to the rest of the body
  - Palpation of head rerears a tense fontanele and separaton of sutures
  - Percussion over the head produces a typical sound called 'crack pot' sign.

v. **Investigations**

X-ray skull will show:

- Separationof suture lines
- Copper beating of the skull
- CECT—to detect the cause of Hydrocephalus
- MRI—when a tumor is seen to determine

A surgical strategy

- When aqueduct stenosis occurs
- To rule out tectalplate tumour when no ther cause, detected by CT scan.

A lumber puncture

Performed in cases of communicating hydrocephalus, even in the presence of raised ICP as both a diagnostic and therapeutic procedure.

vi. **Treatment**

Medical—Acetazolamide a carbonic an hydrase inhibitor and may reduce CSF production around 60%.

- Frusemide has the effect on CSF production
  Truelly speaking drugs are not useful in long term control of hydrocephalusi but these may be used in the short turm

Surgery

Surgical intervention is the ultimate choice for hydrocephalus:

Removalot the cause of obstruction and (b) direct the CSF by :

i. Ventriculoperitoneal (VP) shunt is commonly performed operation.

Others are:

ii. Ventriculoatrial shunt,

iii. Ventriculo - Cysternostomy using polythene catheter called Torkildsen operation

iv. Tapping of lateral ventricles can give temporary relieve.

My patient, Abdul Kalam a 4 years old boy, presented with complains of:

- Mass of left mid abdomen along with discomfort for last 8 months
- Fever off and on for last 3 months.

Eight months back my patient had an experience of abdominal discomfort and mother detected a mass in left mid abdomen which is gradually progressive painless but abdominal discomfort is there off and on.

He has got also a history of fever off and on for last 3 months. The fever is low grade stay for 2/3 days and subsides on medication.

But there is no history of hematuria.

General survey: The patient is thin built, pallor present, pulse 80/min, BP 140/90 mmHg.

On abdominal examination: Presently afebrile, abdomen is scaphoid but there is an obvious bulge at left lumber region, the lump slightly moves with respiration.

On palpation: The retroperitoneal 8 to 6 cm lump is firm in consistency, smooth, mobile at left lumbar region extended above towards left hypochondrium and below towards left iliac fossa. The lump is bimanually palpable and ballotable. Anterior margins are demarcated but posterior margins not well defined and moves with respiration fingers can be insulated between subcostal margin and the lump and it does not cross the midline. Dullness at renal angle and resonant band in front.

Systemic examinations are essentially normal.

So, this is a case of left sided kidney tumor most probably Wilms" tumor of a 4 years old child.

Why are you telling this is a Wilms' tumour?

- Four years old child presented with
- Kidney mass and history of
- Low grade fever and hypertension
- All suggestive of Wilms' tumor

What is the triad of Wilms' tumor?

Renal mass, fever and hematuria.

What are the commonest differential diagnosis?

The component differential diagnoses are:

i. Neuroblastoma
ii. Hydronephrosis
iii. Cystic kidney disease

What are the causes of fever and hematuria in a case of Wilms' tumor?

Fever may be due to tumor necrosis and seen half and hematuria signifies of the cases rupture of tumor into the renal pelvis. It is a grave sign.

Why Wilms' tumor is also called nephroblastoma?

The tumor arises from blast cells of kidney hence called Nephroblastoma.

It arise from embryonic connective tissue containing epithelial and connective tissue elements.

What other anomalies may be associated with Wilms' tumor?

Anomalies may be associated: Up to 12% case the following:

- Glaucoma
- Aniridia
- Beckwith syndrome

What investigations you like to do in this case?

Sir, I will confirm my diagnosis first
I will do,

i. USG abdomen to see the organ of origin of the tumor and whether it is solid or cystic like hydronephrosis. Cortical thickening of kidney to assess the functional status of the kidney.
ii. CECT abdomen

- to stage the disease
- to assess the same and opposite kidney function

Stage I   Tumor is limited to kidney and it is completely resectable

Stage II   Tumor extends beyond kidney but it is completely resectable

Stage III   Residual non-hematogenous tumor confined to abdomen

Stage IV   Hematogenous metastasis to lung, liver, bone

Stage V   Bilateral tumor at the time of diagnosis.

iii. Intravenous pyelography(IVP): It will show distortion and displacement of pelvicalyceal system. But in good CECT scan shows the same picture so IVP is not required all the time.

What is the role of Renal Angiography in this case?

Sir, Renal angiography is only indicated in case of bilateral Wilms' tumor where at least one sided partial nephrectomy is mandatory

What other investigations you would like to do?

I will do,

- X-ray PA view to exclude pulmonary metastasis (as lung is the commonest site for metastasis chest)
- X-ray abdomen typical 'Egg Shell' peripheral calcification is diagnostic
- All base line investigations to make the patient fit for anaesthesia and surgery.

What is the treatment protocol of a case of Wilms' tumor?

Treatment protocol

- < 4 cm Wilms' tumor and patient is asymptomatic - follow-up the patient frequently (3 monthly)
- Symptomatic patients even < 4 cm tumor or > 4 cm tumor
- Unilateral tumor—nephrectomy followed by radiotherapy with or without chemotherapy.

Bilateral tumor

- If possible Bilateral partial nephrectomy
- Partial nephrectomy in less affected side and nephrectomy in more affected side
- If both the side is affected grossly at least one sided Nephron sparing surgery (hemi/partial) to be done
- All of the above followed by Radiotherapy with or without chemotherapy

What are the chemotherapy agents can be used.

Actinomycin B, Vincristine, Doxorubicin.

What is the role of renal artery embolization in a case of Wilms' tumor?

In a large Wilms' tumor renal artery embolization is an effective procedure to reduce the tumor size, thereby, nephrectomy will be relatively easier.

Where does Wilms' tumor metastases?

The Wilms' tumor spreads by hematogenous route and mainly it goes to lung.

Liver metastasis is a late feature bone metastasis and lymph node metastasis is rare.

What are the prognostic factor of wilms' tumor?

The prognostic factors are:

- Age—less age good prognosis
- Size of tumor > 4 cm bad prognosis
- Presence of hematuria suggests grave prognosis spread of tumour
- Histological type—anaplastic features worst prognostic factor.

What are the types of Wilms' tumor?

There are two types of Wilms' tumor:

i. FH Willms'—favorable histology without anaplastic features

ii. Un FH Wilms'—unfavorable histology means with anaplastic features

What are the histological types of Wilms' tumors?

Histological types are:

- Cystic
- Mesoblastic
- Nephroblastoma

What is the prognosis of Wilms' tumour

Five years survival of patients with favorable histology now approaches about 90%.

Mostly recurrence occurs within 1 year.

Tell me, the types of Nephrectomy

There are three types of nephrectomy:

i. Radical—whole kidney fascia of gerota along with lymph nodes clearance

ii. Simple—removal of kidney without lymph node clearance.

iii. Nephron sparing nephrectomy—either partial or heminehrectomy.

Is there any role of MRI in the case of Wilms' tumor?

MRI can provide important information in defining the extent of tumor into the inferior vena cava, including those with intracardiac extension. Good CT scan also provide the same information so, MRI is rarely indicated.

What is the role of needle biopsy?

Pre operative biopsy is indicated in large tumor only for safe primary surgical resection or for which preoperative chemotherapy or radiotherapy is planned.

SHORT NOTES ON WILMS' TUMOR

WILMS' TUMOR (SYNONYM NEPHROBLASTOMA)

It is a mixed tumor containing epithelium and connective tissue elements from embryonic nephrogenic tissue.

- Characteristic features
  - Usually discovered during 4 years of life
  - It is located one or other pole of one kidney
  - Bilateral tumor occurs in 5% cases only
- Clinical features
  - Both sexes are equally affected
  - Classical trial is abdominal mass, fever and hematuria
  - Abdominal discomfort, pain, distension
  - Anorexia, nausea, vomiting
  - Hypertension 25-60% cases (caused by elevated renin levels)
- Investigations
  - USG abdomen
  - CECT Scan
  - IVP
  - Renal angiography
  - Already described
  - Others urine
    RE to exclude hematuria and all routine investigations ME
- Differential diagnosis
  i. Intrarenal neuroblastoma
  ii. Hydronephrosis
  iii. Cystic disease

NEUROBLASTOMA

- Third most common neoplastic disease
- It occur usually in first 2 years of life
- Presentations are abdominal mass, symptoms related to metastasis include fever, malaise, bone pain, failure to thrive, constipation or diarrhea and hypertension

- The mass is at lumber and towards hypochondrial area. The mass is bosselated, nodular, does not move with respiration and it crosses the midline
- Evidence of metastases to skull, liver bone, may be noted
- Laboratory findings—anaemia common norepinephrine, epinephrine, urinary vanillylmandelic acid (VMA) levels may be high.
- Bone marrow aspiration may reveal tumor cells.

Investigations

USG/CT scan may show that tumors size and extent.

Here displacement of pelvicalyceal system may be there but not distortion (both seen in Wilms' tumor)

Treatment

Stage I and II—surgical excision with or without chemotherapy

Stage III and IV—neoadjuvant chemotherapy followed by surgery and radiotherapy (Neuroblastoma is a radiosensitive tumor).

(ii) Hydronephrosis

Unilateral Cases

- Congenital PUJ obstruction and calculus are the most common causes M:F = 2:1
- Right kidney is more commonly affected
- Dull aching loin pain, dragging sensation or history of renal colic
- Mass at lumber region which is smooth, mobile, ballotable, dullness at renal angle and band of colonic resonant in front, moves with respiration
- Dietls' crisis: After an acute attack of renal colic, swelling appears in the loin and following a passage of large volume of urine, the swelling disappears.

In bilateral cases

From bilateral upper urinary tract obstruction:

- Loin pain, mass in the loin, renal colic in severe obstruction. Features of renal failure like oliguria, edema, etc.

From lower urinary tract obstruction:

- Loin pain, features of bladder outlet obstruction frequency, hesitancy, poor stream etc. features of renal failures in persistent cases
- USG abdomen is the investigation of choice which can diagnose cause of obstruction, site of obstruction, thickness of parenchyma, etc.

[Details written in the case of Hydronephrosis]

(iii) Cystic disease

Solitary cyst

- Almost always acquired
- History of trauma or infection may be there
- It presents as unilateral renal mass, which is smooth, may be tender - features of kidney swelling.

Polycystic kidney:

- Presents in third decade
- Bilateral palpable renal mass which is lobular, firm, mobile, moves with respiration, ballotable, dullness at renal angle and resonant in front

- Loin pain (due to stretching of renal capsule or hemorrhage into a cyst)
- Hematuria (due to over distended cyst rupturing into renal pelvis)
- Infection due to stasis of urine
- Hypertension—75% case
- Uraemia occurs in a late stage due to renal failure
- USG abdomen is the investigation of choice

STAGES OF NEUROBLASTOMA

Stage I Tumors confined to structure of origin

Stage II Tumors extending in continuity beyond the organ but not crossing the midline. Ipsilateral lymph node may be involved

Stage III Tumors extending in continuity beyond the midline. Regional lymph nodes may be involved

Stage IV Remote disease involving skeletal organs, soft tissue, and distant lymph nodal groups.

Stage V Stage I and II patients with remote spread of tumor confined to one or more organs like liver, skin, bone marrow etc.

CASE 48 — Congenital Hernia

My patient, Suman a 2 years old male child mother states that the child having a swelling in the right grain since birth.

The swelling increases in size, disappears on lying and becomes prominent on crying or on strains.

On examination the child is comfortably sitting on mother's lap general examination is normal.

Local examination: The right sided inguinoscrotal swelling showing expansible impulse on crying the swelling is reducible.

So, this is case of right sided congenital hernia in a 2 years old child.

Why congenital hernia appears, i.e. what is the basic defect in congenital hernia?

The failure of obliteration of processus vaginalis is the basic congenital defect for this hernia.

What is the basic difference between congenital hernia and hydrocele?

In congenital hernia, processus vaginalis remains patient throughout communicating with the abdomen and the deep ring is larger enough to pass the bowel or omentum through it.

But, in congenital hydrocele deepring is to narrow to admit the bowel or omentum it only admits the escape of fluid.

What is the anatomy of inguinal canal in a child?

In new born and up to first 2 years of life inguinal canal does not develop and superficial and deep ring lie close to each other. Two years onwards the deep ring moves laterally and inguinal canal proper starts developing.

What will you do in this patient?

Sir, I will do base line investigations like hemogram, urine RE, ME and do Herniotomy, i.e. excision of hernia sac only under general anesthesia.

What will you do after dissecting the sac from cord structure?

After dissecting the sac from cord structure, the sac is opened and content is milk into the peritoneal cavity. The sac is transacted distal to the superficial inguinal ring and proximal sac is held by a hemostatic forcep and dissected proximally up to internal inguinal ring. The sac is ligated by transfixation at the neck and the redundant sac is excised.

What is the incision?

Sir, just a transverse incision is made over the deep inguinal ring.

Will you prefer to do opposite sided herniotomy in same sitting?

Actually Sir, this is still debatable few surgeons like to do opposite sided herniotomy as because there is a fair chance (5-10%) of developing hernia in the opposite side but most of the surgeons do not interfere the normal side at the same sitting.

In which case bilateral herniotomy is logical even though manifestation is only in one side?

Sir, the processus vaginalis closes earlier in females, around 6 months of gestation; hence, there are more chances bilateral patient processus if unilateral hernia is present in female child.

The processus vaginalis closes earlier in left side than the right. So if a left sided hernia present, there are more chance of a patent right processus vaginalis.

Also, in an infant the contralateral sac is present about 50% cases so, most of the Bilateral hernias present at less than one year of age.

So, bilateral herniotomy is logical in a female infant under 1 year of age.

What is 'silk glove' sign?

In a case of congenital indirect inguinal hernia the spermatic cord may feel thickened or 'rustle' on palpation as the contagious folds of peritoneum slide over one another this is called 'silk glove' sign.

What are the approaches for congenital inguinal hernia?

There are two approaches:
  i. Inguinal approach
  ii. Preperitoneal approach

In inguinal approach the incision is made in the lower most transverse inguinal skin crease (not parallel to inguinal ligament like in adult). The superficial inguinal ring is not to be opened.

In neonate superficial inguinal ring lies over the deep inguinal ring so the incision is to be kept limited to the medical portion of skin crease.

Preperitoneal approach a standard grid iron incision is used to reach the preperitoneal plane. The deep ring and hernia sac are identified lateral to inferior epigastric vessels.

How will you take irreducible obstructed congenital inguinal hernia?

Congenital hernia is likely to get complicated with obstruction and even strangulation. It occurs when the intestine gets stuck at the internal inguinal ring.

The treatment of obstructed hernia includes:
- Cold fomentation to reduce edema
- A gently pressure is applied to reduce the hernial contents (but not in presence of peritonitis). Adequate sedation, analgesic to calm the child
- Child to be observed hourly to notice any damage intestine or testis has occurred.

Herniotomy is preferably done after 48 hours when tissue oedema has subsided.

In case of strangulated hernia an urgent surgery is essential.

What are the signs of triangulation?

There will a history of sudden increase in size with severe pain and symptoms of bowel obstruction.

On examination there is a tense, tender and fixed in the groin:
- Bowel sounds increased
- It may be confused with torsion of testis, acute inguinal lymphadenitis or infected hydrocele.

What are the likely post operative complications?

The post operative complications may be:
- Scrotal swelling
- Ascending testis
- Injury to vas

- Testicular atrophy.
- Intestinal injury and chance of recurrence is up to 20%.

NOTES ON CONGENITAL HERNIA AND HYDROCELE

Congenital inguinal hernia:

- Incidence 8 to 9.9%
- Male : Female 6:1

The patient processus vaginalis present 80% of male child at birth. 40% at 2 years and 20% in adult male.

In children, hernia is almost always indirect inguinal hernia, i.e. hernia sac is lateral to inferior epigastric vessels.

Most of the inguinal hernias are present before 6 months of age. The swelling usually noticed by parents when the child cries. The swelling disappears when the child lying down.

A reliable history is enough to establish the diagnosis, though there is no evidence of such an abnormality when the baby is examined.

How to diagnosis:
- Cough/cry impulse positive
- A soft bulge which is reducible on digital pressure [Remember—hernia in neonates may be transilluminate so it is not a reliable test to differentiate between congenital hernia and hydrocele]
- Spermatic cord may feel thickened as the continuous folds of peritoneum slide over one another called 'silk glove' sign.
Hernia fills from above downwards.

Differential Diagnosis

- Hydrocele—which fills from below upwards
  - No cough/cry impulse
  - Takes long time to get reduced (Inverted Ink effect) on lying down
  - Hydrocele transilluminate (Neonates hernia is also transilluminate)
  - Spermatic cord feels normal i.e. no 'silk glove' sign
  - Hydrocele is light blue color through skin
- An encysted Hydrocele of the cord mimics like a irreducible inguinal hernia. Traction test may differentiate the pro. In encysted hydrocele of the cord will move up and down but hernia does not move.

Remember: Niddle aspiration is contraindicated in inguinal swelling, white suspecting hernia because there is chance of intestinal perforation.

SHORT NOTES ON CONGENITAL HYDROCELE

The neck of the sac is so narrow at deep ring that intestine or omentum cannot pass through on fluid can pass and forms the hydrocele.

Accumulation of fluid in the scrotum due to persistent communication via patient processus vaginalis from the peritoneal cavity.

Left sided hydrocele is more common as it takes longer for the left processus vaginalis to close and it remains patient with the peritoneal cavity.

Ninety percent cases spontaneous resolution occurs within 2 years of life.

If the hydrocele persists more than 2 years simple herniotomy to be done like hernia but no attempt to excise the sac completely.

My patient, Gourav, a 6 months old full-term male baby. Mother presented with complain of swelling in the lower back since birth.

The swelling is gradually increasing in since, painlessly and attained its present size 4 × 3 cm approximately. The swelling becomes more prominent when the baby coughs or cries.

The child moving both upper and lower limbs normally. There is no history of maternal abnormality during pregnancy and delivery.

On examination

Baby sitting comfortably in mother's lap. General examinations are essentially normal. Head circumferences— – 40 cm (normal).

On local examination

- There is a 4 × 3 cm cystic swelling at lumbosacral region
- Presence of impulse in the swelling while child cries
- Overlying skin is free from the swelling
- The swelling compressible
- Fluctuation positive
- Trans illumination brilliantly positive.
- The edge of the bony defect is palpable or bony indentation is palpable of the margin of the swelling
- No other congenital abnormalities notice
- No neurological deficit i.e. both sensory and motor deficit absent.

So this is a case of lumbosacral meningocele of a 6 months old baby.

Why it is not meningomyelocele?

- In meningomyelocele, etc. bony defect usually extend over three or more segments.
  - i. In meningomyelocele–neurological deficits are almost always present in the form of both sensory

and motor deficits like bladder, incontinence, flaccid paraparesis, etc.
  - ii. Transillumination test will show opaque bands within the red glow. The opaque brands are due to presence of nerve fibers.

Why do you in ensure the head circumference of the body?

In around 80% cases hydrocephalus is associated with meningocele. If it is present that is to be treated prior to excision of meningocele.

How will you manage this case?

- First I will confirm the diagnosis
- First I will do simple X-ray lumbosacral region. X-ray will show the bony defect.
- CT scan head establish the causes of obstruction.
- MRI lumbosacral region may show:
  - Clear delineation of the swelling
  - Relation of the swelling to neural structures
  - To see the end of spinal cord and any cord tethering.
- MRI at craniovertebral spine to exclude Arnold Chiari malformation.

What is Arnold Chiari syndrome and how will you manage it?

When meningocele is associated with hydrocephalus the condition is called Arnold Chiary syndrome and due to obstruction at the level of foramen magnum. Decompression of foramen magnum, durotomy and duroplasty are treatments OK.

Next what will you do?

Sir, I will make the baby feet for surgery by doing HB, TLC, DLC BT, CT and urine–RE and ME. As there is no hydrocephalus I will do nothing for that—I will do:

- Excision of meningocele and
- Repair of the defect under general anesthesia.

Can you tell me the operative procedure in short please?

Sir, Longitudinal incision is made over three swelling skin flaps are raised.

- Meningeal sac is dissected and excised
- Covering of dura mater is repaired
- The bony defect is covered with erector spinae muscle
- Skin margins are opposed (If margins are not opposed, a lateral release incision is made to oppose the margins).

If there is hydrocephalus how would you manage?

Sir, I would manage hydrocephalus, before the excision of meningocele as the excision may aggravate the hydrocephalus, so a ventriculoperitoneal shunt is to be done to mange hydrocephalus first. Though most of the paediatric surgeons like to do both the procedure in a same sitting.

What may be the complications of the surgery for meningocele?

- The procedure itself may cause neurological deficit this is the important complication of this surgery.
- Other complication, may be hemorrhage hematoma formation would dehiscence
- Wound infections CST leakage, meningitis, etc.

Tell me, what is meningocele and what is meningomyelocele?

Meningocele is a protrusion of meninges through the gap in the neural arch posteriorly giving rise a cystic swelling containing cerebrospinal fluid.

Whereas meningomyelocele is a protrusion of the spinal cord or nerve fibres of cauda equina along with the meninges.

What are the complications of meningocele and meningomyelocele?

Complications of meningocele are:

- Rupture
- Infection and
- Ulceration
- Hydrocephalus and its complication.

But the complications of meningomyelocele are more, besides repture, infection, ulceration.

- Urinary bladder dysfunction, i.e. infection, hydronephrosis, incontinence, etc.
- Musculoskeletal abnormalities scoliosis, kyphosis.

Can spina bifida be diagnosed antenatally?

Yes sir, severe spina bifida can be diagnosed antenatally by the both of the following over 80% of fetus:

- Ultrasound scan
- By alpha fetoprotein assays in blood or in amniotic fluid by aminocentesis.

What are other sites neural tube defects?

Lumbosacral region is the most common site.

Other common sites are:

- Root of nose
- Occipital region

  Higher the lesion, more serious the defect and worse the neurological condition.

SHORT NOTES ON NEURAL TUBE DEFECTS

Neural tube defect is the most common problem of spinal column. Failure of closure of neural tube fully produces one of many types of neurospinal dysrophism or so called spina bifida.

Spina bifida is three types:

1. **Souba bifida aperta**: The neural tube is open with moskin coverage, through a defect a defect in the posterior vertebral arch. As CSF leakage is a common features so chance of meningitis is very high.

2. **Spina bifida cystic**: Meningocele is the example meninges comes out through the neural arch posteriorly and is covered with skin which contains CSF.

If the neural tissue lames along with meninges, that forms meningomyelocele.

3. **Spina bifida occulta**: Here the defect is within posterior vertebral arch and there is no herniation of the neural tube.
   - Found in 10% of the children population
   - Various skin changes found over the defect like harry patch, pigmentation, fatty lump, dermal sinus, etc.
   - There may be intradural lesions like dermoids, lipomas, epidermoid tumors, etc.
   - Tethering of the cord with thickening of the filum terminate
     Also may be associated abnormality.

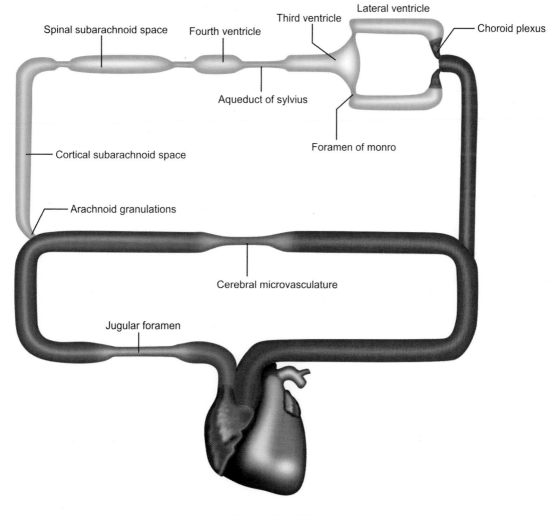

Pathway of CSF flow

How to mange neural tube defects.

Meningocele management already discussed.

Management of Meningomyelocele

The treatment of meningomyelocele includes—treatment of the local condition—treatment for the associated problems like hydrocephalus, musculoskeletal abnormalities, bowel, bladder dysfunctions, etc.

The operation should be done as early as possible after birth with the view of smaller sac, pliable skin, fewer adhesions between the sac and nervous tissue. Less chance of infection as skin flora not established and more over neurological deficit can be reduced to a minimum.

The procedure in short :
- SAC is opened
  - Redundant membrane to be excised.
  - Neural elements are to be separated from the membrane and replaced in the spinal canal
  - Cut margins of the membranae are to be sutured over the cord
  - The defect is to be covered by erector spine muscle with the overlying fascia
  - The wound may be reinforced with the flaps of deep fascia from the erector spine muscle.
  - Skin to be closed without any tension.

Postoperative follow-up

Regular follow-up to see the development of hydrocephalus if any and developmental milestones.

X-ray skull, entire spine, hips along with consultations with urologist, orthopedician, neurosurgeon, physiotherapist may be required.

Know about
1. **Syringomyelocele:** The protrusion of spinal cord along with dilatation of the central canal of the cord to forma cavity filled up with fluid.
   Some neurological deficits are almost always present.
   Clinically it is very difficult to distinguish from meningomyelocele except that trans illumination test is negative is syringomyelocele.
2. **Myelocele:** Exposure of spinal cord and its central canal to the exterior of body surface due to development failure of dorsal wall of neural tube.
   The partial defect through which the spinal cord and its central canal are exposed called Myelocele
   The defect may be complete, through it is rage.

Features

- Constant dribbling CSF through the defect
- Chance of infection is too high to cause meningitis that the baby dies soon.

Notes on Stapler, GI Stapler and Sutures

PRIMARY GOALS OF THE SURGICAL TECHNIQUES

- Restoration of the function of affected organs
- Effective hemostasis
- Reduction of morbidity, infection and sepsis
- Reduction of tissue trauma
- Reduction of mortality.

HUTL'S STAPLING PRINCIPLES

- A "B-shaped" staple eliminates knotting problems when using surgical steel suture

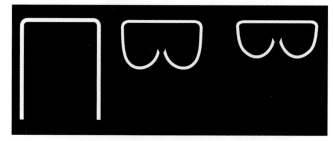

Configuration of surgicals stapler

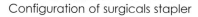
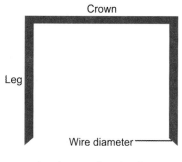

Anatomy of a staple

- "B-shaped" staple
- Use of fine-diameter wire reduces the quantity of foreign objects inserted in the tissues
- Use of fine-diameter wire
  A double-staggered staple line provides hemostasis and leak proof.

HISTORY OF SURGICAL STAPLING

- In 1908, Dr Humer Hütl, Hungarian surgeon, first used surgical stapling device. Those incorporate several stapling principles still in us.
- In 1924, Dr Petz Aladar, another Hungarian surgeon, discovered gastrointestinal stapling device. Each staple was individually loaded. One firing per surgery and reusable which accepted Globally.
- In 1934, Dr H Friedrich, German Surgeon, modifies the "Von Petz" instrument, creates the concept of reuse of stapler in surgery, designs a reusable cartridge, allowing multiple uses of one instrument in one surgical procedure.

Russian Contributions

- 1940, USSR starts a surgical staplers development program
- "Scientific Institute for Experimental Surgical Apparatus and Instruments"
- The concept of surgical stapling advances significantly
- Complicated instruments.

USA Contributions

- In 1960s of the Russian instruments are introduced, rapid improvements of design
- Stapling devices become lighter, simpler, and reliable
- Introduction of the disposable stapler cartridge

Ethicon Contributions

- In 1978, Ethicon introduces the first disposable stapling device
- The concept and advantages of the disposable instrument become a standard
  - Time savings
  - Cost control
  - Reliability
  - Less potential for infection, etc.

ADVANTAGES OF SURGICAL STAPLING

- The use of surgical staplers-especially disposables-can be faster than traditional techniques for suturing and anastomosis, thus reducing total operating times
- Speed
- Less tissue manipulation due to the speed and ease of use of disposable staplers, which reduces tissue trauma
- Surgical staplers allow for reach into areas of difficult access, allowing procedures that otherwise could not be performed (low anterior resection)
- Access
- Stapled tissue and anastomoses heal as reliably and rapidly as sutured anastomoses
- Reliability
- Quality control-instrument by instrument
  - Sterilization
  - Assembling
  - Packaging
- Uniform quality
- Nosocomial infection control
  - Cross-contamination
  - Process errors
- Cost control.

ANASTOMOSIS

Side-to-side Gastrojejunostomy

- Skeletonization of the gastric greater curvature
- Elevation of a jejunal loop
- Gastrostomy
- Jejunostomy
- Introduction of a TLC55 or TLC75 linear cutter

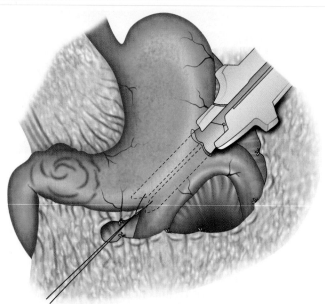

Side-to-side gastrojejunostomy by linear cutter stapler

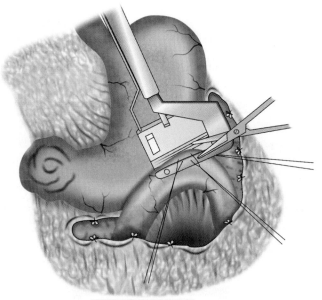

Closure of the common opening using a TL60 linear stapler

- Firing of the device
- Placement of three traction and guide sutures
- Closure of the common opening using a TL60 linear stapler
- Elimination of excess tissue
- Procedure to be completed

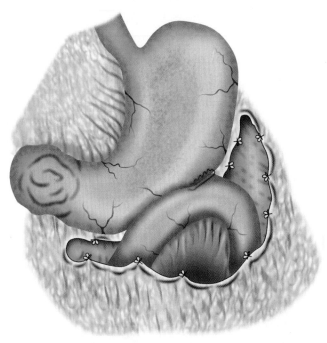

Side-to-side Gastrojejunostomy completed

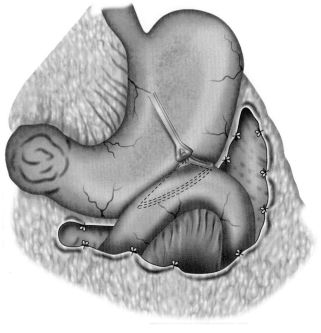

Gastrojejunostomy stoma

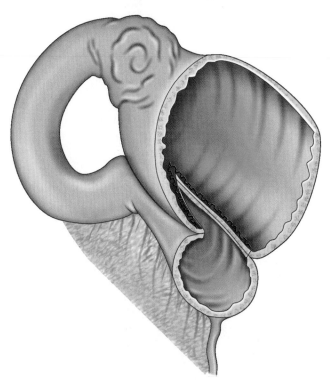

Interior view gastrojejunostomy

ANASTOMOSIS: END-TO-END FUNCTIONAL

- Closure of a temporary colostomy.
- The closed colostomy is detached from the abdominal wall.
- A window is opened in the mesocolon.
- Both segments are occluded using an intestinal clamp. Two antimesenteric colostomies
- Introduction of the jaws of a TLC55 or TLC75 linear cutter
- Placement of a seromuscular traction and guide suture closure and firing of the device
- Introduction of the jaws of a TLC55 or TLC75 linear cutter
- Placement of a seromuscular traction and guide suture closure and firing of the stapler
- Closure of the common opening using a TL60 linear stapler
- Colon section using the device as a cutting guide
- Specimen retrieval
- Completed procedure

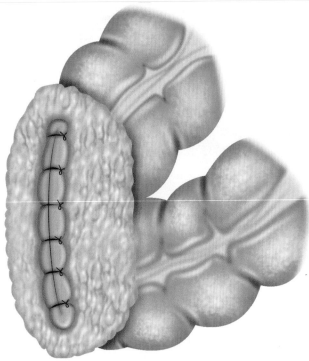

Closure of a temporary colostomy

ANASTOMOSIS

End-to-side Ileocolostomy

- Terminal ileectomy
- Right hemicolectomy
- A purse-string suture is placed in the terminal ileum

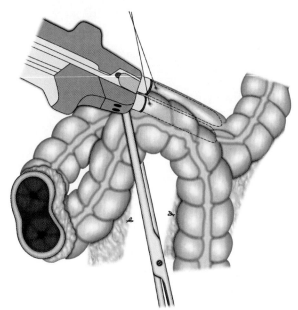

Closure and firing on the stapler

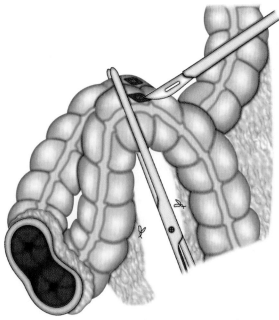

Introduction of linear cutter stapler

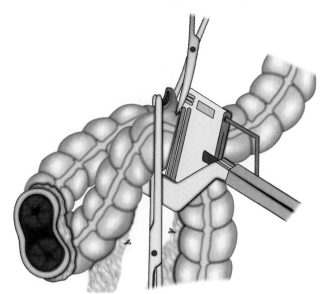

Closure of the common opening using a TL60 linear stapler

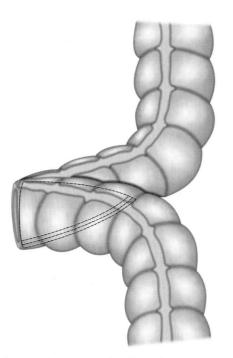

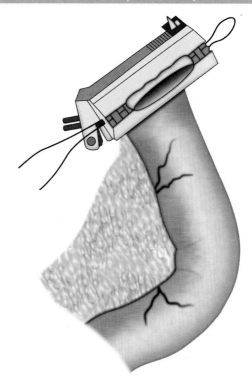

The image shows a projection of the stoma of the functional end-to-end

A purse-string suture is placed in the terminal ileum

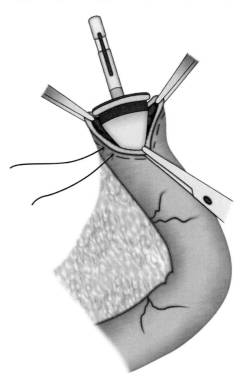

The anvil of a CDH25 or CDH29 circular stapler is introduced in the ileal end

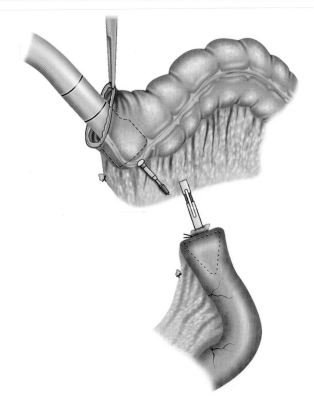

Introduction of the device through the proximal colonic end

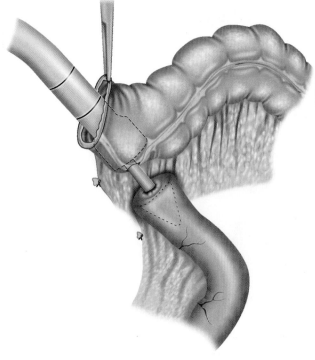

Closure and firing of the instrument

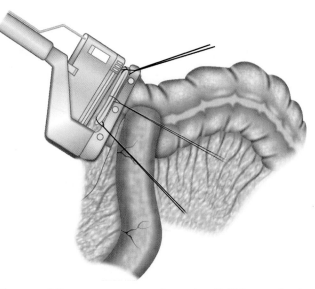

Closure of the common opening using TL60 linear stapler

TYPES OF SURGICAL STAPLERS

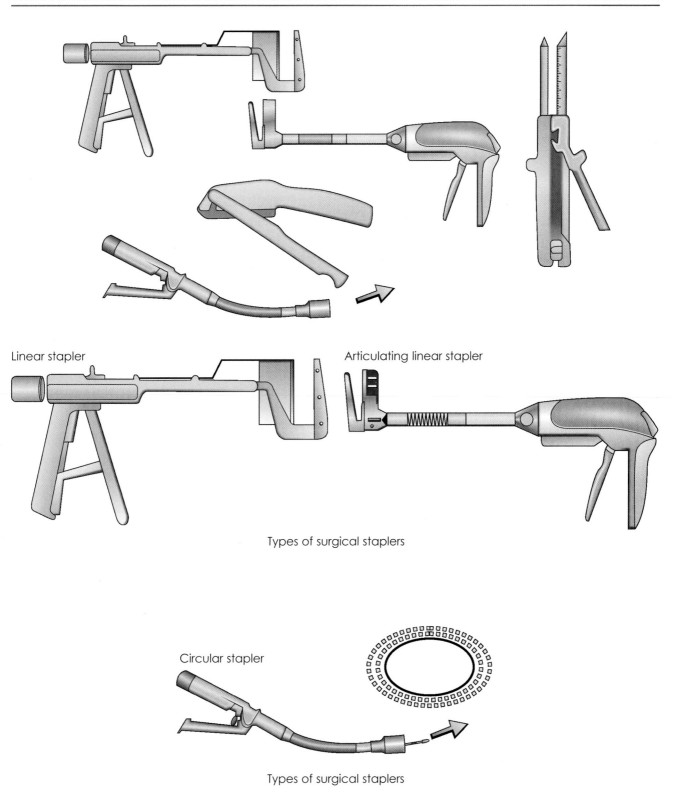

Linear stapler

Articulating linear stapler

Types of surgical staplers

Circular stapler

Types of surgical staplers

Skin stapler

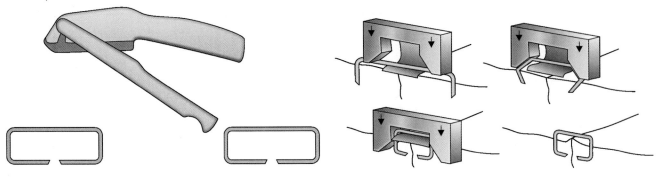

Skin stapler: staple formation

- The anvil of a CDH25 or CDH29 circular stapler is introduced in the ileal end
- Closure of the purse-string suture on the integral trocar
- Elimination of excess tissue
- Introduction of the device through the proximal colonic end
- Perforation of the antimesenteric border with the integral trocar
  A purse-string suture is placed
- The instrument is assembled
- Closure and firing of the instrument
  The integrity of the anastomosis to checked
- Placement of three traction and guide sutures
- Closure of the common opening using a TL60 linear stapler
- Procedure completed

GASTRIC SURGERY

Antrectomy with a Billroth Type I

Gastroduodenal Reconstruction

- Skeletonization of the lesser and greater curvatures
- Proximal transection using a TLC75 linear cutter of stomach. If needed, the device can be reloaded for a second firing to complete the duodenal transection using a TLC55 linear cutter
- The distal line of transection can be made first
- Alternative: Duodenal transaction using a purse-string device and a Doyen intestinal clamp.
- Preparation for a triangulation anastomosis
- A gastrotomy is made in the distal staple line, toward the greater curvature
- Placement of guide sutures

- Stabilization of the line to be sutured with a Babcock clamp
- Posterior wall anastomosis using a TL60 linear stapler
- Elimination of excess tissue
Placement of an additional
- The device is reloaded
- Closure of the anterosuperior edge of the anastomosis using the same TL60 linear stapler
- Elimination of excess tissue
- The device is reloaded
- Closure of the anteroinferior edge of the anastomosis using the same TL60 linear stapler
  Elimination of excess tissue and completed procedure
- **Alternative:** Gastroduodenal anastomosis using a CDH25 or CDH29 circular stapler
- Placement of the anvil in the duodenum
- Closure of the purse-string suture around the integral trocar and elimination of excess tissue
- Gastrostomy with a TLC55 linear cutter
- Perforation of the posterior gastric wall
- Joining of the instruments
- The device is closed
- The device is fired
- Verification of anastomotic site
- Placement of traction and guide sutures
- Closure of the gastrostomy with a TL60 linear stapler
- Completed procedure
- **Alternative technique** using a circular stapler
- Duodenal transection
- Placement of the anvil in the duodenum
- Alternative technique using a circular stapler
- Duodenal transection
- Placement of the anvil in the duodenum
- Closure of the purse-string suture around the integral trocar and elimination of excess tissue

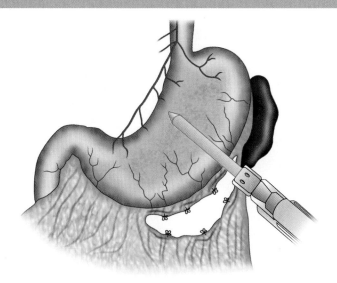

Proximal transection of stomach using TLC75 linear cutter

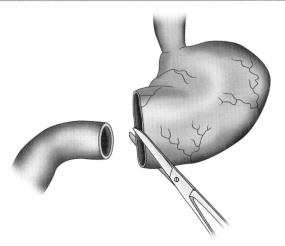

A gastrotomy is made in the distal staple line, toward the greater curvature

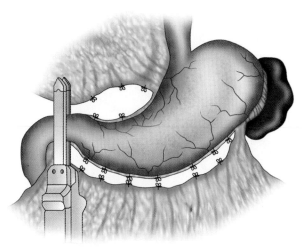

Duodenal transection using a TLC55 linear cutter

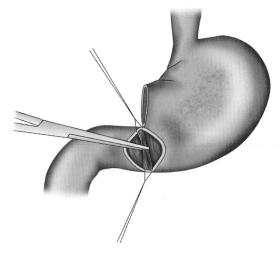

Stabilization of the line to be sutured with a Babcock clamp

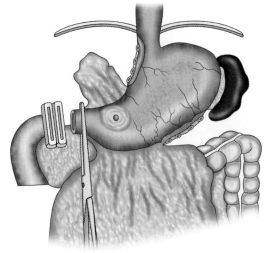

Preparation for a triangulation anastomosis

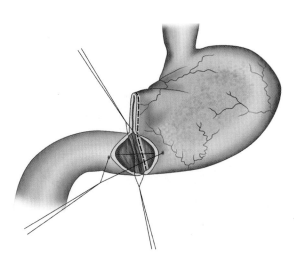

Placement of guide sutures

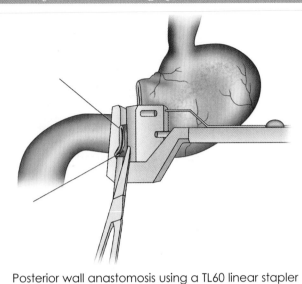

Posterior wall anastomosis using a TL60 linear stapler

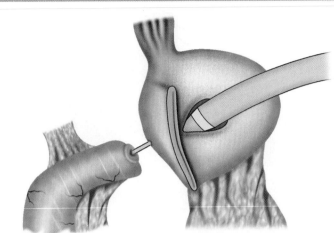

The divice is placed for firing

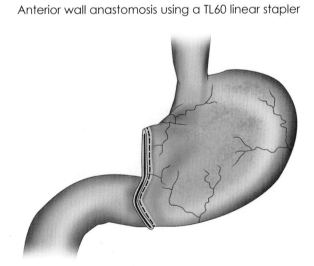

Anterior wall anastomosis using a TL60 linear stapler

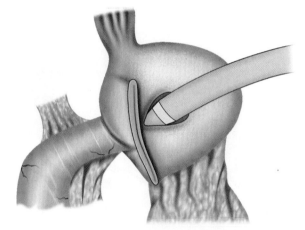

The divice is closed and fired

Completed procedure

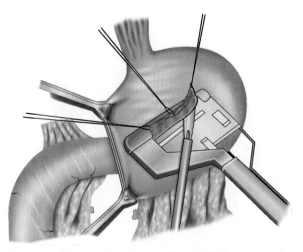

Closure of the gastrostomy with a TL60 linear stapler

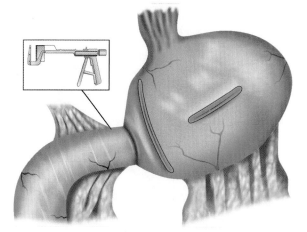

The procedure is completed

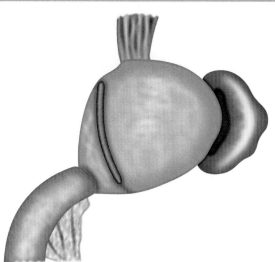

The procedure is completed

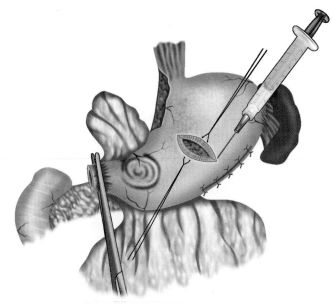

Alternative technique using a circular stapler

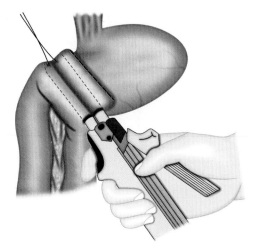

Gastrojejunal anastomosis with the firing of a TLC75 linear cutter

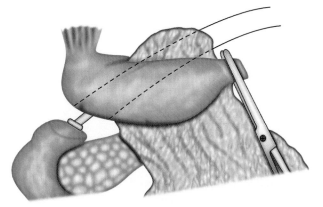

Use of CDH25 or CDH29 circular stapler through the gastrostomy

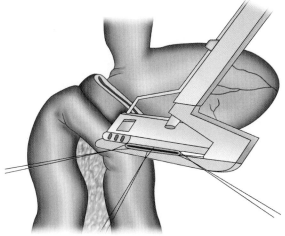

Closure of the common opening using a TL60 linear stapler

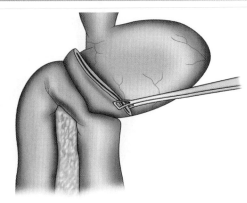

The procedure is completed

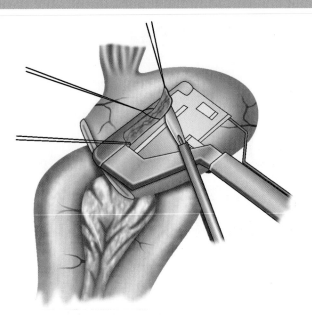

Closure of the common opening using a TL60 linear stapler

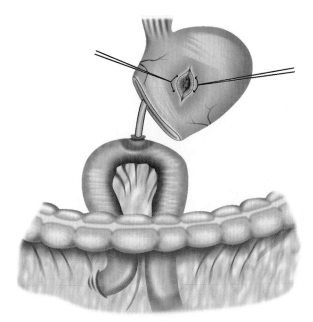

Alternative technique using a CDH25 or a CDH29 circular stapler

A gastrostomy is made
- Introduction of the body of the CDH25 or CDH29 circular stapler through the gastrostomy
- Perforation of the posterior wall of the stomach
- Joining of the device components
- Firing of the device
- Check the integrity of the anastomosis
- Gastric transection using one or two firings of a TLC75 linear cutter
- The specimen contains the gastrostomy
- Finished procedure
- The antrectomy has been made
- A jejunal loop is selected
- Antimesenteric jejunostomy
- Gastrostomy in the posterior gastric surface
- Gastrojejunal anastomosis with the firing of a TLC75 linear cutter
- Placement of traction and guide sutures
- Closure of the common opening using a TL60 linear stapler
- Elimination of excess tissue
- Completed procedure
- Alternative technique using a CDH25 or a CDH29 circular stapler
- A jejunal loop is passed retrocolic
- Jejunostomy and placement of the anvil
- Closure of a purse-string suture around the integral trocar and elimination of excess tissue

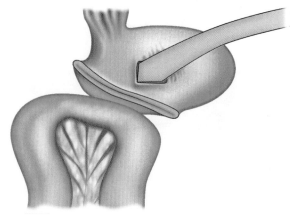

Introduction of the body of the stapler through the gastrostomy

A gastrostomy is made using
- Introduction of the body of the stapler through the gastrostomy
- Perforation of the posterior wall of the stomach
- Joining of the device components
- Firing of the device

Check the integrity of the
- Placement of traction and guide sutures
- Closure of the common opening using a TL60 linear stapler
- Elimination of excess tissue.

TOTAL GASTRECTOMY WITH ROUX-EN-Y ANASTOMOSIS

- Skeletonization of the greater and lesser curvatures
- Duodenal transection with a TLC55 linear cutter
- Placement of a purse-string suture and esophageal transection
- Specimen retrieval
- Jejunal transection distal to the ligament of Treitz
- The jejunal loop is passed retrocolic and a purse-string suture is placed on its proximal end
- Placement of the anvil of a CDH21 or a CDH25 circular stapler in the esophagus
- Closure of a purse-string suture around the integral trocar and elimination
- Distal jejunostomy
- Retrograde introduction of the device through the jejunostomy
- Joining of the device components
- Firing of the device
- Check the integrity of the esophagojejunal anastomosis
- Antimesenteric jejunostomy in the distal end of the proximal jejunal segment
  The jejuno-jejun anastomosis is made with one firing of a TLC55 linear
- Placement of traction and guide sutures
- Closure of the common opening using a TL60 linear stapler
- Elimination of excess tissue

  Alternative technique:
- Placement of the anvil of a CDH25 circular stapler in the distal end of the proximal jejunal segment
- Placement of the anvil of a CDH21 circular stapler in the distal esophagus
- Closure of the purse-string sutures around the integral trocars and elimination of excess tissue
- Anterograde introduction of the device through the proximal end of the distal jejunal segment

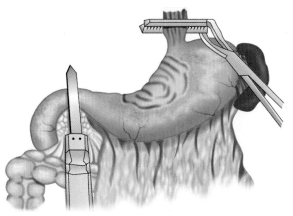

Duodenal transcetion with a TLC55 linear cutter

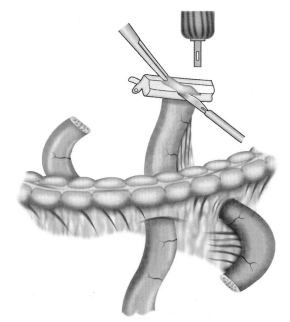

Placement of the anvil of a CDH21 or a CDH25 circular stapler in the esophagus

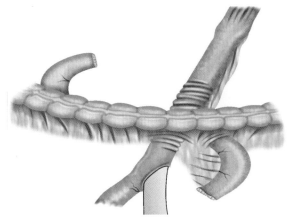

Retrograde introduction of the divice through the jejunostomy

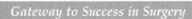

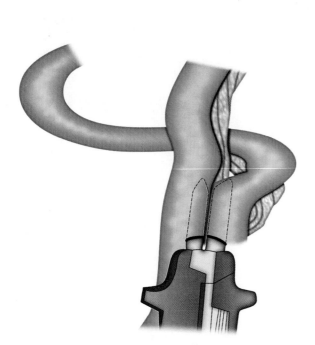

The jejuno-jejunonal anastomosis is made with firing of a TLC55 linear stapler

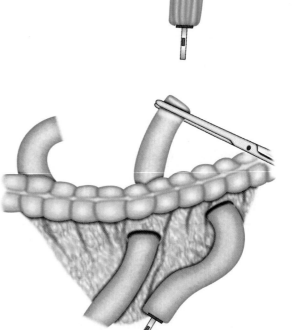

Placement of anvil CDH25 at proximal jejunal end CDH21 in distal esophagus

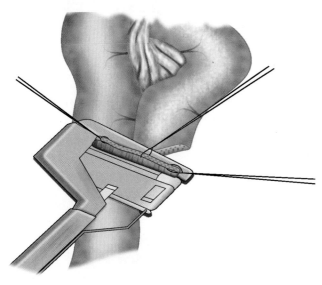

Closure of the common opening using a TL60 linear stapler

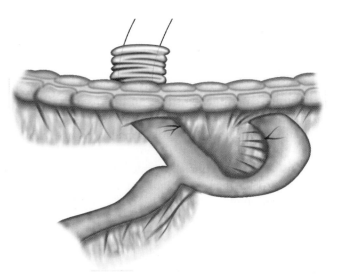

Joining of the components and firing of the divice

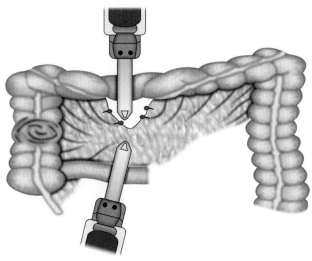

Ileal transcetion with a TLC75 linear cutter

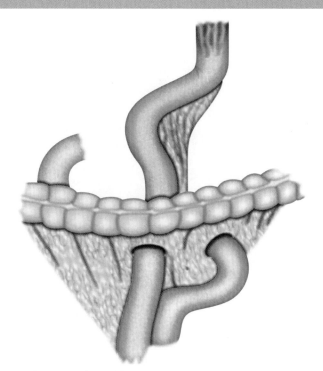

Closure of the jejunostomy and complete the procedure

- Joining of the components and firing of the device
- Jejunostomy and retrograde introduction of a CDH21 circular stapler
- Joining of the components and firing of the device
Verification of the integrity
- Closure of the jejunostomy with a TL60 linear stapler
- Elimination of excess tissue
- Completed procedure

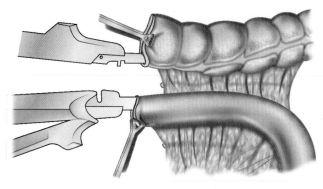

Placement of a TLC75 linear stapler

COLORECTAL SURGERY

Right Hemicolectomy

Side-to-side Ileocolostomy

- Side-to-side ileocolostomy
- Mobilization of the right colon
- Mobilization of the hepatic flexure
- Ileal transection with a TLC75 linear cutter
- The instrument is reloaded
- Transection of the transverse colon using the same device
- Antimesenteric enterotomies
- Stabilization of the tissues with Babcock forceps
- Placement of a TLC75 linear
- Firing of the TLC75 device

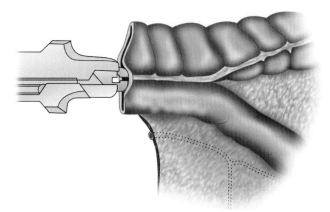

Firing of the TLC75 divice

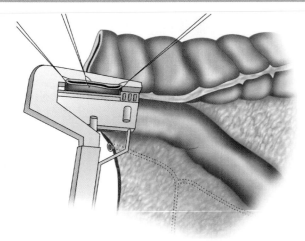

Closure of the common opening using a TL60 linear stapler

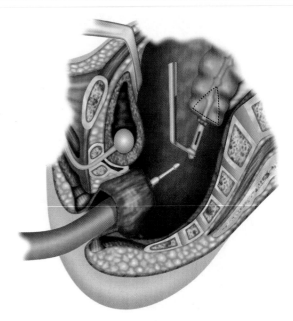

Transanal introduction of the body of the instrument

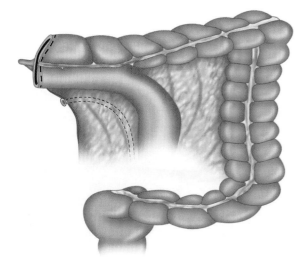

Closure of the mesenteric defect and complete the procedure

- Distraction of the staple lines using three traction sutures
- Closure of the common opening with a TL30 or TL60 linear stapler
- Closure of the mesenteric defect
- Completed procedure

LOW ANTERIOR RESECTION WITH END-TO-END ANASTOMOSIS

- Colorectal mobilization
- Closed specimen extraction: Proximal and distal transections with a TLC55 linear cutter
- Placement of proximal and distal purse-string sutures
  Alternative: Use of a rigid or articulating linear stapler for the creation

- Removal of the proximal line of staples
- Placement of the anvil of a CDH29 or CDH33
- Closure of the purse-string suture over the integral trocar
- Elimination of excess tissue
- Transanal introduction of the body of the instrument
- Alternative: If a distal line of staples is present, then the integral trocar is introduced passing through it, thus eliminating the need for a distal purse-string suture
- Closure of the purse-string suture around the integral trocar
- Elimination of excess tissue
- The tissues must be taut over the anvil and body of the instrument
- Completed procedure

COLOPROCTECTOMY WITH ILEAL "J"

Pouch and Ileoproctostomy

- Creation of the rectal stump
- Placement and firing of an ACCESS55 articulating linear stapler 2 cm superior to the line of the crypts
- Rectal transection using the instrument as a cutting guide
- Creation of the ileal pouch
- Distal enterotomy at the end of the "J" loop
- Introduction and firing of a TLC55 or TLC75 linear cutter
- The instrument is reloaded

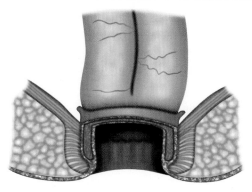

Coloproctectomy with ileal "J" pouch and ileoproctostomy

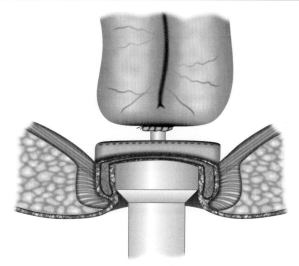

Placement of the anvil of a CDH29 or CDH33 circular stapler in the enterotomy

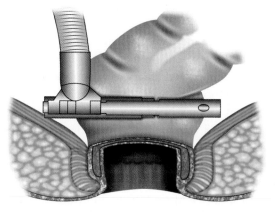

Placement and firing of an ACCESS55 articulating linear stapler

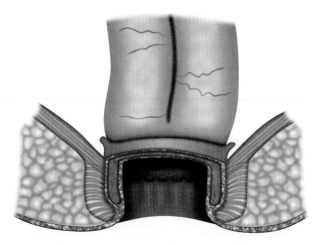

Ileoproctostomy completed

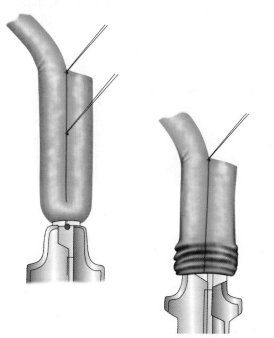

Introduction and firing of a TLC55 or TLC75 linear cutter and distal enterotomy at the end of the "J" loop

- The instrument is introduced again, allowing the tissues to "bunch" over the shoulders of the device, and fired again
- A purse-string suture is placed on the enterotomy in preparation for the anastomosis
- Placement of the anvil of a CDH29 or CDH33 circular stapler in the enterotomy
- Closure of the purse-string suture and elimination of excess tissue
- Transanal introduction of the circular stapler body
- The integral trocar must perforate the rectal staple line
- The instrument is fired and the integrity of the staple line is verified
- Completed procedure

GI STAPLING

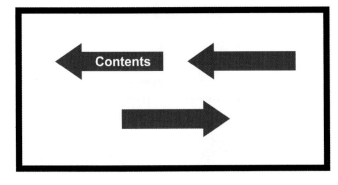

anastomosis or an esophageal anastomosis. Stapling should, therefore, be part of the modern surgeon's armoury and you should be equally adapt with a staple gun as with a needle holder and suture.

HISTORICAL PRINCIPLES

There are many types of stapling devices that may be used on the bowel, but these may be broadly categories into those which:

- Produce a linear staple line
- Cut between two linear staple lines
- Cut and result in a circular staple line

In all cases it is essential to be sure of what you wish to achieve with the mechanical stapler and to then select the appropriate instrument. In many cases there are different sizes of instrument and the correct one must be chosen for the correct procedure. Similarly, the size of the staples may be different or may be changeable depending upon the instrument and the manufacturer - clearly this must be gauged by the surgeon, again depending upon the task in hand.

Because the actual anastomosis is performed with a mechanical device instead of the individual placement of

INTRODUCTION

Until now in the course you have been using suturing techniques in different situations, however the development of mechanical stapling devises means that there are alternative ways of performing many anastomoses.

The few trials that have been conducted have not shown any benefit in terms of outcome for either a sutured or a stapled anastomotic techniqueThere is no doubt, however, that stapling techniques are quicker to perform, particularly in situations where access is difficult such as a low colorectal

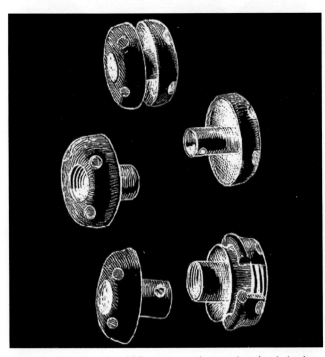

Murphy's Button in 1892 as an early mechanical device for GI anastomoses

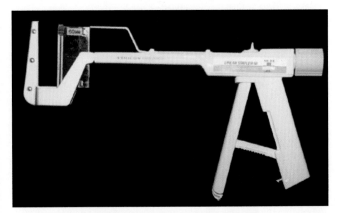

Linear stapling device

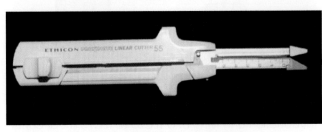

Linear stapler and cutting device

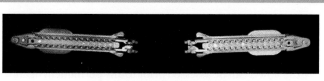

Note the two cartridge sizes

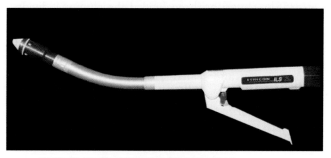

Circular stapling device

sutures, it does not mean that you afford to be any less meticulous in the setting up of the anastomosis and in the performance of the procedure.

A stapled anastomosis will fail in the same way that a sutured anastomosis will, ie if the bowel ends are not well vascularized, are under tension or there is a technical failure in the performance of the anastomosis.

Clearly the application of each of these points will be dependent upon the site of the anastomosis, ie whether this is a small bowel, a colorectal or oesophago-gastric anastomosis. For the purposes of this course we will describe the reconstruction following a total gastrectomy using a stapling technique. Instead, emphasis will be given to stages of the reconstruction in which stapling devices are frequently utilised.

DIVISION OF THE DUODENUM

The duodenum is divided at least 2 cm distal to the proximal border of the tumour. Care should be taken in the mobilization of the duodenum to ensure that the small vessels between the first part of the duodenum and the pancreas are ligated or coagulated as these may bleed profusely. When the site of the duodenal transection has been decided upon, ensure that the common bile duct will not be compromised. A clean and reliable method of transection of the duodenum is to use a linear cutting stapler such as the PLC (Ethicon, UK) or GIA (Autosuture, UK)

Division of the Duodenum

The advantage of this technique is that the duodenum is divided cleanly and both the gastric and duodenal margins

are sealed with a row of staples. Many surgeons will then invert the duodenal stump using a continuous 3/0 PDS suture although this may not be necessary.

Formation of a Roux-en-Y Loop

There are many ways of reconstruction after a total gastrectomy but the use of a Roux-en-Y loop is perhaps the most widely utilised. It has the advantage of providing a loop of jejunum without any tension on the anastomosis and at the same time reducing the risk of bile reflux into the oesophagus. The preparation of the jejunal loop has to be undertaken with the utmost care always ensuring that the vascularity is maintained. There are certain technical aspects to this:

- The division of the peritoneum over the mesentery using a scalpel may aid in the visualisation and subsequent division of vessels
- Care must be taken in the application of ligatures to vessels such that the feeding vessels to the bowel are not compromised. The use of Lahey's forceps to place the sutures and then tying in continuity helps in this regard

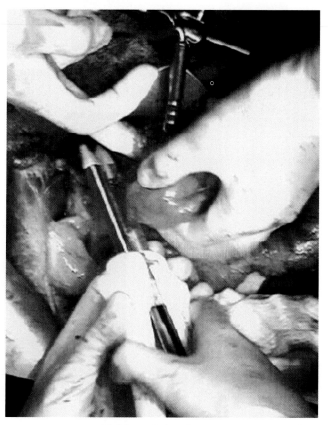

Division of duodenum

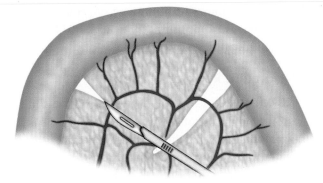

Division of the peritoneum covering the mesentery facilities visualization of the underlying vessels

- Where a long loop of jejunum is required and several arcades of vessels have to be ligated it may be useful to apply a soft clamp to the vessels so that the vascularity of the bowel can be assessed prior to any permanent ligation and division.

Once the mesentery has been divided, the jejunum is divided. This is conveniently performed using a short linear cutting stapling device the smaller size of staple being favoured for most cases (blue cartridge). After firing the stapler the jejunum is cut and sealed. However, the ends must be inspected to ensure that there is good vascularity or, alternatively, they are not bleeding.

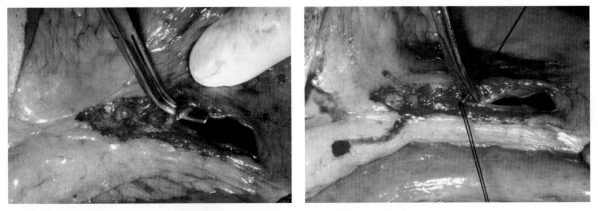

Ligation of mesenteric vessels in continuity

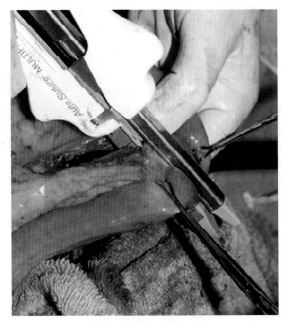

Division of the jejunum

The distal limb of the jejunum is now brought retro-colically to the level of the eventual esophagojejunal anastomosis.

Esophagojejunal Anastomosis

This can be a very difficult anastomosis to perform as access may be difficult, a long segment of jejunum may be required, and its vascularity may, therefore, be difficult to maintain so the esophagus may not be well vascularized. Care must be taken in your set up and preparation to circumvent these problems. The anastomosis can be performed using a sutured technique but a stapled anastomosis will be described in this situation.

The site of the anastomosis should be on the anti-mesenteric border of the jejunal loop at a site that easily reaches to the divided end of the esophagus, approximately 2-5 cm away from the divided end of the jejunum.

Prior to the division of the esophagus stay sutures should be placed at the right and left sides of the esophagus. After division, further stay sutures placed anteriorly and posteriorly will allow the anvil of a circular stapling device to be inserted into the oesophagus.

Care must be taken at this stage to ensure that the anvil is of the appropriate size and that the esophagus is not split/torn by its insertion. A purse string suture is inserted around the circumference of the esophagus and tied snugly against the anvil.

Attention is now focused on the jejunal loop. At a distance 45-50 cm proximal to the intended site for the anastomosis an enterotomy is made and the circular stapling gun is inserted into the jejunum.

It should be well lubricated and gently advanced, concertinaing the jejunum over this until the chosen point for the anastomosis is reached. The jejunum is held taught

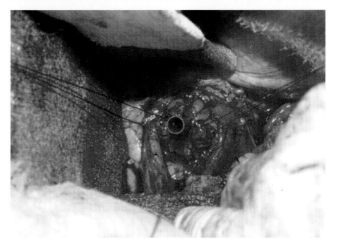

A purse-string suture has been tied around the anvil of a circular stapler in the esophagus

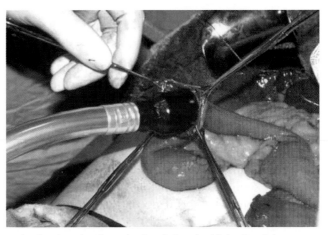

A circular stapling device is inseted into the jejunum

over the end of the gun and an assistant advances the spike through the bowel wall. Care is taken not to tear the jejunum and often a small incision over the advancing spike is helpful.

Different staplers have different mechanisms but the anvil and stapler should be joined together.

Now the stapling gun should be tightened so that the jejunum and the esophagus are approximated. Ensure that the jejunum lies well, ie untwisted and with no other tissues interposed between the esophagus and jejunum. Most devices will have an indicator as to when the anvil and stapling gun are close enough together; only when this is reached can the gun be fired. After the stapler has been fired it should be loosened (usually two full twists of the tightening mechanism). The whole stapler is now gently rotated and then removed. Inspection of the cartridge should reveal two complete circles of jejunum and oesophagus. The staple line should also be inspected to ensure that it is complete.

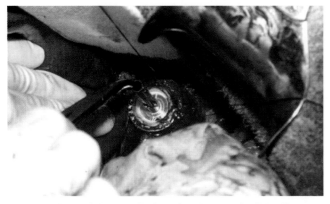

Insertion of the anvil of a circular stapler into the esophagus

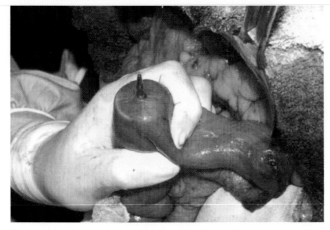

The spike of a circular stapling device is shown emerging through the anti-mesenteric border of the jejunum at the proposed site of an esophagojejunal anastomosis

Jejuno-Jejunostomy

The final stage of the reconstruction is to join the proximal divided jejunum to the jejunal loop. To ensure that there is adequate biliary diversion this should be 45-50 cm distal to the esophagojejunostomy. The enterotomy site used for the insertion of the staple gun is a suitable site for the anastomosis. The proximal jejunal loop should be brought to lie adjacent to the existing enterotomy. It may be useful to insert stay sutures both at the site of the enterotomy and distally. An enterotomy is made on the proximal loop of jejunum and a linear stapling device inserted into the two limbs of jejunum.

Care must be taken to ensure that the two components of the stapler are correctly fitted back together and that the jejunum is held up against the proximal end of the stapler - thereafter the stapler can be fired. After removal of the stapler the enterotomy wounds can be closed with a sero-submucosal continuous PDS suture as described previously.

Key Points

- When using stapling devices ensure you are familiar with their assembly and function
- Careful preparation and meticulous set up of the anastomotic site is as essential when stapling as when suturing
- Ensure that you select the correct sized instrument for the task required

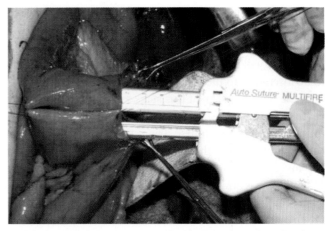

Side-to-side jejunostomy using a linear cutting stapler

KNOW FEW IMPORTANT THINGS ABOUT SUTURE MATERIALS

Ideal Suture Material-Criteria

- Adequate tensite strength
- Minimal tissue reaction
- Good knotting capacity
- Nonallergic, noncarcinogenic
- Easy handling quality
- Less memory
- Easily available
- Relatively cheaper

Classification

A. Absorbable
   i. Natural
   ii. Synthetic
B. Nonabsorbable
   i. Natural
   ii. Synthetic

Examples of different sutures:
   i. Natural
       a. Plain Catgut
       b. Chromic Catgut
   ii. Synthetic
       a. Polyglactic acid (Vicxyl)
       b. Polyglycocolic acid (Dexon)
       c. Polydioxanone suture (PDS)
       d. Polyglecaprone (Monocryl)
       e. Glycomer (Sisyn)
       f. Polyglyconate (maxon)

Note: Catgut is synthesized from the submucosa of sheeps intestine or serosa of beefs intestine, not cats intestine plain catgut is treated with 20% chromic acid called chromic catgut.

Uses of Absorbable Suture

- In bowel anastomosis, cholecystojejunostomy, choledo-chojejunostomy, pancreas jejunostomy, etc.
- To suture muscosa, subcutaneous tissue muscle, fascia, peritoneum
- Base of the appendix, stump of the appendix
- Chosure of subcostal incision rectus sheath, external, oblique aponeurosis
- In ligating pedicles
- In circumcision.

(Remember—absorbable suture should not be used in vascular anastomosis, vessels, tendon and nerve)
Nonabsorbable suture:
a. Natural
   i.   Silk
   ii. Linen
   iii. Cotton
b. Systhetic
   i.   Polypropylene (Prolene)
   ii. Polyethylene (Ethylene)
   iii. Polymide
   iv. Steel
   v.   Polyester (Ethybond)
   vi. Nylon, etc.

Uses of nonobsorbable suture:
- Closuer of abdomen
- In herniorrhaphy for repairing posterior wall of inguinal ligament
- Repair of incisional heria
- In tendon injury
- Vascular anastomoses
- Suturing of skin
- Posterior seromuscular suture in small gut anastomosis,gastrojejunostomy, pancreas ticojejunostomy, etc.

Monofilament and Polyfilament Suture

Monofilament

Suture is made of a single strand of fiber. So the surface of this suture is smooth.

Usually these suture are strong and chance of bacterial contaminations are less but knot holding capacity is poor. So 4/5 knot to be tied.

Examples polypropylene, polymide catgut, polyglecaprone (Monocryl), etc.

Polyfilaments—Surture is made of multiple srrands of fibers.

Surface is not smooth but knot holding capacity is excellent chance of bacterial contaminations is more due to presence of crevices. So infections.
Example—Silk, linen, polyglactin (Vicryl), Polyglycocolic acid (Dexon), Braised polymide, braises, polyester suture.

Numbering of Suture Materials

2 - Thick suture

1,	0,	1-0,	2-0,	3-0,	4-0,	5 - 0 ,
6-0,	7-0,	8-0,	9-0.			

No - 2 is used usually for pedicle ligation

2-0, 3-0 for bowel suturing.

5-0, 6-0 for vascular anatomosis, nerve repair etc.

9-0 is used under microscopic vision. Usually used in ophthalmic surgery.

The number indicates thickness of the suture. Higher the number, thicker is the suture.

When o is used suffixed , higher the number, finer the sutures.

Example - 4,0 is thinner than 3,0 sutures.

Mechanism of Absorption of Suture

Absorbable Suture

These suture get absorbed in the tissue, either enzymatic digestion or by phagocytosis except polyglactin (Vicryl), Polyglecaprone—Which digested by (Monocryl) hydrolysis. So the sutures leave behind the scar mark over the skin. For this why absorbable suture usually is not used in cosmetic area like face, neck, etc.

Nonabsorbable suture remain in the tissue for indefinite period for this why it is used for Henia repair. In body surface it is removed at face at 4 days, neck 4-5 days, abdomen 7-10 days, upper limbs 10-12 days and lower limbs 12-14 days.

Example of Tensile Strenghth

	Tensile strength	Absorbed by
Polygloctin (Vicryl)	28-30 days	80-90 days
Vicryl Rapid	10-12 days	40-45days
Polyglecaprone (Monocryl)	18-21 days	90-120 days

PDS (Polydioxanone suture) - It maintains tensile strength for a longer period, i.e, about 56 days

At 2 weeks tensile strength 5% maintained

At 4 weeks -----------50% maintained

At 6 weeks -----------25% maintained

At 8 weeks it loses its all tensile strength.

Atraumatic Suture

When the suture is attached with an eyeless needle called atraumatic suture. Chance of tissue injury is less here.

THE CARE WORLD

- Brings colours to life

World Population Control (WPC)

Population growth is the change in population overtime and can be qualified as the change in the uumber of individuals in a population using 'per unit time" for measurement.

Over population has a negative impact on the environment due to pollution and over crowding. The more people are there, more resources they use and the more pollution that results.

- Air pollution is due to increased fossil fuel emissions from vehicles.
- Land or water pollution due to increased amounts of waste.

Population increased as people are born or immigrate into a country and decrease as people die or emigrate.

Rate, of population growth, usually expressed as a percentage, very greatly.

Our aim to control world population by preventing unwanted new born and make the world a more happier place for ever.

Index

Page numbers followed by *f* refer to figure and *t* refer to table